MEDICAL CARE OF THE PREGNANT PATIENT

For a catalogue of publications available from ACP–ASIM, contact:

Customer Service Center
American College of Physicians–American Society of Internal Medicine
190 N. Independence Mall West
Philadelphia, PA 19106-1572
215-351-2600
800-523-1546, ext. 2600

Visit our Web site at www. acponline.org

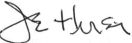

Medical Care of the Pregnant Patient

Edited by

Richard V. Lee, MD, FACP

Karen Rosene-Montella, MD, FACP

Linda Anne Barbour, MD, FACP

Peter R. Garner, MB, FACP

Erin Keely, MD

Women's Health Series Editor

Pamela Charney, MD, FACP

American College of Physicians

Philadelphia

Clinical Consultant: David R. Goldmann, MD
Acquisitions Editor: Mary K. Ruff
Manager, Book Publishing: David Myers
Administrator, Book Publishing: Diane McCabe
Editorial Assistant, Book Publishing: Alicia Dillihay
Production Supervisor and Editor: Allan S. Kleinberg
Interior Designer: Patrick Whelan
Cover Designer: Jeanette Jacobs

Printed in the United States of America
Composition by Fulcrum Data Services, Inc.
Printing/binding by McNaughton & Gunn

American College of Physicians (ACP) became an imprint of the American College of Physicians—American Society of Internal Medicine in July 1998.

Library of Congress Cataloging-in-Publication Data

Medical Care of the Pregnant Patient / Richard V. Lee . . . [et al.].
   p. cm. — (Women's health series)
   Includes bibliographical references and index.
   ISBN 0-943126-81-9
   1. Pregnant women—Medical care. 2. Pregnancy—Complications. 3. Pregnant women—Health and hygiene. 4. Prenatal care. I. Lee, Richard V., 1937–. II. Series: Women's health series (Philadelphia, Pa.)
   [DNLM: 1. Pregnancy Complications—therapy. 2. Internal Medicine. 3. Drug Therapy—in pregnancy. WQ 240 M4858 2000]
   RG571.M382 2000
   618.3—dc21
   DNLM/DLC
   for Library of Congress   99-12514
                                       CIP

The authors and publisher have exerted every effort to ensure that the drug selection and dosages set forth in this volume are in accordance with current recommendations and practice at the time of publication. In view of ongoing research, occasional changes in government regulations, and the constant flow of information relating to drug therapy and drug reactions, the reader is urged to check the package insert for each drug for any change in indications and dosage and for added warnings and precautions. This care is particularly important when the recommended agent is a new or infrequently used drug.

00 01 02 03 04/9 8 7 6 5 4 3 2 1

Editors

Richard V. Lee, MD, FACP, FRGS
Professor of Medicine, Pediatrics, and Obstetrics
Adjunct Professor of Anthropology and Social Preventive Medicine
Director, Division of Maternal Medicine
Department of Medicine
State University of New York at Buffalo
Buffalo, New York

Karen Rosene-Montella, MD, FACP
Chief of Medicine
Women & Infants Hospital of Rhode Island;
Associate Professor of Medicine and Obstetrics & Gynecology
Brown University School of Medicine
Providence, Rhode Island

Linda Anne Barbour, MD, MSPH, FACP
Associate Professor of Medicine and Obstetrics & Gynecology
Department of Medicine
Division of General Internal Medicine
University of Colorado Health Sciences Center
Denver, Colorado

Peter R. Garner, MB, BCHIR, FRCPC, FACP
Professor
Departments of Medicine and Obstetrics & Gynecology
University of Ottawa
Ottawa Hospital
Ottawa, Ontario, Canada

Erin Keely, MD, FRCPC
Associate Professor
Departments of Medicine and Obstetrics & Gynecology
University of Ottawa
Ottawa Hospital
Ottawa, Ontario, Canada

Women's Health Series Editor

Pamela Charney, MD, FACP
Associate Professor of Medicine
Assistant Professor of Obstetrics and Gynecology and Women's Health
Jacobi Medical Center
Albert Einstein College of Medicine
Bronx, NY

Contributors

Isabelle Bence-Bruckler, MD
Assistant Professor of Medicine
Department of Medicine
University of Ottawa
Ottawa Hospital
Ottawa, Ontario, Canada

Janis Bormanis, MD
Division of Hematology
Ottawa Civic Hospital
Ottawa, Ontario, Canada

Gerard N. Burrow, MD
Special Advisor to the President of
  Health Affairs
Davis Paige Smith Professor of Medicine
Professor of Medicine and Obstetrics &
  Gynecology
Yale University School of Medicine
New Haven, Connecticut

Elizabeth A. Burrows, BA, MBA
Department of Obstetrics and
  Gynecology
Clayton Campus
Monash University
Clayton, Victoria, Australia

Robert F. Burrows, MD, FRCSC, FRACOG
Professor and Chair
Maternal–Fetal Medicine Group
Clayton Campus
Monash University
Clayton, Victoria, Australia

Michael P. Carson, MD
Department of Medicine
University of Medicine and Dentistry
Robert Wood Johnson Medical School
St. Peter's Medical Center
New Brunswick, New Jersey

Malcolm C. Champion, MD
Division of Gastroenterology
University of Ottawa
Ottawa Civic Hospital
Ottawa, Ontario, Canada

Donald R. Coustan, MD
Department of Obstetrics & Gynecology
Brown University School of Medicine;
Obstetrician and Gynecologist-in-Chief
Women & Infants Hospital of Rhode
  Island
Providence, Rhode Island

Susan Z. Cowchock, MD
Department of Obstetrics and
  Gynecology
Division of Maternal–Fetal Medicine
New York University School of Medicine
New York, New York

John M. Davison, MD
Professor of Obstetric Medicine
Consulting Obstetrician and Gynecologist
Royal Victoria Infirmary
University of Newcastle upon Tyne
Newcastle, England

Susan Diaz, MD
Division of Women's Behavioral Health
Women & Infants Hospital of Rhode
  Island
Providence, Rhode Island

Lorraine Dugoff, MD
Assistant Professor
Department of Obstetrics and Gynecology
University of Colorado Health Sciences
  Center
Denver, Colorado

Janice I. French, CNM, MS
Department of Obstetrics and Gynecology
Division of Obstetrics and Gynecology
University of Colorado Health Sciences
  Center
Denver, Colorado

Henry L. Galan, MD
Assistant Professor of Obstetrics and
  Gynecology
Division of Maternal–Fetal Medicine
University of Colorado Health Sciences
  Center
Denver, Colorado

Ronald Gibbs, MD
Chairman and Professor
Department of Obstetrics and Gynecology
University of Colorado School of Medicine
Denver, Colorado

Kathryn Hassell, MsD
Associate Professor of Medicine
Division of Hematology/Oncology
University of Colorado Health Sciences
  Center
Denver, Colorado

John P. Hayslett, MD
Professor of Internal Medicine
Department of Internal Medicine
Section of Nephrology
Yale School of Medicine
New Haven, Connecticut

**Mary Hepburn, BSc, MD, FRCOG,
MRCGP**
Senior Lecturer in Women's
  Reproductive Health
Department of Obstetrics and
  Gynecology
University of Glasgow
Glasgow Royal Maternity Hospital
Glasgow, Scotland

John C. Hobbins, MD
Chief of Obstetrics
Professor of Obstetrics and Gynecology
Division of Maternal–Fetal Medicine
University of Colorado Health Sciences
  Center
Denver, Colorado

Margaret Howard, PhD
Women & Infants Hospital of Rhode
  Island
Providence, Rhode Island

Neeta Jain, MD
Division of Women's Behavioral
  Health
Brown University School of Medicine
Women & Infants Hospital of Rhode
  Island
Providence, Rhode Island

Oliver W. Jones III, MD
Associate Professor of Obstetrics and
  Gynecology
Division of Maternal–Fetal Medicine
University of Colorado Health Sciences
  Center
Denver, Colorado

Anne Kenshole, MB, FRCPC, FACP
Professor of Medicine
University of Toronto
Women's College Hospital
Toronto, Ontario, Canada

Sandra L. Kweder, MD
Deputy Director
Office of Drug Evaluation
Center for Drug Evaluation and
  Research
Federal Drug Administration
Rockville, Maryland

Steven A. Laifer, MD
Associate Professor of Clinical Obstetrics
Department of Obstetrics and Gynecology
Yale University School of Medicine
Bridgeport Hospital
Bridgeport, Connecticut

Lucia Larson, MD
Assistant Professor of Medicine and
  Obstetrics & Gynecology
Brown University School of Medicine
Division of Obstetric and Consultative
  Medicine
Women & Infants Hospital of Rhode
  Island
Providence, Rhode Island

Lisa M. Latts, MD, MSPH
Associate Medical Director
Blue Cross & Blue Shield of Colorado
Denver, Colorado

Robert D. Legare, MD
Medical Oncologist
Women & Infants Hospital of Rhode
  Island
Providence, Rhode Island

Phyllis C. Leppert, MD, PhD
Professor of Obstetrics and
  Gynecology
Department of Obstetrics and
  Gynecology
State University of New York
  at Buffalo
Buffalo, NY

Kimberly K. Leslie, MD
Associate Professor of Maternal–Fetal
  Medicine
Director of Research for Obstetrics and
  Gynecology
University of Colorado Health Sciences
  Center
Denver, Colorado

Howard Lippes, MD, FACP
Clinical Associate Professor
  of Medicine
Clinical Assistant Professor of
  Gynecology and Obstetrics
State University of New York
  at Buffalo
Chief, Division of Endocrinology
Sisters of Charity Hospital
R&B Medical Group
Williamsville, New York

James A. McGregor, MD
Professor of Obstetrics and
  Gynecology
Department of Obstetrics and
  Gynecology
University of Colorado Health
  Sciences Center
Denver Health Medical Center
Denver, Colorado

Ellen D. Mason, MD
Consulting Internist
Department of Obstetrics and
  Gynecology
Division of Maternal–Fetal
  Medicine
Cook County Hospital
Chicago, Illinois

Philip S. Mehler, MD
Chief of General Internal Medicine
Denver Health Medical Center
Professor of Medicine
University of Colorado Health Sciences
  Center
Denver, Colorado

J. Lee Nelson, MD
Immunogenetics D2-100
Fred Hutchinson Cancer Research
  Center
Seattle, Washington

Catherine Nelson-Piercy, MA, FRCP
Consulting Obstetric Physician
St. Thomas Hospital Trust
Whipps Cross Hospital
London, England

Teri Pearlstein, MD
Assistant Professor of Psychiatry
Brown University School
  of Medicine
Director, Division of Women's
  Behavioral Health
Women & Infants Hospital of Rhode
  Island
Providence, Rhode Island

Jeffrey Pickard, MD
Assistant Professor of Medicine
Department of Medicine
Division of General Internal
  Medicine
HealthOne Affiliated Hospitals and
  University of Colorado Health
  Sciences Center
Denver, Colorado

Athena Poppas, MD
Assistant Professor of Medicine
Department of Cardiology
Director of Echocardiography
  Laboratory
Rhode Island Hospital
Providence, Rhode Island

Raymond O. Powrie, MD
Associate Professor of Medicine and
  Obstetrics & Gynecology
Brown University School of Medicine
Director, Division of Obstetric and
  Consultative Medicine
Women & Infants Hospital of Rhode
  Island
Providence, Rhode Island

Joel Ray, MD, FRCPC
Department of Medicine
Women's College Hospital
Toronto, Ontario, Canada

Caroline A. Riely, MD
Professor of Medicine and
  Pediatrics
Gastroenterology Division
Department of Medicine
University of Tennessee, Memphis
Memphis, Tennessee

Donald Schmidt, MD
Clinical Associate Professor of
  Obstetrics and Gynecology
State University of New York
  at Buffalo
Sisters of Charity Hospital
Buffalo, New York

Linda J. Scully, MD, FRCPC
Associate Professor
University of Ottawa
Department of Medicine
Division of Gastroenterology
Ottawa Civic Hospital
Ottawa, Ontario, Canada

Robert M. Silver, MD
Department of Obstetrics and
  Gynecology
Division of Maternal–Fetal Medicine
University of Utah
Salt Lake City, Utah

Carol A. Stamm, MD
Assistant Professor of Obstetrics and
  Gynecology
Department of Obstetrics and
  Gynecology
Denver Health Medical Center
University of Colorado Health Sciences
  Center
Denver, Colorado

Jami Star, MD
Associate Professor of Obstetrics and
  Gynecology
Brown University School of Medicine
Division of Maternal–Fetal Medicine
Women & Infants Hospital of Rhode
  Island
Providence, Rhode Island

Kai Yang, MD
Clinical Assistant Professor of Medicine
Yale University School of Medicine
New Haven, Connecticut

Caron Zlonick, PhD
Assistant Professor of Psychology
Brown University
Division of Women's Behavioral Health
Women & Infants Hospital of Rhode
  Island
Providence, Rhode Island

Foreword

The Relationship Between the Obstetrician and the Internist—East is East?

Oh, East is East, and West is West,
and never the twain shall meet...
But there is neither East nor West,
border, nor breed, nor birth,
When two strong men stand face to face,
though they come from the ends of the earth!

From "The Ballad of East and West"
—Rudyard Kipling (1889)

Historically, the relationship between the obstetrician and the internist, when jointly unraveling a medically complicated pregnancy, is one of sincere mutual respect, spiced with a hint of suspicion. The obstetrician sees a pregnancy complicated by a medical disorder; the internist notes a medical problem encumbered by a pregnancy. The obstetrician is unsure about how much the internist remembers about the normal physiological changes in pregnancy but is equally uncertain of the recent developments in medical tests, the methods or values of which can change in the blink of an eye. The internist may wonder whether the obstetrician realizes that there is life after delivery but is equally doubtful whether a third heart sound is classified as physiological or pathological in pregnancy. The ensuing dance around the patient is similar to a first waltz, and stepped-on toes and egos may quickly sour the relationship. East remains East and West remains West.

Out of this sometime adversity has recently emerged a medical *glasnost*, with the single end-point being the improved medical care of the pregnant patient. The emergence of the subspecialty of maternal-fetal medicine has successfully produced a new breed of medicine-wise obstetrician who is at ease with the niceties of internal medicine. Belatedly, a new generation of general internist, the obstetric internist, is emerging who is more at home in the labor room than in the coronary care unit. The major beneficiary is of course the pregnant woman and her child. Successful pregnancies now occur in the face of the most daunting medical obstacles.

Some, perhaps with just cause, shake their heads as the evolution of such medical subspecialization continues inexorably onward. Obstetrics/gynecology has sanely, if temporarily, halted the number of subspecialty divisions at three. Internal medicine, with amoebic persistence, has, at last count, replicated fourteen times. The fear has been that such subspecialization builds fences, with superspecialists zealously guarding highly selected patients. Cross-fertilization of ideas and information is then much diminished and attempts at breaching the barriers viewed with Ludditic suspicion. In spite of this view, successful symbiotic subspecialty relationships have thrived. Cardiologists and cardiac surgeons march to the same drum, and neurologists and neurosurgeons unabashedly meet in public. As just described, however, the interface between obstetricians and internists has been decidedly more reserved and cool. There has been a need, then, for alternative avenues through which to cultivate dialogue between the two specialties. To this end, several areas of exchange have emerged.

Clinically, some medical centers have established Medical Problems of Pregnancy clinics, which provide not only excellent joint care but also a stimulating and provocative teaching environment for obstetric and medical staff. The provision of prepregnancy counseling services is also a fruitful area of joint endeavor. Preconception counseling and treatment provide the optimal opportunity for the medically complicated pregnancy with respect to pregnancy timing, drug regimen changes, genetic counseling, and metabolic control. Prepregnancy counseling clinics ideally benefit from joint input by the obstetrician and the internist, with added interaction between other medical specialties and allied staff when required.

In an academic vein, it is certainly encouraging to see the two disciplines together writing and editing textbooks such as *Medical Care of the Pregnant Patient*. The Society of Obstetricians and Gynecologists and the Royal College of Physicians and Surgeons are presenting symposia on obstetric medicine at their annual meetings. In the United States, demand for information about obstetric medicine is so great that the American College of Physicians–American Society of Internal Medicine holds annual courses and workshops for both internists and obstetricians. Further collegial interaction is now provided by organizations such as the Society of Obstetric Medicine, the International Society for the Study of Hypertension in Pregnancy, and the McDonald Society. (The last is named after a Scotsman, Angus McDonald (1836-1885), who in 1867 was the first clinician to obtain a Royal College Fellowship in both Obstetrics and Medicine—FRCS (Ed); FRCP (Ed). In 1878 he published *The Bearings of Chronic Disease of the Heart on Pregnancy*, which was the first textbook on medical matters relating to pregnancy. It remained the authority for the next half century.) As the number of qualified clinicians with expertise in two fields continues to rise, it is now not unusual to find an obstetrician with a subspecialty in critical care medicine. These dual qualifications may lead to a somewhat chameleonic practice, but they certainly will facilitate obstetric/medical consultation!

As internists are welcomed by obstetric colleagues as consultants to their pregnant patients, care must be taken not to rekindle the Cold War. Though interaction between the two specialties is increasing, inevitably pockets of suspicion remain and King Ludd occasionally rears his head. Respectful consultation that teaches without condescension is required. An order from an internist to an obstetrician for immediate delivery will not be well received. A suggestion that the patient's medical condition will benefit from delivery when obstetrically feasible may be quite helpful.

Fortunately, in North America internists have been welcomed unreservedly by their obstetrician counterparts, which bodes well for future maternal and fetal care. With continued joint clinical, educational, and research initiatives, obstetric medicine may prove to be one of the most fruitful crossroads where East finally meets West.

Peter R. Garner

Preface

Medical care of the pregnant patient is a topic that has consumed the major portion of our professional lives. Obstetric medicine arose out of the need created when pregnant patients with medical illness were often orphaned by the health care system. The internist often saw the pregnancy as an impediment to the care of the patient's medical problem, and the obstetrician generally viewed the woman's medical illness as an impediment to her pregnancy. Both physicians were motivated by a desire to serve the pregnant woman and her unborn child, but a hesitancy to do harm to either sometimes resulted in inadequate care or incomplete investigation.

Our goal in this volume of ACP's Women's Health series is to provide a framework with which to approach the medically complicated pregnant patient that will assist the provider in the care of this very special population. Nothing is more rewarding than being involved in a successful outcome for both mother and baby. Primary care physicians are in the unique position of having access to patients with whom they can discuss the relationship of medical illness to pregnancy before the pregnancy occurs. Obstetricians are often not afforded this luxury, because they usually do not encounter patients until after the time in gestation when most teratogenic effects will already have occurred. We urge primary care physicians to talk openly about reproductive plans with all women of childbearing age and to involve obstetric and genetic expertise early in those discussions when appropriate.

The editors first began working together in 1989, when Drs Lee, Garner, Rosene, and Barron met to discuss starting an American Society of Obstetric Medicine. Dr Lee, who as a professor of pediatrics and medicine has dedicated his career to the care of pregnant women with medical problems, served as host and mentor. Dr Garner, an endocrinologist who was the only internist ever to serve as chairman of an obstetrics department, had already founded such a society in Canada. He graciously agreed to merge it into what later became the North American Society of Obstetric Medicine, which works with similar societies in the United Kingdom (the McDonald Club) and Australia (the Australasian Society of Obstetric Medicine). Dr Rosene-Montella, who as an internist had also completed a fellowship in maternal fetal medicine, was heading a medical consultation service at a large women's hospital and had started a fellowship, now directed by Dr Powrie, in obstetric medicine. She joined Drs Lee and Barron the following year to comprise the faculty for the Medical Problems in Pregnancy workshop at the Annual Session of the American College of Physicians. The course, later joined by Dr Garner and subsequently by Drs Barbour, Keely, Pickard, and Powrie, is now in its 15th year. Dr Barbour had come to obstetric medicine via a collaborative effort between the Medicine and Ob-Gyn Departments at the University of Colorado, and Dr Keely had become involved through her endocrine fellowship with Dr Garner. During our tenure as faculty for this very interactive workshop, the need for a clinically based book that would perform much as would a consultation with a colleague became clear to us all.

Medical Care of the Pregnant Patient is designed for the busy clinician. Most chapters begin with a table of key values, the normals for diagnostic tests that reflect the physiologic changes of pregnancy. At the end of appropriate chapters is a drug table to be referred to in a clinical context when use of one of the medications is indicated. Decisions about medication in pregnancy should be made on the basis of a benefit-to-risk ratio, never forgetting that fetal well-being depends on maternal well-being. Because the Food and Drug Administration is currently working on a new classification system of medications used in pregnancy, we have placed them in one of three categories:

Data Suggest Drug Use May be Justified When Indicated
When data and/or experience supports the safety of the drug.

Data Suggest Drug Use May Be Justified in Some Circumstances
When less extensive or desirable data are reported, but the drug is reasonable as a second-line therapy or may be used on the basis of the severity of maternal illness.

Data Suggest Drug Use Is Rarely Justified
Use drug only when alternatives supported by more experience and/or a better safety profile are not available.

Most of the chapters of *Medical Care of the Pregnant Patient* have been written by multiple authors from different backgrounds, a fact which reflects the true interdisciplinary nature of obstetric medicine. Together, we invite you to join us on a journey through a new understanding of medical illness in pregnancy. It is our sincerest hope that the true recipients of this newfound knowledge will be our pregnant patients, to whom this book is dedicated.

Richard V. Lee
Karen Rosene-Montella
Linda Anne Barbour
Peter R. Garner
Erin Keely

Acknowledgments

RVL: Sometime in 1996 or 1997, the editors began to talk seriously about a book derived from our Medical Complications of Pregnancy workshops at the Annual Session of the American College of Physicians. A compilation of our workshop handouts had received a warm reception; thus encouraged, both the College and we resolved to produce a full-size practitioner-friendly book. Mary Ruff's visionary support of the proposed volume and Diane McCabe's energetic attention to the composition of the book are its *sine qua non*. Without their encouragement, entreaties, and expectations I suspect the editors would still be in the planning stage! Alicia Dillihay became our editorial assistant at the College and her cheerful discipline kept us focused. The team of Diane, Alicia, and Donna Bagdasarian in Karen Rosene-Montella's office managed to coordinate a complex, at times bewildering, array of manuscripts, faxes, letters, and anxious queries from authors and editors. To all of them we owe our thanks and the reassurance that any flaws or inaccuracies that remain in the text are solely our responsibility.

No book escapes the concern of an author's spouse; Susan Lee has kindly tolerated my consuming involvement in the book and has been a gentle critic of the work in progress. For a practitioner of obstetric medicine nothing could be more joyful and symbolic than the safe arrival of a grandchild. The writing of this book coincided with the gestation of Susan's and my first grandchild, Aurora Vaille Guilbert, born March 2, 1999.

My long-time loyal secretary, Susan Rubino, has been the focal point of communication, the sole typist, and the mistress of the computer techniques necessary for a book such as this.

KRM: A great deal of gratitude and my heartfelt thanks go to Drs Powrie and Larson, who both always believed in me and without whose expert coverage during those long summer months my contribution to this book would not have been possible; my husband, Mark, and my children, Brian and Julia, who have so lovingly shared me with obstetric medicine for all these years; my dear friend and business manager, Leslie Macksoud, for her never-ending support of me and of obstetric medicine; and Donna Bagdasarian, whose friendship and editorial and secretarial assistance made this project happen.

LAB: My deep gratitude to my children, who provided the inspiration for this book; my husband, for his constant support; and my parents, whose lifelong nurturing has made me a better physician and mother.

PRG: I would like to thank my wife, Pamela, for her support and help.

EK: To my husband, Rick, and children, Jennie, Allison, Laurie, and John, for their unconditional love even when the conditions get tough, and to my secretary, Nadea Saikaley, for her ability to get things done no matter how much there is to do.

Contents

Chapter 3 Behavioral and Emotional Health in Pregnancy

Chapter 4 Hypertension and Renal Disease

Chapter 5 Endocrine Problems

CHAPTER 6   CARDIOVASCULAR DISEASE

CHAPTER 7   PULMONARY DISEASE

CHAPTER 8   HEMATOLOGY

CHAPTER 9 RHEUMATOLOGIC DISORDERS AND THE ANTIPHOSPHOLIPID ANTIBODY SYNDROME

CHAPTER 10 GASTROINTESTINAL AND LIVER DISEASE

CHAPTER 11 ONCOLOGY

CHAPTER 12 NEUROLOGIC DISORDERS

CHAPTER 13 INFECTIOUS DISEASE

Editors Note—For the convenience of the reader, a table summarizing the physiologic changes that take place during pregnancy is given on the following two pages.

Table of Normal Physiologic Changes During Pregnancy

	Physiologic Changes
Alimentary system	
Gallbladder function	Decreased emptying; increased size
Gastric secretion	Increased mucous production
Gastrointestinal motility	Decreased lower esophageal sphincter tone
	Delayed gastric emptying
	Decreased peristaltic force and frequency
Liver function	Increase in alkaline phosphatase
Cardiovascular system	
Blood pressure	Decreases; gradually returns to prepregnancy level by term
Cardiac output	Increases
Heart rate	Increases
Organ perfusion	
Brain	No change
Breasts	Increases
Gastrointestinal tract	Slightly increases
Kidneys	Increases
Skin	Increases
Uterus	Increases
Peripheral resistance	Decreases
Renal system	
Creatinine clearance	Increases
Glomerular filtration rate	Increases
Renin and angiotensin levels	Increase
Ureteral peristalsis	Decreases
Respiratory system	
Tidal volume	Increases
Respiratory rate	No change
Peak expiratory flow	No significant change
Functional residual volume	Decreases
Arterial P_{CO_2}	Decreases
Arterial P_{O_2}	Increases
Hematologic system	
Blood volume	Increases
Plasma volume	Increases
Viscosity	Decreases
Biochemistry	
Albumin	Decreases
Alkaline phosphatase	Increases (produced by placenta)
Antithrombin III	Decreases (in preeclampsia)
Bicarbonate	Decreases

Table of Normal Physiologic Changes During Pregnancy—*continued*

	Physiologic Changes
Biochemistry—*continued*	
Calcium	
Ionized	Unchanged
Total	Decreases due to decreased serum albumin
Ceruloplasmin	Increases
Cholesterol	Increases
Clotting factors (fibrinogen VII-XII)	Increases
Copper	Increases
Creatinine	Decreases
Glucose	Variable
Hepatocellular enzymes (AST, ALT,...)	No change; occasional slight increase
Triglycerides	Increase
Urea	Decreases
Uric acid	Decreases
Endocrine system	
ACTH	Increases
Aldosterone	Increases
Calcitonin	No change
Catecholamines	No change to small increase
Cortisol	Increases
FSH, LH	Suppressed
HCG	Increases
HGH	Decreases or no change
HPL	Increases
Prolactin	Increases
PTH	Slightly increases
Relaxin	Increases
TBG	Increases
Total T_4	Increases
Free T_4	No change
TSH	Decreases early, then returns to baseline
Hematology	
Hematocrit	Decreases
Hemoglobin	Decreases
Sedimentation rate	Increases
Serum folate	Decreases
Serum iron	Decreases
Transferrin	Increases

CHAPTER 1

Preparing for Pregnancy: The Internist's Role

I. Preconception Counseling
Linda Anne Barbour, MD, MSPH, and Steven A. Laifer, MD

II. Effective Birth Control for Women with Medical Disorders
Carol A. Stamm, MD, Linda Anne Barbour, MD, MSPH, and James A. McGregor, MD

III. Genetic Counseling
Lorraine Dugoff, MD

IV. Normal Labor and Delivery
Phyllis C. Leppert, MD, PhD

V. Symptoms Produced by Normal Physiologic Changes in Pregnancy
Richard V. Lee, MD

VI. Prescribing for the Pregnant Patient
Sandra L. Kweder, MD, and Richard V. Lee, MD

I. Preconception Counseling
Linda Anne Barbour and Steven A. Laifer

The counseling and care of all pregnant women, especially those with medical illness, should ideally begin before conception. This is a daunting task because almost 50% of pregnancies in the United States are unplanned. Brief inquiries about sexual history, pregnancy, and contraceptive plans should be a routine component of the medical care of all women of reproductive age. Because so many pregnancies are unplanned, primary care providers should routinely initiate discussions about preconception care with all women of childbearing age.

The U.S. Public Health Service recommends a preconception visit to a physician for all women of childbearing age (1). The purpose of a preconception evaluation is to identify any medical, psychosocial, or genetic problems that might pose risk to a pregnancy. Frequently, patients are unaware of these risks. Patients need to be assessed fully for medical conditions, substance abuse problems, psychiatric conditions, high-risk behaviors, and genetic conditions before pregnancy obscures a diagnosis or limits diagnostic and therapeutic options. Most medical, behavioral, and genetic conditions associated with adverse pregnancy outcomes can be identified by an appropriate history (which should incorporate medical, immunization, obstetric, social, and family history) and physical examination. If problems are identified, the physician may have an opportunity to intervene in some way to reduce or eliminate risks. Alternatively, after receiving counseling, patients and couples may elect to defer or avoid pregnancy.

It is estimated that approximately 15% of women entering prenatal care have underlying medical problems (2). Internists and other primary care providers are uniquely positioned to see patients with chronic medical conditions before conception. Preconception counseling and care have been conclusively shown to improve pregnancy outcomes in women with specific chronic medical disorders, such as diabetes and phenylketonuria, and may almost double the likelihood of a live birth, according to one series (3). Furthermore, increasing numbers of women elect to have children later in their reproductive life. In addition to having a higher risk for children with chromosomal abnormalities, these women are more likely to have underlying medical conditions that may complicate pregnancy.

One of the most important ways in which the internist can affect pregnancy outcomes is by eliminating the use of medications that may be teratogenic. It is critical that this be done before conception because organogenesis begins only 17 days after conception, before most women realize that they are pregnant (4).

Organogenesis is completed within 8 weeks of conception in the organs most vulnerable to defects caused by drugs or maternal medical conditions. Most women do not enter prenatal care until after organogenesis is complete, and 50% of women with planned pregnancies do not access prenatal care until the third trimester (5). Many major congenital malformations and adverse fetal outcomes can be prevented if medical management is modified appropriately during the periconceptional period (6). All medications, including over-the-counter agents and herbal remedies, should be reviewed, and use of noncritical medications should be avoided during the period of organogenesis.

It is not uncommon for women, upon discovering that they are pregnant, to abruptly discontinue the use of medications that are vital to their health because of concern about the fetus. It is important that patients be informed before conception about the possible teratogenic effects of the medications that they use and about the relative safety of many necessary medications. All health care providers who care for women of childbearing age should have ready access to a reference on medications and pregnancy, such as that by Briggs and colleagues (7), and should carefully review the risks and benefits of treatment with the patient and with the other physicians involved in the patient's care. Home pregnancy tests can be helpful if a patient is using a teratogenic agent, such as warfarin, whose use should be discontinued before organogenesis.

A preconception evaluation has six essential components that should be addressed in all women with medical illness (Box 1-1). These are 1) a full assessment of the patient's pathologic state; 2) an evaluation of the likelihood that the pregnancy will adversely affect the patient's health; 3) an evaluation of the effect of the mother's underlying medical condition on pregnancy and fetal outcomes; 4) appropriate modification of pharmacologic or other therapies; 5) counseling of the patient about the best time for conception; and 6) emphasis of the importance of early prenatal care. The following section briefly discusses some of the more common medical conditions likely to be seen in women of childbearing age. Box 1-2 lists these conditions and appropriate preconception interventions for them. In-depth discussions of the spe-

---

Box 1-1 Components of Preconception Counseling

- Fully assess the woman's pathophysiologic state (e.g., Are there diagnostic tests that should be completed before pregnancy?)
- Discuss the likelihood that pregnancy will adversely affect the mother's health
- Explain the likelihood that any medical condition will adversely affect pregnancy outcome and explain any risk for transmission to the baby
- Modify pharmacologic and other therapies (e.g., Should a drug be discontinued or its dosage reduced? Should a drug be substituted for one currently used?)
- Discuss the optimal timing for conception versus avoidance of pregnancy (e.g., Is the patient using appropriate and effective contraception?)
- Emphasize the need for early care and discuss home pregnancy tests

Box 1-2 Common Medical Condition and Preconception Interventions

- Type 1 or Type 2 Diabetes Mellitus
    Normalize Hb A_{1c} levels; screen for DM if history of gestational diabetes
    Obtain remission of proliferative retinopathy; evaluate for renal disease
    Emphasize need to discontinue ACE inhibitors after first missed period
    Discuss probable need to decrease insulin during first trimester if type 1 DM
- Chronic Hypertension or Renal Disease
    Discuss changing ACE inhibitor if not needed for renal disease
    Evaluate extent of end-organ disease and quantify glomerular filtration rate and proteinuria
    Rule out secondary causes of hypertension if appropriate
    Discuss risk for superimposed preeclampsia and drugs of choice for blood pressure in pregnancy
    Discuss risks for moderately severe renal disease and rule out reflux nephropathy
- Epilepsy
    Determine whether antiepileptic drug is needed and whether patient is a candidate for withdrawal
    Attempt monotherapy with most effective agent at lowest possible dose
    Prescribe preconception folate at 1-4 mg per day
    Discuss ineffectiveness of low-dose oral contraceptives and Norplant with certain antiepileptic drugs
- Cardiac Disease
    Obtain echocardiography if congenital disease, stenotic lesion, or pulmonary hypertension suspected
    Evaluate for coronary artery disease in women with multiple risk factors
- Asthma
    Ensure that the patient has an asthma action plan and uses a peak flow meter
    Discuss relative safety of all asthma medications except leukotriene modifiers
- Thromboembolic Disease
    Consider evaluation for factor V Leiden mutation or other thrombophilia
    Discuss need to discontinue warfarin by 4 weeks of gestation or begin heparin prophylaxis
    Discuss strategy to convert women with prosthetic valves to therapeutic unfractionated heparin or low-molecular-weight heparin
    Discuss options to combined oral contraceptives
- Systemic Lupus Erythematosus and Autoimmune Disease
    Evaluate for renal and cardiopulmonary disease and antiphospholipid and other autoantibodies
    Avoid pregnancy if disease active; discuss relative safety of most immunosuppressants
- Transplantation
    Counsel about need for contraception after transplantation
    Delay conception for a minimum of 6 months after transplantation

cific medical conditions and their effects on maternal and fetal outcomes can be found later in this book.

General Considerations

All women of childbearing age should receive at least 0.4 to 1 mg of folic acid per day to decrease the incidence of neural tube defects (8). To reduce the risk for neural tube defects, folic acid must be present between day 1 and day 28, when the posterior neuropore closes. The U.S. Public Health Service recommends 0.4 mg of folic acid per day for all women of childbearing age and recommends 4 mg/d for women with a previous child with neural tube defects. Women who regularly exercise can safely continue to do so during pregnancy, although adequate hydration, periods of rest, and avoidance of supine positioning should be encouraged. It may be prudent to avoid immersion in hot tubs because hyperthermia has been associated with a twofold increase in spontaneous loss. Caffeine is probably safe at modest levels, but amounts greater than 300 mg/d should be avoided (5, 9).

Diabetes Mellitus

Diabetes is associated with an increased risk for miscarriage, congenital malformations, accelerated or restricted fetal growth, preeclampsia, and preterm delivery. Studies have shown a direct correlation between glycemic control at the time of conception and during organogenesis and the frequency of congenital anomalies and spontaneous abortions (10). Other studies have conclusively shown that optimizing glucose control and normalizing the hemoglobin A_{1c} (Hb A_{1c})level at the time of conception and during early pregnancy can significantly reduce the risk for miscarriage and congenital abnormalities from as high as 30% to close to the baseline risk of 2% to 3% seen in the general population. Included in this risk are major cardiac, neural tube, renal, and gastrointestinal malformations (11). Insulin doses should be adjusted to achieve fasting glucose concentrations less than 5.5 mmol/L (<100 mg/dL) and 2-hour postprandial glucose concentrations less than 7.7 mmol/L (<140 mg/dL). Patients must understand that, depending on the previous level of control and the previous intensity of insulin therapy, it may take several months to achieve optimal control. Therefore, appropriate contraception is necessary until the Hb A_{1c} level is normalized. With the intensification of insulin therapy, episodes of hypoglycemia are more likely to occur.

First- and second-generation hypoglycemic agents are probably not teratogenic, but their use should be discontinued if control is suboptimal or when pregnancy is confirmed. Data on the use of metformin or thiazolidinediones during embryogenesis are insufficient, so the use of these agents should be discontinued in women who desire pregnancy. Angiotensin-converting enzyme (ACE) inhibitors are renal sparing for women with type 1 diabetes and are probably not teratogenic. However, their use must be discontinued as soon as pregnancy is confirmed because chronic exposure during the second and third trimesters creates risk for irreversible fetal anuria, oligohydramnios, and pulmonary hypoplasia (12). Mild renal disease (creatinine concentration <1.4 mg/dL) is probably not adversely affected by pregnancy, but moderate or severe renal disease does carry a risk for progression and is associated with a high risk for superimposed preeclampsia, especially in women with underlying hypertension (13). Proliferative retinopathy can progress in pregnancy, so identification and remission with laser therapy are indicated before conception (14). Patients with type 1 diabetes are at high risk for life-threatening hypoglycemia during the first trimester, especially if they have prolonged fasting and morning sickness. Many women need to have their insulin doses reduced by one third during the first trimester and need to move their evening dose to bedtime to avoid early-morning hypoglycemia.

Women with a previous history of gestational diabetes have a 50% risk for developing type 2 diabetes within 5 to 10 years. They should be screened after pregnancy for glucose intolerance and should be treated appropriately. If they have not been evaluated for glucose intolerance, their preconception evaluation should include measurement of the Hb A_{1c} concentration in order to avoid undiagnosed hyperglycemia during organogenesis (15).

Chronic Hypertension

Women with mild hypertension tend to do well during pregnancy, although their risk for superimposed preeclampsia, at 10% to 15%, is higher than that of women without this condition. Women with more severe hypertension (diastolic blood pressure >110 mm Hg) have a risk for superimposed preeclampsia as high as 50%, and this risk is associated with intrauterine growth restriction, prematurity, placental abruption, and perinatal death (16). Unfortunately, neither optimal control of blood pressure nor use of low-dose aspirin during pregnancy has been convincingly shown to reduce the risk for preeclampsia (17). Hypertension must be controlled to prevent adverse maternal consequences, and some blood pressure agents are favored during pregnancy based on the amount of fetal outcome data (18). However, because no antihypertensive agents have been shown to be teratogenic, it is usually not necessary to switch agents before conception in a woman with well-controlled blood pressure. If a woman is using an ACE inhibitor and does not need it for its renal-sparing properties, it may be reasonable to switch her to a different agent, especially if there is concern that she may not access prenatal care until the second or third trimester. Underlying causes of hypertension must be ruled out in women in whom they are suspected because conditions such as renal artery stenosis, parenchymal renal disease, Cushing syndrome, primary hyperaldosteronism, and coarctation of the aorta may be difficult to diagnose in pregnancy and are associated with elevated maternal and fetal morbidity and mortality rates. Undiagnosed pheochromocytoma is associated with a maternal mortality rate as high as 50% (19).

Renal Disease

Chronic renal disease portends a poor pregnancy outcome if severe renal insufficiency (creatinine concentration >2.5 mg/dL) is present, but women with mild renal disease (creatinine concentration <1.4 mg/dL) tend to have favorable pregnancy outcomes, especially if they do not have underlying hypertension (20, 21). Women with renal disease should have their children early in their reproductive years because advanced renal disease with creatinine clearances less than 50 cc/min is associated with an 85% likelihood of pregnancy complications, a 50% rate of a successful pregnancy outcome, and a 30% likelihood of more rapid progression (20). Hemodialysis is associated with a very high risk for superimposed preeclampsia, preterm delivery, intrauterine growth restriction, and fetal loss (22). In contrast, women who have well-preserved renal function after renal transplantation have much better pregnancy outcomes, even though they require immunosuppressive medications (23). Proteinuria that is present before conception can be expected to worsen during pregnancy, and women may become nephrotic. Unless proteinuria is severe (protein excretion >8 to 10 g) or associated with renal dysfunction or hypertension, pregnancy outcome is usually favorable and unlikely to be irreversibly affected by pregnancy. Women with progressive renal deterioration or worsening proteinuria of unknown cause should have biopsy done to determine whether a reversible renal lesion is present. Patients with reflux nephropathy and recurrent urinary tract infections (UTIs) have a higher incidence of pyelonephritis, which is associated with preterm delivery and urosepsis during pregnancy. These women must be evaluated and definitively treated before pregnancy.

Heart Disease

Patients with cardiac disease should be fully evaluated with echocardiography or functional testing because some cardiac lesions are very poorly tolerated during pregnancy (24). Stenotic lesions, pulmonary hypertension, right-to-left shunts, the Marfan syndrome with aortic root involvement, and complicated coarctation are associated with high mortality rates during pregnancy (25). Patients with congenital heart disease should be made aware that their offspring have a higher risk for congenital heart defects (26). Fetal echocardiography is generally recommended during the second trimester for detection of fetal cardiac abnormalities. Women at high risk for underlying coronary artery disease, especially those with advanced age, hyperlipidemia, diabetes, chronic hypertension, a history of smoking, or strong family histories should be appropriately evaluated because the increased oxygen demands of pregnancy can result in myocardial infarction (15).

Thyroid Disease

Autoimmune thyroid disease may flare during the first trimester and the postpartum period, and undiagnosed hyperthyroidism may cause maternal heart failure, spontaneous fetal loss, fetal growth restriction, prematurity, and perinatal death (27). Radioactive iodine scanning to identify the cause of hyperthyroidism and the possible definitive treatment should be done before conception because radioactive iodine is avidly taken up by the fetal thyroid by 12 weeks and thus is contraindicated during pregnancy. Both propylthiouricil and methimazole cross the placenta. (Although propylthiouricil can be safely used in pregnancy, it can cause fetal hypothyroidism at high doses.) Thyroxine requirements increase with pregnancy, and women with hypothyroidism must have TSH measurements taken frequently and their thyroxine level adequately maintained before and during pregnancy.

Epilepsy

Epilepsy is associated with at least a twofold increase in the occurrence of major fetal malformations, especially neural tube and cardiac defects, and each drug used to control epilepsy doubles the risk again (28, 29). Whether the new antiepileptic drugs (AEDs) are safer has yet to be determined (30). Polypharmacy carries a much higher risk for malformations, many of which seem to be dose related. Poorly controlled generalized seizures not only carry intolerable maternal risks but can also result in fetal hypoxia and acidosis. Because all of the AEDs have been associated with malformations or neurobehavioral abnormalities, a single drug used at the lowest dose that controls seizures is the treatment of choice (28, 29). However, some women are candidates for drug withdrawal because they have not had a seizure for more than

2 years. Withdrawal must be done very slowly, starting at least 6 months before conception, and should be done in conjunction with a neurologist. In the Medical Research Council Antiepileptic Drug Withdrawal Study, 12% of patients had relapse during the first 6 months of drug withdrawal, 32% had relapse during the first year, and 41% had relapse during the first 2 years. Predictors of relapse included need for polytherapy, prolonged seizures, awakening seizures, myoclonic seizures, and grand mal epilepsy (28). The patient should refrain from driving during the drug withdrawal period.

Periconceptional folic acid supplementation has been conclusively shown to decrease the risk for neural tube defects (31). Larger dosages (4 mg/d) are recommended to prevent recurrent abnormalities in women with a previous affected child, and smaller dosages (0.4 to 1 mg/d) are advocated for prevention of neural tube defects in all patients considering pregnancy. Although the higher dosage is recommended by some (29) for women using AEDs, it is not clear that folic acid provides the usual protection against neural tube defects in these women. There is concern that high doses of folic acid may increase the metabolism of AEDs and reduce their efficacy; therefore, AED levels should be monitored if high folic acid doses are given.

Venous Thromboembolism

Thromboembolic disease is five to six times more common during pregnancy, and women with a previous thromboembolic event or a mechanical heart valve are at increased risk for thrombosis or embolic events during pregnancy (32). Women with a history of thromboses and underlying hypercoagulable states may require therapeutic anticoagulation during pregnancy (33). Up to 50% of women with a history of deep venous thrombosis during pregnancy may be positive for the factor V Leiden mutation (34) and a common mutation in the prothrombin gene was recently found in 30% of women with such a history (35).

Warfarin can cause an embryopathy between 5 and 12 weeks of gestation and is associated with an increased risk for fetal hemorrhagic complications throughout pregnancy. Heparin is the anticoagulant of choice during pregnancy. However, heparin has been associated with thromboprophylaxis failures, especially in women with mechanical valve prostheses in the mitral position, because of difficulty in maintaining adequate therapeutic anticoagulation throughout pregnancy (36). Low-molecular-weight heparin (LMWH) may be an alternative because of its longer half-life, but trials of this agent in pregnancy are inadequate (37, 38). Hypercoagulable states should be diagnosed before pregnancy and heparin prophylaxis should be started after conception in patients with a previous thromboembolic event. In patients using therapeutic warfarin, it is important to emphasize 1) the need to diagnose pregnancy early and 2) that patients must not discontinue warfarin therapy on their own. Conversion to therapeutic heparin must be highly supervised.

Systemic Lupus Erythematosus

Women with active lupus at the time of conception are at high risk for flares during pregnancy. Additional risks associated with SLE include preeclampsia, fetal loss, intrauterine growth restriction, and preterm birth, especially in patients with active renal disease (39). Women with systemic lupus erythematosus and the antiphospholipid antibody syndrome are also at significant risk for venous thromboembolism and require heparin and baby aspirin throughout pregnancy. Patients with quiescent SLE at conception who do not have significant renal disease or the antiphospholipid antibody syndrome do not seem to be more likely to have lupus flares during pregnancy (40). Women with progressive systemic scleroderma, especially those with pulmonary hypertension and cardiac disease, have a prohibitive risk for maternal and fetal complications and should be advised not to conceive.

Asthma

Asthma that is poorly controlled during pregnancy increases risk for preterm birth, intrauterine growth restriction, and perinatal death. The vast majority of asthma medications, including prednisone, are safe. Patients should be discouraged from discontinuing their medications, with the exception of the leukotriene modifiers, for which no reports about safety in pregnancy exist (41, 42).

Transplant Recipients

Sexual dysfunction, menstrual dysfunction, and amenorrhea are often present in the setting of chronic liver, kidney, or heart disease (43). With restoration of health after transplantation, normal menstrual function and ovulation are likely to resume, and conceptions have occurred as early as 3 weeks after transplantation (44). This possibility should be reviewed with patients before or shortly after transplantation so that appropriate contraception is used.

The optimal timing of conception after transplantation has not been clearly determined. Some recommend a delay of 2 years before conception in renal transplant recipients (45). However, this delay has not been shown to improve pregnancy outcomes or to optimize graft health. Infectious complications are a major cause of morbidity and mortality in transplant recipients. Infections caused by herpesviruses and, especially, cytomegalovirus (CMV) are common and occur primarily in the first several months after transplantation, coincident with the period of maximal immunosuppression. In addition to causing graft failure and death, CMV infection is associated with fetal complications, including hydrops, death, compromised growth, preterm delivery, and long-term neurologic sequelae in survivors. Thus, it seems prudent to avoid pregnancy during the 6 months after transplantation, the period when CMV infections are most likely to occur (46). Because the dose of immunosuppressants can often be decreased 1 to 2 years after transplantation, it may be reasonable to delay pregnancy for 1 to 2 years.

Immunosuppressive medications must be continued during pregnancy, and dose adjustments may be needed because of physiologic changes in pregnancy that can alter the metabolism of cyclosporine and tacrolimus. Complications of pregnancy that occur more often in transplant recipients include prematurity, low birthweight, and preeclampsia (43). Limited data in a small series of women with liver transplants suggest that pregnancy outcome is improved in patients primarily immunosuppressed with tacrolimus compared with patients primarily immunosuppressed with cyclosporine (47).

Infectious Diseases

Infections are important causes of adverse pregnancy outcome. Maternal infections can be classified as those that can cause fetal infection and fetal disease (the TORCH infections) and those that are transmitted to the baby during labor and delivery (perinatal acquisition), although there may be some overlap. Fetal infections are primarily toxoplasmosis, syphilis, varicella, parvovirus infection, CMV infection, and rubella. Perinatal infections are primarily hepatitis B, hepatitis C, HIV infection, herpes, and group B streptococcal infection. It is standard in the practice of prenatal care to screen patients for immunity to rubella, and many practitioners now screen patients (those who have not had or cannot recall having had chickenpox) for immunity to varicella. The purpose of screening is twofold: to identify patients at risk for infection during pregnancy and to identify candidates for vaccination after pregnancy. Both the rubella and varicella vaccines are live attenuated virus vaccines and should not normally be given to pregnant women. A preconception visit is the better setting for serologic screening and vaccination of susceptible patients because potential pregnancy risks can be eliminated. Similarly, vaccination against hepatitis B in appropriate patients can prevent infection during pregnancy and risk for perinatal transmission during delivery.

Psychosocial or Nutritional Problems and Substance Abuse

Women with a history of depression or bipolar disorders must be identified so that appropriate psychological support and medical therapy can be instituted (5). Lithium, valproic acid, and carbamazepine should be avoided during the first trimester if possible, although the psychological well-being of the mother is paramount. Serotonin-reuptake inhibitors are the antidepressants of choice during pregnancy, and their use does not need to be stopped (48). Postpartum depression is a serious disorder, and women with any psychological history should be carefully followed during pregnancy and the postpartum period. Eating disorders are common, and obese women have a higher incidence of infants with neural tube defects, gestational diabetes, infections, hypertension, cesarean section, and stillbirths. Underweight persons are at risk for low-birth-weight infants (49). Domestic violence resulting in maternal trauma is still a leading nonobstetric cause of fetal death. Adolescent mothers account for 13% of all live births in the United States and have an increased risk for low-birth-weight and premature infants who die in the first year of life (9).

Abuse of alcohol or other recreational drugs occurs in 10% to 15% of women of childbearing age. Alcohol is the leading cause of mental retardation in the United States, and prenatal effects may occur in as many as 1 in 10 babies whose mothers drink 1 to 2 oz of alcohol per day (50). It is estimated that 3% to 17% of women use cocaine, which decreases uteroplacental blood flow and causes placental abruption and numerous congenital anomalies (51). Smoking is the leading cause of low birthweight in the United States, and it is estimated that 25% of women of reproductive age smoke. Smoking is thought to account for 10% of perinatal deaths and is associated with placental abruption, early fetal loss, preterm delivery, the sudden infant death syndrome, and respiratory disorders in the neonate. Unfortunately, most women who smoke continue to smoke during pregnancy, and smoking cessation programs that use nicotine replacement or bupropion hydrochloride are not yet approved for use during pregnancy (52).

Occupational or household hazards include exposure to organic chemicals, including tetrachloroethylene, styrene, and anesthetic gases that can cause spontaneous fetal loss (9). Women should avoid exposure to heavy metals and solvents, including those in oven cleaners, wood-finishing products, paint, and bleach.

Family History and Genetic Disorders

Carrier screening for genetic disorders may be offered to special populations with an increased frequency of a particular disease. For example, African

Americans should be screened for sickle-cell trait; Ashkenazi Jews should be screened for Tay-Sachs disease (TSD), Canavan disease, Gaucher disease, Niemann-Pick disease, and Fanconi anemia; Mediterranean and North African populations should be screened for beta-thalassemia; Mediterranean and Asian populations should be screened for alpha-thalassemia; and women with family members with cystic fibrosis (CF) should have their DNA analyzed. These patients should be offered a referral to a genetic counselor. To avoid spontaneous loss, congenital heart disease, mental retardation, and low birthweight, women with phenylketonuria should be placed back on phenylalanine-restricted diets with control at least as strict as that used during infancy (5, 9).

Obstetric History

Women with two or more fetal losses are candidates for evaluation for chromosomal abnormalities or, possibly, the antiphospholipid antibody syndrome and other thrombophilias (5, 9, 37). Women of advanced maternal age (>34 years) are at increased risk for infants with chromosomal abnormalities and may be candidates for amniocentesis or chorionic villous sampling (CVS). Women with a history of babies larger than 8 lb should be screened for diabetes, and women with small infants may have had complicating uteroplacental insufficiency, which can be associated with smoking, vascular insufficiency, thrombophilia, autoimmune disease, hypertension, preeclampsia, substance abuse, or certain sexually transmitted diseases. Women with histories characterized by recurrent poor obstetric outcomes and women with advanced maternal age who are concerned about the risk for chromosomal abnormalities should be referred for appropriate perinatal evaluation or genetic counseling.

Contraception

In prenatal counseling, it is imperative that the caregiver document that any woman of childbearing age is using an adequate birth control method if she does not desire pregnancy or if the timing for conception is suboptimal because of an underlying medical or psychosocial condition. Estrogen-containing oral contraceptives are not optimal for women with a history of thromboembolism or women with antiphospholipid antibodies or other thrombophilias (53). However, progesterone-only contraceptives do not seem to increase thromboembolic risk (54, 55). Low-dose birth control pills are insufficient protection in women receiving phenytoin, phenobarbital, or carbamazepine because these agents increase the estradiol metabolism and sex-hormone binding globulin levels (56). At least a 50-µg estradiol pill should be used. Levonorgestrel implants are not an effective alternative; more than 30 accidental pregnancies have occurred with Norplant in women who were using AEDs that induce the cytochrome P-450 system (56). However, intramuscular medroxyprogesterone given every 2 to 3 months is likely to be effective. Women with controlled hypertension who have no other risk factors for coronary artery disease, women with mild hyperlipidemia without hypertriglyceridemia, and diabetic women without vascular disease are candidates for low-dose combination oral contraceptives (55, 57). Women who are not monogamous must use condoms to avoid acquiring sexually transmitted diseases. The caregiver should discuss contraception alternatives, such as intrauterine devices (IUDs), diaphragms, subdermal levonorgestrel, and emergency postcoital contraception, or make appropriate referral to an obstetrician–gynecologist (58). It is recommended that women using oral contraceptives or IUDs use another form of birth control for at least one cycle before becoming pregnant. Women who desire pregnancy and have a history of more than 1 year of unprotected intercourse without conception should be considered for an infertility evaluation.

Infertility and Assisted Reproduction

Approximately 8.4% of women 15 to 44 years of age have an impaired ability to have children (59); of these women, 45% have primary infertility and 55% have secondary infertility. Medical conditions likely to be associated with infertility include obesity, autoimmune disease, thyroid disease, chronic renal disease, hyperprolactinemia, cancer treated with chemotherapy or pelvic irradiation, and inflammatory bowel disease. Treatment of infertility depends on the cause of infertility. Conventional approaches include 1) induction of ovulation with clomiphene citrate, 2) use of gonadotropins or pulsatile GnRH, 3) tubal surgery, 4) ablation of endometriosis, 5) intrauterine insemination, and 6) luteal-phase support with progesterone supplementation.

Assisted reproduction has revolutionized the treatment of infertility. Assisted-reproduction techniques include in vitro fertilization, gamete intrafallopian transfer, zygote intrafallopian transfer, and intracytoplasmic sperm injection. With the additional use of donated gametes and surrogate mothers, many women and couples with previously untreatable infertility can now successfully have pregnancies and children. Pregnancies have even been reported in women in the sixth and seventh decades of life (60, 61). The application of the various assisted-reproduction techniques has, in some cases, raised troubling ethical dilemmas (62), and the economic considerations in assisted reproduction are significant (63). Perhaps the most serious obstetric consequence of assisted reproduction is the increased frequency of multiple gestations and high-order (more than two fetuses) multiple gestations. Multiple-gestation pregnancies are at increased risk for preterm delivery, preeclampsia, gestational diabetes, and fetal growth disorders. Because high-order multiple gestations have such a high risk for previable preterm delivery, the option of fetal reduction is available. This procedure, done toward the end of the first trimester, results in the demise of one or more fetuses and reduces the total number of fetuses to decrease the risk for preterm delivery.

The internist is likely to encounter infertility, and it is especially common in women older than 40 years of age because these women are more likely than younger women to have medical illnesses. We know of no guidelines used in the selection of women in their 50s and 60s for assisted-reproduction technologies, but an evaluation of cardiovascular function and lipid levels should be strongly considered. It should also be noted that despite a lack of supportive data, many women use heparin and aspirin in association with assisted reproduction once conception is established, sometimes with unfortunate consequences (64). Caregivers should be familiar with the ovarian hyperstimulation syndrome. This syndrome is a complication of ovulation induction and ovarian hyperstimulation in assisted reproduction and occurs in its severe form in as many as 10% of patients undergoing these treatments (65). It is characterized by cystic enlargement of the ovaries and marked fluid shifts that can lead to hypovolemia, hypotension, hemoconcentration, electrolyte disturbances, renal insufficiency, and thromboembolic events. Deaths have been reported (65). Various mediators have been suggested in the pathophysiology of the increased vascular permeability that characterizes this syndrome, but the precise cause of this syndrome has not been elucidated (65). Patients present initially with abdominal distention, nausea and vomiting, and dyspnea. Hemodynamically unstable patients may require hospitalization and intensive care support.

Summary

Advances in the medical management of pregnant women, in prenatal diagnosis and treatment, and in assisted reproduction now offer a growing number of women the opportunity to conceive and have good pregnancy outcomes. Preconception counseling and care may be as important as optimal prenatal care and is the responsibility of all health care providers who care for women of childbearing age.

REFERENCES

1.   **Adams MM, Bruce FC, Shulman HB.** Pregnancy planning and preconception counseling. Obstet Gynecol. 1993;82:955-99.

2.   **Jones EF, Forrest JD, Henshaw SK, Silverman J, Torres A.** Unintended pregnancy, contraceptive practice and family planning services in developed countries. Fam Plann Perspect. 1988;20:53-67.

3.   **Cox M, Whittle MJ, Byrne A, Kingdom JCP, Ryan G.** Prepregnancy counseling: experience from 1075 cases. Br J Obstet Gynaecol. 1992;99:873-6.

4.   **Lee RV, Barron WM.** J Gen Int Med. 1988;3:602-4.

5.   **Grimes DA.** Unplanned pregnancies in the US. Obstet Gynecol. 1986;67:438-42.

6.   **Kuller JA, Laifer SA.** Preconception counseling and intervention. Arch Intern Med. 1994;154:2273-80.

7.   **Briggs GC, Freeman RK, Yaffe SJ.** Drugs in Pregnancy and Lactation, 5th ed. Baltimore: William & Wilkins; 1998.

8.   **Czeizel AE, Dudas I.** Prevention of the first occurrence of neural-tube defects by periconception vitamin supplementation. N Engl J Med. 1992;327:1832-5.

9.   **Leuzzi R, Scoles K.** Preconception counseling for the primary care physician. Med Clin North Am. 1997;24:559-74.

10. **Greene MF, Hare JW, Cloherty JP, et al.** First trimester hemoglobin A1 and the risk of major malformation and spontaneous abortion in diabetic pregnancy. Teratology 1989;39:225-31.

11. **Kitzmiller JL, Gunderson E.** Preconception counseling: rationale for evaluation and management of diabetes prior to pregnancy. Current Obstetric Medicine. 1991;1:1-16.

12. **Piper JM, Ray WA, Rosa FW.** Pregnancy outcome following exposure to angiotensin-converting enzyme inhibitors. Obstet Gynecol 1992;80:429-32.

13. **Kimmerle R, Zass RP, Cupisti S.** Pregnancy in women with diabetic nephropathy: long-term outcome for mother and child. Diabetologia. 1995;38:227-35.

14. **Garner P.** Type I diabetes mellitus and pregnancy. Lancet. 1995;346:157-61.

15. **Mason E, Rosene-Montella K, Powrie R.** Medical problems during pregnancy. Med Clin North Am. 1998;82:249-69.

16. **Sibai BM.** Treatment of hypertension in pregnant women. N Engl J Med. 1996;335:257-65.

17. **Collaborative Low-dose Aspirin Study in Pregnancy Collaborative Group.** CLASP: a randomized trial of low-dose aspirin for the prevention and treatment of pre-eclampsia among 9364 pregnant women. Lancet. 1994;343:619-29.

18. **National High Blood Pressure Education Program Working Group Report on High Blood Pressure in Pregnancy.** Am J Obstet Gynecol. 1990;163:1689-712.

19. **Keely EJ.** Pheochromocytoma in pregnancy. In: Current Obstetric Medicine, v 3. Chicago: Mosby–Year Book; 1995:73-94.

20. **Davison JM, Lindheimer M.** Renal disease in pregnancy. Current Obstetric Medicine. 1991;1:197-228.

21. **Jones DC, Hayslett JP.** Outcome of pregnancy in women with moderate or severe renal insufficiency. N Engl J Med. 1996;35:226-32.

22. **Hou S.** Frequency and outcome of pregnancy in women on dialysis. Am J Kidney Dis. 1994;23:60-3.

23. **Sturgiss SN, Davison JM.** Effect of pregnancy on long-term function of renal allografts: an update. Am J Kidney Dis. 1995;26:54-6.

24. **Sermer M, Siu S, Seaward G.** Pregnancy complicated by congenital heart disease. Curr Obstet 1995;3:117-46.

25. **Perloff J.** Congenital heart disease and pregnancy. Clin Cardiol. 1994;17:579-87.

26. **Nora JJ, Nora AH.** Maternal transmission of congenital heart disease: new recurrence risk figures and the questions of cytoplasmic inheritance and vulnerability to teratogens. Am J Cardiol. 1987;59:459.

27. **Mestman JH, Goodwin TM, Montoro MM.** Thyroid disorders of pregnancy. Endocrinol Metab Clin North Am. 1995;24:41-71.

28. **Delgado-Escueta AV, Janz D.** Consensus guidelines: preconception counseling, management, and care of the pregnant woman with epilepsy. Neurology. 1992;42(Suppl 5):149-60.

29. **Malone FD, D'Alton ME.** Drugs in pregnancy: anticonvulsants. Semin Perinatol. 1997;21:114-23.

30. **Malone MJ.** The new antiepileptic drugs and women: efficacy, reproductive health, pregnancy, and fetal outcome. Epilepsia. 1996;37(Suppl 6):34-44.

31. **MRC Vitamin Study Research Group.** Prevention of neural tube defects: results of the Medical Research Council Vitamin Study. Lancet. 1991;338:131-7.

32. **Barbour LA, Pickard J.** Controversies in thromboembolic disease during pregnancy: a critical review. Obstet Gynecol. 1995;86:621-33.

33. **Montella KR.** Hypercoagulable states in pregnancy. In: Current Obstetric Medicine v 2. Chicago: Mosby–Year Book; 1993:141-62.

34. **Dizon-Townson DS, Nelson LM, Jung H, Varner MW, Ward K.** The incidence of the factor V Leiden mutation in an obstetric population and its relationship to deep venous thrombosis. Am J Obstet Gynecol. 1997;176:883-6.

35. **Grandone E, Margaglione M, Colaizzo D, D'Andrea G, Cappucci G, Brancaccio V, Di Minno G.** Genetic susceptibility to pregnancy-related venous thromboembolism: roles of factor V Leiden, prothrombin G20210A, and methylenetetrahydrofolate reductase C677T mutations. Am J Obstet Gynecol. 1998;179:1324-8.

36. **Barbour LA.** Current concepts of anticoagulant therapy in pregnancy. Obstet Gynecol Clin North Am. 1997;24:499-521.

37. **Nelson-Piercy C, Letsky EA, de Swiet M.** Low molecular weight heparin for obstetric thromboprophylaxis: experience of sixty-nine pregnancies in sixty-one women at high risk. Am J Obstet Gynecol. 1997;176:1062-8.

38. **Lee LH, Liaun PCY.** Low molecular weight heparin for thromboprophylaxis during pregnancy in 2 patients with mechanical heart valve replacement. Thromb Haemost. 1996;76:628-31.

39. **Silver RM, Branch DW.** Autoimmune disease in pregnancy: systemic lupus erythematosus and antiphospholipid syndrome. Clin Perinatol. 1997;291-320.

40. **Petri M.** Systemic lupus erythematosus and pregnancy. Rheum Dis Clin North Am. 1994;20:87-115.

41. **Witlin AG.** Asthma in pregnancy. Semin Perinatol. 1997;21:284-97.

42. **Dombrowski MP.** Pharmacologic therapy of asthma during pregnancy. Obstet Gynecol Clin North Am. 1997;24:559-74.

43. **Laifer SA.** Pregnancy after transplantation. Current Obstetric Medicine. 1993;2:1-23.

44. **Laifer SA, Darby MJ, Scantlebury VP, Harger JH, Caritis SN.** Pregnancy and liver transplantation. Obstet Gynecol. 1990;76:1083-8.

45. **Davison JM.** Renal transplantation and pregnancy. Am J Kidney Dis. 1987;9:374-80.

46. **Laifer SA, Ehrlich GD, Huff DS, Balsan MJ, Scantlebury VP.** Congenital cytomegalovirus infection in offspring of liver transplant recipients. Clin Infect Dis. 1995;20:52-5.

47. **Casele HC, Laifer SA.** Association of pregnancy complications and choice of immunosuppressant in liver transplant patients. Transplantation. 1998;65:581-3.

48. **Kulin NA, Pastuszak A, Sage SR, Schick-Boschetto B, Spivey G, Feldkamp M, et al.** Pregnancy outcome following maternal use of new selective serotonin-reuptake inhibitors: a prospective controlled multicenter study. JAMA. 1998;279:609-10.

49. **Chattingius S, Bergstrom R, Lipworth L, Kramer M.** Prepregnancy weight and the risk of adverse pregnancy outcomes. N Engl J Med. 1998;338:147-52.

50. **Committee on Substance Abuse and Committee on Children with Disabilities.** Fetal alcohol syndrome and fetal alcohol effects. Pediatrics. 1993;91:1004-6.

51. **Slutsker L.** Risks associated with cocaine use during pregnancy. Obstet Gynecol. 1992;79:778-89.

52. **Mainous AG, Hueston WJ.** The effect of smoking cessation during pregnancy on preterm delivery and low birthweight. J Fam Pract. 1994;38:262-6.

53. **Anderson BS, Olsen J, Nielsen GL, Steffensen FH, Sorenson HT, Baech J, Gregersen H.** Third generation oral contraception and heritable thrombophilic as risk factors of non-fatal venous thromboembolism. Thromb Haemost. 1998;79:28-31.

54. **Jones KP, Wild RA.** Contraception for patients with psychiatric or medical disorders. Am J Obstet Gynecol. 1994;170:1575-80.

55. **Corson SL.** Contraception for women with health problems. Int J Fertil. 1996;41:77-84.

56. **Krauss GL, Brandt J, Campbell M, Platel C, Summerfield M.** Antiepileptic medication and oral contraceptive interactions: a national survey of neurologists and obstetricians. Neurology. 1996;46:1534-9.

57. **Kjos SL.** Contraception in diabetic women. Obstet Gynecol Clin North Am. 1996;23:243-58.

58. **Glasier A.** Emergency postcoital contraception. N Engl J Med. 1997;337:1058-64.

59. **Jones HW, Toner JP.** Current concepts: the infertile couple. N Engl J Med. 1993;329:1710-5.

60. **Borini A, Bafaro G, Violini F, Bianchi L, Casadio V, Flamigni C.** Pregnancies in postmenopausal women over 50 years old in an oocyte donation program. Fertil Steril. 1995;63:258-61.

61. **Paulson RJ, Thornton MH, Francis MM, Salvador HS.** Successful pregnancy in a 63-year-old woman. Fertil Steril. 1997;67:949-51.

62. **Annas G.** The shadowlands—secrets, lies, and assisted reproduction. N Engl J Med. 1998;339:935-9.

63. **Callahan TL, Hall JE, Ettner SL, Christiansen CL, Greene MF, Crowley WF.** The economic impact of multiple-gestation pregnancies and the contribution of assisted-reproduction techniques to their incidence. N Engl J Med. 1994:244-9.

64. **Centers for Disease Control and Prevention.** Pregnancy-related death associated with heparin and aspirin treatment for infertility, 1996. MMWR Morb Mortal Wkly Rep. 1998;47:368-71.

65. **Beerendonk CCM, van Dop PA, Braat DDM, Merkus JMWM.** Ovarian hyperstimulation syndrome: facts and fallacies. Obstet Gynecol Surv. 1998;53:439-49.

II. Effective Birth Control for Women with Medical Disorders
Carol A. Stamm, Linda Anne Barbour, and James A. McGregor

One of every two pregnancies in the United States is unintended (1), and fully 50% of these unintended pregnancies result in abortion (2). Thus, there is a compelling need to provide effective and safe contraception to all women and men who desire contraception. Further, pregnancy may involve substantial risks for medically high-risk patients, and these risks can be mitigated by safe and effective contraception. Contraceptive counseling must be specifically tailored to the patient with co-existing medical diseases. The health care provider must help the patient choose an effective contraceptive method that does not exacerbate her underlying medical condition and is easy to use.

Choices of Contraceptive Methods

Oral Contraception

Oral contraceptives are effective and safe and are cost saving when used appropriately. The progestin dose in the combination oral contraceptive and the progesterone-only oral contraceptive is sufficient to inhibit ovulation; the estrogen stabilizes the endometrium to prevent breakthrough bleeding and increases the effectiveness of ovulation inhibition. In addition, progestins make the cervical mucus hostile to sperm.

Other noncontraceptive benefits of oral contraceptives include decreased benign breast disease, decreased dysmenorrhea, decreased pelvic inflammatory disease (PID) (3), decreased risks for ovarian (4) and endometrial cancer (5), and alleviation of acne (6). The best data available today show that oral contraceptives probably have no significant effect on risk for breast cancer (7).

The dangers of oral contraceptive use include an increased risk for thromboembolic disease, particularly during the first 2 years of use, but this risk is significantly less than the risk for thromboembolic disease seen in pregnancy. The risk for myocardial infarction in nonsmoking women who use birth control pills is negligible (8). The data linking oral contraceptive use with cervical cancer are not conclusive. The American College of Obstetricians and Gynecologists (ACOG) recommends that every woman using oral contraceptives have annual Papanicolaou (Pap) smear screening.

Injectable Hormonal Contraceptives

Depo-Provera effectively inhibits ovulation for 3 months. The side effects also last for 3 months. Injectable hormonal contraceptives work very well for patients who cannot remember to take a pill each day. However, patients who wait more than 3 months for their next injection place themselves at increased risk for pregnancy. Depo-Provera is one of the least obtrusive methods of birth control. The noncontraceptive benefits of Depo-Provera include a decreased risk for endometrial cancer, less menstrual blood loss, and decreased risk for dysmenorrhea. Depression may be exacerbated by progestin use in a small percentage of women. The abnormal bleeding (spotting or menometrorrhagia) seen with Depo-Provera use regresses in 80% of women after two injections. Depo-Provera should not be given to women with unexplained vaginal bleeding. Depo-Provera confers no increased risk for breast cancer (9, 10).

The Norplant system—six silastic stalks of polymer-coated levonorgestrel that slowly release a constant low level of this potent progestin—inhibits ovulation and thickens cervical mucus. Norplant is 99% effective and is therefore as effective as tubal ligation. It is ideal for women who do not like to take a pill every day and who wish to avoid pregnancy for up to 5 years. The adverse effects of Norplant are similar to those of Depo-Provera and include menometrorrhagia, depressive symptoms, and headache (11).

Intrauterine Device

The IUD is a spermicidal contraceptive that makes the endometrium hostile to sperm. Because of the risk for PID, it is best used in monogamous patients. The risk for PID is greatest within 21 days of insertion (12), so it may be reasonable to offer antibiotic prophylaxis around the time of insertion. Because PID may be an important cause of infertility, the IUD is not preferred in nulliparous women. Many patients have increased menstrual blood loss, approximately 15 cc more than usual, and increased dysmenorrhea. Both of these conditions respond well to nonsteroidal anti-inflammatory drugs (NSAIDs). The progesterone IUD lasts for 1 year and has a first-year failure rate of approximately 3%; the copper IUD lasts for 10 years and has a first-year failure rate of approximately 0.5% (13).

Barrier Methods

The diaphragm is a barrier method of contraception that is used in conjunction with another barrier, spermicide. A motivated patient is necessary to maintain efficacy: The diaphragm must be set in place before intercourse and remain in place for 8 hours after intercourse. Because the diaphragm is a risk factor for UTI, it is not recommended for women with frequent UTIs. Urinating after coitus does not decrease risk for UTIs as it does in the absence of diaphragm use.

The condom is the most commonly used barrier contraceptive. Because it must be applied before intercourse, like the diaphragm, it requires motivated users. Efficacy is increased if a spermicide is also used. Condoms are useful for preventing sexual transmission of diseases in addition to pregnancy.

Surgical Method (Sterilization)

Sterilization seems to be the method of choice for married patients (11). There are various ways to disrupt tubal continuity to prevent the ovum and sperm from uniting. The Nurses Study indicates that female sterilization is associated with a decreased risk for ovarian cancer (14). Female sterilization should be considered permanent. The patient should be advised that this surgical procedure has a 1 in 50 failure rate and that one third of pregnancies after tubal sterilization are ectopic (15). Many women receive their annual Pap smear screening for cervical cancer in conjunction with renewal of their birth control prescriptions, and these patients should be reminded to continue regular Pap smear screening after tubal sterilization. Heterosexual women are the fastest group of patients who are acquiring HIV infection through sexual intercourse, so it is prudent to remind all sterilized patients that a barrier method may still be necessary to prevent disease. Male sterilization is another choice for permanent contraception.

Emergency Contraception

Emergency contraception is defined as postcoital contraception. Situations may arise in which a woman with pre-existing medical disease may seek help in preventing pregnancy after an unprotected act of intercourse. Many options exist and, as with contraception in general, choices must be tailored to the needs of the individual patient. Precise mechanisms of action depend on the phase of the menstrual cycle in which the agents are administered.

Many of the unpleasant cardiovascular changes associated with oral contraceptives occur over time. Therefore, it may be reasonable to offer emergency contraception with combination oral contraceptives to a patient who would not ordinarily be a candidate for oral contraception, such as a smoker older than 35 years of age. The dosage is 2 Ovral tablets taken twice at a 12-hour interval within 72 hours of a single act of unprotected intercourse; Ovral administration is usually preceded by administration of an anti-emetic (16). Most patients have menses within 5 to 7 days of receiving this regimen. Other regimens are shown in Table 1-1 (17). In general, it is prudent to use only those oral contraceptives listed in Table 1-1 because the necessary ingredients seem to be levonorgestrel or norgestrel and ethinyl estradiol. Administration of an antinausea agent before each dose may be beneficial.

Table 1-1 Emergency Contraception Options*

Agent	First Dose	Repeat Dosage
Within 72 Hours of a Single Unprotected Act of Intercourse		
Ovral	2 white tablets	2 tablets in 12 hours
Lo/Ovral	4 white tablets	4 tablets in 12 hours
Levlen	4 orange tablets	4 tablets in 12 hours
Novette	4 orange tablets	4 tablets in 12 hours
Plan B	1 white tablet	1 tablet in 12 hours
Preven	2 blue tablets	2 tablets in 12 hours
Tri-Levlen	4 yellow tablets	4 tablets in 12 hours
Triphasil	4 yellow tablets	4 tablets in 12 hours
Within 48 Hours of a Single Unprotected Act of Intercourse		
Ovrette	20 tablets	20 tablets in 12 hours
Within 5 Days of a Single Unprotected Act of Intercourse		
Insertion of Paragard IUD		

*Adapted from U.S. Food and Drug Administration. Prescription drug products: certain combined oral contraceptives for use as emergency postcoital contraception. Federal Register. 1997;62:8610-2.

Patients who should avoid estrogen may be offered the alternative of 20 Ovrette tablets taken 12 hours apart within 48 hours of a single act of unprotected intercourse (18). Both combination oral contraceptives and progesterone-only contraceptives have an efficacy of 75%. This does not mean that they result in a 25% rate of pregnancy; it means that the chance of pregnancy is reduced by 75% (19). Recall that not every act of coitus results in conception.

In a monogamous patient who plans to obtain an IUD in the future and has no sexually transmitted disease, an IUD can be placed up to 5 days after a single act of unprotected intercourse. As with hormonal contraception methods, a pregnancy test should be done if menses do not occur within 21 days with all postcoital contraception methods. The efficacy of postcoital IUD placement is 99% (20, 21).

In the future, antiprogestins may also be available for use.

Contraception in Specific Medical Problems

AIDS

The only method of contraception that should be avoided in patients with AIDS is the IUD, which increases menstrual blood loss and therefore theoretically increases risk for transmission of HIV. In addition, the IUD provides no barrier against transmission of HIV, which should be a part of contraception for HIV-infected patients. Evidence suggests that women with AIDS may have a higher incidence of unexplained vaginal bleeding, and this may complicate their use of hormonal contraceptive methods (22). Recently, the efficacy of nonoxynol 9 in decreasing sexual transmission of diseases was questioned (23). However, condoms and diaphragms are mechanical barriers that are thought to be effective in reducing transmission of HIV.

Gynecologic Cancer

Patients with breast cancer are generally advised to avoid the use of estrogen-containing contraceptives. Depo-Provera seems to be a reasonable alternative, although it is interesting that mitotic activity in the breast is increased in the luteal or progesterone-dominant phase of the cycle (11). For a patient concerned about the theoretical implications of this fact, the IUD, the diaphragm, foam and condoms, and male or female sterilization are all reasonable choices.

Patients with early germ-cell cancer of only one ovary who wish to delay childbearing may use any method of birth control because hormonal stimulation is not related to the disease process.

Oral contraceptives, Depo-Provera, Norplant, and the IUD are all good choices for the patient who had gestational trophoblastic disease during the 6 months after diagnosis and dilation and curettage while trying to detect persistent or metastatic disease.

Nongynecologic Cancer

Some evidence suggests that malignant melanoma is hormonally influenced. In a randomized trial, megestrol acetate seemed to confer a survival advantage in patients with malignant melanoma (24). This suggests that combination oral contraceptives may not be the best choice for patients with this disease.

Anticoagulation

Patients who are anticoagulated and have artificial heart valves are often excellent candidates for oral contraceptives because the irregular bleeding of the endometrium caused by warfarin can be stabilized with the addition of the hormones. An added benefit is the reduction in hemorrhage from corpus luteal cysts (25). In patients without a history of other abnormalities, this approach does not lead to an increase in thromboembolism (25). Menstrual blood loss can often be substantially reduced with oral contraceptives in patients with anticoagulation or von Willebrand disease (26).

Hypertension

Approximately 25% of the population has hypertension (defined as a blood pressure reading of 140/90 mm Hg). Fortunately, low-dose oral contraceptives seem to have little influence on hypertension (26). In a small prospective study, 61 patients with a history of hypertension were compared with a women without such a history, and only 5 patients (8.2%) had to discontinue oral contraceptive use because of the re-emergence of hypertension (27). For the patient who does not smoke and who has regular blood pressure monitoring, oral contraceptives are reasonable (26). If blood pressure increases significantly, oral contraceptive use may need to be discontinued.

Mitral Valve Prolapse

Mitral valve prolapse generally has only a minimal effect on pregnancy outcomes or contraceptive choices. In the absence of symptomatic heart disease or thrombosis, it is unreasonable to withhold any contraceptive from patients with mitral valve prolapse.

Mental Impairment

Often, health care workers and the parents of patients with mental impairment ignore the sexual and contraceptive needs of these patients (28). Oral contraceptives are a good choice if patients can be compliant with a daily pill requirement. It is also possible to use Depo-Provera and Norplant, but mentally impaired patients may be more intolerant than other patients of the bleeding or spotting that may result. There are specific criteria for sterilization in patients with mental handicaps; these include legal emancipation, current or anticipated sexual activity, evidence of ovulation, inability to tolerate or use reversible methods of contraception, permanent mental handicap, evidence of a thoughtful decision-making process, and self-guardianship (29). Barrier methods of contraception are probably not a prudent choice.

Sickle-Cell Disease

No solid data suggest that oral contraceptives are harmful to patients with sickle-cell disease who have no other diseases or risk factors (30). However, two cases of thromboembolism were reported in a small study of 156 patients in London (31). Depo-Provera remains the contraceptive agent of choice for patients with sickle-cell disease. It reduces the frequency of crises, presumably by stabilizing the erythrocyte membrane (32).

Diabetes Mellitus

For many women with diabetes, combination oral contraceptives are an acceptable contraceptive option, particularly given the increased risks of pregnancy (including the risk for an infant with congenital abnormalities) in women with poor periconceptional glucose control. It has been suggested that oral contraceptives may provide an opportunity to institute tight glucose control before conception to minimize the risk for congenital abnormalities (33). Patients with uncontrolled diabetes, end-stage renal disease, coronary heart disease, or untreated proliferative retinopathy should avoid pregnancy (25). A small study of 27 insulin-dependent diabetic patients beginning oral contraceptives compared glucose and lipid values at 2 and 6 months and found no significant differences in glucose control or lipid profile (34). Combination oral contraceptives, progesterone-only contraceptives, Depo-Provera, Norplant, IUDs, sterilization, and barrier contraceptives may all be reasonable choices for patients with controlled type 1 and type 2 diabetes who do not have vascular disease (25). There seems to be no increased risk for accelerated retinopathy or nephropathy in diabetic patients who use combination oral contraceptives (33). Some evidence suggests that the estrogens in combination oral contraceptives may provide some protection against coronary atherosclerosis (35). Progesterone-only contraceptives should be used in place of combination oral contraceptives for patients who desire hormonal contraception but have vascular disease (25). Baseline and periodic laboratory values, including glucose levels, glycosylated hemoglobin levels, lipid levels, blood pressure, and body weight, should be obtained in all patients with diabetes (26).

In addition, oral contraceptive users seem to have no increased risk for diabetes according to data obtained by the Royal College of General Practitioners' oral contraceptive study (relative risk, 0.8) (36). This lack of risk was also noted in the Nurses' Health Study (37). No difference in the prevalence of diabetes was seen among 230 postpartum patients with gestational diabetes who were randomly assigned to receive various oral contraceptives (38). The strongest risk factor for type II diabetes after gestational diabetes seemed to be the need for insulin during pregnancy.

No problems have been reported with other types of contraceptives in diabetic patients who require insulin. The opportunity to provide birth control for members of this high-risk patient population is also an opportunity for preconception counseling.

Crohn Disease

A recent study of 152 patients showed that among women with Crohn disease, those who smoke or use oral contraceptives are at increased risk for relapse compared with those who do not smoke and those who do not use oral contraceptives (39). However, there does not seem to be synergism between these two factors; rather, the effects seem to be additive. The study was small, and the findings are not yet conclusive.

Headache

Tension headaches are generally unaffected by contraceptive choices. Migraine headaches can make it difficult for the patient and the clinician to select an appropriate form of contraception. Common migraines (characterized by throbbing head pain, sensitivity to light, nausea, and, sometimes, vomiting but no neurologic symptoms) are not a reason to withhold combination oral contraceptives (40). Classic migraines, characterized by aura with or without focal neurologic symptoms, are a reason to choose contraceptives other than combination oral contraceptives. The focal neurologic symptoms may be a marker for increased risk for cerebrovascular accident (40).

Tobacco Use

The risks for patients older than 35 years of age who smoke and use oral contraceptives include an unacceptably high risk for stroke and myocardial infarction. Progestin-only contraceptives, the IUD, or barrier methods are acceptable options. Of course, cessation of tobacco use should be encouraged. Although many of the adverse cardiovascular changes seen with tobacco use reverse shortly after cessation of smoking, it may be prudent to wait about 6 months before initiating combination oral contraceptive use because recidivism rates are high.

Dyslipidemia

Hypertriglyceridemia with fasting serum triglyceride levels greater than 250 mg/dL is a contraindication to combination oral contraceptives because of increased risk for pancreatitis. Progestin-only contraceptives are preferred if the patient desires hormonal contraception (25).

Thromboembolism

Patients with a history of thromboembolism are usually not considered to be candidates for combination oral contraceptives, given the twofold to fourfold increase in thrombosis seen in women who use these agents (41–43). A rare exception to this is the woman receiving therapeutic anticoagulation who requires oral contraceptives to manage heavy menstrual bleeding (26). Mechanisms for thrombosis include an estrogen-related 10% to 20% increase in fibrinogen levels, a 10% to 20% decrease in protein S levels, an increase in levels of fibrinopeptide A (a marker of activated hemostasis), and an acquired resistance to activated protein C (44, 45). Combination oral contraceptives also seem to activate thrombin because levels of prothrombin fragments 1 and 2 and thrombin–antithrombin complexes are significantly elevated in women who use these agents (46).

Whether the new third-generation progestins (desogestrel and gestodene) in combination oral contraceptives are more thrombogenic than the first-generation (norethindrone-type) and second-generation (norgestrel group) progestins continues to be debated. Users of low-estrogen combined oral contraceptives containing levonorgestrel had a 3.5-fold risk of thrombosis compared with nonusers versus a 9.1-fold risk for users of third-generation combined oral contraceptives (47). However, this study has been criticized for confounding by indication related to differences in prescribing behaviors. Higher-risk women may have been preferentially given third-generation oral contraceptives because these agents were thought to reduce risk for arterial thrombosis and to have favorable effects on lipid and carbohydrate metabolism. Confounding by indication, first-time use, and underlying hypercoagulable states (including presence of the factor V Leiden mutation) have all been examined in post hoc reanalyses of the data, and less impressive risks have been estimated (43). However, it is still unclear whether the new progestational agents carry a higher risk for thrombosis (48–51). In one meta-analysis (41), women using combination oral contraceptives that contained a third-generation progestin had a pooled risk ratio for thrombosis of 5.0 compared with nonusers.

Women receiving combination oral contraceptives who carry the factor V Leiden mutation are at increased risk for thrombosis (52) (Table 1-2). However, it is not cost effective to check for this mutation before giving combination oral contraceptives unless the patient has a strong family history of thrombosis (53). Although users of combination oral contraceptives who have the factor V Leiden mutation are at increased risk for thrombosis, the absolute risk is small (28.5 events per 10,000 woman-years), much smaller than the 2% risk for a first deep venous thrombosis during pregnancy (54).

Depomedroxyprogesterone (DMPA), medroxyprogesterone acetate tablets (the minipill), and levonorgestrel implants (Norplant) are all reasonable options for contraception in women with thromboembolism. No increases in the incidence of thromboembolism and no alterations in the clotting cascade have been documented with the use of progestational agents alone. Unfortunately, the package labeling of DMPA indicates that DMPA is contraindicated in women with a history of thromboembolism. The reason for this is that thrombotic complications were seen when DMPA was used in higher doses for women with gynecologic cancer in the 1960s. However, these women probably had an underlying hypercoagulable state resulting from their cancer, and

Table 1-2　Risk for Thrombosis in Women with Factor V Leiden Mutation Who Use Oral Contraceptives Pills (OCP)

	Relative Risk	Incidence/10,000 Woman-Years
No OCP and no factor V Leiden mutation	1.0	0.8
OCP only	3.8	3.0
Factor V Leiden mutation only	7.9	5.7
OCP and factor V Leiden mutation	34.7	28.5

Adapted from Vandenbroucke JP et al. Increased risk of venous thrombosis in oral-contraceptive users who are carriers of the factor V Leiden mutation. Lancet. 1994:344:1453–7.

Table 1-3　Antiepileptic Drugs and Liver Microsomal Cytochrome P-450

Inducers of Liver Microsomal Cytochrome P-450	Noninducers of Liver Microsomal Cytochrome P-450
Phenobarbital	Valproic acid
Primidone	Benzodiazepines
Phenytoin	Gabapentin
Carbamazepine	Lamotrigine
Ethosuximide	

they received doses much higher than those used for contraception (55). In women with a history of thrombosis, ACOG considers progestin-only contraceptives to be appropriate (56).

Other contraceptive methods, including barrier methods and IUDs, are compatible with a history of thromboembolism. However, women receiving chronic therapeutic anticoagulation may have problems with excessive vaginal spotting with IUDs or levonorgestrel implants.

Epilepsy

Low-dose estrogen combination oral contraceptives are unlikely to exacerbate epilepsy, but the contraceptive failure rate is increased fourfold in patients who use some AEDs (57). Of the established AEDs, phenobarbital, primidone, phenytoin, ethosuximide, and carbamazepine induce the cytochrome P-450 system, enhancing steroid hormone metabolism; reduce levels of ethinyl estradiol in combination oral contraceptives by about 40% (58); and decrease free progestin levels, probably as a result of the increased synthesis of sex hormone–binding globulins. Valproic acid, benzodiazepines, gabapentin, and lamotrigine do not have these effects and do not seem to decrease the efficacy of combination oral contraceptives (Table 1-3). If combination oral contraceptives are used, a 50-µg pill should be prescribed, although infrequent failures have also been reported with this dose (58). If breakthrough bleeding is noted

Table 1-4 Summary of Contraceptive Choices

Medical Problem	Estrogen-Progestin OCP	Progesterone-only OCP	DMPA	Norplant	Sterilization	Vasectomy	IUD	Barriers
					Contraceptive Option			
Tobacco use (> 35 years old)	No	Yes	Yes	Yes	Yes	Yes	Yes	Yes
Well-controlled diabetes without retinopathy or nephropathy	Yes	Yes	Yes	Yes	Yes	Yes	Yes	Yes
Well-controlled diabetes with retinopathy or nephropathy	No	Yes	Yes	Yes	Yes	Yes	Yes	Yes
Thromboembolic disease	No	Yes	Yes	Yes	Yes	Yes	Yes	Yes
Tension headache	Yes	Yes	Yes	Yes	Yes	Yes	Yes	Yes
Common migraine	Yes	Yes	Yes	Yes	Yes	Yes	Yes	Yes
Classic migraine	No	Yes	Yes	Yes	Yes	Yes	Yes	Yes
Breast cancer	No	?	?	?	Yes	Yes	Yes	Yes
HIV infection	Yes	Yes	Yes	Yes	Yes	Yes	No	Yes
Thyroid disease	Yes	Yes	Yes	Yes	Yes	Yes	Yes	Yes
Gestational trophoblastic disease	Yes	Yes	Yes	Yes	Yes	Yes	Yes	Yes
Epilepsy	Yes	Yes	Yes	Yes	Yes	Yes	Yes	Yes
Hepatitis or cirrhosis	No	No	No	No	Yes	Yes	Yes	Yes

Adapted from Family and Reproductive Health Programme. Improving Access to Quality Care in Family Planning. Medical Eligibility Criteria for Contraceptive use. Geneva: World Health Organization; 1996.

or women desire very high effectiveness, barrier contraceptives or spermicidal gel or foam should be added. Barrier contraceptives should be used initially until it is confirmed that ovulation is being consistently suppressed by oral contraceptives. Use of the new ovulation kits for the first several months after beginning use of oral contraceptives may help confirm this (57). Despite the effects of AEDs on sex hormone levels, combination oral contraceptives are still usually more effective than barrier methods (57). The IUD is also an option for women seeking high effectiveness.

The AEDs that induce the cytochrome P-450 system may also decrease the effectiveness of levonorgestrel implants. More than 30 accidental failures have been reported with Norplant in women using AEDs (58). Depo-Provera has not been associated with contraceptive failures due to AEDs, probably because it contains higher levels of progesterone (58). Depo-Provera may also confer a therapeutic benefit with respect to the incidence of seizures. Progesterone seems to increase the seizure threshold, and small studies have shown that it improves seizure control (26).

A summary of contraceptive choices for patients with various medical problems is given in Table 1-4.

REFERENCES

1. **Forest JD.** Epidemiology of unintended pregnancy and contraceptive use. Am J Obstet Gynecol. 1994;170:1485-9.

2. **Henshaw SK.** Unintended pregnancy in the United States. Fam Plann Perspect. 1998;30:24-9, 46.

3. **Mishell DR Jr.** Non-contraceptive health benefits of oral steroidal contraceptives. Am J Obstet Gynecol. 1982;142:809.

4. **The Cancer and Steroid Hormone Study of the Centers for Disease Control and the National Institute of Child Health and Human Development.** The reduction in risk of ovarian cancer associated with oral-contraceptive use. N Engl J Med. 1987;316:650-5.

5. **The Cancer and Steroid Hormone Study of the Centers for Disease Control and the National Institute of Child Health and Human Development.** Combination oral contraceptive use and the risk of endometrial cancer. JAMA. 1987;257:798-800.

6. **Redmond GP, Olson WH, Lippman JS, Kafrissen ME, Jones TM, Jorizzo JL.** Norgestimate and ethinyl estradiol in the treatment of acne vulgaris: a randomized, placebo-controlled trial. Obstet Gynecol. 1997;89:615-22.

7. **Romieu I, Willett WC, Colditz GA, Stampfer MJ, Rosner B, Hennekens CH, et al.** Prospective study of oral contraceptive use and risk of breast cancer in women. J Natl Cancer Inst. 1989;81:1313-21.

8. **Rosenberg L, Palmer JR, Lesko SM, Shapiro S.** Oral contraceptive use and the risk of myocardial infarction. Am J Epidemiol. 1990;131:1009-16.

9. **World Health Organization.** Depo-medroxyprogesterone acetate (DMPA) and cancer: memorandum from a WHO meeting. Bull World Health Organ. 1986;64:375.

10. **Skegg DCG, Noonan EA, Paul C, et al.** Depot medroxyprogesterone acetate and breast cancer: a pooled analysis of the World Health Organization and New Zealand studies. JAMA. 1995;273:799-804.

11. **Herbst A.** Comprehensive Gynecology. St. Louis: Mosby–Year Book; 1992.

12. **Farley TMM, Rosenberg MJ, Rowe PJ, et al.** Intrauterine devices and pelvic inflammatory disease: an international perspective. Lancet. 1992;339:785-8.

13. **Sivin I, Schmidt F.** Effectiveness of IUDs: a review. Contraception. 1987;36:55-84.

14. **Hankinson SE, Hunter DJ, Colditz GA, et al.** Tubal ligation, hysterectomy, and the risk of ovarian cancer. JAMA. 1993;270:2813-8.

15. **Peterson HB, Xia Z, Hughes JM, et al.** The risk of pregnancy after tubal sterilization: findings from the U.S. Collaborative Review of Sterilization. Am J Obstet Gynecol. 1996;174:1161-70.

16. **Yuzpe AA, Lancee WJ.** Ethinyl estradiol and dl-norgestrel as a postcoital contraceptive. Fertil Steril. 1977;28:932-6.

17. **U.S. Food and Drug Administration.** Prescription drug products: certain combined oral contraceptives for use as emergency postcoital contraception. Federal Register. 1997;62:8610-2.

18. **Ho PC, Kwan MSW.** A prospective randomized comparison of levonorgestrel with the Yuzpe regimen of emergency contraception. Fam Plann Perspect. 1996;28:58-64.

19. **Trussell J, Ellertson C, Stewart F.** The effectiveness of the Yuzpe regimen of emergency contraception. Fam Plann Perspect. 1996;28:58-64.

20. **Trussell J, Ellertson C.** Efficacy of emergency contraception. Fertil Control Rev. 1995;4:8-11.

21. **Fasoli M, Parazzini F, Cecchetti G, LaVecchia C.** Post-coital contraception: an overview of published studies. Contraception. 1989;39:459-68.

22. **Shah P, Smith R, Kitchen V, Wells C, Barton S, Kitchen VS, et al.** Menstrual symptoms in women infected by the human immunodeficiency virus. Obstet Gynecol. 1994;83:397-400.

23. **Roddy RE, Zekeng L, Ryan KA, Tamoufe U, Weir SS, Wong EL.** A controlled trial of nonoxynol 9 film to reduce male-to-female transmission of sexually transmitted diseases. N Engl J Med. 1998;339:504-10.

24. **Creagan ET, Ingle JN, Schutt AJ, Schaid DJ.** A prospective, randomized controlled trial of megestrol acetate among high-risk patients with resected malignant melanoma. Am J Clin Oncol. 1989;12:152-5.

25. **Jones KP, Wild RA.** Contraception for patients with psychiatric or medical disorders. Am J Obstet Gynecol. 1994;170:1575-80.

26. **Corson SL.** Contraception for women with health problems. Int J Fertil. 1996;41:77-84.

27. **Tsai CC, Williamson HO, Kirkland BH, Braun JO, Lam CF.** Low-dose oral contraception and blood pressure in women with a past history of elevated blood pressure. Am J Obstet Gynecol. 1985;151:28-32.

28. **Kreutner AK.** Sexuality, fertility, and the problems of menstruation in mentally retarded adolescents. Pediatr Clin North Am. 1981;28:475-80.

29. **Elkins TE, Hoyle D, Darnton T, et al.** The use of a societally-based ethics/advisory committee to aid in decisions to sterilize mentally handicapped patients. Adolesc Pediatr Gynecol. 1988;1:190-4.

30. **Goldzieher JW, Zamah NM.** Oral contraceptive side-effects: where's the beef? Contraception. 1995;52:327-35.

31. **Guillebaud J.** Sickle cell disease and contraception. BMJ. 1993;307:506-7.

32. **De Ceulaer K, Gruber C, Hayes R, et al.** Medroxyprogesterone acetate and homozygous sickle cell disease. Lancet. 1982;ii:229-31.

33. **Garg SK, Chase HP, Marshall G, et al.** Oral contraceptives and renal and retinal complications in young women with insulin-dependent diabetes mellitus. JAMA. 1994;271: 1099-102.

34. **Skouby SO, Mølsted-Pedersen L, Kuhl C, Bennet P.** Oral contraceptives in diabetic women: metabolic effects of four compounds with different estrogen/progestogen profiles. Fertil Steril. 1986;46:858-64.

35. **Mishell DK Jr.** Contraception. N Engl J Med. 1989;320:777.

36. **Hannaford PC, Kay CR.** Oral contraceptives and diabetes mellitus. BMJ. 1989;299: 1315-6.

37. **Rimm EB, Manson JE, Stampfer MJ, et al.** Oral contraceptive use and the risk of type 2 (non-insulin-dependent) diabetes mellitus in a large prospective study of women. Diabetologia. 1992;35:967-72.

38. **Kjos SL, Shoupe P, Douyan S, et al.** Effect of low-dose oral contraceptives on carbohydrate and lipid metabolism in women with recent gestational diabetes: results of a controlled, randomized, prospective study. Am J Obstet Gynecol. 1990;163:1822-7.

39. **Timmer A, Sutherland LR, Martin F.** Oral contraceptive use and smoking are risk factors for relapse in Crohn's disease. The Canadian Mesalamine for Remission of Crohn's Disease Study Group. Gastroenterology. 1998;114:1143-50.

40. **Family and Reproductive Health Programme.** Improving Access to Quality Care in Family Planning. Medical Eligibility Criteria for Contraceptive Use. Geneva: World Health Organization; 1996.

41. **Douketis JD, Ginsberg JS, Holbrook A, Crowther M, Duku EK, Burrows RF.** A reevaluation of the risk for venous thromboembolism with the use of oral contraceptives and hormone replacement therapy. Arch Intern Med. 1997;157:1522-30.

42. **Farmer RDT, Lawrenson RA, Thompson CR, Kennedy JG, Hambleton IR.** Population-based study of risk of venous thromboembolism associated with various oral contraceptives. Lancet. 1997;349:83-8.

43. **Suissa S, Blais L, Spitzer WO, Cusson J, Lewis M, Heinemann L.** First-time use of newer oral contraceptives and the risk of venous thromboembolism. Contraception. 1997;56:141-6.

44. **Comp PC.** Thrombophilic mechanisms of OCs. Int J Fertil. 1997;42:170-6.

45. **Hellgren M, Svensson PJ, Dahlback B.** Resistance to activated protein C as a basis for venous thromboembolism associated with pregnancy and oral contraceptives. Am J Obstet Gynecol. 1995;173:210-3.

46. **Levine AB, Teppa J, McGough B, Cowchock S.** Evaluation of the prethrombotic state in pregnancy and in women using oral contraceptives. Contraception. 1996;53:255-7.

47. **World Health Organization Collaborative Study of Cardiovascular Disease and Steroid Hormone Contraception.** Effect of different progestagens in low oestrogen oral contraceptives on venous thromboembolic disease. Lancet. 1995;346:1582-8.

48. **Anderson BS, Olsen J, Nielsen GL, Steffensen FH, Sorenson HT, Baech J, Gregersen H.** Third generation oral contraceptives and heritable thrombophilia as risk factors of non-fatal venous thromboembolism. Thromb Haemost. 1998;79:28-31.

49. **Vandenbroucke JP, Helmerhorst FM, Bloemenkamp KWM, Rosendaal FR.** Third-generation oral contraceptive and deep venous thrombosis: from epidemiologic controversy to new insights in coagulation. Am J Obstet Gynecol. 1997;177:887-91.

50. **Bloemenkamp KWM, Rosendaal FR, Helmerhorst FM, Buller HR, Vandenbroucke JP.** Enhancement by factor V Leiden mutation of risk of deep vein thrombosis associ-

ated with oral contraceptives containing a third-generation progestagen. Lancet. 1995;346:1593-6.

51. **Spitzer WO, Lewis AL, Heinemann LAJ, Thorogood M, Mac Rae KD, the Transitional Research Group on Oral Contraceptives and the Health of Young Women.** Third generation oral contraceptives and risk of venous thromboembolic disorders: an international case-control study. BMJ. 1996;312:83-8.

52. **Vandenbroucke JP, Koster T, Briet E, Reitsma PH, Bertina RM, Rosendaal FR.** Increased risk of venous thrombosis in oral-contraceptive users who are carriers of factor V Leiden mutation. Lancet. 1994;344:1453-7.

53. **Price DT, Ridker PM.** Factor V Leiden mutation and the risks for thromboembolic disease: a clinical perspective. Ann Intern Med. 1997;127:895-903.

54. **Middeldorp S, Henkens CMA, Koopman MMW, van Pampus ECM, Hamulyak K, van der Meer J, et al.** The incidence of venous thromboembolism in family members of patients with factor V Leiden mutation and venous thrombosis. Ann Intern Med. 1998; 128:15-20.

55. **Frederiksen MC.** Depot medroxyprogesterone acetate contraception in women with medical problems. J Reprod Med. 1996;41:414-8.

56. **American College of Obstetricians and Gynecologists.** Hormonal contraception. ACOG Technical Bulletin. 1994;198:1-11.

57. **Shuster EA.** Epilepsy in women. Mayo Clin Proc. 1996;71:991-9.

58. **Krauss GL, Brandt J, Campbell M, Plate C, Summerfield M.** Antiepileptic medication and oral contraceptive interactions: a national survey of neurologists and obstetricians. Neurology. 1996;46:1534-9.

III. Genetic Counseling
Lorraine Dugoff

Recent technological advances in genetics and prenatal diagnosis have made it possible to identify persons who are at risk for having children with a variety of genetic disorders and, in many cases, to diagnose these disorders in the fetus before birth. Currently, many genetic disorders can be diagnosed as early as the first trimester. Conditions that can be detected before birth include fetal chromosomal abnormalities, Mendelian disorders (including autosomal-recessive, autosomal-dominant, and sex-linked conditions), and certain fetal structural abnormalities (including ventral wall defects and neural tube defects). It is important that health care providers know how to identify couples who should be offered genetic counseling or testing.

This section discusses specific situations in which persons or couples should be offered genetic counseling, genetic screening, or prenatal diagnosis. Recommendations on screening for Down syndrome and neural tube defects and on carrier screening for cystic fibrosis (CF), sickle-cell anemia, alpha- and beta-thalassemia, and Tay-Sachs disease (TSD) are reviewed.

Genetic Screening History

It is impractical to screen all couples and pregnancies for every condition that might be diagnosable before birth. A genetic history may help identify couples who would benefit from genetic counseling or testing. Ideally, in any situation in which there is an abnormality or a significant family history, confirmation should be made by reviewing pertinent medical records, including karyotype results, laboratory results, and pathology reports. Screening women of childbearing age by history provides an opportunity for evaluation before conception. Box 1-3 lists some of the most common indications for genetic counseling and prenatal screening.

Most indications for an offer of genetic counseling can be identified from a complete genetic history. In certain cases, such as maternal insulin-dependent diabetes mellitus, maternal phenylketonuria, or a maternal history of thrombosis or pulmonary embolism that may be associated with the factor V

Box 1-3 Indications for Genetic Counseling and Prenatal Screening

- Advanced maternal age (35 years of age or older at delivery)
- Advanced paternal age (50 years of age or older at conception)
- Abnormal biochemical screening result
- Patient, father, or previous child with known or suspected genetic disorder (e.g., cystic fibrosis, sickle-cell anemia, Tay-Sachs disease, muscular dystrophy), chromosomal defect (e.g., Down syndrome), birth defect (e.g., cleft lip, cleft palate, spin bifida, congenital heart defect), or mental retardation
- Positive family history of a known or suspected genetic disorder, chromosomal defect, or mental retardation
- Patient/family with multiple miscarriages or stillbirths
- Known or suspected teratogenic exposures, including exposure to parental medications, exposure to drugs, occupational and environmental exposures (e.g., to alcohol and recreational drugs), exposure to maternal illness (e.g., diabetes, phenylketonuria, epilepsy), or exposure to maternal infections (e.g., cytomegalovirus, rubella, toxoplasmosis)
- At-risk ethnic background for specific disorders
- Consanguinity (e.g., parents are first cousins)
- Suspected abnormality of the fetus on ultrasonography
- Positive family history of blood clots, pulmonary embolism, or stroke

Leiden mutation, it may be helpful to have an internist or perinatologist participate in the genetic counseling session.

Down Syndrome

Down syndrome occurs in 1 of 800 live births (1). In 95% of cases, it is a result of meiotic nondisjunction of the chromosome 21 pair, usually in the mother's gamete, resulting in a 47, +21 karyotype (Figure 1-1). The incidence of a fetus with Down syndrome increases with maternal age. The incidence of Down syndrome at birth in relation to maternal age is shown in Table 1-5. Four percent of cases of Down syndrome result from a translocation; about 1% result from mosaicism. These cases are not related to advanced maternal age.

Both ACOG and the American Academy of Pediatrics (AAP) state that women younger than 35 years of age should be offered serum screening to assess risk for Down syndrome. They do not consider multiple-marker screening to be equivalent to cytogenetic diagnosis in women who are 35 years of age or older (2).

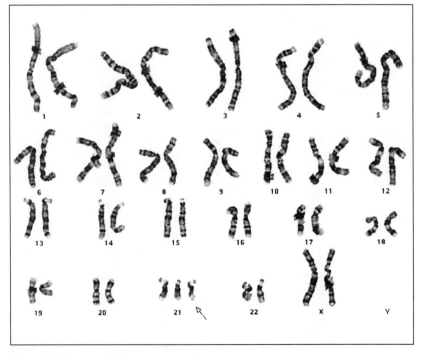

Figure 1-1 Trisomy 21 (Down syndrome).

Multiple-marker testing should ideally be offered between 15 and 18 weeks of gestation, although it can be done between 15 and 22 weeks. It is critical to know the precise gestational age because the median values for the biochemical markers and thus, the risk ratios, are based on gestational age. Prenatal screening for Down syndrome is most accurately done by chromosomal studies that require tissue obtained with amniocentesis or CVS. To avoid these invasive procedures, combinations of serum markers have been explored.

Various combinations of serum biochemical markers have been used to screen for Down syndrome since 1984, when it was found that low maternal

Table 1-5 Incidence of Down Syndrome in Live Births in Relation to Maternal Age

Maternal Age (years)	Incidence of Down Syndrome at Birth
20	1/1667
21	1/1667
22	1/1429
23	1/1429
24	1/1250
25	1/1250
26	1/1176
27	1/1111
28	1/1053
29	1/1000
30	1/952
31	1/909
32	1/769
33	1/625
34	1/500
35	1/385
36	1/294
37	1/227
38	1/175
39	1/137
40	1/106
41	1/82
42	1/64
43	1/50
44	1/38
45	1/30
46	1/23
47	1/18
48	1/14
49	1/11

Data from Hook EB. Rates of chromosome abnormalities at different maternal ages. Obstet Gynecol. 1981;58:282.

serum alpha-fetoprotein (MSAFP) levels were associated with Down syndrome (3). The combination of maternal age and MSAFP, human chorionic gonadotropin (hCG), and unconjugated estriol levels gives a sensitivity of about 58% with a 5% false-positive rate in women younger than 35 years of age (4). In women 35 years of age and older, one large study found that the same serum markers yielded a sensitivity for Down syndrome of 89% with a 25% false-positive rate (5). Biochemical screening may have a role in women 35 years of age and older who wish to avoid the risks associated with an invasive prenatal diagnostic procedure. Some women may use the result of this screening to decide whether to have amniocentesis. If a woman 35 years of age or older decides to undergo serum screening, she should be informed of the higher false-positive rate in her age group and of the decreased ability of the test (compared with fetal cytogenetic analysis) to detect fetal aneuploidy. In the future, first-trimester biochemical screening for Down syndrome may become available. A sensitivity of 60% was reported with a combination of maternal age and two markers: free beta-hCG levels and pregnancy-associated plasma protein-A levels (6).

Ultrasonographic markers for Down syndrome in both the first and second trimester may prove to be useful adjunct noninvasive screening tools. Subcutaneous edema in the neck region, visualized on ultrasonography as a thickened nuchal translucency measurement, is a common finding in the first trimester in fetuses with Down syndrome. Extensive studies in the United Kingdom have shown that the combination of maternal age and nuchal translucency is an effective screening test for Down syndrome between 10 and 14 weeks of gestation; the sensitivity is approximately 80% with a false-positive rate of 5% (7). Numerous ultrasonographic markers, including shortened humeri (8, 9), shortened femora (10, 11), pyelectasis (12), duodenal atresia (13), hypoplasia of the middle phalanx of the fifth digit (14), congenital heart anomalies (15), and nuchal skinfold (16), have been associated with Down syndrome in the second trimester.

Neural Tube Defects

All women with singleton or twin gestations should be offered serum screening for neural tube defects. Women at increased risk for a fetus with a neural tube defect include those with epilepsy or diabetes, those receiving valproic acid or carbamazepine, and those with a previous affected child or a family history of neural tube defects. Both ACOG and the AAP state that serum screening for neural tube defects should be offered to all women, ideally between 15 and 18 weeks of gestation and optimally at 16 weeks (2). Although screening for neural tube defects is most accurate when done between 16 and 18 weeks of gestation, it can be done between 15 and 22 weeks.

Screening for fetal neural tube defects is done by assaying maternal MSAFP levels. Elevated MSAFP levels were first reported to be associated with fetal neural tube defects in 1973 (17, 18). MSAFP screening can detect approximately 85% of all open neural tube defects, including about 90% of cases of anencephaly and 80% of cases of open spina bifida. Most laboratories use a cutoff value of 2.5 multiples of the median, which is associated with a 3% to 4% false-positive rate. The most common reason for a false-positive result is the underestimation of gestational age; thus, patients with elevated MSAFP levels should have ultrasonography to date the pregnancy and to rule out multiple gestation and fetal demise, which can be associated with an elevated MSAFP level. If the gestational age is correct, a comprehensive ultrasonographic examination should be done to seek evidence of neural tube defects or other abnormalities that have been associated with elevated MSAFP levels, including some of the conditions listed in Box 1-4. In some cases, amniocentesis may be done. Amniotic fluid alpha-fetoprotein levels, acetylcholinesterase levels, and fetal karyotype may be assessed to help clarify a diagnosis (4).

Cystic Fibrosis

Cystic fibrosis, an autosomal-recessive condition, is one of the most common genetic diseases in white persons, with an incidence of approximately 1/3300 and a carrier frequency of 1/29. It is less common in persons of other ethnic backgrounds; the incidence is 1/9500 in Hispanic persons and 1/50,000 in native Africans and native Asians. Although more than 600 mutations have been identified in the CF gene, it is possible to detect significant percentages of CF mutations in selected populations. This is because of the prevalence of a small number of specific mutations in these populations. The ΔF508 mutation accounts for approximately 70% of the CF alleles in the white population. Combining detection of this mutation with that of other mutations common to specific ethnic groups results in 90% to 95% sensitivity in Ashkenazi Jews, French Canadians from Quebec, Celtic Bretons, and some Native Americans. The overall detection rate for white persons approaches 90% when screening is done for F508 and several other mutations (19).

A National Institutes of Health (NIH) consensus statement published in April 1997 (19) recommended that several groups be offered carrier testing. These groups are 1) persons with a positive family history of CF, 2) partners of persons with CF, 3) couples planning a pregnancy, and 4) couples seeking prenatal care. The American College of Medical Genetics (ACMG) (20) supports offering testing to couples in which one or both partners has CF or has a relative with CF. However, the ACMG has stated that it is premature to offer CF testing to all couples who are planning a pregnancy or who are pregnant. The NIH and

---

Box 1-4   Conditions Associated with Elevated MSAFP (Maternal Serum α-Fetoprotein Level)

Neural tube defects
Multiple gestation
Fetal demise
Ventral wall defects
    Gastroschisis
    Omphalocele
Urinary tract disease
    Renal agenesis
    Congenital nephrosis
    Polycystic kidney disease
    Obstructive lesion
Integumental defects
    Epidemolysis bullosa
    Congenital ichthyosiform erythroderma
Cystic hygroma
Hydrops or ascites
Esophageal or duodenal atresia
Placental abnormalities
    Retroplacental hemorrhage
    Placental lakes
    Hemangiomas of placenta and cord
Selective fetal reduction
Maternal hepatoma

---

the ACMG agree that only a provider who is familiar with the tests, the interpretation of the tests, and the limitations of testing should offer genetic testing for CF. If a couple with no family history of CF requests testing, it is appropriate to arrange for genetic counseling followed by carrier testing if the couple wishes it. Prenatal testing is done by using fetal DNA obtained through CVS, amniocentesis, or percutaneous umbilical blood sampling (PUBS).

Sickle-Cell Anemia

Sickle-cell anemia is an autosomal-recessive disorder that affects approximately 1 in 600 black Americans. The carrier rate in this population is approximately 8% (1). Ideally, all persons of African, Middle Eastern, Mediterranean, Indian, Caribbean, or Latin American descent should be offered carrier testing before conception (21). Persons at high risk for a hemoglobin disorder should have electrophoresis. Although useful as a screening test solely for sickle-cell anemia, solubility tests, such as Sickledex, are inadequate in assessing reproductive genetic risk because they may give negative results in persons with a variety of hemoglobin gene abnormalities, including beta-thalassemia trait and hemoglobin C trait. Carriers with these and other genotypes may be asymptomatic. However, if a woman has a partner with sickle-cell trait or another hemoglobinopathy, she is at risk for offspring with more serious hemoglobinopathies, including hemoglobin S/beta-thalassemia and hemoglobin sickle-cell disease (22).

It is reasonable to offer genetic counseling to all women at risk for a child with sickle-cell anemia. If a woman declines genetic counseling, carrier testing, or prenatal diagnostic testing, this should be documented in her chart. Prenatal diagnosis for sickle-cell anemia may be done on fetal DNA obtained through CVS, amniocentesis, or PUBS. If a mother is a carrier for sickle-cell anemia and the father declines carrier testing, prenatal testing for sickle-cell anemia may be appropriate (23). If the father is a black American, the risk for an affected fetus may be as high as 2%.

Thalassemias

The thalassemias are most prevalent in persons from the Mediterranean region and parts of Africa and southeast Asia. They are a heterogeneous group of hereditary anemias in which the common feature is decreased synthesis of one or more of the globin chains of hemoglobin. The two main types are the alpha-thalassemias, in which alpha-chain synthesis is reduced or absent, and the beta-thalassemias, in which beta-chain synthesis is deficient (24). Many hemoglobinopathies, including beta-thalassemia, are autosomal recessive.

All pregnant women should be screened for thalassemia traits with a complete blood count with erythrocyte indices and routine prenatal laboratory tests. An underlying thalassemia syndrome should be suspected in a patient with microcytosis, hypochromia, and a mean corpuscular hemoglobin concentration less than 27% in the absence of iron-deficiency anemia. If ferritin studies are normal, hemoglobin electrophoresis may be done to detect heterozygous beta-thalassemia that is associated with mild increases in hemoglobin A2. In patients with a consistently low mean corpuscular hemoglobin concentration, normal iron study results, and normal results on hemoglobin electrophoresis, DNA-based testing can be used to detect heterozygous alpha-thalassemia (23).

Carrier testing of the partner should be strongly recommended if a woman is a carrier for beta-thalassemia, alpha-thalassemia, or another hemoglobinopathy. Erythrocyte indices and hemoglobin electrophoresis should both be done (23).

Prenatal diagnosis should be offered to all couples in which both partners are carriers for an autosomal-recessive hemoglobinopathy. Prenatal diagnosis may be done on fetal DNA obtained through CVS, amniocentesis, or PUBS. If the results of prenatal testing are positive, it may be helpful for the couple to consult with a hematologist.

Tay-Sachs Disease

Tay-Sachs is an autosomal-recessive lysosomal storage disease that results from deficiency of an enzyme called *hexosaminidase A*. Gangliosides accumulate in the central nervous system, causing progressive neurologic deterioration and death in early childhood. The frequency of TSD is 100 times higher in Ashkenazi Jews (1/3600) than in most other populations (1/360,000) (1). The carrier rate for TSD is 1/27 in Ashkenazi Jews. Three alleles account for approximately 97% of all TSD mutations in this population. Persons of French-Canadian and Cajun descent also have a greater prevalence of TSD compared with the general population.

Carrier screening for TSD is done by measuring hexosaminidase A activity. A higher rate of false-positive test results is seen in women who are pregnant or using oral contraceptives when the serum is assayed for hexosaminidase A. Therefore, these women should have leukocyte testing. Prenatal diagnosis may be done by measuring hexosaminidase A activity in both CVS and amniocentesis samples. The ACOG Committee on Genetics published recommendations on TSD in 1995 (Box 1-5) (25).

Mental Retardation

If a couple has a family history of mental retardation, the cause of the condition should be identified if possible. It is helpful to determine whether the condition is genetic or acquired (from infection, trauma, asphyxia, alcohol use, or toxin exposure). Down syndrome is the most common genetic cause; it accounts for an estimated one third of cases of moderate mental retardation. Other chromosomal abnormalities account for only 1% to 5% of cases. The most common inherited and second most common genetic cause of mental retardation is the fragile X syndrome, which affects approximately 1 in 1000 males (26). When a woman is a known carrier of the fragile X permuta-

---

Box 1-5 Recommendations for Screening for Tay-Sachs Disease

- Offer testing before pregnancy if both members of a couple are Ashkenazi Jews or of French-Canadian or Cajun descent. Screen those with a family history consistent with TSD.
- Offer testing to the member of a couple who is at high risk (i.e., Ashkenazi Jew, of French-Canadian or Cajun descent, or a family history consistent with TSD). If the high-risk partner is determined to be a carrier, then the other partner should also be screened. If the woman is already pregnant, consider screening both partners simultaneously so that the results are obtained quickly and to ensure that all options are available to the couple.
- Ambiguous or positive screening tests in persons not at high risk should be confirmed by molecular analysis for the most common mutations. This will detect patients who carry genes associated with mild disease or pseudo-deficiency states.
- For TSD screening in women who are pregnant or using oral contraceptives, leukocyte testing must be used.
- If both partners are determined to be carriers of TSD, genetic counseling and prenatal diagnosis should be offered.

Recommendations from American College of Obstetricians and Gynecologists, Committee on Genetics. Screening for Tay-Sachs disease. Committee opinion. 1995; 162.

---

tion or mutation, prenatal diagnostic testing for fragile X with amniocentesis should be offered (27).

Teratogen Exposure

If a pregnant woman has been exposed to a drug or substance that may be teratogenic, it is appropriate to refer her for genetic counseling and subsequent fetal ultrasonographic examination, if indicated. Gestational age, dose, and duration of exposure should be determined. If a patient has been exposed to a potentially teratogenic virus, such as rubella, CMV, or toxoplasmosis, consultation with a perinatologist may be appropriate. Maternal conditions such as pregestational diabetes mellitus, epilepsy, congenital heart disease, and phenylketonuria are associated with potential birth defects. Women with these conditions should receive preconception counseling if possible. Pregnant women with pregestational diabetes mellitus should be referred for a comprehensive ultrasonographic evaluation to rule out fetal anomalies, including cardiac and neural tube defects.

REFERENCES

1. **Thompson MW, McInnes RR, Willard HG, eds.** Thompson & Thompson: Genetics in Medicine, 5th ed. Philadelphia: WB Saunders; 1991:70, 215, 248-263.

2. Guidelines for Perinatal Care, 4th ed. American Academy of Pediatrics, American College of Obstetrics and Gynecology; 1997:79-80.

3. **Merkatz IR, Nitowshy HM, Macri JN, Johnson WE.** An association between low maternal serum alpha-fetoprotein and fetal chromosomal abnormalities. Am J Obstet Gynecol. 1984;148:886-94.

4. **American College of Obstetricians and Gynecologists.** Maternal serum screening. ACOG Technical Bulletin. 1996;228.

5. **Haddow JE, Palomaki GE, Knight GJ, Williams J, Polkkinen A, Canich JA, et al.** Prenatal screening for Down syndrome with use of maternal serum markers. N Engl J Med. 1992;327:588-93.

6. **Haddow JE, Palomaki GE, Knight GJ, Williams J, Miller WA, Johnson A.** Screening of maternal serum for fetal Down's syndrome in the first trimester. N Engl J Med. 1998;338:955-61.

7. **Snijders RJM, Noble P, Sebin NJ, Souka AP, Nicolaides KH.** UK Multicentric project on assessment of risk for trisomy 21 by maternal age and fetal nuchal translucency at 10-14 weeks of gestation. Lancet. In press.

8. **Fitzsimmons J, Droste S, Shepard TH, Pascoe-Mason J, Chinn A, Mack LA.** Longbone growth in fetuses with Down syndrome. Am J Obstet Gynecol. 1989;161: 1174-7.

9. **Johnson MP, Michaelson JE, Barr M Jr, Treadwell MC, Isada NB, Dombrowski MP, et al.** Sonographic screening for trisomy 21: fetal humerus:footlength ratio, a useful new marker. Fetal Diagn Ther. 1994;9:130-8.

10. **Lockwood C, Benacerraf BR, Krinsky A, et al.** A sonographic screening method for Down syndrome. Am J Obstet Gynecol. 1987;157:803-8.

11. **Cuckle H, Wald N, Quinn J, Royston P, Butler L.** Ultrasound fetal femur length measurement in the screening for Down's syndrome. Br J Obstet Gynaecol. 1989;96:1373-8.

12. **Benacerraf BR, Mandell J, Estroff JA, Harlow BL, Frigoletto FD.** Fetal pyelectasis: a possible association with Down syndrome. Obstet Gynecol. 1990;76:58-60.

13. **Nyberg DA, Resta RG, Luthy DA, Hickok DE, Mahony BS, Hirsch JH.** Prenatal sonographic findings of Down syndrome: review of 94 cases. Obstet Gynecol. 1990;76:370-7.

14. **Benacerraf BR, Harlow BL, Frigoletto FD.** Hypoplasia of the middle phalanx of the fifth digit: a feature of the second trimester fetus with Down's syndrome. J Ultrasound Med. 1990;9:389-94.

15. **Copel JA, Pilu G, Kleinman CS.** Congenital heart disease and extracardiac anomalies: associations and indications for fetal echocardiography. Am J Obstet Gynecol. 1986;154:1121-32.

16. **Crane JP, Gray DL.** Sonographically measured nuchal skinfold thickness as a screening tool for Down syndrome: results of a prospective clinical trial. Obstet Gynecol. 1991;77:533-6.

17. **Leek AE, Ruoss CF, Kitau MJ, Chard T.** Raised alpha-fetoprotein in maternal serum with anencephalic pregnancy. Lancet. 1973;2:385.

18. **Brock DJH, Bolton AE, Monaghan JM.** Prenatal diagnosis of anencephaly through maternal serum alpha-fetoprotein measurement. Lancet. 1973;2:923-4.

19. **National Institutes of Health.** NIH Consensus Statement. Genetic Testing for Cystic Fibrosis, v 15. 1997.

20. **American College of Medical Genetics.** ACMG Statement on Genetic Testing for Cystic Fibrosis; 1997.

21. **American College of Obstetricians and Gynecologists.** Preconceptional care. ACOG Technical Bulletin. 1995;205.

22. **American College of Obstetricians and Gynecologists, Committee on Genetics.** Genetic screening for hemoglobinopathies. Committee opinion. 1996;168.

23. **American College of Obstetricians and Gynecologists.** Hemoglobinopathies in pregnancy. ACOG Technical Bulletin. 1996;220.

24. **Gelehrter TD, Collins FS.** Molecular genetics of human disease: hemoglobinopathies. In: Principles of Medical Genetics. Baltimore: Williams & Wilkins; 1990:97-121.

25. **American College of Obstetricians and Gynecologists, Committee on Genetics.** Screening for Tay-Sachs disease. Committee opinion. 1995;162.

26. **Robinson A, Linden MG.** Clinical Genetics Handbook, 2d ed. Blackwell Scientific Publications; 1993:71-5.

27. **American College of Obstetricians and Gynecologists, Committee on Genetics.** Fragile X syndrome. Committee opinion. 1995;161.

IV. Normal Labor and Delivery
Phyllis C. Leppert

Modern scientific knowledge of normal labor and delivery shows that these processes are part of a physiologic continuum that begins at conception (Figure 1-2). Current understanding of the complex biochemical events culminating in birth shows that labor and delivery are not initiated at one isolated point in time. Neither are they triggered by one factor alone. A series of complex but carefully orchestrated modulations in reproductive tract anatomy and physiologic function seems to commence at the onset of pregnancy. The biological mechanisms that maintain the fetus in utero are followed gradually by specific, sequentially triggered pathways that facilitate the safe passage of the newborn from the uterus through the cervix and vagina. These physiologic pathways are not only gradual in timing but often overlap. Therefore, even a meticulous clinician sometimes finds it difficult to determine exactly when the process of parturition begins. Often, the diagnosis of labor is made in retrospect.

Phase 0	Phase 1	Phase 2	Phase 3
Prelude to parturition	*Preparation for labor*	*Process of labor*	*Postpartum*
Relative contractile paralysis	CRH and CRH binding protein increases 50-fold	Uterine contractions Cervix dilates	Involution persistent
Refractory to oxytocin	Oxytocin receptors increase		Uterine contractions
Few oxytocin receptors	Contractile response increases	Increased contractile response to prostaglandin, oxytocin, and other hormones and proteins	
Progesterone effect	Number and size of gap junction increase		
	Progesterone withdrawal		
↑	↑ Uterine preparedness for labor	↑ Active labor (3 stages of labor)	↑
Conception	Initiation of parturition	Onset of labor	Delivery

Figure 1-2 Functional phases of the uterine fundus and lower segment throughout child-bearing. Adapted from Cunningham FG, et al. William's Obstetrics, 20th ed. Stanford, CT: Appleton & Lange; 1997:280.

Definition of Clinical Labor

The most widespread and useful definition of labor encompasses the concept of regular, rhythmic uterine contractions that lead to cervical changes. Four or more contractions per hour in a multiparous woman or six or more contractions per hour in a nulliparous woman are seen. These contractions, however, must cause progressive changes in the consistency, effacement, or dilation of the cervix or the cervix must be dilated 2 cm or more for labor to be diagnosed. Many pregnant women have palpable regular uterine contractions during the last 4 weeks of pregnancy, making the clinical presentation of labor confusing to the practitioner. The digital cervical examination is semiquantitative (Table 1-6). Several authors have shown vaginal-probe ultrasonography to be effective in elucidating cervical change, but this approach currently seems to be best used in situations of abnormal parturition, such as preterm labor or prolonged preterm rupture of fetal membranes. Vaginal-probe ultrasonography is not routinely used in normal labor at term (1, 2).

Physiology

During gestation, the uterus (composed of smooth muscle and connective tissues) must enlarge to contain the growing fetus. At the same time, it must remain relatively quiescent and unresponsive to contractile stimuli so that the

Table 1-6 Bishop Score for Digital Cervical Examination*

Factor	Points			
	0	1	2	3
Dilatation of cervix, cm	0	1-2	3-4	5+
Effacement of cervix, %	0-30	40-50	60-70	80+
Consistency of cervix	Firm	Medium	Soft	
Position of cervix in vagina	Posterior	Middle	Anterior	
Station[†]	−3	−2	−1	+1/+2

*A score of 9 or more indicates that the cervix will easily dilate upon onset of regular uterine contractions.
†This factor is somewhat confusing because old criteria are used (station below or above the ischial spine divided into *thirds*). Newer criteria divide the station above or below the spine into *fifths*.
Adapted from Oxon H. Oxon-Foote's Human Labor and Birth, 5th ed. Norwalk, CT: Appleton & Lange; 1986.

pregnancy is maintained for the average 40 weeks of gestation. The uterine cervix is softer in early and mid-gestation than it is in nonpregnant women, but it must remain resistant enough to uterine contractions to remain closed, allowing the fetus to remain in the uterus until birth (3). The uterus and cervix prepare for parturition from conception through mid-gestation to a transitional phase that begins at about 35 weeks of gestation.

The muscles of the myometrium are organized in thick and thin filaments found in random, long bundles throughout the cells. These smooth muscle cells are capable of greater shortening during contractions than striated muscle cells are. Forces can be exerted in any direction in smooth muscle, although skeletal striated muscles have a contraction force aligned with the axis of the muscle fibers. Contractions of myometrial cells are involuntary.

Uterine contractions in laboring women are painful. The degree of pain felt varies in individual women. Psychological stress, such as fear and anxiety, can increase the pain felt; thus, educational preparation before labor is offered to childbearing women. The reason for the pain of contractions is unclear. Suggested causes are hypoxia of the myometrium, compression of nerve ganglia of the cervix and lower uterine cervix, stretching of the dilating cervix, and stretching of the peritoneum over the fundus (1). When the cervix is stretched mechanically by an examining finger, uterine contractions are enhanced. This is known as the *Ferguson reflex* and is probably caused by the release of prostaglandin $F_{2\alpha}$ metabolite from the fetal membranes.

During labor, the upper portion of the uterus (fundus) contracts and thickens as labor progresses. The lower portion is passive and becomes thin as labor advances. Thus, the upper part of the uterus expels the fetus while the lower segment and cervix dilate. As labor progresses, the fundus does not relax to its original length but remains shorter, decreasing the volume of the uterine cavity. The fetus is gently forced toward the cervix and vagina with each contraction and remains in position until the next contraction. When the cervix is dilated fully to 10 cm, increased maternal intra-abdominal pressure created by a voluntary contraction of the abdominal muscles with the glottis closed, along with the involuntary contraction of the myometrium, allows for expulsion of the infant. This force is similar to the force involved in defecation but is much more intense.

The cervix changes as it is effaced or obliterated. As the presenting part or fetal membranes are forced against the internal os of the cervix, the smooth muscle cells, cervical collagen, and elastin become aligned and thinned out. It becomes impossible to determine where the cervix begins and the lower uterine segment ends.

Clinical Progress of Labor

Regardless of his or her medical specialty, every physician must understand the process of childbirth because this experience affects women on many levels: physiologic, emotional, and spiritual. Although the exact details of the events of each woman's labor and delivery are unique and may be forgotten over time, the overall experience is indelible. Childbirth and motherhood alter a woman's perception of herself forever. The alterations that the physiologic process makes to her body can lead to changes that may cause health problems in both the immediate and distant future. Internists must appreciate that birth may affect the functioning of the urinary tract both acutely postpartum and many decades later. Hormonal changes in the postpartum period may be a precipitating factor in postpartum depression. Birth affects a woman's relationship to her family and to her sexual partner. Domestic violence and abuse are often initiated during or after the first pregnancy.

Stages of Labor

First Stage

The first of the three stages of labor begins when regular rhythmic contractions of the uterine fundus are strong and coordinated enough to cause dilation and effacement. At term, before the onset of parturition, the cervix softens. The first stage of labor ends when the cervix is fully dilated to 10 cm and can be evaluated by using the semiquantitative Bishop score (see Table 1-6). This stage takes the longest period of time and lasts, on average, 5 hours in multiparous women and 8 hours in nulliparous women. It can be shorter or longer but, by definition, labor shorter than 3 hours or longer than 18 hours is not considered to be normal physiologic labor.

Most women describe the sensation of irregular Braxton Hicks contractions that increase in intensity and frequency as pregnancy approaches term (36 to 41 weeks of gestation). These contractions may masquerade as labor contractions but do not cause dilation of the cervix. Over several hours, the Braxton Hicks contractions decrease in intensity and frequency and then disappear completely. This pattern of contractions constitutes false labor, a phenomenon that can be exceedingly frustrating to the woman and her physician. Other signs of impending labor include a sudden spurt of energy that usually occurs 24 hours before the onset of contractions that may signify true labor and result in cervical dilation.

Labor, or phase 2 of parturition, begins as a series of mild but regular uterine contractions that start approximately 20 or 30 minutes apart. Women experience these contractions as pressure; cramps; and, sometimes, backache. Over several hours, these regular contractions become stronger, closer together, and painful. As labor progresses to an active phase, the digestive system slows and most women are not hungry. The laboring woman at this point stops her activity, begins to focus her energies on labor, and begins to concentrate inwardly.

The first stage of labor is subdivided into the latent phase and the active phase. The latent phase varies in length and starts with the onset of regular rhythmic contractions that are strong and coordinated enough to cause effacement and dilation of the cervix. In nulliparous women, the average length of the latent phase is 8.6 hours; in multiparous women, it is 5.3 hours (Figure 1-3) (4). The normal limit of the latent phase is 20 hours in nulliparous and 14 hours in multiparous women.

The active phase of the first stage of labor starts when the cervix is dilated 3 to 4 cm. The connective tissue of the cervix has been changed, allowing for more rapid dilation. The contractions are stronger and more frequent, occurring about 5 to 6 minutes apart. This active phase is normally 12 hours in nulliparous and 6 hours in multiparous women.

A transition phase of varied but very short duration occurs between the first and second stages. This transition phase from stage one to stage two corresponds to the time between 8 cm and 10 cm or full dilation. During transition, normal laboring women may experience a full gamut of emotions and may feel overwhelmed by the intensity of these feelings. Rigors and vomiting are common during transition.

Second Stage

The second stage of labor begins with complete dilation of the cervix and ends with the birth of the baby. The second stage is the expulsion stage. The laboring woman feels an instinctive urge to push or bear down. Pushing, accomplished by the Valsalva maneuver, extends the force of the contraction by 20% to 30% to allow the infant to pass through the vagina and pelvis. Progress of the second stage of labor is measured by the station of the presenting part (the distance above or below the ischial spine).

The fetal membranes usually rupture spontaneously in the active phase. In some cases at term, membranes rupture before the onset of labor. In most of these cases, contractions begin spontaneously within 12 hours. The time between spontaneous rupture of the membranes and onset of labor usually does not exceed 24 hours.

The normal mechanisms of labor that allow the fetus to pass the pelvic bone are descent, flexion, internal rotation, extension, restitution, and external rotation, followed by delivery. These classic mechanisms occur because the force of the mother's expulsive efforts and of the contractions causes the fetal presenting part to meet the resistance of the pelvis. The fetal presenting part passively turns as it makes its way through the pelvic canal. The birth process can be aided by gentle maneuvers by the physician or midwife. An episiotomy may be done but is not always indicated.

Third Stage

The third stage of labor is the delivery of the placenta. The upper limit of this stage is 30 minutes. The placenta should be removed manually under anesthesia after 30 minutes, although many obstetricians do this removal sooner.

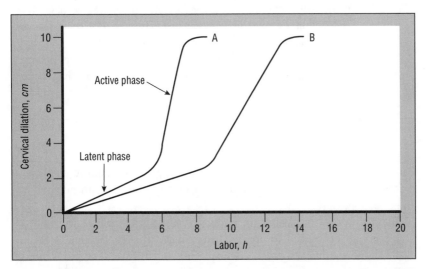

Figure 1-3 Friedman curves in first stage of labor in multiparous (A) and nulliparous (B) women.

Box 1-6 Abnormalities in Fetal Heart Rates

- Fetal Bradycardia (Baseline fetal heart rate less than 120 beats/min lasting 15 min or more)
    - *Mild*—100 to 119 beats/min for 50 min
    - *Moderate*—80 to 100 beats/min for 3 min
    - *Severe*—80 beats/min for 3 min or more
- Fetal Tachycardia
    - *Mild*—161 to 180 beats/min
    - *Severe*—181 beats/min or more
- Beat-to-Beat Variability (Baseline fetal heart rate normally exhibits oscillating form)
    - *Short-term*—Measures time interval between cardiac systoles
    - *Long-term*—Oscillatory changes over time; normally there are three to five wave cycles per minute
    - *Decreased*—Absent short-term variability, then two cyclic changes per minute in long-term variability
- Periodic Fetal Heart Rate (Deviation from baseline related to uterine contraction)
    - *Acceleration*—Increases above baseline
    - *Deceleration*—Decreases below baseline based on timing of deceleration in relation to contraction
    - *Early*—Decreases with uterine contractions (the form mirrors the uterine contraction thought to be due to physiologic head compression)
    - *Late*—A symmetrical decrease beginning at or after the peak of the uterine contraction; return to baseline after the contraction has ended; uniform in shape; descent and return of fetal heart rate is gradual and smooth; sign of uteroplacental insufficiency
    - *Variable*—Most common in labor; abrupt, jagged-appearing deceleration; heart rate decreasing to less than 70 beats/min lasting more than 60 sec is significant; a sign of cord compression

---

Care must be taken to ensure that the complete placenta is delivered because even small portions of retained placenta can cause postpartum hemorrhage and infection.

After the third stage of labor, the physician must ensure that the new mother's uterus is well contracted to prevent hemorrhage. This contraction is accomplished by giving the mother Pitocin (oxytocin) 20 U in 1 L of fluid intravenously or 10 U intramuscularly, or by putting the infant immediately to breast, or both.

Maternal and Fetal Monitoring

During labor, there are two persons to be monitored: the woman and the fetus. The mother is observed carefully for fatigue, an abnormal uterine contraction pattern, and hemorrhage. Vital signs, including blood pressure, are checked frequently (at least hourly in a normal first stage of labor).

In the second stage of labor, vital signs should be recorded every 15 minutes. Normally, the maternal temperature is taken and recorded every 4 hours. These statements reflect guidelines, and adherence to them does not replace constant attention, observation, and good judgment about when to change routines. Laboring women should never be alone for many reasons, not the least of which is that they require companionship and assistance in maintaining physiologic labor.

The fetus must also be monitored carefully. In most clinical situations, fetal monitoring means continuous electronic fetal heart rate monitoring. Auscultation, if done properly by skilled, educated attendants, has produced satisfactory results. However, proper auscultation is expensive because of the need for the constant attendance of the physician or midwife, so labor in the United States is usually monitored by continuous electronic fetal monitoring. The fetal heart rate shows frequent periodic variations and, at term, the normal average fetal heart rate is 120 to 160 beats/min.

Abnormalities in fetal heart rates are listed in Box 1-6. Interpretation of electronic fetal monitoring can be difficult and is always best left to experts.

REFERENCES

1. **Cunningham FG, MacDonald PC, Gant NF, Leveno KJ, Gilstrap LC, Hankins GDV, Clark SL, eds.** William's Obstetrics, 20th ed. Stamford, CT: Appleton & Lange; 1997:261-317.

2. **Dyson DC, Danbe KH, Bamber MSD, Crites YM, Field DR, Maier JA, et al.** Monitoring women at risk for preterm labor. N Engl J Med. 1998;338:15-9.

3. **Leppert PC.** Cervical softening, effacement and dilation: a complex biochemical cascade. Journal of M-F Medicine. 1992;1:213-23.

4. **Friedman EA.** Labor: Clinical Evaluation and Management. 2d ed. New York: Appleton-Century-Crofts; 1978:45-59.

V. Symptoms Produced by Normal Physiologic Changes in Pregnancy
Richard V. Lee

Physicians and patients expect that gestation will be accompanied by normal emotional and physical symptoms, and most pregnant women do not complain about these expected aberrations. In some patients, however, the anatomic, physiologic, and social changes produced by normal gestation profoundly alter perceptions of well-being. The common complaints related to gestation are of four types, each with a distinct pattern of onset and intensity:

1. Complaints beginning early in pregnancy and persisting until delivery.
2. Complaints usually confined to the first half of pregnancy.
3. Complaints beginning in mid-pregnancy and increasing or persisting until delivery. (The anatomic and physiologic effects of the enlarging gravid uterus are responsible for many of these discomforts.)
4. Complaints related to labor, delivery, and lactation.

Complaints Beginning Early in Pregnancy and Persisting until Delivery

In questionnaire-based surveys of pregnant women and their husbands, the symptoms that most reliably appear in early pregnancy are nausea, vomiting, easy fatigability, and concern about weight (Box 1-7) (1).

Box 1-7 Complaints Beginning Early in Gestation

Sensory dysphoria (changes in taste and smell)
Nausea and vomiting
Concern about weight
Ptyalism
Nasal stuffiness
Esophageal reflux
Change in voice
Dyspnea and hyperventilation symptoms
Skin changes
  Telangiectasia
  Increased pigmentation
Fatigability

Weight and Shape

Many pregnant women in North America "eat for two" and exceed the recommended weight gain of 12 to 14 kg. There has been a proscription against weight loss during pregnancy, so there is a tendency to feed overweight women the same amounts as lean pregnant women and expect them to gain the same amount of weight. This practice is abetted by liberal dietary recommendations of 2200 to 2600 kcal/d, which are based on the calculation that pregnancy and lactation increase caloric requirements by 300 to 400 kcal/d. However, the assumption that a healthy woman has a basal caloric requirement, varying with body weight, of 1600 to 2100 kcal/d is not supported by recent data that indicate basic caloric requirements of 1200 to 1500 kcal/d (2).

Stricter definition of or closer adherence to recommended weight gain and more emphatic instruction about a diet of 1800 to 2200 kcal/d may diminish the burden of and the medical risks inherent in pregnancy-related obesity. Modest limitations in diet (1400 to 1600 kcal/d) may be indicated for obese women (3). Recent studies in pregnant women with type 1 insulin-dependent diabetes suggest that ketonemia, especially excess beta-hydroxybutyrate, may be associated with developmental delay (4). However, occasional ketonuria (usually acetoacetate) in the absence of acidosis is common in normal pregnancy and is not associated with adverse fetal outcome.

Changes in Gastrointestinal Motility and Secretion

Upper Gastrointestinal Tract Complaints
Successful implantation and placentation are accompanied by relaxation of smooth muscle. Every muscular tube in a woman's body has reduced tone and frequency and force of peristalsis. Vasodilatory prostaglandins, progesterone, and vascular endothelial substances have been shown to contribute to this loosening of tubes. Decreased lower esophageal pressures, decreased gastric peristalsis, delayed gastric emptying, and decreased colonic motility are responsible for two prominent complaints during pregnancy: heartburn and constipation.

Decreased lower esophageal pressures can be seen throughout gestation. Esophageal reflux is frequent but often asymptomatic. Reflux is aggravated by vomiting in early pregnancy and by the expanded uterus later in pregnancy. All pregnant women are at risk for aspiration pneumonia, and this risk is not confined to the period of labor and delivery.

Excessive salivation (ptyalism or sialorrhea) is less common, and its pathophysiology is not well known. The constellation of morning sickness, sialorrhea, esophageal reflux with heartburn, and constipation can make even the hardiest woman miserable. Esophageal reflux may exacerbate sialorrhea, or

"water brash." Pregnant patients with ptyalism describe their copious oral secretions as thin, watery, and bitter (5). Swallowing them may induce nausea
and vomiting and may not relieve heartburn.

As pregnancy progresses, diminished gastrointestinal motility combines
with the enlargement of the gravid uterus to produce persistent esophageal
reflux. During late pregnancy, some women are obliged to sleep in a sitting or
semirecumbent posture because of reflux and intense pyrosis. These patients
may present with recurrent cough, wheezing, and aspiration pneumonia.
Avoiding meals after 6:00 P.M. and elevating the head of the bed with bed
blocks may be useful to the patient.

Lower Gastrointestinal Tract Complaints

Constipation is an annoyance associated with pregnancy that often is the subject of humor and is frequently attributed to the use of prenatal vitamins or
iron pills. Annoyance can be transformed into discomfort with the appearance
of hemorrhoids with bleeding, itching, and pain with defecation. A high-fiber
diet, increased water intake, use of stool softeners (such as dulcusate
sodium), and careful attention to vulvar and perianal hygiene are helpful but
often insufficient. Sitz baths and hemorrhoidal preparations (hydrocortisone-
containing suppositories and creams) may give temporary relief. Postural
changes are important—for example, the uterine obstruction to venous flow
can be relieved by assumption of the lateral decubitus position. The squatting
posture or a semisquatting position can be achieved by using footstools to elevate the legs. Labor and delivery usually produce transient exacerbation of
hemorrhoids, which gradually resolve postpartum. Surgical management of
protruding or thrombosed hemorrhoids may be required.

Changes in Mucosae of the Nose and Oropharynx

Nasal stuffiness, hoarseness or changes in voice quality, and cough are common in pregnant women. During pregnancy, the nasal mucosa undergo mucous gland hypertrophy, increased connective tissue ground substance, and
increased vascular pooling related to general vasodilatation (6).

A substantial minority of women have nasal stuffiness during pregnancy
(7, 8). Many of these patients have had symptoms of atopic or obstructive
rhinitis before pregnancy (8). All gravid women have an enhanced risk for superimposed bacterial sinusitis and Eustachian tube dysfunction (8), which
predisposes to barotrauma. Pregnant women should be cautioned about air
travel and underwater sports. Recognition of sinusitis may be difficult, with
nasal congestion in the absence of rhinitis or in the woman who had allergies
before pregnancy. Ear, nose, and throat evaluation, followed by vigorous therapy with antibiotics and topical vasoconstrictors and steroids, is indicated if
sinusitis is suspected. The indications for sinus radiography are unchanged in

pregnancy. The classic history and findings for sinusitis are not present in many patients with documented purulent sinusitis (8).

There are few therapeutic options for the nasal congestion of pregnancy (9). Topical and systemic decongestants should be avoided, especially if the patient has labile or elevated blood pressure. Chronic maternal use of systemic antihistamines has caused some cases of neonatal withdrawal symptoms. It is unclear whether antihistamines can cause congenital malformations, but given that antihistamines do not relieve pregnancy-induced nasal stuffiness, it is probably best to avoid their use during pregnancy. Women with pre-existing allergic or obstructive rhinitis may continue to use topical intranasal cromolyn and corticosteroids without undue risk.

The changes that occur in the nasal mucosa predispose to epistaxis. Occasionally, a pregnant patient may develop a vascular polyp similar to the vascular granuloma gravidarum that develops on the gingivae (10). In the absence of infection or thrombosis, these lesions disappear spontaneously shortly after delivery. Treatment, except for excision for intractable bleeding, is unnecessary.

Mucosal changes in the larynx and trachea may contribute to alterations in voice and the presence of a bothersome nonproductive cough (11), symptoms that can be exacerbated by esophageal reflux. Vocal performers may note changes in timbre, pitch, and breathing that can inhibit practice and performance.

Dyspnea

Progestational hormones stimulate central ventilatory drive and increase tidal volume so that the pregnant woman, very soon after conception, develops hypocapnia; the normal arterial PCO_2 for pregnancy is 28 to 32 mm Hg. The respiratory alkalosis is compensated for by increased metabolism from the fetoplacental unit and by maternal renal mechanisms. Pregnant women often note dyspnea; as many as 60% to 70% have dyspnea at some point during pregnancy (12, 13). The genesis of dyspnea in pregnancy is not entirely clear (14). The physiologic hyperventilation and reduced arterial PCO_2 and the increased circulating blood volume that accompany gestation seem to be consistently important factors. Increased work of breathing is probably less important. Symptoms most often begin during the first or second trimester, coinciding with maximal increases in maternal blood volume and central ventilatory stimulation and preceding enlargement of the uterus beyond the pelvis and any substantial increase in abdominal girth.

Persistent dyspnea during pregnancy requires exclusion of other causes. Serious heart and lung disease can be excluded by careful auscultation and percussion of the heart and lungs and by a few other, simple procedures. Observation of neck vein distention during inspiration and expiration can give useful hemodynamic information. Measurement of peak expiratory flow, which should not be reduced by pregnancy, can exclude asthma or obstructive lung disease. Chest radiographs give information about heart size and the pleuropulmonary anatomy. Evaluation of heart murmurs or abnormal heart sounds in the dyspneic pregnant patient often requires electrocardiography and echocardiography, especially if pulmonary hypertension is a possibility.

Symptoms of the hyperventilation syndrome (15, 16) are common in pregnant women. Because pregnant women have a reduced resting $Paco_2$, even a modest increase in rate or depth of respiration can induce symptoms. An extra bag of groceries carried up an extra flight of stairs can make a pregnant patient lightheaded, numb, breathless, and anxious about her thumping heart. Because many patients are not conscious of their increased breathing, some present with hyperventilation syndrome but do not mention dyspnea. It is diagnostically useful to have patients hyperventilate on command while they are partially supine and while their vital signs or electrocardiogram are monitored. Patients with the hyperventilation syndrome almost always report the reproduction of their symptoms, including the appearance of premature atrial or ventricular contractions, after 30 to 60 seconds of voluntary hyperventilation.

The presence of systolic murmurs complicates the clinical assessment of dyspneic pregnant patients with symptoms of hyperventilation. Because of the similarity between panic attacks and hyperventilation, and their association with mitral valve prolapse (16), we find it useful to perform echocardiography to exclude structural heart disease and pulmonary hypertension.

Management of hyperventilating patients includes reassurance and rebreathing with a paper bag. Anxiolytic medications are neither desirable nor effective for pregnancy-related hyperventilation.

Changes in the Skin

The largest organ, the skin, can show three obvious changes beginning early in pregnancy: increased hyperpigmentation, telangiectasia, and striae gravidarum.

Hyperpigmentation

Increased pigmentation often accompanies pregnancy. Melanin hyperpigmentation is usually localized, especially in pre-existing areas of pigmentation, such as nevi, freckles, the aureole and nipple, the vulvar and perianal areas, the umbilicus, and the linea alba, which becomes the linea nigra. Melasma, "the mask of pregnancy," is an irregular, blotchy melanin hyperpigmentation on the forehead, temples, cheeks, and lips. None of these pigmentary changes are due to melanocyte-stimulating hormone; estrogen and progesterone seem to be the hormones principally responsible for the pigmentary changes of pregnancy (17). Similar changes can be seen in women who have used combination oral contraceptives.

There is no satisfactory treatment for hyperpigmentation other than camouflaging cosmetics. Skin bleaches, such as topical hydroquinone, should not be used during gestation. In fair-complected women, pigmentary changes fade after delivery, but women with darker complexions may have some degree of permanent extra pigmentation.

Telangiectasia

Pregnancy causes vascular proliferation as well as vasodilatation. Spider telangiectasias appear as early as 8 weeks of gestation and continue to appear until after delivery. Palmar erythema, indistinguishable from that seen with cirrhosis, begins early in pregnancy and may become more prominent as pregnancy proceeds. Capillary hemangiomas of the head and neck have a similar course (18). Pre-existing hemangiomas may increase in size during pregnancy. The spiders, hemangiomas, and palmar erythema typically recede after delivery. However, the vascular anomalies that existed before pregnancy do not resolve.

As with pregnancy hyperpigmentation, there is no therapy for telangiectasia other than camouflage. Because most facial telangiectasias recede after delivery, laser excision is best considered several months after birth. For bleeding hemangiomas of the mucosae during pregnancy, cautery or excision may be necessary.

Striae Gravidarum

Stretch marks, usually on the breasts, the anterior axillary fold, or the lower abdomen, are common during pregnancy. They begin as purple or pink striae that ultimately become irregular, white, and depressed. It has been assumed that the striae are caused by stretching of the skin, but their appearance before large changes in the volume of the breasts and uterus suggests other mechanisms. The similarity of striae gravidarum to the skin changes seen with the Cushing syndrome and the skin changes that follow the use of topical steroids with occlusive dressings suggests that corticosteroid hormones are important in the genesis of striae. Poidevin (19) showed that striae gravidarum were not related to the degree of skin distention and could develop in the absence of skin stretching. Topical lotions and vitamin E have been part of obstetric practice and folklore for years. However, no satisfactory maneuvers to prevent striae gravidarum exist.

Complaints Usually Confined to the First Half of Pregnancy

Altered senses of taste and smell are regular companions to early pregnancy (20). The bizarre food cravings and aversions, or "pregnancy pica," that are often joked about are expressions of changed taste and smell perception (21,

22). Nausea and vomiting, better known as *morning sickness*, often accompany these symptoms. Most women have morning sickness during the early stages of most of their pregnancies. Nausea and vomiting may be precipitated by odors and flavors sickeningly transformed from previously appetizing stimuli. It is more than just curious that the outcome of a pregnancy is more favorable when the pregnancy is accompanied by the nausea and vomiting of morning sickness (23, 24).

The genesis of the nausea and vomiting of early pregnancy is not well understood. Several biological associations, however, are clinically important because they indicate that nausea and vomiting are not caused by emotional disarray.

Morning sickness usually begins 2 to 4 weeks after conception, is maximal during placentation, and resolves (sometimes abruptly) after 12 to 16 weeks of gestation. Relaxation of the gastrointestinal tract with delayed gastric emptying and esophageal reflux is an essential component of the problem. It has been claimed that elevated levels of steroid hormones, free thyroxine, and hCG are associated with morning sickness (25). Mori and colleagues (26) have shown a correlation between pregnancy-related nausea and vomiting, and a pattern of elevated hCG and free thyroxine, and decreased thyrotropin measured in the serum. Previous studies had failed to document a consistent correlation between serum and urinary hCG levels and the presence and severity of nausea and vomiting in normal and molar pregnancies. When contemporary thyroid function tests are done and hCG is measured in early pregnancy, however, there is a good correlation between the presence and severity of nausea and vomiting and the amount of thyrotropin suppression and elevation of free thyroxine levels produced by hCG (or a cogener) stimulating the thyroid gland (27). These studies may explain the clinical association between hyperemesis gravidarum and transient hyperthyroidism. Altered expression or function of membrane receptors for odor and taste, associated with immunologic events, has been suggested as another factor in the origin of morning sickness (28).

Odor and olfaction are determined genetically and are highly specific (29). The relation between odor and histocompatibility genes has been documented in rodents and canines (30). Genetically determined conditions, such as the Kallmann syndrome (characterized by anosmia and gonadotropin hyposecretion) and the ability to taste phenylthiocarbamide, suggest that in humans, the closely related senses of taste and smell are modulated genetically (21). Patients with an altered immune capacity that accompanies iatrogenic or acquired immunosuppression and chemosensation suggest that taste and smell can be influenced by immunologic events.

Successful pregnancy requires maternal accommodation of fetoplacental antigens that are linked closely to histocompatibility leukocyte antigen loci.

These maternal immunologic events may be signaled by changes in chemosensation that produce dysgeusia and dysosmia and may trigger nausea and vomiting. It seems possible that the connection between a favorable pregnancy outcome and morning sickness resides in the connection between successful maternal modulation of the immune response producing altered chemosensory function (21, 28).

For most women with morning sickness, dietary discretion and simple maneuvers are usually sufficient. Many patients are reassured and comforted to learn that their queasy stomachs, malaise, and vomiting are a positive, not a negative, component of normal gestation. Antiemetics are rarely necessary and they are often ineffective. Dystonic reactions are most common with phenothiazine antiemetics.

Persistent vomiting becomes hyperemesis gravidarum when the patient loses weight, develops persistent ketonuria, and cannot maintain adequate hydration. The anxiety and dismay caused by hyperemesis in the past brought attention to the psychological aspects of the condition. The association of transient hyperthyroidism with hyperemesis gravidarum indicates the biological origin of the condition. Although we do not wish to minimize the important psychological effects of persistent, pernicious vomiting and their psychiatric management, we believe that clinicians should emphasize that hyperemesis gravidarum is a biological response to pregnancy. Hyperemesis should not be a cause of maternal guilt.

Complaints Beginning in Midpregnancy and Increasing or Persisting until Delivery

Complaints beginning in midpregnancy and increasing or persisting until delivery are given in Box 1-8 and discussed below.

Dependent Edema, Varicose Veins, and Leg Cramps

The physiologic decline in serum albumin levels and the uterine impedance to venous flow from the legs (31) result in the appearance of edema and superficial varicosities of the perineum and tributaries of the femoral and saphenous veins. The edema and varicosities can be unsightly and uncomfortable, and they increase the risks and complications of minor trauma, including ecchymosis, superficial thrombophlebitis, and infection. Elastic pantyhose or elastic graded compression stockings are imperative to improve venous return, and avoidance of the supine or sitting positions is a mainstay of management. The lateral decubitus position and walking are the best postural manipulations. Occasionally, the patient's edema and varicosities may be unbearable and un-

---

Box 1-8 Complaints Beginning in Midpregnancy

Constipation and hemorrhoids
Musculoskeletal syndromes
  Backache
  Pelvic, pubic symphysis, and sacroiliac pain
  Instability
Nerve entrapment syndromes
  Carpal tunnel syndrome
  Abnormal wall syndrome
Varicose veins
Dependent edema
Muscle cramps
Flank pain secondary to dilation and distention of urinary tract

---

manageable, short of delivery. These patients can suffer from exquisitely un-comfortable vulvar edema, painful superficial thrombophlebitis, and serous weeping from stretch marks of the abdomen, buttocks, and thighs with risk for secondary skin infection. In these extreme circumstances and in patients at bedrest, low-dose heparin seems advisable. If the edema is copious, diuretics are a last resort because of the risk for decreasing intravascular volume. Although usually not very helpful in antepartum patients, they may promote postpartum recovery.

The anatomic changes of pregnancy include distortion of the pelvic, lymphatic, and venous drainage and, thus, may predispose patients to episodes of vulvar or lower-extremity cellulitis. Recurrent cellulitis of the lower extremities can be confused with deep or superficial thrombophlebitis. A syndrome of repetitive cellulitis, often caused by group A or group B streptococci and temporally associated with coitus, has been described in women with underlying distortion of the pelvic lymphatics (32).

Painful muscle cramps of the legs occur in a surprisingly large minority of pregnant women (33). They almost always occur at night or when the patient is reclining or recumbent. The calf pain is exquisite, catapulting the woman out of bed. The muscle is hard and tender, and the foot and toes may be tonically plantar flexed. Calf-muscle cramps associated with pregnancy are often repetitive, protracted, and severe, producing tender, palpable areas of persistent contraction that can be confused with deep thrombophlebitis.

Painful leg cramps have been attributed to pregnancy-induced changes in calcium and phosphate metabolism, to venous stasis and varicose veins, and to vasodilatation (34). Nonpregnant patients using vasodilating drugs, such as beta-adrenergic agonists, calcium-channel blockers, and hydralazine, may have similar painful muscle cramps; this suggests that vascular dilatation is the cause of the cramps. Pregnancy increases ventilation, and carpopedal spasm is a common manifestation of hyperventilation.

Pregnant patients with painful, perhaps asymmetrically edematous, calves generate considerable clinical anxiety because of fears about thrombophlebitis. Properly performed noninvasive venous studies in a pregnant patient in whom calf pain and swelling are the only clinical findings suggesting deep venous thrombophlebitis are useful in clinical management. A careful evaluation documenting the history of calf cramps in a patient with negative results on venous plethysmography or serial Doppler studies may help stifle the impulse to perform x-ray venography and to start anticoagulation (33).

Doppler and impedance plethysmography performed by technicians inexperienced with the effects of the gravid uterus on venous function of the lower extremities can be unreliable. These studies are less accurate and sensitive in demonstrating thrombosis of calf veins as opposed to thrombosis of the popliteal and iliofemoral veins. When the clinical diagnosis of calf-muscle cramps is established, management includes the use of elastic-fitted pantyhose or graded compression stockings, stretching exercises, and frequent assumption of the lateral decubitus position. Calcium supplementation for women consuming inadequate amounts of calcium may help. Restricting dairy excess may be helpful in patients who consume large amounts of milk and milk products.

Changes in the Urinary Tract

Dilatation of the renal pelvis and ureters during pregnancy is well documented. The combination of decreased frequency and force of ureteral peristalsis and mechanical impedance to ureteral flow produced by the expanding uterus lead to enhanced susceptibility to acute UTIs and to overdistention, even rupture, of the renal pelvis (35, 36).

Because of the increased risk for ascending UTIs, even minor symptoms of cystitis or urethritis must be evaluated carefully and treated vigorously. We advise women with established acute pyelonephritis to assume a lateral decubitus posture, which fosters drainage and clearance of bacteria from the affected kidney. The dangers of the supine position for women who have been pregnant for more than 18 to 20 weeks are not always recognized by general medical and surgical staffs. If a pregnant patient, ill with sepsis related to acute pyelonephritis, is admitted to an intensive care unit, it is prudent to remind the staff and consultants about the mechanical effects of the gravid uterus on the cardiovascular system and urinary tract.

The overdistention syndrome is probably more common than we think. The affected patient has bothersome episodes of flank and upper abdominal pain, usually on the right side, so that gallbladder disease may be suspected (35). The discomfort may mimic that of ureteral colic or cholelithiasis, but the colicky pain is often related to position. Acute discomfort can be precipitated by abrupt increases in ureteral or renal pelvic pressure caused by diuresis or changes in fetal and maternal position. The patient finds relief by assuming and maintaining either the lateral decubitus position with the affected side uppermost or the knee–chest position. Renal ultrasonography shows hydronephrosis and hydroureter exceeding the usual expectations for pregnancy. Urinalysis may show no erythrocytes, leukocytes, or bacteriuria. The variation of symptoms with postural changes and the sonographic demonstration of marked distention of the urinary collecting system are hallmarks of the overdistention syndrome.

Infection is a common complication of pregnancy. Occasionally, the renal pelvis may rupture, resulting in the leakage of urine into the perirenal tissue and the appearance of hematuria (35, 36). Blunt abdominal trauma, perhaps considered to be only minor, may contribute to increased pain or rupture. Women who have infection, rupture, or persistent severe pain—especially if they are remote from term—may require the insertion of ureteral stents.

Musculoskeletal Syndromes

The hormonal milieu of pregnancy foster laxity of joints, connective tissue, and cartilage (37). These changes, in synergy with the postural and mechanical effects of the enlarging uterus, are responsible for many of the common aches and pains of pregnancy. As the gravid uterus expands in volume, especially after it extends above the pelvis, the woman's posture and gait are altered and her abdominal wall is stretched, increasing stress and strain on the spine and pelvis when the woman is upright.

Trauma
The bulging abdomen not only changes posture and gait but also interferes with visual cues when walking and, thus, contributes to a tendency for minor trauma: bumps and falls. Fort and Harlin (38) followed 3675 pregnant women for 3 years with repetitive queries about minor trauma at each antenatal visit. They found 242 instances of trauma in 212 patients. More than 50% of the traumatic events occurred in the third trimester, and 40% occurred in the second trimester. Pregnant women were more likely to fall on their buttocks or their sides than on their abdomen. With the increased risk for falling, exaggerated lordosis, and relaxation of collagenous structures, there is an increase in intervertebral disk injury and back symptoms during pregnancy.

Backache

Long-term studies involving more than 1000 women found that 49% of pregnant women experienced backache and that, of these, about 20% to 30% considered the backache severe or persistent enough to interfere with their usual activities (39). Symptoms were reported more often by women who had falls, women performing physically strenuous work (farming, cleaning, nursing, and industrial work with much lifting), women with previous low back pain or injury, and women who were older and multiparous. Pre-existing orthopedic conditions, such as scoliosis and spondylolisthesis, increased the risk for pregnancy-induced exacerbations or exaggerations of back and pelvic pain (Box 1-9).

Two distinct but overlapping entities of back and pelvic girdle pain in pregnant women can be defined: the musculotendinous insufficiency associated with the chronic low-back syndrome and the relaxation of pelvic joints that is associated with pregnancy.

With musculotendinous insufficiency, the patient has low backache, stiffness and movement discomfort of the low back and hips, and fatigability. Paravertebral muscle tenderness and "trigger points" are common, but there are no neurologic signs of radiculitis and the range of motion of the back and hips is normal. Paresthesias, changes in reflexes, and reduction in strength or sensory perception suggest nerve compression (see Section IV of Chapter 12) and require further evaluation. Heat, avoidance of high-heeled shoes, firm back support, and a nonsagging bed are the essentials of management. The usual exercises for abdominal and back muscles prescribed for low-back syndrome are not performed easily after the first trimester, but gentle stretching and flexibility exercises can be gratifying.

Several characteristic pain syndromes are caused by the relaxation of pelvic joints and ensuing pelvic instability (37, 39). The symptoms may be referable to the pubic symphysis, the sacroiliac joints, or both.

Box 1-9 Factors Contributing to Low-Back Pain During Pregnancy

---

Exaggerated lumbar lordosis and "pelvic tilt"
Loosening of the pelvic girdle
  Pubic symphysiolysis
  Sacroiliac joint laxity and dysfunction
Low-back pain or injury before pregnancy
Physically strenuous work
Increasing age and parity
Trauma

Pubic symphysiolysis is the most common of this set of complaints, and pubic symphysis pain or tenderness is the most common complaint (37). Palpation of the symphysis not only demonstrates marked localized tenderness but also reveals separation and movement of the pubic rami. Pubic mobility and pain should be assessed. The discomfort is exacerbated by beginning to move, and especially to bear weight, after sitting or lying; by climbing stairs; or by performing a Valsalva maneuver when defecating. The pain is occasionally referred down the insides of the thighs. Some patients may have a sensation of grinding or movement of the pubic bones when walking. Most patients cannot walk normally. Almost half of women with pubic pain also have sacroiliac joint dysfunction.

The principal sacroiliac symptoms are backache and sacroiliac joint pain. Sciatic-type pain, referred down the leg, is rare. Walking is invariably uncomfortable, and patients tend to waddle rather than walk. Asymmetry of the pelvic bony landmarks with abnormal movement of the landmarks on forward flexion can be found on examination. The Trendelenburg sign can often be demonstrated: When the patient stands on one leg, she has pain and is unable to hold the pelvis horizontal, and the opposite buttock drops (37). A useful provocative test is to place a heel on the opposite knee and, with the patient recumbent, rotate the leg outward; pain suggests sacroiliac joint dysfunction. Tenderness in the sacroiliac region may be found with low back pain not related to sacroiliac joint dysfunction. Maneuvers to show sacroiliac pain and laxity, therefore, are helpful in clinical diagnosis. Two thirds of affected patients have the onset of sacroiliac joint dysfunction during the second trimester (37). Patients with the most severe symptoms have complaints and physical findings referable to both the pubic symphysis and sacroiliac joints.

The general management of patients with musculoskeletal backache consists of changes in work status and function and conservative physical therapy. Injection of lidocaine and a small amount of repository steroid into the pubic symphysis region produces only transient relief. For patients with severe discomfort resulting from pelvic instability, use of a trochanteric belt to minimize the movements of the sacroiliac joint and the pubic symphysis has had some value. Some patients are so disabled that bedrest with pelvic support is necessary. Heat, massage, and soaking in a hot tub can provide transient symptomatic relief. Immersion in a swimming pool may also provide considerable relief by reducing gravity-induced musculotendinous and joint stresses. Regardless of the responses to antepartum treatment, many women with severe back and pelvic pain have persistent postpartum symptoms that require continued orthopedic attention.

Pregnancy predisposes to lumbar intervertebral disk disease. One review found that 39% of 179 women of childbearing age had symptoms of disk prolapse during pregnancy: back and radicular pain, paresthesias, and diminished ipsilateral reflexes (40). Magnetic resonance imaging has facilitated the diagnosis of disk prolapse in pregnant patients and is indicated clinically in patients with progressive radicular symptoms and signs. In the absence of progression, conservative symptomatic management is advised and surgical intervention is reserved until after delivery. During the latter weeks of pregnancy, patients may be unable to maintain the supine position that is usually recommended. The left lateral decubitus position on the floor or on a nonsagging bed, such as a futon, is a satisfactory alternative.

Complaints Related to Labor, Delivery, and Lactation

Complaints related to labor, delivery, and lactation are given in Box 1-10 and discussed below.

Postpartum Backache

The orthopedic miseries of gestation are tolerated because they are expected to go away after delivery. Backache beginning after delivery can be depressing and disabling. In one recent retrospective study of 11,701 women, 23.3% of women reported backache lasting more than 6 weeks beginning within 3 months of delivery (41). A smaller prospective study of 917 women found that 37% had postpartum back pain (42). In both of these studies, a substantial minority of women with postpartum back complaints had a history of back complaints before or during pregnancy. Persistent or recurrent back pain after delivery was associated with previous back injury and physically heavy or monotonous work.

In the larger study (41), 1634 women (14%) reported the onset of new back pain after delivery. In this group, 903 women had undergone epidural

---

Box 1-10 Complaints Related to Labor, Delivery, and Lactation

Compression neuropathies
Superficial phlebitis
Postpartum backache
"Valsalva purpura"
Breast engorgement and pain

anesthesia. These women had a statistically significant positive correlation between backache and labor under epidural anesthesia. Women having elective cesarean section (in other words, no labor) under epidural anesthesia had fewer back complaints than did women laboring under epidural anesthesia, and they had no more backaches than women having elective cesarean section under general anesthesia. The authors of this study suggest that the musculoligamentous and postural stresses of labor may be exaggerated because of the muscular relaxation and abolition of pain after epidural anesthesia. Careful attention to posture, position, and the course of labor during epidural anesthesia may help reduce the frequency of postpartum backache. Studies of this are underway.

"Valsalva Purpura"

The petechial rash, almost always confined to the head and neck of women undergoing prolonged and vigorous pushing with labor, is well recognized. We look for hemostatic defects but almost always find none. The rash may be more common in women with facial edema and fades rapidly with no residual dermal abnormality.

Postpartum Hair Loss

Postpartum hair loss is a common cause of referral to an internist or endocrinologist. Even women experiencing repetitive postpartum hair loss are distressed, despite previous reassurances and regrowth of the hair. An individual hair has a 2- to 6-year growing phase (anagen). Eventually, the hair bulb involutes and the hair follicle enters a resting phase (telogen). After about 3 months, a new hair bulb forms within the follicle and, as the new hair shaft grows out, the old hair bulb is ejected. Each hair lost is replaced by a new hair. Normally, 15% to 20% of scalp hair is in the telogen phase (43).

During the last half of pregnancy, the percentage of telogen-phase hair follicles declines; thus, many pregnant women notice a fuller and thicker head of hair. However, after delivery, a larger-than-normal number of hair follicles enters the telogen phase. In one study (44), 30% of hair follicles were in the telogen phase 9 weeks after delivery, a phase which continues up to 20 to 26 weeks (45).

Postpartum hair loss begins 2 to 4 weeks after delivery and may last up to 6 months (rarely more than a year). Hair is lost diffusely and, because it takes several weeks for the new hair to reach an acceptable length, there is great consternation about "going bald." Within 2 to 3 months, however, appearance of the new hair reassures the patient and her family. No special evaluation or therapy is necessary, except in the unusual event that the patient has another pathologic process.

Painful Breasts

Transient postpartum breast engorgement and discomfort are expected and managed simply. Persistent breast and nipple pain can be discouraging and frightening for the nursing mother. Puerperal mastitis, often caused by *Staphylococcus aureus*, and the formation of breast abscess require appropriate antibiotics and sometimes surgical drainage. Persistent nipple and breast pain in a nursing mother, however, requires consideration of *Candida albicans* infection of both mother and infant (46). A careful history usually reveals the presence of thrush or monilial diaper rash in the child of a mother with burning nipple pain and mastalgia. Often, *C. albicans* can be cultured from fissures of the nipple. Treatment with antibiotics for presumed bacterial mastitis may be accompanied by worsening symptoms in the mother and spread of monilial infection in the baby. Correct management of candidal mastitis includes topical antifungal therapy and oral nystatin when indicated. Treatment should be continued for several weeks. Relapses are common because the mother–infant dyad is highly susceptible to infection by *C. albicans*.

Summary

Pregnancy can produce a variety of aches and pains. Fortunately, although these aches and pains mimic those of serious medical or surgical disease, they indicate complaints that resolve spontaneously without serious or chronic residua. The problem for the clinician is distinguishing between the benign commonplace nuisance and the unusual ominous problem. Simple clinical diagnostic procedures, especially history taking and physical examination, are valuable screening techniques.

REFERENCES

1. **Lips HM.** Somatic and emotional aspects of the normal pregnancy experience: the first five months. Am J Obstet Gynecol. 1982;142:524-9.
2. **Owen OE.** Resting metabolic requirements of men and women. Mayo Clin Proc. 1988;63:503-10.
3. **Gregory PB, Rush D.** Iatrogenic caloric restriction in pregnancy and birthweight. Am J Perinatol. 1987;4:365-71.
4. **Rizzo T, Metzger BE, Burns WJ, et al.** Correlations between antepartum maternal metabolism and intelligence of offspring. N Engl J Med. 1991;325:911-6.

5. **Van Dinter MD.** Ptyalism in pregnant women. J Obstet Gynecol Neonatal Nurs. 1991; 20:206-9.

6. **Mortimer H, Wright RP, Collip JB.** The effect of oestrogenic hormones on the nasal mucosa: their role in the naso-sexual relationship and their significance in clinical rhinology. Can Med Assoc J. 1936;35:615-21.

7. **Mohun M.** Incidence of vasomotor rhinitis during pregnancy. Arch Otolaryngol. 1943; 37:699-709.

8. **Incaudo GA.** Diagnosis and treatment of rhinitis during pregnancy and lactation. Clin Rev Allergy. 1987;5:325-37.

9. **Mabry RL.** Intranasal steroid injection during pregnancy. South Med J. 1980;73:1176-9.

10. **Kent DL, Fitzwater JE.** Nasal hemangioma of pregnancy. Ann Otol Rhinol Laryngol. 1979;88:331-3.

11. **Brodnitz FS.** Hormones and the human voice. Bull N Y Acad Med. 1971;47:183-91.

12. **Gilbert R, Auchincloss JHJ.** Dyspnea of pregnancy: clinical and physiological observations. Am J Med Sci. 1966;252:270-6.

13. **Milne JA, Howie AD, Pack AI.** Dyspnoea during normal pregnancy. Br J Obstet Gynaecol. 1978;85:260.

14. **Rubin A, Russo N, Goucher D.** The effect of pregnancy upon pulmonary function in normal women. Am J Obstet Gynecol. 1956;72:963-9.

15. **Magarian GJ.** Hyperventilation syndromes: infrequently recognized common expression of anxiety and stress. Medicine (Baltimore). 1982;61:219-35.

16. **Cowley DS, Roy-Byrne PP.** Hyperventilation and panic disorder. Am J Med. 1987;83: 929-37.

17. **Snell RS, Bischitz PG.** The effect of large doses of estrogen and progesterone on melanin pigmentation. J Invest Dermatol. 1960;35:73-9.

18. **Letterman G, Schwiter M.** Cutaneous hemangiomas of the face in pregnancy. Plast Reconstr Surg. 1962;29:293-8.

19. **Poidevin LOS.** Striae gravidarum: their relation to adrenal cortical hyperfunction. Lancet. 1952;2:436-8.

20. **Jarnfelt-Samsioe A, Samsioe G, GV.** Nausea and vomiting in pregnancy—a contribution to its epidemiology. Gynecol Obstet Invest. 1983;16:221-9.

21. **Lee RV.** Olfaction—and the smell of summer. J Chron Dis. 1987;40:819-21.

22. **Ackerman D.** A Natural History of the Senses. New York: Random House; 1990.

23. **Medalie JH.** Relationship between nausea and/or vomiting in early pregnancy and abortion. Lancet. 1957;2:117.

24. **Tierson FD, Olsen CL, Hook EB.** Nausea and vomiting of pregnancy in association with pregnancy outcome. Am J Obstet Gynecol. 1986;155:1017-22.

25. **Soules MR, Hughes CL, Garcia JA, et al.** Nausea and vomiting of pregnancy: role of human chorionic gonadotropin and 17-hydroxyprogesterone. Obstet Gynecol. 1980; 55:696-700.

26. **Mori M, Amino N, Tamaki H, et al.** Morning sickness and thyroid function in normal pregnancy. Obstet Gynecol. 1988;72:355-9.

27. **Goodwin TM, Mestman J, Montoro M, et al.** Role of chorionic gonadotropin as a thyroid stimulator in hyperthyroidism of hyperemesis gravidarum. Clin Res. 1991;39: 207A.

28. **Lee RV.** Possible immunologic factors in nausea and vomiting of pregnancy. J Allergy Clin Immunol. 1988;81:935.

29. **Beauchamp GK, Yamazaki K, Boyse EA.** The chemosensory recognition of genetic individuality. Scientific American. 1985;253:86-92.

30. **Beauchamp GK, Yamazaki K, Wysocki CJ, et al.** Chemosensory recognition of mouse major histocompatibility types by another species. Proc Natl Acad Sci U S A. 1985;82: 4186-8.

31. **Milsom I, Forssman L.** Factors influencing aortocaval compression in late pregnancy. Am J Obstet Gynecol. 1984;148:764-71.

32. **Ellison RT, McGregor JA.** Recurrent postcoital lower extremity streptococcal erythroderma in women. JAMA. 1987;257:3260-2.

33. **Lee RV, McComb LE, Mezzadri FC.** Pregnant patients, painful legs: the obstetrician's dilemma. Obstet Gynecol Surv. 1990;45:290-8.

34. **Page EW, Page EP.** Leg cramps in pregnancy. Obstet Gynecol. 1953;1:94-100.

35. **Meyers SJ, Lee RV, Munschauer RW.** Dilatation and nontraumatic rupture of the urinary tract during pregnancy. Obstet Gynecol. 1985;66:809-15.

36. **Van Winter JT, Ogburn PL, Engen DE, et al.** Spontaneous renal rupture during pregnancy. Mayo Clin Proc. 1991;66:179-82.

37. **Abramson D, Roberts SM, Wilson PD.** Relaxation of the pelvic joints in pregnancy. Surg Gynecol Obstet. 1934;58:595-613.

38. **Fort AT, Harlin RS.** Pregnancy outcome after noncatastrophic maternal trauma during pregnancy. Obstet Gynecol. 1970;35:912-5.

39. **Berg G, Hammar M, Moller-Nielsen J, et al.** Low back pain during pregnancy. Obstet Gynecol. 1988;71:71-5.

40. **O'Connell JEA.** Lumbar disc protrusions in pregnancy. J Neurol Neurosurg Psychiatry. 1960;23:138-41.

41. **MacArthur C, Lewis M, Knox EG, et al.** Epidural anesthesia and long term backache after childbirth. BMJ. 1990;30:9-12.

42. **Ostgaard HD, Anderson GBJ.** Postpartum low back pain. Spine. 1992;17:53-9.

43. **Kligman AM.** Pathological dynamics of human hair loss. Arch Dermatol. 1961;83:175-98.

44. **Lynfield YL.** Effect of pregnancy on the human hair cycle. J Invest Dermatol. 1960; 35:323-7.

45. **Schiff BL, Kern AB.** A study of postpartum alopecia. Arch Dermatol. 1963;87:609-11.

46. **Amir LH, Pakula S.** Nipple pain, mastalgia, and candidiasis in the lactating breast. Aust N Z J Obstet Gynaecol. 1991;31:378-80.

VI. Prescribing for the Pregnant Patient
Sandra L. Kweder and Richard V. Lee

Prescribing or administering drugs to pregnant women is a task that many physicians would prefer to avoid. The information needed to assess individual drugs may not be readily available and, when it is, the data often do not seem applicable to the clinical circumstances of the patient at hand. Moreover, as gestation proceeds, maternal physiology and fetal development change constantly. The need to make treatment decisions elicits anxiety in both the prescriber and the patient about the potential effects of medications on the developing fetus. The potential emotional, legal, and economic consequences of a perceived bad outcome are a glaring reminder of the uncertainties inherent in clinical medicine. Many of us find ourselves indecisive in its light, and this makes otherwise simple management and prescribing decisions seem insurmountable. Ironically, the result is often that the pregnant patient is incompletely studied, misdiagnosed, or not treated at all.

We believe that this does not have to be the case. Armed with some basic considerations and with knowledge about where to seek additional information, physicians can develop a rational, prospective approach to prescribing in pregnant patients. This contrasts with the retrospective consideration of risks in women who have already been exposed to drugs during pregnancy, although many of the same principles apply.

A rational approach to the pregnant patient who may need medication (or any intervention) begins with an appreciation of the clinical elements operative in decision making (Figure 1-4). Clinical and scientific considerations—the medical condition or conditions of concern; issues specific to pregnancy; and individual medications and their interrelations, each of which requires direct assessment—form a core triad of interrelations. This dynamic triad exists within the contextual envelope of the perspectives and communications of the patient, her family, and her medical care providers.

Many therapeutic decisions in the care of pregnant women do not lend themselves to closure. The physiology of pregnancy is dynamic, making it best to consider prescribing decisions to be dynamic and subject to periodic reassessment. It is important to conduct such reassessments in a focused and orderly manner, beginning with, and always returning to, a basic understanding of the patient herself.

Where To Begin: Know the Patient

Cultural beliefs and practices surround pregnancy and lactation. The use of natural and synthetic chemicals as medicines and foods is common and culturally defined. For example, traditional herbal treatments are widely available and, as natural products, are often not perceived to have potential toxicity. On the other hand, prescription medications are often suspected of being potent and dangerous, and their use is often discontinued by patients. In the past two decades, societal and cultural pressures in the United States have encouraged women to avoid exposing their unborn babies to any poten-

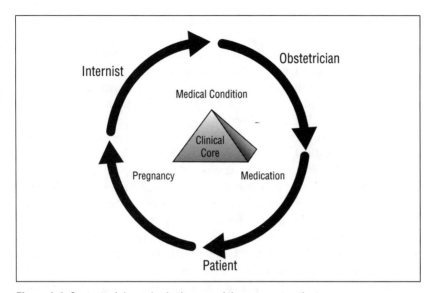

Figure 1-4 Contextual dynamics in the care of the pregnant patient.

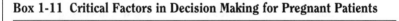

Box 1-11 Critical Factors in Decision Making for Pregnant Patients

Patient's understanding of disease or condition
Patient's need for certainty
Patient's tolerance for possible outcomes
Physician's tolerance of uncertainty and risk

---

tial toxins. Generally, this is good public health advice. However, although it is true that all chemicals can adversely affect pregnancy if given in high-enough doses at a susceptible period of gestation, it is not true that all medications should be avoided during pregnancy. The treatment of illness in the mother may be vital for a successful pregnancy outcome.

Critical factors that lay the foundation for prescribing decisions for pregnant patients are shown in Box 1-11. It is far better to consider them early rather than late in the process.

First, it is critical to assess what the patient understands about her disease. The patient should understand the risks of lack of treatment, both for her and for her baby, and the risk for an adverse pregnancy outcome conferred solely by the disease. Misperceptions in these areas are common and can have substantial implications for the patient's collaboration in her own care and for her perceptions about her care providers and their advice.

The second consideration is the patient's need for certainty. Pregnant women and their families may demand certainty about the risks of medications to the fetus. For the physician, an understanding of what underlies their need is essential. Patients often do not appreciate the normal risk that pregnancy carries for fetal malformations and complications. Sometimes, they are frightened by a particular bad outcome, and this fear may not be warranted. For example, the patient or her family may fear a particular untoward effect of a medicine in the absence of any plausible connection to the patient's condition or medications (e.g., they may fear that a medication used in the third trimester will lead to limb reduction or anencephaly, or they may fear that a drug will increase the likelihood of sickle-cell disease).

Related to certainty is the patient's tolerance of possible outcomes of pregnancy. This is especially important for the patient being evaluated and treated early in pregnancy. How does she view the possibility of a very complicated pregnancy that may require repeated courses of medication? If a medication is clearly indicated for her treatment but is associated with untoward fetal effects, how would she balance this information? For example, a pregnant woman with a mechanical heart valve who had a life-threatening pulmonary embolus while using heparin during a previous pregnancy may be so intolerant of the possibility of coumarin fetopathy that she would choose to use heparin again and risk another embolism. An appreciation of the personal perspectives of the patient and of her life circumstances is invaluable for the physician who cares for her and makes recommendations about pharmacologic interventions.

The physician's understanding of his or her own risk tolerance and need for certainty can be as important as his or her understanding of the patient's. There may be no area of medicine where this comes into play more dramatically than in caring for a pregnant patient. In many areas of medicine, studies and data are abundant, but the medical literature on prescribing for the pregnant woman often seems to be an abyss. Ironically, in a situation where the physician seeks the most certainty, data are scant. Furthermore, caring for a pregnant woman often forces the physician to confront his or her own views on matters that are emotionally charged. There is little question that the physician must be open to the possibility that his or her own views or feelings may be so strong (even if they are concordant with those of the patient) that it is in the best interest of all concerned that the patient be referred to another caregiver. When the prescribing physician needs a high level of certainty and confidence in recommending specific pharmacologic interventions and that confidence is not inspired by the data available, the patient will likely perceive this. In such circumstances, offering to refer the patient to a knowledgeable source for a second opinion will serve all parties well.

The Clinical Core

It is necessary to have a basic understanding of the medical condition at hand before implementing any pharmacologic intervention. As a practical matter, three general adages apply to the decision-making process in prescribing for the pregnant patient; these are listed in Box 1-12. Life-threatening conditions, such as overwhelming infections, almost always require treatment. On the other hand, patients may seek treatment for conditions that many would consider merely annoyances, such as cutaneous acne or other asymptomatic dermatoses. If a condition will not worsen without treatment, it is difficult to justify systemic pharmacotherapy. However, the vast majority of patients do not fall tidily at the ends of the spectrum of clinical medicine.

When, how, and what to prescribe for the pregnant patient are determined by judgment based on the patient's needs in combination with the answers to three clinical questions. First, what is known about the maternal condition itself, its natural history, and how pregnancy is likely to affect it? Second, how will the maternal condition affect the expected course of pregnancy, including maternal, fetal, or neonatal morbidity? Third, what are the therapeutic options for management of the maternal condition? Evaluation should include an exploration of the pros and cons of treatment itself, including the choice of no pharmacologic treatment. It should also include an honest assessment of the short- and long-term goals of any intervention. A review of all pharmacologic options for treatment, with a careful evaluation of how each might affect fetal development and outcome and the mother's risk for toxicity, can then be done.

How Will Pregnancy Affect the Mother's Medical Condition?

Many conditions are known to be exacerbated by pregnancy and therefore are likely to require treatment during gestation, even in patients who did not

---

Box 1-12 Clinical Perspectives on Prescribing for Pregnancy

- It is easy to justify pharmacologic treatment for progressive acute and chronic maternal conditions.
- It is hard to justify pharmacologic treatment for nonprogressive chronic maternal conditions and harder still to justify it for acute, self-limited maternal conditions.
- Medical assessment of the patient and her condition must incorporate how the pregnancy affects the condition and how the condition affects the pregnancy as well as a consideration of the full range of therapeutic options.

need treatment in the past (Box 1-13). For instance, approximately one third of asthmatic patients will have exacerbations during pregnancy. Women with mitral valve stenosis are at increased risk for congestive heart failure because of physiologic changes of pregnancy, particularly pregnancy-induced hypertension. Systemic lupus erythematosus may flare during pregnancy. Knowing what to expect about the course of a medical condition during pregnancy will influence decisions about when and whether to intervene pharmacologically. Other chapters in this book and other texts are excellent resources for exploration of these considerations.

How Will the Mother's Medical Condition Affect the Pregnancy?

Numerous medical conditions place the pregnant woman at substantial risk for morbidity related to the pregnancy outcome itself, a fact that most nonobstetricians are not accustomed to considering. These conditions may be self-limited, progressive, disabling, or life-threatening complications, and intervention may or may not prevent them. Nonetheless, it is critical for the physician to understand any potential effect of the maternal condition on the pregnancy and its outcome. In some cases, the obstetrician will be able to provide such information to the internist; in other situations, the obstetrician may look to the internist for guidance. For example, maternal diabetes mellitus has a strong association with fetal macrosomia and related complications in mother and infant. Some maternal infections, such as HIV infection, carry a risk for vertical transmission but may not necessarily affect pregnancy itself. On the other hand, maternal hypertension and diabetes each increase the risk for a pregnancy complicated by preeclampsia, which is associated with both maternal and fetal morbidity. Maternal antiphospholipid antibody syndrome

---

Box 1-13 Conditions That Require Treatment During Pregnancy

Asthma
Autoimmune conditions
Cancer
Cardiac arrythmia
Congestive heart failure
Diabetes mellitus
Endocrinopathies (e.g., thyroid, adrenal, parathyroid)
Infection
Seizures
Transplantation

is associated with an increased risk for midtrimester fetal loss and maternal thromboembolic events during pregnancy.

What Are the Therapeutic Options?

The third core clinical element in decision making for the pregnant patient is the spectrum of treatment options for a particular condition (Box 1-14). In some cases, the alternative of no pharmacologic intervention is the safest option and still offers potential benefit (for example, in mild essential hypertension). Box 1-15 lists the risks of withholding drug therapy, and the only addition to this list in considering the categorical risks of any active treatment is that of a toxic reaction (maternal or fetal) to the treatment itself; this is discussed in more detail later in this chapter. However, it is often instructive to actively consider these risks in the context of no treatment. Nonpharmacologic but active interventions, such as diet in the management of

---

Box 1-14 Therapeutic Options

No treatment
Nonpharmacologic treatment
Current pharmacologic standard of care
Older pharmacologic treatment
New therapies

Box 1-15 Risks of Withholding Drug Therapy

Progressive maternal disease
  Death
  Disability
  Inanition
Fetopathy
  Impaired fetal growth and development (e.g, due to maternal inanition or placental compromise)
  Transplacental infection
Prematurity
Unfulfilled parenteral expectations
Untoward outcome perceived as due to failure to treat

diabetes and physical therapy in the management of back pain or sciatica, may be attractive. Older drugs (those that have been marketed for many years) should be explored. Many have been used extensively in obstetrics even though they are rarely used by internists. For instance, methyldopa is rarely prescribed by internists but is the traditional drug of choice for obstetricians treating hypertension in pregnant women. Occasionally, new treatments may be most attractive, especially when their therapeutic margin is wide or when their expected safety profile in the developing fetus is better than that of alternative treatments. For example, inhaled rather than long-term systemic corticosteroids may be preferred in the management of asthma.

On the other hand, it is important that interventions not be made by default. Any intervention should be fully assessed, and this assessment must consider risks to both mother and fetus (see Box 1-15). This is especially true for the choice of no treatment. Indecision, whatever its roots, is easily masked by watchful waiting.

In considering the therapeutic alternatives, it is useful to continually reassess the goal of any intervention, whether it is for short-term management or to prevent long-term morbidity. For the pregnant woman with mild essential hypertension, several months without pharmacologic treatment are unlikely to alter the long-term risk for vascular disease. In the severely hypertensive patient, lack of pharmacologic treatment may place the pregnancy at risk. The patient with longstanding endogenous depression requiring medication may reasonably try a course of psychological counseling alone during the first trimester to carry her through the period of organogenesis; reassessment can be done in the second trimester. On the other hand, the short-term potential for depression if this is not effective may outweigh the risk for continuing or starting medication use.

Evaluating Pharmacologic Agents for Use in Pregnancy

Chemicals can adversely affect pregnancy by interfering with conception, implantation, placentation, organogenesis, fetal growth and development, placental function, parturition, or maternal health. The thalidomide experience of the 1950s, in which a seemingly innocuous agent was found, after widespread use in Europe, to be responsible for severe fetal malformations, has had a substantial effect on perceptions of prescription drugs in the United States. First and foremost, it has led to an intense, exclusive focus on teratogenesis as the toxicity of greatest concern. It has also prompted the belief that every drug has the potential to be another thalidomide (1), even though most known human teratogens are associated with much lower rates of malformations than is thalidomide.

The safety of each therapeutic option for the pregnant patient should be examined comprehensively for its potential adverse effects on mother and fetus, including, but not limited to, teratogenic or developmental effects.

Fetal Risk

Four major factors to be weighed in a consideration of the risks posed to the fetus by pharmacologic intervention are listed in Box 1-16. These include the risk of withholding maternal treatment, the risk for teratogenesis, the risk for other fetal toxicity, and how fetal development and pharmacokinetics may alter these.

Fetal Morbidity Resulting from Lack of Maternal Treatment

The maternal and fetal effects of treatment or no treatment of maternal illness are intricately related and often difficult to separate. Some untreated maternal conditions, such as tension headache or eczema, will have no substantial consequences for the fetus. At the other end of the spectrum are maternal conditions that, untreated, can cause substantial morbidity in the fetus. Maternal hyperparathyroidism can cause neonatal tetany. Uncontrolled maternal epilepsy can result in severe fetal neurodevelopmental effects due to the maternal hypoxia known to occur with seizures. Most conditions fall somewhere along the continuum between these ends of the spectrum, leaving the clinician to factor in other elements of risk and benefit.

Teratogenesis

Strictly speaking, a teratogen is an agent that, under certain conditions of exposure, causes anatomic or developmental abnormalities. According to some definitions, teratogenesis also leads to functional abnormalities (2). Of the thousands of drugs on the market in western countries, many have demonstrated teratogenesis in animal models. Fewer than 30 have been confirmed as human teratogens, but these drugs and others may be associated with fetal

---

Box 1-16 Fetal Risk Considerations for Maternal Treatment

Risk of no maternal treatment

Teratogenic effects

Fetal toxicity

Fetal development and pharmacokinetics (including neurodevelopmental [long-term] effects)

growth impairment or may otherwise be fetotoxic. Some better-known teratogens are listed in Table 1-7 (1, 3). Recent information can be obtained from the references given in Table 1-8.

Despite the small number of agents known to be teratogenic (nearly all of which are well known to obstetricians), the clinician often faces difficult decisions about individual drugs that are suspected of being teratogenic. Examples of agents that were initially thought to be teratogenic but for which large epidemiology studies have not shown teratogenicity include diazepam, oral contraceptives, spermicides, salicylates, and the combination product Bendectin (doxylamine plus pyridoxine) (2).

Understanding the basis of a suspicion of teratogenicity is essential in deciding how risk is to be weighed for a particular fetus of a particular mother. Key questions to ask when weighing the information available are given below:

1. *Is the concern based on controlled clinical or epidemiologic data or another large body of human experience?* Clinical trials that include a control group inspire the most confidence in determining causality of a drug and adverse effects, but one must remember that very large studies are needed to show increases in rates of rare events. When such studies are unavailable, epidemiology studies can detect associations (or lack thereof) between a drug and an adverse event or outcome.

2. *Is the suspicion based on a case report, case series, or other anecdotal experience?* Such reports are the least reliable form of scientific evi-

Table 1-7 Drugs Known or Suspected To Be Teratogenic or Fetotoxic in Humans

Drug	Teratogenic Effect
ACE inhibitors	Decreased skull ossification
	Renal dysgenesis
Alcohol	Neurodevelopmental defects
Carbemazepine	Neural tube defects
Cyclophosphamide	CNS malformations
	Secondary cancers
Androgens	Masculinization
Diethylstillbesterol	Vaginal carcinoma
	Genitourinary defects
Lithium	Ebstein anomaly
Methimazole	Aplasia cutis
Methotrexate	CNS and limb malformations
Phenytoin	CNS defects
Retinoids (systemic)	CNS, craniofacial, and cardiovascular defects
Tetracycline	Anomalies of bone and teeth
Thalidomide	Limb-reduction defects
	Internal organ defects
Valproic acid	Neural tube defects
Warfarin	Skeletal and CNS defects

Table 1-8 Reference Sources in Assessment of Fetal Risk

Source	Type	Description
TERIS (www.weber.u.washington.edu); also in Micromedix's TOMES Reprorisk Module	On-line subscription or diskette	Comprehensive evaluations of all available human and animal data on individual drugs by a panel of experts. Provides specific judgements of risk in pregnancy and lactation with rationales. Excellent reference.
Friedman JM, Polifka JE. Effects of Drugs on the Fetus and Nursing Infant: A Handbook for Health Care Professionals. Baltimore: Johns Hopkins Univ Press; 1996.	Paperback book	Succinct summaries of risk based on more comprehensive reviews of TERIS. Practical book that focuses on the most clinically relevant aspects of TERIS reviews. Excellent and convenient resource.
FDA Pregnancy Categories (found in most prescription-drug package inserts and labeling; also in Physicians' Desk Reference)	Drug labels	Well-known categories A, B, C, D, and X. Focus on teratogenesis. Inconsistently applied and rarely updated. Best used in combination with other reference sources.
REPROTOX (www.REPROTOX.org); also in Micromedix's TOMES Reprorisk Module	On-line subscription or diskette	Comprehensive evaluation of all available human and animal data on individual environmental hazards and drugs. All aspects of human reproduction are considered. Similar to TERIS but less direct in linking risk to management. Excellent resources that is updated often and provides selected references.
Briggs GS, Freeman R, Yaffe S. 5th ed. Drugs in Pregnancy and Lactation, Baltimore: Williams & Wilkins; 1998.	Hardcover book	Good resources for data on human and animal experience with drugs in pregnancy and lactation. Summaries not as organized as those in other resources, but thoughtful commentary geared to the clinician is provided.
Coustan DR, Mochizuki TK. Handbook for Prescribing Medications Drug Pregnancy, 3rd ed. Philadelphia: Lippincott-Raven; 1998.	Pocket-size paperback book	Discusses individual drugs with summary considerations for mother and fetus, including less common uses. New section on antineoplastic agents and an updated vaccine section. Less extensive referencing and analysis than other sources but convenient and reliable.

dence of cause and effect. Unfortunately, because they are considered newsworthy, abnormal cases are more likely than normal outcomes to be reported. Single reports or small series of any outcome, abnormal or normal, should be viewed with skepticism, unless the series suggest an unusual pattern of findings or confirm findings predicted by animal studies.

3. *Is the suspicion based on animal data? If so, do the data constitute a reasonable reflection of human risk?* For most clinicians, this is where drug safety assessment becomes overwhelming. It is often wrongly assumed that animal studies are not useful, and their interpretation requires more expertise and time than most practicing physicians have. References on animal and human data on teratogenesis that we recommend to busy clinicians are listed in Table 1-8.

In assessing risk for teratogenesis for any particular agent in an individual patient, it is helpful to remember that human organogenesis occurs predominantly during gestational weeks 3 through 12. Avoiding unnecessary medications during this period, which is essentially the first trimester, is a good general rule. However, fetal growth and physiology and placental function are susceptible to pharmacologic and toxic effects throughout gestation.

Fetal Toxicity
Risk for fetal toxicity is usually independent of teratogenic risk. All the reference sources listed in Table 1-8 address fetal toxicity issues as well as teratogenesis. Some fetotoxic effects can be predicted on the basis of a drug's pharmacology. Some, such as growth restriction or hypothyroidism, are reversible but are nonetheless potentially associated with morbidity. In general, any agent that is pharmacologically active in the mother should be considered to be similarly active in the fetus and to possess the potential to cause similar toxicities. Among the most important examples of this are psychoactive agents that are known to be associated with acute withdrawal syndromes and are associated with neonatal withdrawal after regular in utero exposure during the third trimester (Box 1-17). Irreversible fetal toxicities resulting from in utero exposures include renal failure associated with ACE inhibitors and fetal hypoxic damage related to maternal hypotension. Unfortunately, some of the potential fetal and neonatal effects of intrauterine exposures are not well studied, particularly neurodevelopmental effects that may not manifest until well after the neonatal period.

Fetal Development and Pharmacokinetics
The fetal toxicity of a drug may be predicted by the intensity of fetal exposure in utero, which may depend equally on the maternal and fetal pharmacoki-

---

Box 1-17 Drugs Associated with Neonatal Withdrawal

Benzodiazepines
Opiates
Cocaine
Sympathomimetics
Antihistamines

---

netics of the drug. Fetal pharmacokinetics can often be extrapolated from animal models and human adult data. Drug metabolism by the fetal liver, including most enzymatic processes, early in the first trimester has been documented but at lower levels than in adults (3). As the fetal kidney develops, it is able to excrete increasing amounts of renally cleared agents and their active metabolites into the amniotic fluid. This can increase the concentration of substances in the fetoplacental compartment and, because the fetus continuously ingests amniotic fluid, increase fetal exposure to drugs that are renally cleared. The specific clinical implications of this phenomenon are not well developed, but the phenomenon should increase the level of caution for the prescriber and for pediatricians caring for the newborns of mothers who have been treated with such products, especially if treatment was given in the third trimester.

Physical and chemical factors influence the transfer of pharmacologic agents across the placenta. Large molecules (such as heparin) and compounds that bind to protein (such as insulin) do not readily cross the placenta. Lipid-soluble drugs are likely to diffuse across the placenta more readily than water-soluble drugs do. The pH of fetal umbilical cord blood is 0.1 to 0.15 pH units lower than the pH of maternal blood. After crossing from the maternal to the fetal circulation, basic drugs (those with a higher pH) become ionized. Because compounds cross biological membranes more readily in the nonionized state, these drugs may have a propensity to accumulate in the fetal compartment. Fetal acidosis, already present relative to maternal pH, may be augmented during physiologic stress and can amplify this effect. The opposite applies to acidic drugs: Fetal concentrations are likely to be lower than concentrations in the maternal compartment (3). Although these factors are difficult to balance in terms of fetal risk from a chronically administered drug, it may be important to discuss them with a neonatologist when a drug will be given chronically. Some agents may need to be tapered to protect the soon-to-be-delivered baby. The pediatrician who cares for the newborn who has been subjected to physiologic stress before and during delivery must know of the baby's exposures to maternal medications.

Maternal Risk

The assessment of the maternal risks of drugs is similar to that of the fetal risks. Considerations include the risk of withholding drug therapy (this is similar to the risk of the untreated disease itself) and the risk for maternal toxicity. Fetal pharmacokinetics are important in an assessment of risk to the fetus from maternal drug therapy, but the pharmacokinetic properties of drugs in the mother are often forgotten in weighing maternal risk. Maternal pharmacokinetics and pharmacodynamics should be considered in dosing decisions once a therapeutic agent has been selected and re-evaluated often.

In the interplay of pregnancy and drugs, maternal toxicity may be the factor least often considered. In part, this may be a byproduct of the lack of clinical studies of drugs in pregnant women. The effects of gender and hormonal changes on the safety and efficacy of drugs are only beginning to be systematically considered and explored. For example, women have a higher risk for the cardiovascular effects of certain nonsedating antihistamines; this risk is not explained by dose or pharmacokinetics but may be a complex manifestation of hormonal effects (4). Although data are conflicting, it has long been suspected that pregnant women have a greater risk for isoniazid-related hepatotoxicity than do nonpregnant women. Such examples are clues to the likelihood that pregnancy, with its dramatic physiologic changes, may alter drug safety and effectiveness profiles in ways that go beyond simple pharmacokinetics.

Another aspect of maternal toxicity that should be considered is the predictable side-effect or adverse-event profile of a given product on the course of pregnancy. For example, some antihypertensive agents and systemic steroids have diabetogenic effects; systemic steroids have hypertensive effects; and antiretroviral agents are associated with anemia. Predictable adverse events to be considered should include those that many clinicians usually consider nuisances or annoyances but that may be intolerable or unsafe in pregnant patients. For example, many pregnant women have severe, hormonally mediated gastroesophageal reflux. Medications that tend to increase such reflux not only are unlikely to be complied with but can contribute to asthma exacerbation and aspiration.

Rational Prescribing for the Pregnant Woman

Weighing the Alternatives: A Model

Deciding whether to treat a particular condition in a pregnant woman requires an integrated consideration of all of the factors outlined in this section.

The condition being treated, its consequences to the mother and the pregnancy, and the fetal and maternal risks of each possible intervention (including no treatment) must be considered. All risk profiles are subject to change as the pregnancy progresses, depending on the mother's health, intervening complications or conditions, and the stage of pregnancy. The greater the impairment of maternal physiologic function, the greater the risk for gestational decompensation and the greater the need to initiate and continue medication use. A model for weighing alternatives in decision making about drug use in pregnancy is shown in Figure 1-5.

The role of teamwork and communication among all health professionals who care for a pregnant woman taking medications is paramount in the decision-making process. Most critical is open and frequent communication between the obstetric provider, the consulting physicians, and other health care providers who might influence the patient's decisions about which, if any, treatment course to start. As indicated earlier in this section, the risk tolerance and need for certainty on the part of the influencing physicians should be addressed openly so that these factors are considered but not substituted for the patient's needs.

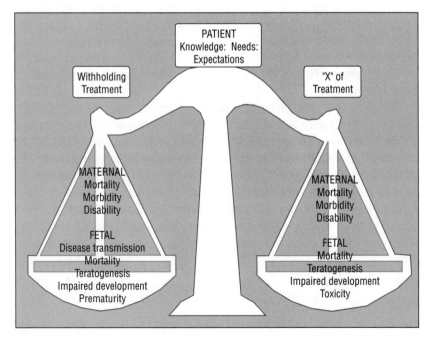

Figure 1-5 Weighing risks of alternative therapies in pregnancy.

Dose Management

Once a decision is made to initiate a pharmacologic therapy, it is critical to ensure that dosing is appropriate, that careful follow-up and reassessment are done, and that the obstetrician is engaged in the prescribing plan. A reasonable starting point for dosing most drugs in pregnancy is to use the lowest dose known to be effective in adults. Too often, however, the assumption that less is better for pregnant patients incorrectly leads to the use of doses far lower than those that have been shown to be effective. The result is that the mother receives little or no benefit and yet she and the fetus are exposed to potential toxicity. Situations in which it is reasonable to decrease or increase doses relative to standard dosing for a particular drug are best identified by considering the drug's pharmacokinetic profile and the ways in which pregnancy can be expected to influence this profile.

Pregnancy decreases gastrointestinal motility and can lead to delays in oral drug absorption and lower peak maternal plasma concentrations. The increases in maternal blood volume (approximately 50%), cardiac output (30% to 50%), body fat content, and glomerular filtration rate (50%) in pregnancy produce variations in the pharmacokinetics of many drugs (4). Such changes are particularly relevant for drugs that are renally cleared; these drugs may need to be given at higher doses or given more frequently. The gestational decline in serum albumin levels, which is only partly due to increased plasma volume, results in increases in unbound drug concentrations for agents that bind to albumin. Unbound or free drug is more accessible for transfer across the placenta. This may be particularly relevant in the management of patients taking AEDs, especially in the third trimester, when physiologic changes are most dramatic.

The most common pharmacokinetic effect of maternal physiologic changes in pregnancy is lower serum drug concentrations. Thus, increased dosing or increased dose frequency may be required, in opposition to the clinician's first instinct, which is to minimize dosing during pregnancy. The examples listed in Table 1-9 are excellent reminders of this. Unfortunately, most drugs have not been studied in pregnant women. The decision about whether to increase a dose will depend on the therapeutic window and on a careful clinical assessment of the patient's response. In very few cases do pregnant women require doses lower than those that are effective in non-pregnant patients.

Communication with the Obstetrician

The relationship between a pregnant woman and her obstetric care provider is a very special one. Even the internist who cared for the woman before her pregnancy often finds that she or he is suddenly a consultant once the pregnancy is known. The internist should expect this and recognize that it may take extra effort to work as a member of a triad. This is especially important in making recommendations and decisions about drug prescribing. Obstetricians may or may not be familiar with treatments for less common conditions or with new treatments for common conditions. Most appreciate and expect an opportunity to discuss anticipated risks and benefits with the consultant, preferably before the patient's next obstetric visit. Such discussions can be very valuable for the internist who is considering maternal and fetal physiology and toxicities. Even more important, it is certain that the patient will seek the counsel of the obstetrician in deciding whether to initiate therapy and, if so, which one(s).

Table 1-9 Effects of Pregnancy on Pharmacokinetics of Common Drugs

Drug	Pharmacokinetics and Physiology	Clinical Relevance
Ampicillin	Reduced serum half-life; increased clearance	Dosing at higher end of spectrum appropriate
Phenytoin	Increased clearance; altered free and bound fractions	May require higher doses; monitoring of free and total levels warranted
Digoxin	Increased clearance	Serum levels almost twofold lower in pregnancy; therapeutic drug monitoring essential

Box 1-18 Guidelines for Prescribing for Pregnant Patients

- Do not start any medication unless it is clearly indicated.
- Do not discontinue any medications that successfully maintain the maternal condition unless there are clear indications to do so.
- Whenever possible, use principles of clinical pharmacology to make decisions about dosing (e.g., obtain and consider concentrations of bound and unbound drug).
- Always ask about and document the patient's use of nonprescription remedies and dietary supplements.
- Very few drugs are absolutely contraindicated because of pregnancy.
- Know the patient.

Practical Application

The core triad of clinical and scientific considerations introduced in this section are critical for prescribing decisions in the pregnant patient. Sound decision making is best fostered by clear and open communication among all persons involved in the patient's care, especially the patient herself. With that as a given, we offer some final, self-explanatory, practical advice for the potential prescriber (Box 1-18).

REFERENCES

1. **Koren G, Postuszak A, Ito S.** Drugs in pregnancy. N Engl J Med. 1998;338:1128-32.
2. **Moore KL, Persaud TVN.** The Developing Human: Clinically Oriented Embryology, 6th ed. Philadelphia: WB Saunders; 1998.
3. **Koren G, ed.** Maternal-Fetal Toxicology, 2d ed. New York: Marcel Dekker; 1994.
4. **Scialli AR.** A Clinical Guide to Reproductive and Developmental Toxicology. Boca Raton, FL: CRC Press; 1992.

CHAPTER 2

Obstetric Monitoring: Maternal and Fetal Testing

I. Antepartum Fetal Surveillance
Henry L. Galan, MD, and John C. Hobbins, MD

II. Chorionic Villus Sampling and Amniocentesis
Oliver W. Jones III, MD

III. Diagnostic Imaging
Karen Rosene-Montella, MD, and Lucia Larson, MD

In the first of the three sections in this chapter, uterine and fetal growth, maternal recording of fetal kick counts, and fetal activity are reviewed. In addition, more complex techniques of obstetric monitoring, including nonstress tests (NSTs), biophysical profiles (BPPs), contraction stress tests (CSTs), and Doppler ultrasonography (assessment of the umbilical and middle cerebral arteries), are described. The second section discusses invasive fetal surveillance using chronic villus sampling or amniocentesis. The third section moves from fetal monitoring to a review of maternal diagnostic imaging in pregnancy.

I. Antepartum Fetal Surveillance
Henry L. Galan and John C. Hobbins

Numerous techniques are available for fetal surveillance. Although controversy surrounds the prognostic value of these techniques, whether used alone or in combination, antepartum fetal surveillance in high-risk pregnancies remains the standard of care in North America.

Many maternal and fetal conditions may result in fetal or neonatal death during the perinatal period (22 weeks of gestation through 28 days after birth). Since the advent of electronic fetal heart rate (FHR) monitoring, intrapartum fetal death has been almost eliminated, making antepartum fetal loss a greater determinant of perinatal mortality rates (1, 2). Currently, stillbirths account for approximately 50% of all perinatal deaths, and approximately 80% of stillbirths occur before term (37 to 42 weeks of gestation) (3).

Antepartum risk factors can be identified in 50% of stillbirths, and up to 70% of these risk factors are amenable to antenatal intervention (4). According to the American College of Obstetricians and Gynecologists (ACOG), the primary goal of antepartum fetal surveillance is to prevent fetal death in pregnant women at risk for fetal death (5). A secondary goal is to prevent fetal and neonatal asphyxia and their sequelae; this has become possible as a result of recent technological advances in fetal imaging.

Indications for Testing

Identifying persons who would benefit from fetal surveillance involves identifying risk factors by using history, physical examination, and serial clinical assessment of pregnancy status (e.g., blood pressure, fundal height increase, and laboratory data). Box 2-1 lists the major causes of fetal death. A substantial proportion of stillbirths occur in women who have identifiable risk factors for uteroplacental insufficiency, which is defined as placental or uterine dysfunction that results in an inadequate supply of oxygen and nutrients to the fetus and inadequate removal of waste products (carbon dioxide, nitrogen compounds, and fixed acids) from the fetus. Uteroplacental insufficiency is the pathologic basis for antepartum testing. Any maternal condition that could impair the normal exchange that occurs across the uterus and placenta warrants antenatal testing. Box 2-2 lists the maternal and obstetric conditions that are indications for antepartum testing (5).

Box 2-1 Major Causes of Fetal Death

Uteroplacental insufficiency	Congenital anomalies
Hydrops fetalis	Umbilical cord accidents
Congenital infections	Unknown

Surveillance Techniques

Assessment of Uterine and Fetal Growth

Uterine growth should be determined at each prenatal visit, particularly during the third trimester. In general, the distance in centimeters from the pubic symphysis to the fundus of the uterus corresponds to the weeks of gestation (i.e., a fundal height of 28 cm is consistent with a gestational age of 28 weeks). Maternal obesity, uterine fibroids, multiple gestation, polyhydramnios, and fetal macrosomia may cause the fundal height to be greater than expected; intrauterine fetal growth restriction (IUGR), oligohydramnios, and a low fetal lie may make the fundal height less than expected. Although a clinical diagnosis of IUGR by fundal measurement has been shown to be a poor predictor of IUGR at birth (6), any gross discrepancy between fundal height and gestational age should be studied with real-time ultrasonography so that fetal and amniotic fluid status can be determined. If a disturbance in fetal growth or amniotic fluid is present, further testing of the fetus is indicated. Decreased amniotic fluid volume is a reflection of fetal oliguria and may indicate compromised fetal renal or placental blood flow.

Box 2-2 Indications for Antepartum Testing

Maternal conditions
Chronic renal disease
Collagen vascular disease
Cyanotic heart disease
Diabetes mellitus
Hemoglobinopathies
Hypertensive disorders
Hyperthyroidism
Isoimmunization
Thrombophilias

Obstetric conditions
Decreased fetal movement
Discordant multiple gestation
Intrauterine growth restriction
Oligohydramnios
Postdates pregnancy (>42 weeks of gestation)
Previous unexplained stillbirth

Uterine growth may provide clinical clues to fetal compromise, and the maternal and obstetric conditions listed in Box 2-2 place the fetus at risk for disturbances in growth or amniotic fluid volumes. It is therefore recommended that if these conditions are present, real-time ultrasonographic assessment of the fetus should be done to exclude fetal compromise. Results should be plotted against normative data for comparable populations.

Fetal Kick Counts and Fetal Activity Records

Numerous studies have shown that fetal movement as determined by the mother is useful in assessing the well being of the fetus (7–9). Several factors, including gestational age, maternal sensitivity and anxiety, fetal sleep cycles, fetal neurologic anomalies, certain depressant medications, and amniotic fluid volume, influence the maternal perception of fetal movement. The first maternal perception of fetal movement ("quickening") often occurs between 16 and 20 weeks of gestation, but this varies widely, and parous patients may experience quickening earlier in gestation. Maximal fetal movement has been reported to occur between 28 and 32 weeks and to decrease gradually until term (10).

One randomized study compared routine maternally recorded fetal activity with no monitoring in a high-risk population and showed that recording led to a reduction in antepartum fetal demise (7). A similar randomized, multicenter trial failed to show a benefit from routine monitoring (11). Another recent, large, prospective, but nonrandomized study showed that fetal activity recording reduced the rate of fetal demise from 8.7% to 2.1% (8). The last two studies (8, 11), however, used different fetal-movement counting techniques, with one (8) having more stringent criteria for additional testing.

Numerous ways to count fetal movements have been described. An easy one is for the mother to lie on her side and count distinct movements. If 10 movements are counted within 2 hours, this is considered reassuring (8). The mother can stop counting once 10 movements have occurred. If 10 movements do not occur within 2 hours, the fetus should be evaluated immediately with an NST or BPP. Although it is unclear whether fetal activity monitoring is beneficial in low-risk populations, the simplicity, low cost, and patient involvement associated with this monitoring make it a reasonable tool to use in all pregnancies. There is little dispute about the daily use of activity monitoring in high-risk pregnancies. Daily fetal activity counts should be started at approximately 28 to 30 weeks of gestation in all high-risk pregnancies.

Nonstress Tests

Nonstress testing is dependent on the normal neurologic and cardiac development of the fetus. The normal FHR is 120 to 160 beats/min. The baseline FHR progressively decreases during gestation as a result of the normal development of the parasympathetic nervous system. Increases in the FHR above baseline generally develop by approximately 25 weeks of gestation. The duration and degree of acceleration increases as gestation progresses (12,13). Several studies have shown good fetal outcome in association with FHR accelerations that occur in conjunction with fetal movement (14–16).

Numerous definitions for reactivity have been described. The ACOG defines an NST as reactive if two accelerations with a minimum acceleration of 15 beats/min occur and are sustained for 15 seconds within a 20-minute period (5). If this does not happen within 40 minutes, the NST is nonreactive and further investigation is required. A reactive NST carries a high negative predictive value for adverse fetal outcome. A good perinatal outcome is expected with a reactive NST in more than 95% of cases (17). Given that the frequency and amplitude of FHR accelerations increase with gestational age, it is not surprising that reactivity also increases (18). The ideal frequency with which NSTs should be done remains to be determined, but several studies support the twice-weekly use of NSTs in high-risk populations (19, 20). These studies have shown a reduction in the perinatal mortality rate from a range of 0.11% to 0.61% to a range of 0.027% to 0.19%. Therefore, if the NST is the physician's choice for antenatal testing, it is recommended that it be done twice weekly.

The NST is done while the mother is in the lateral recumbent position. A Doppler transducer of approximately 2.5 MHz is applied to the abdomen over the uterus. The high-frequency sound waves are reflected at a frequency different from that of moving objects, such as the ventricles of the fetal heart, and are detected by a receiver that is in the same unit as the transducer. The FHR is then traced on a strip-chart recorder. Maternal blood pressure should be recorded and supine hypotension avoided.

Biophysical Profile

The biophysical profile is an antepartum test that consists of the NST and four observations made on real-time ultrasonography (5). Each of the five components of the BPP receives a score of 0 (abnormal) or 2 (normal), depending on whether the criteria for each component are met (Table 2-1). Manning and colleagues (21) first described the BPP in 1980. When the BPP is used as a primary antenatal surveillance test, the antepartum fetal death rate has been reported to be as low as 0.73 per 1000 patients; the CST is associated with an antepartum fetal death rate of 0.4 per 1000 patients (22, 23).

Modified Biophysical Profile

The modified BPP comprises the NST and measurement of amniotic fluid volume. Like the BPP, the modified BPP tests for both the acute (NST) and the

Table 2-1 Biophysical Profile

Component	Score*
Reactive nonstress test	2
Fetal breathing movements: 1 episode of breathing of 30 seconds or more within 30 minutes	2
Fetal movements: 3 discrete body or limb movements within 30 minutes	2
Fetal tone: 1 episode of extension of a fetal extremity with return to flexion	2
Amniotic fluid†: either 1) a single amniotic fluid pocket of 2 × 2 cm or 2) an AFI > 5 cm	2

*Interpretation: A total score of 8 to 10 is a normal result; a total score of 6 is an equivocal result (retest in 12 to 24 hours); and a total score of 4 is an abnormal result (delivery should be considered).
†Oligohydramnios warrants further evaluation.

chronic (amniotic fluid volume) status of the fetus and placenta. The person performing the modified BPP does not need as much training as the sonologist who performs the BPP does. As a primary antenatal surveillance test, the modified BPP is similar to the CST in predicting fetal well being (24).

Contraction Stress Test

The contraction stress test is a test of placental reserve. Its role is similar to that of an exercise treadmill in determining cardiac reserve. Uterine contractions normally cause a transient paucity of blood flow to the fetus. If a fetus is marginally but adequately oxygenated, the addition of uterine activity may unmask placental dysfunction as reflected by late FHR decelerations occurring at the end of a contraction. (In nonhuman primates, late decelerations reliably reflect suboptimal fetal oxygenation (25).) The test may also reveal variable decelerations due to a nuchal cord, which may indicate oligohydramnios. Box 2-3 gives the procedure and interpretations for the contraction stress test.

Doppler Techniques

Doppler depends on the ability of an ultrasound beam to change in frequency when it encounters a moving object. For example, if one were to intersect an umbilical cord with an ultrasound beam, the refracted echos would be altered in frequency depending on the velocity of the blood encountered during systole and diastole. After some cosmetic manipulation, a waveform would be generated that would have clear systolic and diastolic components. In general, the greater the resistance downstream, the less the amplitude of the end-diastolic flow and the higher the systolic peak. Conversely, in a low-

---

Box 2-3 Contraction Stress Test

Procedure

Supine position with lateral tilt

Abdominal monitor for fetal heart rate and contractions

Induction of contractions by oxytocin or nipple stimulation

Contraction goal: ≥ 3 40-sec contractions per 10 min

Interpretation

Negative result: No late decelerations

Positive result: Late deceleration in 50% of contractions

Equivocal result: Intermittent late or significant variable decelerations

Unsatisfactory result: <3 contractions per 10 min or poor-quality tracing

---

resistance circulation (such as that of the placenta), high end-diastolic flow would be expected.

Waveforms can be assessed in various ways. One can simply "eyeball" the waveform and make an indirect "guesstimate" of the distance between systole and diastole. One can also use the ratio of systole to diastole. Two other quantitative measures are the pulsatility index (systole divided by diastole over the mean across the cardiac cycle) and the resistance index (systole minus diastole over the mean across the cardiac cycle).

In any case, the higher the number in any of the above indices, the greater the resistance downstream. Each vessel in the maternal and fetal circulation has a different resistance for which normative data are available.

Umbilical Artery

The umbilical artery was the first fetal vessel to be sampled. Although the early investigation involved the "blind" acquisition of umbilical artery wave forms with primitive continuous Doppler equipment, today's techniques allow angle corrections, which enhance reliability and accuracy.

The umbilical arteries split at the placental insertion and run along the chorionic plate. These arteries, in turn, give off many "radial arteries" that drive down into the placental substance. Each radial artery feeds a complex of arterioles and capillaries, which form by becoming the functional aspect of the fetal cotyledons. They are responsible for nutrient and gas exchange in the terminal and intermediate villi.

If the villi are developmentally defective (if fewer terminal villi are present) or damaged by infarction, resistance in the villus circulation is increased.

This is reflected in a lower diastolic component of the umbilical artery waveform.

In fetal hypoxia, the umbilical artery waveform becomes abnormal (systole-to-diastole ratio >3 after 30 weeks of gestation) before a change appears on the NST (26). In more than modest hypoxia, the waveform is devoid of end-diastolic flow, and growth-restricted fetuses with severe hypoxia may even show reverse end-diastolic flow. End-diastolic flow in IUGR can sometimes be improved by maternal rest in the lateral recumbent position.

Middle Cerebral Artery

In the early stages of hypoxia, the fetus distributes his or her blood flow in an effort to "spare" the brain. Preferential shunting to the brain is accomplished via increased flow through the carotid arteries. The middle cerebral artery can be sampled with little difficulty because the angle is generally ideal for accurate waveform generation (along the ultrasound beam). The artery supplies a principal portion of the cerebral cortex.

The usual systole-to-diastole ratio of the middle cerebral artery is about 6 because resistance in this artery is normally high. In IUGR, the ratio is often as low as 2.5 to 3.

Increased end-diastolic flow, although it is a sign of IUGR, is designed to protect the brain, and fetuses with IUGR and increased end-diastolic flow often escape neurologic sequelae (27). Unfortunately, while the brain is being spared, other areas of the fetus are not; this is why fetuses with IUGR are predisposed to necrotizing enterocolitis and, later in life, diabetes and cardiovascular disease (28, 29).

Timing and Frequency of Testing

The ideal time to initiate antenatal testing in a high-risk pregnancy remains to be determined. Such testing typically begins by approximately 32 weeks of gestation (5). However, the severity of the disease process or a previous early fetal demise may warrant testing as early as 26 to 28 weeks.

Similarly, the ideal frequency of testing has yet to be determined. Testing should be done at least once a week, and many authors have recommended twice-weekly testing.

Choice of Antepartum Tests

With advances in ultrasonographic imaging and in our understanding of the pathophysiology of uretoplacental insufficiency, the intensity of investigation of the fetal condition has increased dramatically. It is generally accepted that fetal biophysical responses to acidemia and asphyxia are of two kinds: acute and chronic. Acute responses arise from the central nervous system and regulate FHR (nonreactive tracing), tone, breathing, and movements. Chronic responses arise from aortic body chemoreceptor stimulation, resulting in late decelerations in the FHR and preferential redistribution of blood flow to the brain. This "brain-sparing" redistribution of blood flow is seen as an increase in diastolic flow on pulsed-wave Doppler (30). Furthermore, the redistribution of blood flow away from other organs is reflected by a decrease in the amniotic fluid volume, which is caused by a decrease in renal perfusion.

The BPP and the modified BPP are used to assess acute and subacute fetal responses. However, the modified BPP is less involved than the BPP and seems equally able to exclude the possibility of fetal death (5, 24). Chronic responses will be detected by use of the contraction stress test (late decelerations reflective of uteroplacental insufficiency) or Doppler flow changes reflective of redistribution of blood flow to the brain.

REFERENCES

1. **Shamsi HH, Petrie RH, Steer CM.** Changing obstetrical practices and amelioration of perinatal outcome in a university hospital. Am J Obstet Gynecol. 1979;133:855.

2. **Yeh S-Y, Diaz F, Paul RH.** Ten-year experience of intrapartum fetal monitoring in Los Angeles County/University of Southern California Medical Center. Am J Obstet Gynecol. 1982;143:496.

3. **Copper RL, Goldenberg RL, DuBard MB, Davis RO, the Collaborative Group on Preterm Prevention.** Risk factors for fetal death in white, black, and Hispanic women. Obstet Gynecol. 1994;84:490.

4. **Pitkin RM.** Fetal death: diagnosis and management. Am J Obstet Gynecol. 1987; 157:583.

5. Antepartum fetal surveillance. American College of Obstetricians and Gynecologists Technical Bulletin. 1994;188.

6. **Freeman RK, Dorchester W, Anderson G, et al.** The significance of a previous stillbirth. Am J Obstet Gynecol. 1985;151:7.

7. **Neldam S.** Fetal movements as an indicator of fetal well-being. Lancet. 1980;1:1222.

8. **Moore TR. Piacquadio K.** A prospective evaluation of fetal movement screening to reduce the incidence of antepartum fetal death. Am J Obstet Gynecol. 1989;160:1075.

9. **Rayburn W, Zuspan F, Motley ME, Donaldson M.** An alternative to antepartum fetal heart rate testing. Am J Obstet Gynecol. 1980;138:223.

10. **Rayburn WF.** Clinical implications from monitoring fetal activity. Am J Obstet Gynecol. 1982;144:967.

11. **Grant A. Elbourne D, Valentin L, Alexander S.** Routine formal fetal movement counting and risk of antepartum late death in normally formed singletons. Lancet. 1989;i: 345.

12. **Natale R, Nasello C, Turliuk R.** The relationship between movements and accelerations in fetal heart rate at twenty-four to thirty-two weeks' gestation. Am J Obstet Gynecol. 1984;148:591.

13. **Gagnon R, Campbell K, Hunse C, Patrick J.** Patterns of human fetal heart rate accelerations from 26 weeks to term. Am J Obstet Gynecol. 1987;157:743.

14. **Trierweiler MW, Freeman RK, James J.** Baseline fetal heart rate characteristics as an indicator of fetal status during the antepartum period. Am J Obstet Gynecol. 1976; 125:618.

15. **Rochard F, Schifrin BS, Goupil R, Legrand H, Blottiere J, Sureau C.** Nonstressed fetal heart rate monitoring in the antepartum period. Am J Obstet Gynecol. 1976; 126:699.

16. **Phelan JP.** The nonstress test: a review of 3,000 tests. Am J Obstet Gynecol. 1981; 139:7.

17. **Devoe LD, Castillo RA, Sherline DM.** The nonstress test as a diagnostic test: a critical reappraisal. Am J Obstet Gynecol. 1985;152:1047.

18. **Smith CV, Phelan JP, Paul RH.** A prospective analysis of the influence of gestational age on the baseline fetal heart rate and reactivity in a low-risk population. Am J Obstet Gynecol. 1985;153:780

19. **Boehm FH, Salyer S, Shah DM, Vaughn WK.** Improved outcome of twice weekly nonstress testing. Obstet Gynecol. 1986;67:566.

20. **Schneider EP, Hutson JM, Petrie RH.** An assessment of the first decade's experience with antepartum fetal heart rate testing. Am J Perinatol. 1988;5:134.

21. **Manning F, Platt LW, Sipos L.** Antepartum fetal evaluation: development of a biophysical profile. Am J Obstet Gynecol. 1980;136:787.

22. **Manning F, Morrison M, Lange I, et al.** Fetal biophysical profile scoring: selective use of the nonstress test. Am J Obstet Gynecol. 1987;156:709.

23. **Freeman R, Anderson G, Dorchester W.** A prospective multi-institutional study of antepartum fetal heart rate monitoring. II. Contraction stress test versus non stress test for primary surveillance. Am J Obstet Gynecol. 1982;143:778.

24. **Clark SL, Sabey P, Jolley K.** Nonstress testing with acoustic stimulation and amniotic fluid volume assessment: 5973 tests without unexpected death. Am J Obstet Gynecol. 1989;160:694.

25. **Myers RE, Mueller-Heubach E, Adamsons K.** Predictability of the state of fetal oxygenation from a quantitative analysis of the components of late deceleration. Am J Obstet Gynecol. 1973;115:1083.

26. **Ajayi RA, Soothill PW, Campbell S, Nicolaides KH.** Antenatal testing to predict outcome in pregnancy with unexplained antepartum haemorrhage. Br J Obstet Gynecol. 1992;99:122-5.

27. **Chan FY, Pun TC, Lam P, Lam C, Lee CP, Lam YH.** Fetal cerebral Doppler studies as a predictor of perinatal outcome and subsequent neurologic handicap. Obstet Gynecol. 1996;87:981-8.

28. **Barker DJP, Gluckman PD, Godfrey KM, Harding JE, Owens JA, Robinson JS.** Fetal nutrition and cardiovascular disease in adult life. Lancet. 1993;341:938-41.

29. **Hales CN, Barker DJP, Clark PMS, et al.** Fetal and infant growth and impaired glucose tolerance at age 64. BMJ. 1991;303:1019-22.

30. **Wladimiroff JW, Tonge HM, Stewart PA.** Doppler ultrasound assessment of cerebral flow in the human fetus. Br J Obstet Gynecol. 1986;93:471-5.

II. Chorionic Villus Sampling and Amniocentesis
Oliver W. Jones III

The practice of accessing the intrauterine environment to obtain information about a growing fetus with the intention of continuing the pregnancy began in the 1950s with the collection of amniotic fluid to identify fetal sex (1). This was followed by complete chromosomal analysis (2). In the 1960s, placental tissue was biopsied for the purpose of diagnosing gestational trophoblastic disease (3). As technology has improved, these procedures have become so sophisticated that amniocentesis and, to a lesser degree, chorionic villus sampling (CVS) are now commonly offered to pregnant women for prenatal diagnosis.

Invasive fetal testing is offered to pregnant women with specific characteristics, such as advanced maternal age (usually >35 years), abnormal results on maternal serum testing (of alpha-fetoprotein, estriol, and beta-hCG levels), a previous child with a chromosomal abnormality, recurrent fetal loss, balanced parental chromosomal translocation, abnormal results on fetal ultrasonography, family history of an inherited abnormality that can be detected on prenatal testing, and parental concern. If a pregnant woman elects to have invasive testing, it is important that she be informed of the risks of the various procedures.

The most common method of fetal genetic testing is amniocentesis done at 15 to 16 weeks of gestation (Figure 2-1). First, a pocket of amniotic fluid free of the umbilical cord is identified on direct ultrasonographic visualization. The amniocentesis site is cleaned with an antiseptic solution, and the ultrasonographic transducer is wrapped in a sterile plastic cover so that it can be used to guide the needle into the amniotic space. Typically, a 22-gauge spinal needle is used and approximately 20 cc of amniotic fluid is withdrawn. Fetal urination replaces this fluid over a brief period. In skilled hands, introduction of the needle into the amniotic space, removal of the fluid, and removal of the needle should be done in less than about 30 seconds and in a single attempt. Occasionally, the fetus moves or the pocket of fluid is obliterated by a uterine contraction, necessitating a second puncture.

The advantages of amniocentesis over CVS are a lower complication rate, the ability to test for neural tube defects (by measuring alpha-fetoprotein and acetylcholinesterase levels in the amniotic fluid), and slightly more accurate cytogenetic results. Amniocentesis has potential risks. Leakage of amniotic fluid occurs in less than 2% of procedures (4, 5). One study reported a significantly lower rate of leakage when the placenta was traversed during the procedure than when it was not (0% compared with 0.5%; $P < 0.05$) (6). Vaginal bleeding occurs in less than 1% of procedures (5).

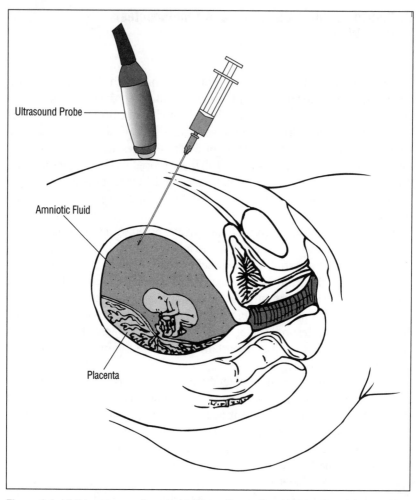

Ultrasound Probe

Amniotic Fluid

Placenta

Figure 2-1 Midtrimester amniocentesis. (From Counseling Aids for Geneticists, 3rd ed. Greenwood, SC: Greenwood Genetic Center; 1995; with permission.)

Fetal loss rates are reported in different ways: 1) additional loss directly related to amniocentesis, 2) total rate of loss in relation to loss in women with fetuses of the same gestational age who do not have amniocentesis, or 3) loss in relation to loss occurring with another method such as early amniocentesis or CVS. Early data on fetal loss were published when amniocentesis was done without ultrasonography or during the early development of ultrasonography. Improvements in ultrasonographic technology and overall amniocentesis technique have probably contributed to decreased fetal loss rates. The excess fetal loss due to midtrimester amniocentesis is commonly cited as

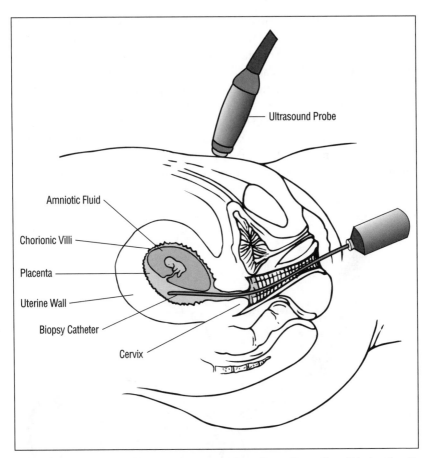

Figure 2-2 Transcervical chorionic villus sampling. (From Counseling Aids for Geneticists, 3rd ed. Greenwood, SC: Greenwood Genetic Center; 1995; with permisison.)

0.5% (7), and the recent literature continues to support this. In a Canadian study comparing early with midtrimester amniocentesis (4), the fetal loss rate after amniocentesis done after 15 weeks of gestation was 0.8%. Similarly, Assel and colleagues (8) and Crandall and co-workers (9) report loss rates of 0.4% and 0.6%, respectively. It is important to recognize that without any intervention there is a natural fetal loss rate in documented live pregnancies. This is 1% to 3% up to a maternal age of 34 years and then increases to about 5% to 7% (10).

The CVS procedures began to be used more often in the early 1980s. The advantage of CVS over standard midtrimester amniocentesis is the early diagnosis of chromosomal abnormalities and, thus, earlier and safer termination of the pregnancy, if the parents desire it. The procedure is currently done 10 to 13 weeks after the last menstrual period. There are two methods of CVS: transcervical (Figure 2-2) and transabdominal (Figure 2-3).

In the transcervical approach, a specialized polyethylene catheter is used. With ultrasonographic guidance, the catheter is passed through the cervical os to the site of the developing placenta (specifically, the chorion frondosum). The chorion frondosum is a site of mitotically active villi and provides tissue that readily allows karyotyping. When appropriate placement of the catheter tip is confirmed, tissue is gently suctioned into an attached syringe that contains collecting media as the catheter is withdrawn from the uterus. Adequate sampling is confirmed by direct inspection of the obtained tissue under a dis-

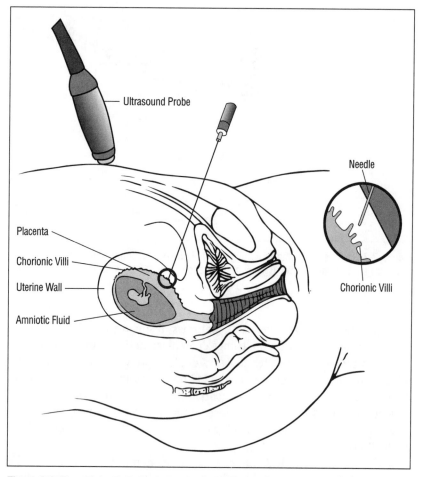

Figure 2-3 Transabdominal chorionic villus sampling. (From Counseling Aids for Geneticists, 3rd ed. Greenwood, SC: Greenwood Genetic Center; 1995; with permisison.)

secting microscope. Chorionic villi have a characteristic bud-and-branch appearance. Contraindications to transcervical CVS are a poor approach to the biopsy site due to placental position, obstruction of the cervical os, and active genital herpes simplex infection.

The transabdominal CVS technique is similar to the technique of amniocentesis. With ultrasonographic guidance, a 20-gauge spinal needle is directed to the chorion frondosum. A syringe containing collecting media is attached to the needle, and the needle is passed back and forth in the chorion frondosum four to five times to obtain enough tissue for analysis. The tissue is then inspected as it is with transcervical CVS. Contraindications to transabdominal CVS are difficult access due to placental position and obstruction of the path of the needle by the maternal bowel. The primary advantage of CVS over amniocentesis is earlier diagnosis of chromosomal abnormalities. Karyotype results can be available in just a few hours, although a more definitive result is usually available in 4 to 8 days. In contrast, karyotyping in an amniocentesis specimen may take 10 days to 2 weeks.

Brambati and colleagues (11) recently published their experience with 10,000 cases of CVS. The overall fetal loss rate up to 28 weeks of gestation was 2.6%. Women older than 40 years of age had a fetal loss rate of 3.8%. This suggests that in very experienced hands, the fetal loss rate due to CVS is similar to the background spontaneous loss rate. Similarly, Chueh and associates (12) reported their experience in 9000 CVS procedures. They noted that with the introduction of transabdominal CVS the overall fetal loss rate (background loss plus procedure-related loss) decreased from 5.12% to 3.07%. They also found that the odds for fetal loss were 2.5 times greater after transcervical CVS than after transabdominal CVS. Although various centers report slightly different fetal loss rates, the commonly cited rates of procedure-related excess loss are 1% for CVS and 0.5% for amniocentesis.

Beginning in the late 1980s, there appeared several case reports of fetal limb defects in mothers who had CVS (13–15). These were transverse limb defects associated with CVS done at less than 66 days of gestation. Recently, Firth (16) reviewed the data on this issue. The hypothesis is that in CVS vascular disruption leads to necrosis of the developing distal limbs. The critical period of limb development is from about the end of the fifth week of gestation to the end of the ninth week (63 days). This information is compelling, but transverse limb defects are so rare (incidence, 3 in 10,000) that current published reports are inadequate to provide a definitive solution to this problem. However, the current recommendation is that CVS be done after about 10 weeks of gestation because there seems to be a gestational age–related risk for this abnormality.

As an alternative to CVS, amniocentesis has been done earlier than the standard 15 to 16 weeks of gestation. Early amniocentesis is typically done at

11 to 14 weeks of gestation. The procedure is technically the same as a standard amniocentesis, but it can be difficult to pass the needle into the amniotic space because the amnion has not always completely fused with the chorion by 14 weeks. In a Canadian study (4), first-attempt success rates were 96.9% for early amniocentesis and 99.6% for midtrimester amniocentesis; the difference was significant. Postprocedural spontaneous loss rates were 2.6% for early amniocentesis and 0.8% for midtrimester amniocentesis. The rate of total fetal loss, including spontaneous and elective abortions, before the procedure was 7.6% for early amniocentesis and 5.9% for midtrimester amniocentesis; the difference was significant. In addition, a higher incidence of club foot was seen in the early amniocentesis group (1.3% compared with 0.1%; $P < 0.0001$). This is presumably due to reduced amniotic fluid volume and compression of the extremities. A similar finding was seen in an earlier study by Sundberg and co-workers (17), who compared CVS with early amniocentesis. Sundberg and co-workers also reported total fetal loss rates due to elective abortion, spontaneous loss, and neonatal death after each procedure. For CVS, the total loss rate was 4.8%; for early amniocentesis, it was 5.4%. The difference was not significant.

In summary, there are three options for fetal genetic testing in early pregnancy: amniocentesis at 15 to 16 weeks of gestation (standard amniocentesis), CVS at 10 to 12 weeks of gestation, and early amniocentesis at 11 to 14 weeks of gestation. Although there are nationally accepted fetal loss rates for each procedure, the loss rates reported in several studies are variable. However, the loss rate is probably lowest with standard amniocentesis and higher for early amniocentesis and CVS. The lowest loss rates are usually associated with centers with the most experience. Counseling patients about the risks and benefits of each procedure is important in allowing each patient to make the choice best suited to her needs.

REFERENCES

1. **Fuchs F, Riis P.** Antenatal sex determination. Nature. 1956;177:330.
2. **Steele MW, Breg WR Jr.** Chromosome analysis of human amniotic-fluid cells. Lancet. 1966;1:382-5.
3. **Alvarez H.** Diagnosis of hydatidiform mole by transabdominal placental biopsy. Am J Obstet Gynecol. 1966;96:38-41.
4. Randomized trial to assess safety and fetal outcome of early and midtrimester amniocentesis. The Canadian Early and Mid-trimester Amniocentesis Trial (CEMAT) Group. Lancet. 1998;351:242-7.
5. **Brumfield CG, Lin S, Conner W, Cosper P, Davis RO, Owen J.** Pregnancy outcome following genetic amniocentesis at 11-14 versus 16-19 weeks' gestation. Obstet Gynecol. 1996;88:114-8.

6. **Giorlandino C, Mobili L, Bilancioni E, D'Alessio P, Carcioppolo O, Gentili P, Vizzone A.** Transplacental amniocentesis: is it really a higher-risk procedure? Prenat Diagn. 1994;14:803-6.

7. **Creasy RK, Resnik R, eds.** Maternal-Fetal Medicine, Principles and Practice, 3d ed. Philadelphia: WB Saunders; 1994:65-65.

8. **Assel BG, Lewis SM, Dickerman LH, Park VM, Jassani MN.** Single-operator comparison of early and mid-second-trimester amniocentesis. Obstet Gynecol. 1992;79:940-4.

9. **Crandall BF, Kulch P, Tabsh K.** Risk assessment of amniocentesis between 11 and 15 weeks: comparison to later amniocentesis controls. Prenat Diagn. 1994;14:913-9.

10. **Cashner KA, Christopher CR, Dysert GA.** Spontaneous fetal loss after demonstration of a live fetus in the first trimester. Obstet Gynecol. 1987;70:827-30.

11. **Brambati B, Tului L, Cislaghi C, Alberti E.** First 10,000 chorionic villus samplings performed on singleton pregnancies by a single operator. Prenat Diagn. 1998;18:255-66.

12. **Chueh JT, Goldberg JD, Wohlferd MM, Golbus MS.** Comparison of transcervical and transabdominal chorionic villus sampling loss rates in nine thousand cases from a single center. Am J Obstet Gynecol. 1995;173:1277-82.

13. **Planteydt HT, van de Vooren MJ, Verweij H.** Amniotic bands and malformation in child born after pregnancy screened by chorionic villus biopsy. Lancet. 1986;2:756-9.

14. **Christians GCML, van Baarlen J, Huber J, Leschot NJ.** Fetal limb constriction: a possible complication of CVS. Prenat Diagn. 1989;9:67-71.

15. **Boyd PA, Keeling JW, Selinger M, MacKenzie IZ.** Limb reduction and chorion villus sampling. Prenat Diagn. 1990;10:437-41.

16. **Firth H.** Chorion villus sampling and limb deficiency—cause or coincidence? Prenat Diagn. 1997;17:1313-30.

17. **Sundberg K, Bang J, Smidt-Jensen S, Brocks V, Lundsteen C, Parner J, et al.** Randomized study of risk of fetal loss related to early amniocentesis versus chorionic villus sampling. Lancet. 1997;350:697-703.

III. Diagnostic Imaging
Karen Rosene-Montella and Lucia Larson

The term *radiation* provokes anxiety in the nonpregnant patient, and this fear is amplified in the pregnant patient, her family, and her care providers. The term connotes atomic bombs, accidents and leaks in nuclear power plants, and the carcinogenic effects of large occupational exposures. Although exposure to events like Hiroshima, Nagasaki, or Chernobyl is very different from exposure to the low-dose ionizing radiation used in diagnostic imaging, they are one and the same to many persons. The task of clinicians who care for pregnant women is to introduce some rationality, both for our patients and our colleagues, into this very emotional area of care.

The approach to diagnostic imaging in pregnancy is similar to the approach to drug prescribing in pregnancy described in the previous chapter. The use of a diagnostic procedure is indicated when its importance to maternal well being outweighs any risk to the mother or fetus. The low doses of radiation used for most diagnostic tests have not been correlated with any human genetic disorder or congenital malformation to date.

Four major categories of imaging exist: ionizing radiation imaging, such as that done with x-rays and gamma rays; ultrasonography; magnetic resonance imaging (MRI); and direct exposure to isotopes used in nuclear medicine. These categories are often lumped together inappropriately. Ionizing radiation, which is used in radiography and computed tomography (CT), is discussed first. Then ultrasonography (the imaging method preferred in pregnancy) and MRI are reviewed. Finally, direct exposure to isotopes used in nuclear medicine is considered.

Ionizing Radiation

The effect of fetal exposure to ionizing radiation is dependent on the level of exposure (most effects require a certain threshold dose) and the gestational age at which the exposure occurs (Table 2-2). During the preimplantation period (0 to 2 weeks of gestation), the embryo is sensitive to the lethal effects of radiation but not to its teratogenic or growth-restricting effects. This means that the outcome after a significant exposure is either a normal conceptus or complete fetal resorption. The cells of the preimplantation stage are pluripotent; if a small number of cells is damaged, other cells multiply and take their place. However, if too many cells are damaged, the embryo does not survive.

Table 2-2 Effects of Radiation in Utero

Gestation (days)	Phase	Possible Effects
1 to 9	Preimplantation	Most likely adverse effect is death; malformation unlikely (18 to 50 rads)
10 to 12	Implantation	Death less likely; malformation still unlikely; growth restriction possible (10 to 50 rads)
13 to 50	Organogenesis	Fetal malformations; growth restriction; (>25 rads)
51 to 280	Fetal growth	Intrauterine growth restriction (≥10 to 50 rads); central nervous system abnormalities (≥10 to 50 rads); possible increased incidence of cancer or leukemia (relative risk; 1.5) (>1 rad)

Adapted from Elkayam U, Gleicher N, eds. Cardiac Problems in Pregnancy: Diagnosis and Management of Maternal and Fetal Disease, 3rd ed. New York: Wiley-Liss; 1998:34.

During organogenesis (2 to 8 of weeks gestation), the embryo is very sensitive to the teratogenic and growth-restricting effects of radiation. Because some limitations on growth can be "made up for" by the infant after birth, the most significant lasting effect in a liveborn infant exposed to radiation at this stage is malformation. The central nervous system is especially sensitive to radiation, and microcephaly and mental retardation are the most common manifestations of exposure to high-dose radiation during organogenesis. Numerous studies indicate that the minimal exposure necessary for any teratogenic effect is 10 rads, and most effects are not seen with less than 100 rads. Because this is 100 to 1000 times the exposure expected from, for example, a single chest film, it is unlikely that simple diagnostic procedures will cause malformation.

During the fetal period (8 weeks to term), the fetus is most sensitive to the growth-restricting effects of radiation, and malformations are unlikely. However, with high doses of radiation (50 to 100 rads), damage to the central nervous system leading to mental retardation may occur. The chance of childhood leukemia is slightly increased with exposures later in gestation, up to a relative risk of 1.5 when the exposure exceeds 1 rad. However, this risk should be viewed in the context of overall risks for childhood leukemia, which are low in the general population (Table 2-3) (1).

Table 2-3 Risk for Childhood Leukemia in Patients with Long-Term Follow-up

Group	Approximate Risk	Increased Risk over Control Population	Occurrence
Identical twin of twin with leukemia	1 in 3	1000	Weeks to months
Patients with irradiation-treated myeloproliferative disorder	1 in 6	500	10 to 15 years
Patients with Bloom syndrome	1 in 8	375	< 30 years of age
Hiroshima survivors who were within 1000 m of the hypocenter	1 in 60	50	Average, 12 years
Patients with Down syndrome	1 in 95	30	< 10 years of age
Patients irradiation-treated with ankylosing spondylitis	1 in 270	10	15 years
Siblings of leukemic children	1 in 720	4.0	To 10 years
Children exposed to pelvimetry in utero (gestational exposure)	1 in 2000	1.5	< 10 years
U.S. white children < 15 years old	1 in 2800	1.0	To 10 years

Adapted from Miller RW: Epidemiologic conclusions from radiation toxicity studies. In: Fry RJM, Grahan ML, eds. Late Effects of Radiation. London: Taylor & Francis; 1970:245-56.

The exposure to ionizing radiation that occurs with common diagnostic procedures is outlined in Table 2-4. Radiation to which the fetus is exposed during procedures done in areas other than the pelvis is secondary radiation that has been redirected or scattered after direct interaction with the area of study. Only about 5% of the primary radiation is scattered to the uterus and absorbed by the fetus. Ways to reduce fetal exposure include using the highest-speed film possible and limiting the exposure time (for example, in fluoroscopy). Most researchers think that having patients wear a lead apron during a procedure has little value because the fetal exposure to radiation is due to indirect scatter. In theory, the risk for secondary radiation may be increased by photons emitted from the lead shield. The maximum radiation exposure currently considered acceptable over the duration of the pregnancy is 5 rads (500 mrad, 0.05 Gy, 5 cGy). Doses of 5 to 10 rads are considered to confer low or questionable risk. Doses greater than 10 rads before the sixth week of gestation confer high risk, and pregnancy termination should be considered (Table 2-5) (2, 3).

Table 2-4 Estimated Fetal Exposure During Diagnostic Radiology Procedures

Procedure	Estimated Fetal Exposure (rads)
Chest radiography	< 0.005
Chest fluoroscopy	0.07
Skull or sinus	≤ 0.004
Hip or femur	0.2 to 0.3
Cervical spine	≤ 0.001
Lumbosacral spine	0.35 to 0.60
Mammography	0.007 to 0.02
Abdominal film	0.3
Intravenous pyelography	0.4 to 0.8
Upper GI	0.1 to 0.56
Barium enema	0.7 to 0.8
Chest/head CT	0.3 to 0.64
Abdominal/pelvic CT	1.3 to 3.2
CT pelvimetry	0.23 to 1.3

Table 2-5 National Commission on Radiation Protection (NCRP) Recommended Pregnancy Exposures

Total Exposure During Pregnancy (rads)	NCRP Recommendations
≤ 5	Acceptable; low likelihood of problem
5 to 10	Low risk for problem
10 to 15 rads (at ≤ 8 weeks of gestation)	Higher-risk; individual consideration of termination
> 15	Termination of pregnancy recommended

Ultrasonography

Pelvic, abdominal, and cardiac ultrasonography should be considered safe in pregnancy and should be used as the initial imaging test if at all possible. It may be necessary to reassure patients that no evidence in animals or humans indicates that sound waves can damage a developing fetus. Most pregnant women are comfortable with ultrasonography because it is widely used in obstetrics for fetal imaging.

Magnetic Resonance Imaging

Magnetic resonance imaging poses no known risk to the developing human embryo or fetus, and considerable experience in humans has failed to show any associated abnormalities or harm. Limited animal data suggest that changes may occur when animals receive exposure over prolonged periods. The National Institutes of Health Consensus Development Conference (1987) and the U.S. Food and Drug Administration have recommended delaying exposure to MRI until after the first trimester, but they do not support this conclusion with any relevant data (4, 5). Their recommendations have resulted in the practice now current in many radiology departments: to offer MRI after 12 weeks of gestation but reserve its use in the first trimester for patients with clinical conditions that cannot be managed with other diagnostic techniques. We clearly need better data to support rational recommendations. There are times when the benefit of MRI at any gestational age will outweigh the theoretical risks—for example, in a case of possible cerebral venous thrombosis or leaking aneurysm. Gadolinium contrast used in MRI crosses the placenta but has not been associated with adverse effects in the fetus.

Nuclear Medicine Techniques and Radioisotopes

A final area of concern is exposure to radiation from the radioisotopes used for various diagnostic procedures. Although we know the absolute dose of radiation per dose of isotope for most agents, the effects of this radiation are not as well described as the effects of external radiation. Further, isotopes may vary with respect to target organs, ability to cross the placenta, metabolism, distribution, and half life. Fetal exposure to radiation from nuclear isotopes results from accumulation of the isotope in maternal tissues (the uterus and bladder) and from placental blood flow.

Maintenance of maternal hydration with frequent emptying of the bladder will limit fetal exposure. Table 2-6 lists isotopes used in diagnostic procedures and the resulting estimated doses of radiation to the embryo, and Table 2-7 lists procedures using isotopes and the resulting estimated doses of radiation to the fetus (6, 7). Estimates of risk depend on the careful calculation of dose and duration of exposure. For most isotopes, with the exception of iodine (Table 2-8), fetal exposure and risk are minimal. The fetal thyroid begins trapping iodine at 10 weeks of gestation and thus is highly sensitive to the ablative effects of radioactive iodine from 10 weeks of gestation to term.

Table 2-6 Estimated Dose to Embryo from Radiopharmaceuticals

Radiopharmaceutical	Embryo Dose (rad/mCi administered)
^{99m}Tc-human serum albumin	0.018
^{99m}Tc-lung aggregate	0.035
^{99m}Tc-polyphosphate	0.036
^{99m}Tc-sodium pertechnetate	0.037
^{99m}Tc-stannous glucoheptonate	0.040
^{99m}Tc-sulfur colloid	0.032
^{123}I-sodium iodide (15% uptake)	0.032
^{123}I-sodium iodide (15% uptake)	0.100
^{123}I-rose bengal	0.130
^{123}I-rose bengal	0.680

From Brent RL. Effects and risks of medically administered isotopes to the developing embryo. In: Fabro S, Scialli AR, eds. Drug and Chemical Action in Pregnancy. New York: Marcel Dekker; 1986:427-39; with permission.

Table 2-7 Fetal Radiation Doses from Various Nuclear Medicine Procedures

Procedure	Radioisotope	Fetal Dose (rads)
Pericardial imaging	^{99m}Tc-human serum albumin	0.18
Placenta imaging	^{99m}Tc-human serum albumin	0.018 to 0.036
Lung perfusion study	^{99m}Tc-lung aggregate	0.105
Brain imaging	^{99m}Tc-pertechnetate	0.555 to 0.74
Bone marrow imaging	^{99m}Tc-sulfur colloid	0.32
Spleen imaging	^{99m}Tc-sulfur colloid	0.096
Liver imaging	^{99m}Tc-sulfur colloid	0.096
	^{131}I-rose bengal	2.04
Thyroid uptake (15% uptake)	^{123}I-iodine	0.0032
Thyroid imaging (15% uptake)	^{131}I-iodine	0.001
Thyroid therapy	^{131}I-iodine	0.05 to 2.0 (thyrotoxicosis) 7.5 to 15.0 (thyroid cancer)

From Brent RL. Effects and risks of medically administered isotopes to the developing embryo. In: Fabro S, Scialli AR, eds. Drug and Chemical Action in Pregnancy. New York: Marcel Dekker; 1986:427-39; with permission.

Table 2-8 Thyroidal Radioiodine Dose to the Fetus*

Gestation Period	Fetal/Maternal Ratio (Thyroid Gland)	Dose to Fetal Thyroid (rad/µCi) from Ingestion by Mother
≤10 to 12 weeks[†]	–	0.001 (precursors)
12 to 13 weeks	1.2	0.7
Second trimester	1.8	6.0
Third trimester	7.5	—
Birth imminent	–	8.0

*The fetal thyroid is able to trap iodine at 10 to 12 weeks of gestation; risk exists for hypothyroidism or ablation of fetal thyroid.

From Brent RL. Effects and risks of medically administered isotopes to the developing embryo. In: Fabro S, Scialli AR, eds. Drug and Chemical Action in Pregnancy. New York: Marcel Dekker; 1986:427-39; with permission.

Box 2-4 Topics for which Information Is Needed To Counsel Pregnant Patients with Radiation Exposure

Last menstrual period

Whether pregnancy is wanted or unwanted

Extent of exposure (type, duration, dose)

Family history

Other risks for congenital malformations and leukemia

Possibility of additional exposures as pregnancy progresses

Concurrent illnesses

Concurrent exposures

Summary

Exposure to ionizing radiation at doses less than 5 rads during pregnancy is not known to increase risk for congenital malformation, growth restriction, embryo resorption, or miscarriage. Counseling of pregnant women requires taking a careful history of the timing, duration, and extent of any exposure (Box 2-4). Recommendations must be made in the context of the clinical situation and the patient's desires and beliefs so that a true risk–benefit analysis is done. Table 2-9, a compilation of available information, is organized by body part or system so that clinicians can use it as a guide in making these recommendations (8–11).

Table 2-9 Radiation Exposure to Pregnant Patient (by Body Part or System)

Part or Region of Body	Imaging Technique	Radiation Exposure (rads)	Other Effects on Pregnancy and Lactation	Comments
Brain	Head CT	< 0.001	Limited data on IV contrast in pregnancy, but theoretical concern about iodine toxicity to the fetal thyroid. Iohexol used to measure GFR in pregnant women had no apparent adverse effect. No harm to rat and rabbit fetuses has been noted. Little information on diatrizoate meglumine in pregnancy. Use of IV contrast should probably be limited to situations in which the necessary information cannot be obtained with other studies. It is recomended that breastfeeding mothers who receive IV contrast bottle feed infants and pump and discard breastmilk for 24 hours.	Test of choice for acute intraparenchymal, subarachnoid, subdural, or epidural hemorrhage. Bony structures well visualized. Unstable patients more easily monitored than during MRI.
	Cerebral angiography	If long fluoroscopy is required, exposure increases significantly.		
	MRI MRV MRA	None	No harm in pregnancy has been shown, but long-term effects are less certain. Because of limited experience with gadolinium in pregnancy, this agent is usually avoided. Gadolinium is transferred to breastmilk in small amounts, and it is recommended that breastfeeding mothers bottle feed infants and pump and discard breast milk for 36-48 hours.	Useful for imaging in preeclampsia and eclampsia, cerebral vein thrombosis, pituitary adenoma, tumor, infarction, AVM, and aneurysm.

Table 2-9 Radiation Exposure to Pregnant Patient—*continued*

Part or Region of Body	Imaging Technique	Radiation Exposure (rads)	Other Effects on Pregnancy and Lactation	Comments
Head and neck	C-spine CT	< 0.001	See discussion of head CT, above.	
	Sinus radiography	< 0.1		
	MRI	None	See discussion of MRI of the brain, above.	The advantages of MRI over CT are limited, and these studies should probably be used as in non-pregnant patients
	Dental (single exposure)	0.01		
	Skull	0.004		
Thyroid	Radioactive uptake scanning	Contraindicated. May result in fetal hypothyroidism, thyroid ablation, and subsequernt cancer.	Breastfeeding mothers should bottle feed infants and pump and discard breastmilk for 24 to 48 hours.	Inadvertent use is not thought to warrant a recommendation for pregnancy termination.
	Ultrasonography	None		
Spine	MRI	None	See discussion of MRI of the brain, above.	Disc extrusion, spinal tumor, fracture, ingfection, syrinx, and AVM.
	C-spine radiography	< 0.01		
	Thoracic spine CT	0.020	See discussion of head CT, above.	
	Lumbar spine	0.408		
	Lumbosacral region	0.639		
	Lumbar spine CT	0.7	See discussion of head CT, above.	
Chest	CXR	< 0.001		
	Chest CT	0.03	See discussion of head CT, above.	
	Chest and abdomen CT	0.450	See discussion of head CT, above.	

Table 2-9 Radiation Exposure to Pregnant Patient—*continued*

Part or Region of Body	Imaging Technique	Radiation Exposure (rads)	Other Effects on Pregnancy and Lactation	Comments
Chest—*cont.*	MRI	None	See discussion of MRI of the brain, above.	Useful for evaluating mediastinal and hilar nodes, coarctation aorta, aortitis, aortic dissection, and atrial myxoma.
	Lung scanning	0.01 to 0.02 (ventilation) 0.01 to 0.03 (perfusion)	Breastfeeding mothers should bottle feed infants and pump and discard breastmilk for 24 to 48 hours. Isotope can be measured in breast milk.	Procedure of choice for evaluation of pulmonary embolism.
	Pulmonary angiography	< 0.050 via brachial route 0.2 to 0.3 via femoral route	See discussion of contrast, above.	
Breast	Mammography	< 0.1 per breast		Less sensitive in pregnant and lactating women because of increased breast density.
	Ultrasonography	None		
Cardiac system	Cardiac echocardiography	None		
	Cardiac catheterization	0.5	IV contrast agents include ioxaglate, which has shown no adverse effects in rabbits and rats. Also used are iohexol and diatrizoate meglumine (see CT scan).	
	Cardiac radionuclide imaging	≤ 0.8	Persantine has not been associated with congenital abnormalities, but concerns about antiplatelet effects may limit use.	Low-level protocol with fetal monitoring is usually recommended. Stress echocardiography is preferred.
	Stress echocardiography	None	Adverse effects of dobutamine have not been described.	Diagnostic procedure of choice for CAD. Low-level protocol with fetal monitoring is usually recommended.

Table 2-9 Radiation Exposure to Pregnant Patient—*continued*

Part or Region of Body	Imaging Technique	Radiation Exposure (rads)	Other Effects on Pregnancy and Lactation	Comments
GI system	Abdominal radiography	0.263		
	RUQ ultrason-ography	None		
	MRI	None	No harm if pregnancy has been shown, but long-term effects are less certain. See discussion of MRI of the brain, above.	Liver, pancreas, retroperitoneum, large lesions such as tumors, pancreatic pseudocysts.
	Abdominal CT	0.240	See discussion of head CT, above.	
	Abdominal/pelvic CT	0.640		
	Upper GI tract	0.048	Oral preparations of barium sulfate are poorly absorbed from GI tract and unlikely to pose risk to the fetus. May be used in breast-feeding mothers.	
	Barium enema	0.822		
Renal system	Ultrasonography	None		Renal size increase by 1 cm. Hydronephrosis and hydroureter occur.
	IVP	0.814 rads (complete series) A "one shot" IVP is often done to reduce the radiation exposure obtained with the complete series.	There is concern about iodine toxicity to the fetal thyroid with use of IV agents. There is little information on diatrizoate meglumine use in pregnancy. Ipamidol has not been shown to have adverse effects in fetuses of rats and rabbits, but it has been associated with postnatal thyroid alterations in very-low-birthweight infants. It has been recommended that breast-feeding mothers bottle feed infants and pump and discard breastmilk for 24 hours.	
	Limited IVP	0.1 to 0.2 rads		

Table 2-9 Radiation Exposure to Pregnant Patient—*continued*

Part or Region of Body	Imaging Technique	Radiation Exposure (rads)	Other Effects on Pregnancy and Lactation	Comments
Pelvis	Ultrasonography	None		
	Pelvic radiography	0.194 rads		
	MRI	None	See discussion of MRI of the brain, above.	Useful in evaluating arterial and venous abnormalities, including thrombosis, and in separating uterine from adnexal abnormalities.
	Pelvic CT	0.730 rads	See discussion of head CT, above.	
Musculo-skeletal system	MRI	None	See discussion of MRI of the brain, above.	Routine evaluation of joints can often be delayed until after birth. Useful for detecting neoplasm and infection.
	Upper-extremity radiography	0.001 rads		
	Lower-extremity radiography	0.001 rads		
	Radiography of hip or femur	0.128 rads		

AVM = arteriovenous malformation; CAD = coronary artery disease; CT = computed tomography; CXR = chest radiography; GFR = glomerular filtration rate; GI = gastrointestinal; IV = intravenous; IVP = IV Persantine-thallium stress test; MRI = magnetic resonance imaging; RUQ = right upper quadrant.

REFERENCES

1. **Barron WM, Lindheimer MD.** Medical Disorders During Pregnancy. St. Louis: Mosby–Year Book; 1995.

2. National Commission on Radiation Protection Report #54. Medical Radiation Exposure of Pregnant and Potentially Pregnant Women. Washington, DC: National Commission on Radiation Protection; 1997.

3. Guidelines for Diagnostic Imaging in Pregnancy. American College of Obstetricians and Gynecologists Committee Opinion. 1995;158.

4. **Colletti PM, Sylvestre PB.** Magnetic resonance imaging in pregnancy. MRI Clinics of North America. 1994;2:291-307.

5. **Kanal E.** Pregnancy and the society of magnetic resonance imaging. MRI Clinics of North America. 1994;2:309-17.

6. **Steenvoorde P, Pauwels EKJ, Harding LK, Bourguignon M, Mariere B, Broerse JJ.** Diagnostic nuclear medicine and risk for the fetus. Eur J Nucl Med. 1998;25:193-8.

7. **Husak V, Wiedermann M.** Radiation absorbed dose estimates to the embryo from some nuclear medicine procedures. Eur J Nucl Med. 1980;5:205-7.

8. **Moore MM, Shearer DR.** Fetal dose estimates for CT pelvimetry. Radiology. 1989;171: 265-7.

9. **Felmlee JP, Gray JG, Leet Zow ML.** Estimated fetal radiation dose from metastatic CT studies. AJR Am J Roentgenol. 1990;154:185-90.

10. **Mayr NA, Wen BC, Saw CB.** Radiation therapy during pregnancy. Obstet Gynecol Clin North Am. 1998;25:301-21.

11. National Commission on Radiation Protection Report #91. Recommendation on Units for Exposure to Ionizing Radiation. Washington, DC: National Commission on Radiation Protection; 1997.

CHAPTER 3

Behavioral and Emotional Health in Pregnancy

I. Grief Counseling after Pregnancy Loss
Susan Z. Cowchock, MD

II. Psychiatric Disorders
Margaret Howard, PhD, Susan Diaz, MD, Neeta Jain, MD,
Caron Zlonick, PhD, and Teri Pearlstein, MD

III. Eating Disorders
Philip S. Mehler, MD

IV. Illicit Drug Use
Ellen D. Mason, MD

V. Tobacco and Alcohol Use
Lisa M. Latts, MD, MSPH

VI. Violence and Pregnancy
Mary Hepburn, BSc, MD

I. Grief Counseling after Pregnancy Loss
Susan Z. Cowchock

Pain, loss, death, grief, mourning. These experiences are universal, an integral part of being human. Physicians most often spend their professional time caring for people who are sick, and these events and feelings are our daily concern. Even when health is restored or a life is saved, and our patient is "out of danger," the threat averted remains in the patient's mind.

Although Freud was the first to distinguish grief from depression, the normal and abnormal courses of grief and mourning have been considered a subject for descriptive study only in the second half of the 19th century. Lindemann's classic 1944 study of survivors of the Coconut Grove fire was the first to detail the symptoms and time course of grief.

Responses to Pregnancy Loss

How does the loss of a born or unborn baby differ from other deaths? Is it a different experience for parents whose baby has died as the result of a maternal medical problem? How can we physicians—both internists and obstetricians—best help our patients heal, both physically and spiritually, after their babies die?

The full effects and consequences of pregnancy loss have been a fairly recent subject of analysis and study (1). Bowlby and co-workers (2) have described four stages of the response to such loss: 1) shock and numbness, 2) searching and yearning, 3) disorientation and disorganization, and 4) reorganization. Like Kubler-Ross's stages of death and dying, these stages are not necessarily sequential or time-limited. The mourner may not experience all of the phases or may move quickly through a stage only to return to it later—for example, at an anniversary.

Shock and Numbness

The first stage of response is a normal defense and may last anywhere from a few days to 2 weeks. Emotions are uncontrollable. The bereaved may be unable to comprehend or recall information given during this period. The person may feel exhausted yet unable to sleep, or he or she may sleep most of the time. The mourner may be completely unable to express feelings, yet waves of fear, anxiety, guilt, and depression can make the mourner feel "out of my mind." As Emily Dickinson wrote (c. 1862): "This is the Hour of Lead – / Remembered, if outlived, / As Freezing persons, recollect the Snow. / First – Chill – then Stupor – then the letting go –".

At the time of diagnosis and during the earliest stage of grief, information will not be retained. But abandonment by the physician is keenly recognized and is often interpreted as an accusation. Obstetricians and ultrasonographers should not immediately leave the room after a diagnosis of fetal death. If the woman is hospitalized, visits should be frequent but need last only 10 to 15 minutes. It is your presence that is needed. Sit, so you will be at eye level.

Physical touch can be very important to some patients. Although protest may be voiced as questions, answers are not really expected at this stage. Statements such as "I am so sorry," "I wish I knew why," and "I don't know what to say, but I want to help" are all responses of empathy.

Searching and Yearning

The second phase of response may last for months, and it is during this time that the bereaved searches for what was lost. It is during this period that the most bizarre behavior is seen. Mothers hear their babies crying, even from the grave, and their arms literally ache. Preoccupation with the experience and intrusive thoughts and memories are common. A search for answers, guilt, and anger are all part of this stage. Review of all events leading up to the loss, including details from any documents (such as pathology and laboratory reports), is very important. One experienced obstetrician advocates making a first postpartum visit 1 to 2 weeks after hospital discharge (3). This is the best time to direct parents to group or individual therapeutic support. Some of the pregnancy loss–specific descriptions in this section come from publications supplied by one such national group (4).

Disorientation and Disorganization

The long third phase of response becomes most severe 4 to 6 months after the loss. Mourners may be depressed and have impaired judgment. In the struggle to be relieved of disorientation, they begin to search for meaning, to integrate the loss into their life story, and to restore self-esteem. Envy and jealousy may be directed toward pregnant relatives and friends or even toward mothers or pregnant women encountered in daily life. This is evident when women angrily recount and dwell on news and personal stories of women who "abused their bodies when they were pregnant" or do not "care for their children." Almost always, significant feelings of guilt center around fantasies of having caused or contributed to the pregnancy loss in some way. Blame and anger often accompany pregnancy loss as a response to intense feelings of helplessness (1). A history of previous elective abortion is often associated with the belief—maintained despite all assurances from the woman's physicians—that the current loss is a punishment or was caused by the earlier termination procedure in some medical way. Elective and most spontaneous abortions occur in the first trimester, which is the narcissistic stage of pregnancy, when the woman experiences the developing fetus as part of herself. Not only are early miscarriages grieved for as loss of one's self rather than of an outside love object, but previous elective abortions may also have been associated with loss of body integrity or self integrity (5).

Reorganization

The fourth, healing phase of response begins at 18 to 24 months. All too often, identification of the loss and movement toward new relationships and enjoyment of life is interrupted by the strains imposed by a new pregnancy. In fact, some studies show that women whose deceased baby has a surviving twin and women who become pregnant again less than 5 months after the death are at higher risk for prolonged grief reactions (6).

Grief recurs at anniversaries, such as the date of the loss or the expected date of delivery. Religious and secular holidays associated with family and children are particularly difficult times. A telephone call from you the week before these dates will be particularly appreciated. If appropriate, the physician can encourage the couple to limit their exposure to painful family gatherings and celebrations.

Abnormal Grief Reactions

Complicated or prolonged grief reactions are associated with a history of previous depression, lack of social and personal coping resources, and an ambivalent attitude toward the lost fetus (6). Delayed grief is uncommon (4% of couples surveyed) and is most often diagnosed in men (6, 7). Pregnancy loss early in gestation (miscarriage or ectopic pregnancy) is associated with more intense acute grieving (8). Grief from previous pregnancy loss may recur during a subsequent pregnancy at the gestational age at which the pregnancy was lost. The period near or at term is a time of extreme anxiety and renewal of grief for patients who have lost a baby at any gestational age. Women may begin to bargain for early delivery as term approaches in an attempt to relieve fear and anticipatory grief. Closure is much more difficult when loss occurs early in pregnancy, both because of the lack of tokens and accessible memories of the child and because of societal failure to recognize and support mourning in these circumstances. Recurrent pregnancy loss is especially likely to be associated with prolonged grief reactions, such as searching behavior that extends over long periods, and includes multiple medical consultations and batteries of diagnostic tests. A woman's submission to repeated invasive and painful diagnostic testing is sometimes a symptom of unresolved guilt. Pathologic mourning is associated with a persistent and unconscious yearning to recover the lost object, persistent anger, unconscious reproach expressed towards various objects (including self), care of vicarious figures, and denial that the object of attachment is really lost (9). Pathologic grief has been estimated to occur in up to one in five pregnancy losses and may be associated with an attempt to repair the loss by trying to conceive again as soon as possible (10).

In one study, miscarrying women who were childless had a significantly increased risk for a first or recurrent episode of major depressive disorder in the 6 months after the loss compared with community controls (11). Recognition of symptoms of significant depression, including suicidal ideation, or failure of the family unit to move through the normal stages of grief should prompt immediate and sensitive referral for psychotherapeutic care.

Pregnancy after a Loss

The emotional tasks of pregnancy after loss of a previous pregnancy differ from those of normal pregnancy (12). They include 1) working with the fear of another abnormal pregnancy, 2) working through the avoidance of attachment caused by fear of future loss, 3) moving past the unwillingness to give up grieving out of loyalty to the baby who died, 4) attaching to the unborn child and separating from the baby who died, and 5) the mother's renewed grieving of the loss of part of herself. These normal reactions during a pregnancy after a loss may be incorrectly viewed by physicians as abnormal. Many women experience these intense feelings of grief and anxiety among strangers because women who have lost a baby often find themselves unable to return to the place and staff associated with their loss ("I could not bear to enter that ultrasound room."). Anticipatory grief for the loss of the unborn baby; constant need for reassurance; or conversely, emotional distance or denial of pregnancy are common. As birth approaches, mothers may refuse to prepare for their baby and fear the approaching delivery with its associated risk for loss. After successful delivery, parents must again relive and grieve their previous loss. Moving on to love and bond with the new baby may feel like betrayal. Parents usually move quickly through this period, as they take on the multiple tasks associated with the care of a newborn. It is important to reassure these new parents that their mixed feelings are normal and that the fact that they are not responding immediately to their child with unalloyed joy does not mean that they are "bad parents."

Loss Associated with Maternal Medical Complications

Women whose pregnancy loss was associated with a maternal medical complication have not been studied as a separate group. After a loss, both men and women have a sense of failure as a parent to their unborn child. However, women alone lose the sense that their womb is a safe place for a baby. When a maternal medical problem, such as a clotting disorder, diabetes, or hypertension, is causally related to the baby's death, maternal feelings of failed parental competence and self-esteem may never be resolved. Fathers fear the loss not only of their child but of their partner. The couple's relationship may be severely stressed by these understandable fears, which are sometimes complicated by an inability to communicate because of defensive emotional distancing from the new pregnancy. The family physicians must be sensitive to signs of stress in the relationship and should encourage fathers to be present during procedures associated with high anxiety, such as ultrasonography and fetal monitoring. The loss of a child is existential, in the sense that parents (and grandparents) are mourning the loss of continuity through the generations. Death without the possibility of children and grandchildren is infinite ("The Lord said to Cain, 'What have you done? Your brother's blood cries out to me from the ground!'" [Genesis 4:10]). When infertility, advanced maternal age, or a serious maternal medical problem are added to the loss of a baby, fear of a permanent loss of generativity adds a profound existential dimension to grief and mourning.

RESOURCES FOR COUPLES AFTER PREGNANCY LOSS

Nationally-Based Support Groups

Resolve, Inc.
1310 Broadway, Somerville, MA 02144
Telephone: 617-623-0744
Focuses on infertility, assisted reproduction, and early miscarriages.

Share National
St. Joseph's Health Center
300 First Capital Drive
St. Charles, MO 63301
Telephone: 314-947-6164
Provides local patient referral support and literature.

Unite National
Jeanes Hospital
7600 Central Avenue
Philadelphia, PA 19111
Telephone: 215-728-3177

Bereavement Services (formerly Resolve Through Sharing)
1910 South Avenue
LaCrosse, WI 54601
Telephone: 608-791-4747

CLIMB (Center for Loss in Multiple Birth)
Jean Kollantai
PO Box 1064
Palmer, AK
Telephone: 907-746-6123 or 907-333-2935

Patient-Oriented Reading Material

Schwiebert P, Kirk P. When Hello Means Goodbye. Portland, OR: Perinatal Loss; 1985.
Particularly good for the period immediately after loss. Short and simple. Discusses decisions that need to be made in the immediate bereavement period.

Lamb JM, ed. Bittersweet...Hello-goodbye. 2d ed. Bellevue, IL: Share; 1989.
Multifaith. Offers practical suggestions for presentation, collections of baby tokens, and examples of funeral, naming, and memorial services. Aimed at the chaplain or counselor.

Ilse S. Empty Arms—Coping with Miscarriage, Stillbirth, and Infant Death. Maple Plain, MN: Wintergreen Press; 1990.
A brief and simply written general discussion.

Gold M. And Hannah Wept. Philadelphia: The Jewish Publication Society; 1988.
A Jewish focus on adoption.

Kohn I, Moffitt PL. A Silent Sorrow: Pregnancy Loss. New York: Dell; 1992.
A broad and non–faith-oriented presentation of information and prose.

Pregnancy and Infant Loss Center
1421 East Wayzata Boulevard, Suite 70
Wayzata, MN 55391
Telephone: 612-473-9372
A clearinghouse for information for parents.

REFERENCES

1. Pregnancy loss and the grief process. In: Woods JR Jr, Woods JL, eds. Loss During Pregnancy or in the Newborn Period. Pitman, NJ: Janetti Publications, Inc.; 1997.
2. **Bowlby J.** Loss: Sadness and Depression—Attachment and Loss. New York: Basic Books; 1940.
3. **Woods JR Jr.** Pregnancy-loss counseling: the challenge to the obstetrician. In: Woods JR Jr, Woods JL, eds. Loss During Pregnancy or in the Newborn Period. Pitman, NJ: Janetti Publications; 1997.
4. **Lamb JM.** Bittersweet...Hello-goodbye. Bellevue, IL: Share; 1989.

5. **Stack J.** The psychodynamics of spontaneous abortion. Am J Orthopsychiatry. 1984;54:162-7.

6. **Lasker JN, Toedter LJ.** Acute versus chronic grief: the case of pregnancy loss. Am J Orthopsychiatry. 1991;61:510-22.

7. **Janssen HJEM, Cuisinier MCJ, Hoogduin KAL.** A critical review of the concept of pathological grief following pregnancy loss. Omega—Journal of Death and Dying. 1996;33:21-42.

8. **Rowe J, Clyman R, Green C, Mikkelson C, Haight J, Ataide L.** Follow-up of families who experience perinatal death. Pediatrics. 1978;62:166-70.

9. **Bowlby J.** Pathological mourning and childhood mourning. In: Frankiel R, ed. Essential Papers on Object Loss. Essential Papers in Psychoanalysis. New York: New York Univ Press; 1994:185-221.

10. **Cole KL.** Pregnancy loss through miscarriage or stillbirth. In: O'Hara MW, Reiter RC, eds. Psychological Aspects of Women's Reproductive Health. New York: Springer-Verlag; 1995:194-206.

11. **Neugebauer R, Kline J, Shrout P, Skodol A, O'Connor P, Geller PA, et al.** Major depressive disorder in the 6 months after miscarriage. JAMA. 1997;277:383-8.

12. **O'Leary JM, Thorwick C.** Impact of pregnancy loss on subsequent pregnancy. In: Woods JR Jr, Woods JL, eds. Loss During Pregnancy or in the Newborn Period. Pitman, NJ: Janetti Publications; 1997.

II. Psychiatric Disorders

Margaret Howard, Susan Diaz, Neeta Jain, Caron Zlonick, and Teri Pearlstein

Normal Psychological Changes in Pregnancy

Historically, pregnancy was often viewed as the apex of a woman's personal and social fulfillment. This view has been eclipsed by recent findings that highlight the complexity and variability of a woman's emotional response to her pregnancy. Pregnancy is a time of considerable physical and endocrinologic upheaval. For most women, normal pregnancy does not produce significant psychological disruption. For some, however, pregnancy is a time of emotional disturbance. It is important for the clinician to recognize the patient's social and cultural background. Pregnancy folklore can influence a woman's behavior in ways that may be misinterpreted as abnormal.

Psychological status has been shown to vary across trimesters. Some common first-trimester reactions center on physiologic changes such as fatigue, nausea, vomiting, headaches, and food aversions (1). Other reactions include ambivalence, mild anxiety, decreased sexual interest, emotional lability, feelings of detachment, and preoccupation with changing body image.

The second trimester can be characterized by relative psychological quiescence and a sense of well being (2). It has been speculated that hormonal factors have an anxiolytic effect during this period (3). Although prenatal bonding is highly variable, many women report an increased sense of attachment after the onset of fetal movement (4) as fears of miscarriage dissipate. During the second trimester, many women report a return of sexual desire, increased body awareness, and a shifting of focus from self to baby. Although many women experience distress about their changing appearance and weight gain, others are pleased with their pregnant appearance and enjoy the attention and recognition elicited by the pregnancy. Relationships with the baby's father and the woman's family of origin, especially her own mother, may take on new salience, and increased conflict or a heightened sense of closeness may develop. Previous losses and associated feelings may resurface. Results of genetic and other diagnostic testing may affect psychological status.

The third trimester has been associated with heightened anxiety relative to the previous trimester, especially as labor and delivery become imminent (5). Third-trimester anxiety has been viewed as an adaptive, realistic response to the approach of delivery and has been shown to bear a positive relation to a positive birthing experience (6). It is not uncommon for pregnant women to note cognitive difficulties, such as forgetfulness, distractibility, and absent-mindedness, although research both supports (7) and refutes these claims (8). Cognitive and affective symptoms of depression, such as changes in feeling of worth and self-esteem, are common (9) and may be associated with changing roles and responsibilities. Somatic symptoms of depression, such as difficulty in sleeping, changes in appetite, and fatigue, are typical and can lead to the misdiagnosis of depression (3). Clinicians must carefully inquire about non-somatic indicators of depression, such as sadness, loss of pleasure, and suicidal ideation.

Psychological status fluctuates during pregnancy and is influenced by many factors, including age, parity, employment status, marital status, planning of pregnancy, psychiatric history, and previous pregnancy experience (1, 10). Furthermore, a factor well-documented to affect psychological status during pregnancy is perceived social support. Social support not only protects against negative mood states but can actually enhance both the physical and psychological aspects of pregnancy, especially when the support is generated by husbands or partners (11, 12).

Psychiatric Disorders During Pregnancy

Some physical and psychological changes during pregnancy are considered normal, but physical and psychological symptoms that meet the criteria for psychiatric disorders, as defined by the *Diagnostic and Statistical Manual of*

Mental Disorders, Fourth Edition (DSM-IV) (13), should not be considered normal and deserve psychiatric attention. Women may experience the onset of psychiatric disorders or exacerbations of previous psychiatric illness during pregnancy. The most common psychiatric diagnosis in women of childbearing age is depression (14). Management will depend on whether the depression is part of bipolar illness; thus, it is critical to determine whether this is the case. Anxiety and panic disorder are common both in the absence of and during pregnancy. This section discusses the course of each of these disorders and their treatment during pregnancy. Then it reviews common postpartum psychiatric disorders and the use of psychotropic medications during breast-feeding.

The rate of major depression during pregnancy is 10%. This rate is equal to the rate of depression in nonpregnant women, suggesting that pregnancy does not protect against depression (15). Risk factors for the development of major depression during pregnancy include a history of depression, poor social support, younger age, marital conflict, ambivalent feelings about the pregnancy, and having more existing children (16). Depression during pregnancy may lead to inadequate prenatal care, poor nutrition, and attempts to harm the self or the fetus. Depression during pregnancy has been linked to higher rates of postpartum depression, prematurity, and low birthweight (LBW) (17).

The course of bipolar illness during pregnancy is unclear, and risk factors for relapse of this illness during pregnancy have not been identified. Some reports suggest that bipolar patients enjoy a relative quiescence of symptoms during pregnancy; others have described psychotic decompensation in bipolar pregnant women (18). Untreated bipolar illness during pregnancy poses considerable risk and may escalate into a psychiatric and obstetric emergency because it may be characterized by poor judgment, impulsive behavior, substance abuse, and delusional beliefs about the pregnancy. Regardless of their course during pregnancy, women with bipolar illness have high rates of relapse (33% to 50%) after delivery.

Few data are available on the course of anxiety disorders during pregnancy, and risk factors for the development of anxiety disorders in pregnancy have not been elucidated. High levels of progesterone in pregnancy were thought to have anxiolytic effects, but recent data do not support this impression. Conversely, increased heart rate and dyspnea in pregnancy may trigger anxiety symptoms. Symptoms of panic disorder in pregnancy improve in some women and worsen in others (19). Symptoms of obsessive–compulsive disorder (OCD) seem to worsen, particularly late in pregnancy (20). Like mood disorders, panic disorder and OCD often worsen after delivery.

The course of schizophrenia during pregnancy has been described as variable; symptoms are alleviated in some women and worsen in others (21).

Pregnant women with chronic mental illness require close follow-up because psychiatric decompensation gravely threatens the pregnancy. In addition, mothers with psychotic illness have an increased rate of children with malformations, independent of medication use (22). Evaluation by a social service team is usually needed to assess housing, custody issues, family support, parenting skills, and need for financial assistance.

Nonpharmacologic Interventions During Pregnancy

For most women who experience psychological fluctuations during pregnancy, support, information, and reassurance are adequate interventions. For women who have more pronounced psychological difficulties, especially if day-to-day functioning is impaired, referral to a mental health professional is indicated.

Because depression is the most common psychiatric illness among women of childbearing age (14) and because it can have such deleterious effects, the accurate identification of depression in pregnancy is essential. Further, it is well documented that women who have depression during pregnancy are at increased risk for postpartum depression (23). Therefore, the early establishment of a relationship with a mental health provider skilled in the treatment of perinatal psychiatric disorders can be a valuable component of a woman's perinatal care.

Many women and their providers prefer to avoid the use of psychotropic medications during pregnancy because of their possible, often unknown effects on the fetus. If the disorder is not severe, nonpharmacologic interventions may be preferred in the first trimester.

Unfortunately, almost no systematic research has been done on the effectiveness of psychosocial treatments for pregnant women. One such treatment that has shown to be beneficial in postpartum depression is interpersonal psychotherapy (IPT) (24). Preliminary data suggest that IPT may have similarly benefit in depression during pregnancy (25). Despite the lack of treatment outcome studies in pregnant, depressed women, well-documented treatment outcome data in nonpregnant patients show that psychosocial treatments, such as cognitive behavioral therapy (CBT) and IPT, are as effective as pharmacotherapy for mild-to-moderate depression. However, for patients with more severe or recurrent depression, research suggests that a combination of psychotherapy and pharmacotherapy is most effective (26).

The treatment of anxiety disorders in pregnant women has not been well studied. Despite the lack of data in pregnant women, research has consistently shown that behavioral therapy, CBT, and relaxation training are effective nonpharmacologic interventions for anxiety disorders. Similarly, meditation, yoga, and biofeedback, although not well studied in pregnant women, may be viable nonpharmacologic treatments for pregnant women with anxiety. Behavioral therapy is the nonpharmacologic treatment of choice for OCD, and referral to a practitioner who specializes in the treatment of OCD is preferred.

Psychotropic Medication Use During Pregnancy

If nonpharmacologic measures do not alleviate severe psychiatric symptoms, psychotropic medication should be considered. Patients may seek consultation about the use of psychiatric medication during pregnancy for several reasons. Nongravid women using psychotropic medication may seek advice about the safety of their medication use with respect to future pregnancies. Some patients may have inadvertently conceived while using a psychotropic medication. For others, recurrence or onset of severe psychiatric symptoms develops during pregnancy.

Some general principles can be used to guide treatment decisions. In patients whose previous course of illness was not severe or in patients who have had prolonged periods of well being while not using medication, attempts should be made to gradually taper and discontinue drug therapy before conception or as soon as a pregnancy is documented. Medication should be particularly avoided during the first trimester. However, in women with histories of severe, recurring affective disorders, anxiety disorders, or psychotic disorders, the risk for relapse in the absence of medication use is substantial, and maintenance therapy throughout pregnancy must be considered. Minimal effective doses should be used to achieve adequate symptom control in the mother and minimal exposure to the fetus. Although lower doses are desirable, higher doses may be required because of increased maternal plasma volume and increased hepatic and renal clearance rates during pregnancy. The prescribing physician should always consult with the obstetrician and the pediatrician about the treatment plan, and treatment decisions should be carefully documented.

Several excellent reviews present current data on pharmacotherapy during pregnancy (21, 27–29). Before administering a medication to a pregnant woman, the clinician should discuss with the patient and her partner 1) the risks associated with medication use during pregnancy and 2) the risks of untreated maternal illness. All psychotropic agents readily diffuse across the placenta, ensuring fetal exposure. For each medication being considered, the clinician should address three areas of potential risk: 1) teratogenicity as a result of first-trimester exposure, 2) neonatal toxicity or withdrawal resulting from third-trimester exposure, and 3) long-term neurobehavioral sequelae in the older child. The clinician should help the patient balance these potential risks against the risks of untreated maternal illness. Untreated illness may lead to poor nutrition, inadequate prenatal care, substance abuse, delusional beliefs about the pregnancy, suicidal tendency, or attempts to harm the fetus.

Antidepressants, mood stabilizers, anxiolytic agents, and antipsychotic agents are specifically discussed below.

Antidepressants

Of the antidepressants, tricyclic antidepressants (TCAs) and the selective serotonin-reuptake inhibitor (SSRI) fluoxetine are the most studied for use in pregnancy and are the treatments of choice during pregnancy. They may be considered for cases of major depression, anxiety disorders, and eating disorders.

First-trimester exposure to TCAs has not been associated with fetal malformations in case series (27). Use of TCAs through the third trimester has been associated with neonatal side effects, including anticholinergic syndromes and tachyarrhythmias. Neonatal withdrawal syndromes, including jitteriness, hyperreflexia, tachypnea, temperature instability, poor suck reflex, and seizures, have been reported (21). The incidence of these syndromes is unknown, although they are thought to be rare, and they usually resolve by the second week. To lessen risk for these syndromes, it is recommended that the clinician use a less anticholinergic TCA (desipramine or nortriptyline) and gradually reduce the dose 1 month before parturition. Discontinuation of antidepressant therapy before delivery is not recommended because the postpartum period is a time of high risk for symptom recurrence.

Studies suggest that first-trimester exposure to fluoxetine does not increase the risk for major congenital malformations (30–32). One case of transient neonatal toxicity subsequent to third-trimester exposure to fluoxetine, characterized by respiratory and neurologic distress, has been reported (33). Two prospective studies did not report neonatal complications associated with fluoxetine exposure close to delivery (31, 34). One recent study (30) found a higher incidence of multiple minor malformations after first-trimester fluoxetine exposure and higher rates of prematurity and perinatal complications after third-trimester exposure. However, this study's methods have been criticized (35), and its findings have not been replicated.

One study examined the long-term neurobehavioral sequelae of in utero exposure to antidepressants (36). It found no significant differences in global IQ, language development, or behavioral development among preschool children exposed to TCAs or fluoxetine in utero compared with a control group of preschoolers whose mothers had not been exposed to any known teratogen.

Limited data are available on the use of SSRIs other than fluoxetine (buproprion, venlafaxine, trazadone, nefazadone, and mirtazepine) during pregnancy; thus, their use is not recommended. One recent report did not find elevated rates of major malformations in infants exposed to paroxetine, sertraline, or fluvoxamine during the first trimester (37). This is reassuring for women who may inadvertently conceive while using these SSRIs. However, this study did not address the potential for neonatal toxicity or behavioral teratogenicity. Single cases of suspected paroxetine withdrawal in a neonate (38) and of sertraline withdrawal (39) have been reported.

Monoamine oxidase inhibitors should not be prescribed in pregnancy because of the risk for induction of a hypertensive crisis and an increased risk for congenital anomalies. Electroconvulsive therapy (ECT) is considered relatively safe in pregnancy (40). It may be considered a treatment alternative for severe depression, mania, or psychosis that is unresponsive to other therapies.

Mood Stabilizers

The three mood stabilizers commonly used to treat bipolar disorder (lithium, carbamazepine, and valproic acid) all confer significant risk when used in pregnancy. Whenever possible, mood stabilizer therapy should be gradually discontinued before conception and should be avoided during the first trimester. However, bipolar women with a history of rapid symptom decompensation in the absence of medication may need to continue use of a mood stabilizer throughout pregnancy.

First-trimester use of lithium is associated with a higher incidence of cardiac anomalies, particularly Ebstein anomaly (a serious cardiac defect of the tricuspid valve). The risk for this defect is 1/20,000 in the general population but 1/1000 in lithium-exposed babies (41). Level II ultrasonography at week 18 can identify this malformation. Lithium exposure through parturition has been associated with "floppy baby syndrome," which is characterized by hypertonia, poor suck reflex, cyanosis, and hypoglycemia. Fetal diabetes insipidus and neonatal hypothyroidism have also been reported (21). No controlled studies have assessed long-term neurodevelopment in children exposed to lithium in utero.

Maternal lithium levels should be checked regularly throughout the pregnancy. Higher lithium doses may be required because of increased plasma volume. However, in the month before delivery, the lithium dose should be reduced by one third to prevent 1) maternal lithium toxicity subsequent to fluid losses at delivery and 2) neonatal toxicity.

Despite the potential risks, lithium is the preferred mood stabilizer for use in pregnancy because anticonvulsants also confer teratogenic risk. A full discussion of antiepileptic agents is presented in Chapter 12.

Anxiolytic Agents

First-trimester use of benzodiazepines, particularly diazepam and alprazolam, has been associated with a slightly increased risk for orofacial clefts. The risk in the general population is 0.06%; benzodiazepine exposure may increase the risk to 0.7% (10). Benzodiazepines should be avoided in gestational weeks 6 through 9, the period of oral cleft closure. Benzodiazepine use in late pregnancy may lead to neonatal toxicity (decreased tone, low Apgar scores, failure to feed, apnea, and temperature dysregulation) and subsequent neonatal withdrawal (irritability, tremors, increased tone and reflexes, and electroencephalogram abnormalities) (21). The incidence of these neonatal syndromes is unknown. When possible, the benzodiazepine dose should be gradually decreased in the third trimester to decrease risk for neonatal effects. Data on the neurodevelopment of children exposed to benzodiazepines in utero are mixed and inconclusive (27).

Buspirone has not been studied for use in pregnancy. Fluoxetine and TCAs are options to be considered in the treatment of anxiety disorders during pregnancy.

Antipsychotic Agents

High-potency neuroleptics (e.g., haloperidol and trifluoperazine) may be considered for the management of psychosis in pregnancy. First-trimester exposure to neuroleptics does not seem to increase the rate of malformations; exposure to low-potency agents (e.g., chlorpromazine) is associated with a slightly increased risk for nonspecific congenital anomalies (27). Low-potency agents may also cause hypotension in the mother and can threaten placental perfusion. Phenothiazines can cause acute extrapyramidal reactions and are to be used only if necessary.

Use of neuroleptics through the third trimester has been associated with neonatal toxicity and withdrawal syndromes. The incidence of these syndromes is unknown. The symptoms reported in neonates have been transient and include tremor, increased tone, motor restlessness, jaundice, abnormal movements, poor feeding, and anticholinergic effects (tachycardia, urinary retention, and functional bowel obstruction) (21).

Long-term neurobehavioral effects from exposure to neuroleptics in pregnancy have not been adequately studied. In animals, the use of neuroleptics during pregnancy does seem to cause behavioral abnormalities in offspring (27).

Little data are available on the newer antipsychotics in pregnancy; thus, their use is best avoided. Three cases of clozapine use throughout pregnancy have been reported. All of the children were born without malformations, but one had a seizure 8 days after delivery (42, 43). No data exist on the use of risperidone or olanzapine in pregnancy.

Medications used to treat neuroleptic-induced extrapyramidal side effects may be needed in pregnancy, especially if patients have acute, severe symptoms. Benztropine, diphenhydramine, and amantadine may increase risk for minor congenital anomalies and produce neonatal side effects. To replace antiparkinsonian agents, the clinician may consider lowering the patient's dose or switching neuroleptics.

Postpartum Psychiatric Disorders

The literature consistently affirms that the postpartum period is a time of increased vulnerability to psychiatric disorders. Kendell and colleagues (44) cite a sevenfold increase in the rate of psychiatric admissions in the first 3 months after childbirth. Most pregnant women are not educated about the possibility of psychiatric illnesses in the puerperium. In addition, obstetricians and pediatricians often fail to screen for these conditions. Most afflicted women may not be forthcoming about their symptoms as shame and negative thoughts unexpectedly replace the anticipated joy and excitement of motherhood.

Postpartum psychiatric disorders include depression, psychosis, and anxiety disorders. It is helpful to perceive these conditions as existing along a continuum, with the blues representing a mild condition and psychosis indicating a severe disorder.

Postpartum Blues

Postpartum blues is not perceived as a psychiatric disorder but as a common mood disturbance; the prevalence rate may be as high as 85% (45). Symptoms include irritability, tearfulness, mood lability, sadness, and anxiety. Typically, symptoms peak on day 3 or 4 after delivery and resolve within 2 weeks with no long-term sequelae. Most women do well with supportive intervention and reassurance that their symptoms will soon cease. Approximately 15% to 20% of women who have the blues develop symptoms consistent with postpartum depression (46).

Postpartum Depression

Postpartum depression is the most common psychiatric illness in the postpartum period. Its prevalence rates are equivalent to those of nonpuerperal depression (i.e., 10% to 15%) (46). The onset of symptoms usually occurs 2 weeks after delivery. Affected women have symptoms indistinguishable from those of major depression at any other point in the life cycle. General symptoms include changes in sleep and appetite, dysphoric mood, anxiety, preoccupation with the infant's health, fatigue, impaired attachment to the infant, and suicidal thoughts.

When excessive preoccupation with the baby's well-being is the primary manifestation of postpartum depression, the physician may easily overlook the symptoms. Symptoms vary in duration and can last anywhere from 3 to 9 months if unrecognized. The effect on the developing infant and social attachment is paramount. Studies have identified delays in motor, language, and cognitive development in infants of depressed mothers (47).

Researchers have determined which women may be more susceptible to postpartum depression. Risk factors include history of psychiatric illness, family history of affective disorders, social stressors, poor support, premenstrual symptoms, depression during pregnancy (especially in the third trimester), and unplanned pregnancy. In addition, women with a history of major depression have a 25% risk for postpartum depression, and women with a previous postpartum depression have a 50% risk for recurrence (48). The Edinburgh Postnatal Depression Scale (49) is a useful screening instrument for postpartum depression (Figure 3-1).

Management of postpartum depression includes various approaches, such as reassurance and support, exclusion of postpartum thyroid disease, psychoeducation, individual and group psychotherapy, and psychopharmacology. As in any episode of major depression, antidepressants should be considered. Experts recommend that, given the high risk for recurrence, women with previous postpartum depression should receive the first antidepressant dose 24 hours after delivery. Anxious patients can benefit from the short-term use of benzodiazepine. In suicidal or psychotic women refractory to pharmacotherapy, ECT is a consideration. Methods of birth control (particularly oral contraceptives, which can exacerbate depressive or anxious symptoms) should be addressed.

Postpartum Psychosis

Postpartum psychosis is a rare but an acute condition that affects 1 to 2 women per 1000 births. Onset is early and rapid and generally occurs within the first 24 to 72 hours after delivery. Affected women may have mood lability, severe agitation, delusions, hallucinations, disorientation, disorganized thoughts, and sleeplessness. Often, the delusions and hallucinations have a religious theme—for example, the mother may believe that the baby is a demon or Jesus or that she is the mother of God. Postpartum psychosis is a risk factor for infanticide.

Risk factors for postpartum psychosis are a previous psychotic episode, bipolar disorder, family history of bipolar disorder, primiparity, and previous history of postpartum psychosis. Women with bipolar disorder or previous psychosis after parturition have a 50% risk for recurrence with subsequent deliveries (48). Women with a history of bipolar disorder have a 40% to 70% risk for recurrence in the postpartum period (50). In women with histories of manic-depressive illness or puerpal psychoses, prophylaxis with lithium or

Figure 3-1 Edinburgh Postnatal Depression Scale

Today's date_____   Baby's age _____
Baby's date of birth_____   Birth weight _____
Mother's age_____   Baby's place in family: 1   2   3   4   5   6   7

In the past 7 days...

1. I have been able to laugh and see the funny side of things.
0 = As much as I always could
1 = Not quite so much now
2 = Definitely not so much now
3 = Not at all

2. I have looked forward with enjoyment to things.
0 = As much as I ever did
1 = Rather less than I used to
2 = Definitely less than I used to
3 = Hardly at all

3. I have blamed myself unnecessarily when things went wrong.
0 = No, not at all
1 = Hardly ever
2 = Yes, sometimes
3 = Yes, very often

4. I have been anxious or worried for no very good reason.
3 = Yes, quite a lot
2 = Yes, sometimes
1 = No, not much
0 = No, not at all

5. I have felt scared or panicky for no very good reason.
3 = Yes, quite a lot
2 = Yes, sometimes
1 = No, not much
0 = No, not at all

6. Things have been getting on top of me.
3 = Yes, most of the time I haven't been able to cope at all
2 = Yes, sometimes I haven't been coping as well as usual
1 = No, most of the time I have coped quite well
0 = No, I have been coping as well as ever

7. I have been so unhappy that I have had difficulty sleeping.
3 = Yes, most of the time
2 = Yes, sometimes
1 = Not very often
0 = No, not at all

8. I have felt sad or miserable.
3 = Yes, most of the time
2 = Yes, quite often
1 = Not very often
0 = No, not at all

9. I have been so unhappy that I have been crying.
3 = Yes, most of the time
2 = Yes, quite often
1 = Only occasionally
0 = No, never

10. The thought of harming myself has occurred to me.
3 = Yes, quite often
2 = Sometimes
1 = Hardly ever
0 = Never

Total Score_____   (A score of 12 or more indicates the likelihood of depression but not its severity.)

From Cox JL, Holden JM, Sagovsky R. Detection of postnatal depression: development of the 10-item Edinburgh Postnatal Depression Scale. Br J Psychol. 1987;150:782-6; with permission.

other mood stabilizers in the acute postpartum period may reduce the risk from 50% to 10% (50). Of note, schizophrenia does not seem to be a significant risk factor.

Treatment often requires inpatient psychiatric hospitalization because women may neglect or abuse their infants and may commit suicide or infanticide. A medical work-up should rule out postpartum thyroiditis, the Sheehan syndrome, HIV infection, intoxication and withdrawal states, pregnancy-related autoimmune disorders, and an intracranial mass. Pharmacologic management for psychosis consists of use of mood stabilizers, benzodiazepines (for agitation), and antipsychotic agents. All antidepressants should be administered with caution because they may precipitate rapid mood cycling. Again, ECT is an alternative for the treatment of psychosis.

Postpartum Anxiety Disorders

Postpartum anxiety disorders include panic disorders and OCD. The rate of anxiety disorders related to childbearing is approximately 20% (46). Currently, data are based on retrospective studies of the prevalence of and risk factors for these illnesses (46). The literature consists primarily of case reports.

Postpartum Panic Disorders

Postpartum panic disorders include panic attacks with the acute onset of feelings of doom and noradrenergic fight-or-flight symptoms. In addition, many women with postpartum onset of panic disorders develop a fear of being alone with the infant or a fear of leaving home. The postpartum course for women with pre-existing panic disorder is variable, with a high rate of recurrence for some women after delivery. Women at risk for postpartum depression may also be vulnerable to comorbid postpartum panic disorder.

Treatment for postpartum panic disorders consists of standard options such as CBT and pharmacologic management with benzodiazepines and antidepressants.

The literature describes postpartum onset of OCD. Women may have intrusive ego-dystonic thoughts of harming their babies that typically begin 2 weeks after delivery. Although these women do not act on their thoughts, they avoid contact with their newborns and change their behaviors. For example, they avoid bathing the baby because of thoughts of drowning it; avoidance of kitchen knives is also common. These women differ from those with postpartum psychosis in that their awareness of reality remains intact. Consequently, they do not voluntarily reveal their disturbing thoughts to health care professionals, and it is imperative that physicians inquire about these symptoms (20). Treatment entails CBT, individual or group, and SSRIs.

Psychotropic Agents and Breastfeeding

The American Academy of Pediatrics (AAP) advocates breastmilk as the only source of nutrition necessary for newborns in the first year of life. Breastmilk not only offers immunologic protection to the neonate but also enhances mother–infant bonding. The excretion of psychotrophic medication in breastmilk has been reviewed and, to date, all psychotrophic medications have been found to pass into breastmilk. Data on the use of psychotrophics during breastfeeding are currently limited to case reports. The use of psychotrophic agents requires a complete assessment of risk and benefit in the infant compared with an analysis of the effects of untreated maternal mental illness. Parents should be cautioned about the unknown long-term neurobehavioral effects of infant exposures to psychotrophic agents in breastmilk.

Guidelines for the use of psychotrophic medications by breastfeeding mothers should include frequent contact between the pediatrician, obstetrician, and psychiatrist. Before drug therapy is started, the pediatrician must assess the infant to establish baseline function with respect to behavior, sleep, feeding, and alertness.

To minimize exposure of the infant, the lowest dose that treats the mother's psychiatric symptoms should be prescribed. Once steady-state has been reached, serum blood levels of both the parent compound and the metabolite should be measured in the infant. Levels are often negligible, but breastfeeding should be discontinued if levels of 5 to 10 ng/mL are found (46). Dosing immediately after breastfeeding, use of shorter-acting agents, and supplementation with bottle feeding all help reduce the infant's exposure.

The use of TCAs during nursing is thought to be relatively safe. A case report described doxepin-associated respiratory depression in one infant. Clomipramine should be avoided in breastfeeding because cases of neonatal seizures have been cited. No studies have assessed neurodevelopment in children who were exposed to TCAs in breastmilk. Among the SSRIs, most studies have focused on sertraline use in breastfeeding. Of the 28 cases reported in the literature, 26 have not shown evidence of drug accumulation and none have shown evidence of acute toxicity. Again, long-term neurodevelopment data are not available. One case report of an infant exposed to fluoxetine during breastfeeding raised concern about high norfluoxetine levels in the infant as well as acute toxicity (colic, irritability, and insomnia) that resolved with termination of breastfeeding (51). More recent studies in 15 infants did not duplicate these findings (52). Data on breastfeeding and the use of paroxetine, fluvoxamine, buproprion, venlafaxine, nefazadone, and mirtazapine are inadequate.

The AAP does not consider benzodiazepines, carbamazepine, or valproate to be contraindicated during lactation. However, significant lithium levels are detectable in breastmilk (53). In addition, infants of mothers using lithium have reportedly had toxic symptoms, such as cyanosis, hypothermia, and hypotonia (53). Lithium use in lactating mothers is contraindicated.

Four case reports of mother–infant dyads in which the breastfeeding mothers were receiving carbamazapine describe infants with total serum carbamazapine levels 19% to 65% of total maternal carbamazapine levels (53). All four infants remained healthy. There are 20 case reports of women who breastfed while taking valproate. Infant serum levels were 4% to 40% of maternal serum levels (53).

Women using antipsychotic agents are advised not to breastfeed because the risk of these agents for the neuroleptic malignant syndrome in the infant is unknown. The long-term neurobehavioral effects on infants exposed to psychotrophics in breastmilk are unknown, and parents should be apprised of this.

REFERENCES

1. **Rofe Y, Blittner M, Lewin I.** Emotional experiences during the three trimesters of pregnancy. J Clin Psychol. 1993;49:3-12.

2. **Kumar R. Robson KM.** A perspective study of emotional disorders in childbearing women. Br J Psychiatry. 1984;144:35-47.

3. **Klein MH, Essex MJ.** Pregnant or depressed? The effect of overlap between symptoms of depression and somatic complaints of pregnancy on rates of major depression in the second trimester. Depression. 1994;2:1994-5.

4. **Davidson J, Robertson E.** A follow-up study of postpartum illness. Acta Psychiatr Scand. 1985;71:451-7.

5. **Lubin B, Gardner SH, Roth A.** Mood and somatic symptoms during pregnancy. Psychosom Med. 1975;37:136-46.

6. **Crowe K, von Baeyer C.** Predictors of a positive childbirth experience. Birth. 1989;16:59-63.

7. **Condon JT, Ball SB.** Altered psychological functioning in pregnant women: an empirical investigation. J Psychosom Obstet Gynaecol. 1989;10:211-20.

8. **Schnieder Z.** Cognitive performance in pregnancy. Aust J Adv Nurs. 1989;6:40-7.

9. **O'Hara MW, Zekoski EM, Phillipps LH, Wright EJ.** A controlled prospective study of postpartum mood disorders: comparison of childbearing and nonchildbearing women. J Abnorm Psychol. 1990;99:3-15.

10. **Stone AB, Brown WA.** Psychological changes during pregnancy: implications for medical care. In: Schatz M, Zeiger RS, Claman HN, eds. Asthma and Immunological Diseases in Pregnancy and Early Infancy. New York: Marcel Dekker; 1998:117-36.

11. **Marks M, Wieck A, Checkley S, Kumar C.** How does marriage protect women with histories of affective disorder from post partum relapse? Br J Med Psychol. 1996;69:329-42.

12. **Paalberg KM, Vingerhoets AJ, Passchier J, Heinen AG, Dekker GA, van Geijn HP.** Psychosocial factors as predictors of maternal well-being and pregnancy-related complaints. J Psychosom Obstet Gynaecol. 1996;17:93-102.

13. **American Psychiatric Association.** Diagnostic and Statistical Manual of Mental Disorders, 4th ed. Washington, DC: American Psychiatric Association; 1994.

14. **Weissman MM, Olfson M.** Depression in women: implications for health care research. Science. 1995;269:799-801.

15. **Gotlib IH, Whiffen VE, Mount JH, Milne D, Cordy NI.** Prevalence rates and demographic characteristics associated with depression in pregnancy and the postpartum period. J Consult Clin Psychol. 1989;57:269-74.

16. **O'Hara MW.** Social support, life events, and depression during pregnancy and the puerperium. Arch Gen Psychiatry. 1986;43:569-73.

17. **Steer RA, Scholl TO, Hediger ML, Fischer RL.** Self-reported depression and negative pregnancy outcomes. J Clin Epidemiol. 1992;45:1093-9.

18. **Althshuler LL, Hendrick V, Cohen LS.** Course of mood and anxiety disorders during pregnancy and the postpartum period. J Clin Psychiatry. 1998;59(suppl 2):29-33.

19. **Cohen LS, Sichel DA, Dimmock JA, Rosenbaum JF.** Impact of pregnancy on panic disorder: a case series. J Clin Psychiatry. 1994;55:284-8.

20. **Diaz SF, Grush LR, Sichel DA, Cohen LS.** Obsessive compulsive disorder in pregnancy and the puerperium. In: Dickstein LJ, Riba MB, Oldham JM, eds. American Psychiatric Press Review of Psychiatry, v. 16. Washington, DC: American Psychiatric Press; 1997:97-112.

21. **Burt VK, Hendrick VC.** Psychiatric disorders in pregnancy. In: Women's Mental Health. Washington, DC: American Psychiatric Press; 1997:31-61.

22. **Rieder RO, Rosenthal D, Wender P, Blumenthal H.** The offspring of schizophrenics: fetal and neonatal deaths. Arch Gen Psychiatry. 1975;32:200-11.

23. **O'Hara MW, Swain AM.** Rates and risk of postpartum depression: a meta-analysis. Int Rev Psychiatry. 1996;8:37-54.

24. **Stuart S, O'Hara MW.** Interpersonal psychotherapy for postpartum depression: a treatment program. Journal of Psychotherapy and Practical Research. 1995;4:18-29.

25. **Spinelli MG.** Interpersonal psychotherapy for depressed antepartum women: a pilot study. Am J Psychiatry. 1997;154:1028-30.

26. **Thase ME, Greenhouse JB, Frank E, Reynolds CF, Pilkonis PA, Hurley K, et al.** Treatment of major depression with psychotherapy or psychotherapy-pharmacotherapy combinations. Arch Gen Psychiatry. 1998;54:1009-15.

27. **Althshuler LL, Cohen LS, Szuba MP, Burt VK, Gitlin M, Mintz J.** Pharmacologic management of psychiatric illness during pregnancy: dilemmas and guidelines. Am J Psychiatry. 1996;154:592-606.

28. **Cohen LS, Rosenbaum JF.** Psychotropic drug use during pregnancy: weighing the risks. J Clin Psychiatry. 1998;59(suppl 2):18-28.

29. **Miller LJ.** Psychiatric medication during pregnancy: understanding and minimizing risks. Psychiatric Annals. 1994;24:69-75.

30. **Chambers CD, Johnson KA, Dick LM, Felix RJ, Jones KL.** Birth outcomes in pregnant women taking fluoxetine. N Engl J Med. 1996;335:1010-15.

31. **Goldstein DJ.** Effects of third trimester fluoxetine exposure on the newborn. J Clin Psychopharmacol. 1995;15:417-20.

32. **Pastuszak A, Schick-Boschetto B, Zuber C, Feldkamp M, Pinelli M, Sihn S, et al.** Pregnancy outcome following first trimester exposure to fluoxetine. JAMA. 1993;269:2246-8.

33. **Spencer MJ.** Fluoxetine hydrochloride toxicity in a neonate. Pediatrics. 1993;92:721-2.

34. **Cohen LS, Grush LR, Bailey JW.** Perinatal outcome following fluoxetine exposure: a preliminary report [Abstract]. In: New Research Program and Abstracts of the 150th Annual Meeting of the American Psychiatric Association, San Diego. 1997:125.

35. **Cohen LS, Rosenbaum JF.** Birth outcomes in pregnant women taking fluoxetine. N Engl J Med. 1997;336:872.

36. **Nulman I, Rovet J, Stewart DE, Wolpin J, Gardner HA, Theis JGW, et al.** Neurodevelopment of children exposed in utero to antidepressant drugs. N Engl J Med. 1997;336:258-62.

37. **Kulin NA, Pastuszak A, Sage SR, Schick-Boschetto B, Spivey G, Feldkamp M, et al.** Pregnancy outcome following maternal use of the new selective serotonin reuptake inhibitors: a prospective controlled multicenter study. JAMA. 1998;279:609-10.

38. **Dahl ML, Olhager E, Ahlner J.** Paroxetine withdrawal syndrome in a neonate. Br J Psychiatry. 1997;171:391-2.

39. **Kent L, Laidlaw J.** Suspected congenital sertraline dependence. Br J Psychiatry. 1995;167:412-3.

40. **Miller LJ.** Use of electroconvulsive therapy in pregnancy. Hosp Community Psychiatry. 1994;45:444-50.

41. **Cohen LS, Friedman JM, Jefferson JW, Johnson EM, Weiner ML.** A reevaluation of risk of in utero exposure to lithium. JAMA. 1994;271:146-50.

42. **Stoner SC, Sommi RW, Marken PA, Anya I, Vaugn J.** Clozapine use in two full-term pregnancies. J Clin Psychiatry. 1997;58:364-5.

43. **Waldman M, Safferman A.** Pregnancy and clozapine. Am J Psychiatry. 1993;150:168-9.

44. **Kendell RE, Chalmers JC, Platz C.** Epidemiology of puerperal psychoses. Br J Psychiatry. 1987;150:662-73.

45. **O'Hara MW.** Postpartum "blues," depression, and psychosis: a review. J Psychosom Obstet Gynaecol. 1987;7:205-27.

46. **Suri R, Burt VK.** The assessment and treatment of postpartum psychiatric disorders. Journal of Practical Psychology and Behavioral Health. 1997;3:2:67-77.

47. **Tronick EZ, Weinberg MK.** Depressed mothers and infants: failure to form dyadic states of consciousness. In: Murray L, Cooper P, eds. Postpartum Depression and Child Development. New York: Guilford Press; 1997:54-81.

48. **Burt VK, Hendrick VC.** Postpartum Psychiatric Disorders. Concise Guide to Women's Mental Health. Washington, DC: American Psychiatric Press; 1997:63-77.

49. **Cox JL, Holden JM, Sagovsky R.** Detection of postnatal depression: development of the 10-item Edinburgh Postnatal Depression Scale. Br J Psychol. 1987;150:782-6.

50. **Cohen LS, Sichel DA, Robertson LM, Heckscher E, Rosenbaum JF.** Postpartum prophylaxis for women with bipolar disorder. Am J Psychiatry. 1995;152:1641-5.

51. **Lester BM, Cucca J, Andreozzi L.** Possible association between fluxetine hydrochloride and colic in an infant. J Am Acad Child Adolesc Psychiatry. 1993;32:1253-5.

52. **Yoshida K, Smith B, Craggs M, Kumar RC.** Fluoxetine in breast-milk and developmental outcome of breast-fed infants. Br J Psychiatry. 1998;172:175-8.

53. **Wisner KL, Perel JM.** Serum levels of valproate and carbamazepine in breastfeeding mother-infant pairs. J Clin Psychopharmacol. 1998;18:167-9.

III. Eating Disorders
Philip S. Mehler

Anorexia nervosa and bulimia nervosa are two eating disorders that have their peak prevalence during the early reproductive years. Bulimia encompasses a spectrum of conditions that includes overeating and binge eating. There is crossover between anorexia and bulimia. Bulimia is more common than anorexia; it affects 5% to 10% of college-age women in the United States. About 1% of the female population is said to have anorexia nervosa. Anorexia has a substantially higher mortality rate than does bulimia, even though it is less common.

The definitions of these eating disorders describe their typical characteristics. According to DSM-IV, anorexia nervosa is characterized by a refusal to maintain body weight at or above 85% of the weight normal for the person's age and height, an intense fear of gaining weight, and an undue influence of body weight and shape on self-image. Missing three consecutive menstrual cycles is also one of the new diagnostic criteria (1). Bulimia is characterized by secretive binge-eating episodes that are followed by purging done using self-induced vomiting, abuse of laxatives or diuretics, or excessive exercise.

Few organ systems are spared the progressive deterioration that can mark the clinical course of these disorders (2, 3). A system-by-system review of the major medical complications of anorexia and bulimia will facilitate the task of caring for these patients during pregnancy (Boxes 3-1 and 3-2). The medical complications of anorexia primarily result from excessive weight loss and malnutrition; those of bulimia are due to binge and purge behaviors. Anorexia is graded as mild if the patient's weight is 0% to 10% below ideal body weight, moderate if it is 10% to 20% below, and severe if it is more than 30% below. Most complications occur with severe disease.

Cardiac Complications

Cardiac complications are the most common cause of death in anorexia nervosa. Left ventricular mass is known to be reduced, and this is associated with systolic dysfunction (4). Sinus bradycardia and systolic hypotension as low as 60 mm Hg may be found. Generally, these changes are related to an energy-conserving reduction in the basal metabolic rate and thus are adaptive in nature. When the pulse rate is less than 40 beats/min, additional investigation is recommended. Prolongation of the Q-T interval is associated with more severe anorexia and may be a marker for increased risk for cardiac arrhythmia and sudden death (5).

Box 3-1 Signs, Symptoms, and Complications of Anorexia Nervosa

Central nervous system
  Enlarged cerebral ventricles and
    sulci
Dermatologic
  Brittle nails
  Lanugo-like facial hair
  Pruritus
Cardiovascular
  Arrhythmias
  Bradycardia
  ECG abnormalities
  Hypotension
  Left-ventricular irregularities
  Reduced work capacity
  Refeeding cardiomyopathy
Immunologic
  Impaired cell-mediated immunity
  Reduced bactericidal capacity of
    granulocytes
  Reduced CD4 and CD8 counts
  Reduced serum complement levels
Hematologic
  Anemia
  Leukopenia
  Reduced ESR

Endocrine
  Amenorrhea/hypogonadism
  Cold sensitivity
  Diabetes insipidus
  Euthyroid sick syndrome
  Hypoglycemia
  Hypothalamic-pituitary-adrenal axis
    dysfunction
  Osteopenia
Gastrointestinal
  Abdominal pain
  Constipation
  Decreased intestinal motility
  Delayed gastric emptying
  Duodenal dilatation
  Early satiety
  Gastric dilatation
  Postprandial fullness
  Refeeding hepatitis
  Refeeding pancreatitis
Metabolic
  Hypercholesterolemia
  Hypocalcemia
  Hypophosphatemia

Because the myocardium of patients with anorexia has reduced capacity, patients are at risk for cardiac decompensation during the first few weeks of refeeding. The *refeeding syndrome* is a potentially catastrophic complication of overly aggressive refeeding. It results from restoration of the circulatory volume due to refeeding while the left ventricular mass is still depleted. Potentiation of starvation-induced hypophosphatemia also contributes to pathogenesis (6). As long as refeeding is started slowly (800 to 1000 kcal/d) and caloric increases are modest for the first few weeks, this syndrome is completely preventable. A sudden sustained increase in the pulse rate or the development of edema may be a harbinger of cardiac failure. Bulimic patients do not usually have cardiac problems, although they have an increased incidence of mitral valve prolapse.

Box 3-2 Selected Complications of Bulimia Nervosa

Oral
  Cheilosis
  Dental caries
  Perimolysis
  Pharyngeal soreness
  Sialadenosis
Cardiovascular
  Arrythmias
  Diet pill toxicity
    Hypertension
    Intracerebral hemorrhage
    Palpitations
  Hypotension
  Ipecac toxicity
    Cardiomyopathy
    Heart failure
    Ventricular arrhythmias
  Mitral valve prolapse
Gastrointestinal
  Cathartic colon
  Constipation
  Diarrhea
  Hematochezia
  Pancreatitis
Endocrine
  Diabetic complications
  Hypoglycemia
  Irregular menses
  Mineralocorticoid excess

Gastroesophageal
  Barrett esophagus
  Dyspepsia
  Dysphagia
  Esophageal rupture
  Esophageal stricture
  Esophagitis
  Hematemesis
  Mallory-Weiss tears
  Sore throat
Pulmonary
  Aspiration pneumonia
Reproductive
  Low-birthweight infant
  Spontaneous abortion
Neuromuscular
  Ipecac toxicity
  Neuromyopathy
Fluid, electrolyte, and acid-base
  Dehydration
  Hyperamylasemia
  Hypochloremia
  Hypokalemia
  Hypomagnesemia
  Hyponatremia
  Idiopathic edema
  Metabolic acidosis
  Metabolic alkalosis
  Pseudo-Bartter syndrome

Endocrine Complications

Euthyroid sick syndrome is often seen with anorexia nervosa. Thyroid-stimulating hormone levels, however, are normal, and thyroid replacement hormone is not indicated. This is an adaptive change intended to conserve calories. The main endocrine change in a pregnant patient with anorexia is the potential for profound osteoporosis. This change has many causes, including progesterone and estrogen deficiencies, cortisol excess, and perhaps abnormalities in the levels of osteotrophic hormones such as interleukin-1 and tumor necrosis factor (7). In severe cases, osteoporosis can lead to fracture. Trabecular bone is affected more than cortical bone, and bone density may not completely return to normal with disease remission (8). The most effective strategy is to encourage weight gain and prescribe calcium 1500 mg/d and vitamin D 400 U/d because pregnancy and lactation impose tremendous stress on the maternal skeleton for mineralization of the fetal skeleton.

Patients with type 1 diabetes may have an increased prevalence of bulimia. Although the causal relation between bulimia and diabetes is debated, the detrimental effects of the combination are clear. Affected patients may deliberately omit or reduce their insulin dose to induce osmotic diuresis and weight loss. They develop end-organ damage at a younger age, have higher glycosylated hemoglobin levels, and are at increased risk for ketoacidosis (9). Physicians must screen for the propensity of the bulimic diabetic patient for unstable metabolic control. If this exists, intervention is necessary to minimize the risk for later complications in mother and fetus.

Gastrointestinal Complications

Women who purge through excessive vomiting are at risk for esophagitis and reflux-associated symptoms. This may become more manifest as pregnancy progresses and causes gastroesophageal reflux to occur in concert with the laxity of the esophageal sphincter induced by repeated bouts of vomiting (10).

Those who purge through the abuse of laxatives often have marked diarrhea and are at risk for dehydration. Self-induced vomiting, laxative abuse, and abuse of diuretics can lead to severe hypokalemia (11) and acid–base disorders (Table 3-1). In addition, abuse of stimulant laxatives can result in the cathartic colon syndrome, which is characterized by refractory constipation due to the loss of nerve plexus function in the colon, which transforms the colon into an inert tube incapable of propagating fecal material. Constipation can also be due to lack of adequate oral intake. Patients should be advised that restoration of normal bowel function requires complete cessation of laxative use, patience, ample hydration, and a judicious amount of dietary fiber.

In anorexia nervosa, gastrointestinal transit can be prolonged. Delayed gastric emptying with its postprandial gastric fullness can be very annoying to a patient, especially one who is also pregnant. It is a direct result of food restriction, which causes gastric atrophy and shrinkage, and it resolves with food restoration. Similarly, the constipation of anorexia is due to lack of oral intake and should be treated as it is in bulimic patients.

Table 3-1 Electrolyte Values Usually Associated with Purging

Purging Method	Serum					Urine		
	Sodium	Potassium	Chloride	Bicarbonate	pH	Sodium	Potassium	Chloride
Vomiting	Increased Decreased Normal	Decreased	Decreased	Increased	Increased	Decreased	Increased	Decreased
Laxative use	Increased Normal	Decreased	Increased Normal	Decreased Normal	Decreased	Decreased	Increased	Normal
Diuretic use	Decreased Normal	Decreased	Decreased	Increased	Increased	Increased	Increased	Increased

Fluids and Electrolytes

As noted above, bulimic patients have characteristic electrolyte disturbances associated with the purging method used. If bulimia is active during pregnancy, these disturbances must be regularly screened for to avert serious sequelae of abnormal serum electrolyte levels. Fluid and electrolyte shifts can increase risk to the pregnancy and the fetus. One syndrome that can be difficult to treat is known as *pseudo-Bartter syndrome* (12). When a bulimic patient abruptly stops purging, the renin-angiotensin-aldosterone axis, which was activated in response to purging, remains stimulated for a week or two and then precipitates a reflexive edema, which can be severe. This can inspire diuretic use to eliminate the edema, leading to a vicious cycle. Patients must be told that the edema will resolve over 2 to 3 weeks with salt-intake restriction and elevation of the legs. Remarkably, the laboratory values of a patient with anorexia nervosa are generally normal aside from mild leukopenia and normocytic anemia, which revert to normal with weight restoration (13).

Pregnancy Outcome

There have been few studies of pregnancy outcome in women with eating disorders. Earlier studies in active anorexia nervosa found an increased risk for prematurity, perinatal mortality, and infants small-for-gestational age, and lower APGAR scores (14). Bulimic pregnancies have been associated with an increased likelihood of fetal loss through miscarriage or neonatal death (15). A recent study demonstrated that women with disordered eating habits were at greatest risks for delivering term small-for-gestational age infants (16). Other retrospective studies similarly suggest that anorectic and bulimic behaviors jeopardize maternal and fetal health (17). These results suggest that good obstetric care should include a history of a woman's eating behavior and body weight. Excessive clinic visits for hyperemesis gravidarum should prompt the clinician to consider the possibility of an eating disorder (18).

When appropriate, a referral must be made to a mental health professional to help the patient progress through pregnancy with a good outcome for herself and her baby. Patients may also benefit from the help of a sensitive nutritionist who can focus on achieving a good nutritional state. It is important that physicians not assume that women with eating disorders wish to know their body weight at each office visit: A substantial proportion of these women may become more preoccupied with their eating disorder when informed of their weight at each visit. A summary of the elements necessary for successful management of these patients is given in Box 3-3.

Box 3-3 Suggestions for Antenatal Care of Women with Eating Disorders

---

1. Inquire about prepregnancy weight and calculate body mass index. If less than 18, assess carefully for presence of an eating disorder.
2. Measure body weight at each visit but share it with patient only she expresses a desire to know it.
3. Assess overall nutritional state and screen for medical complications of anorexia nervosa and bulimia.
4. Encourage involvement of internist, dietitian, and psychiatrist for antenatal and postnatal support.

A related issue concerns the natural history of eating disorders during pregnancy. Because of the shame and denial that are such an integral part of eating disorders, patients are often reluctant to discuss their behaviors with their obstetric caregivers. Unfortunately, little information is available on the effects of pregnancy in women with anorexia nervosa or bulimia. Earlier studies were inconsistent. Some reported that women developed better control over their symptoms during pregnancy, motivated by the desire for healthy children (19–21). A more recent study found that the severity of features of eating disorders decreased early in pregnancy but increased towards the last trimester (22). Of note, it is agreed that most patients will regress and have relapse after delivery and that eating may then be even more disturbed (23, 24). Obstetricians must be aware of this postpartum risk and the potential benefits of psychiatric intervention in antenatal cases.

Conclusions

Pregnancy can be a very challenging time for women with anorexia nervosa or bulimia. Direct questioning about specific eating disorder–related behaviors should be used to determine the extent to which an eating disorder is a problem. Most authorities recommend that pregnancy take place only after an eating disorder has been resolved (25). However, if a patient with an eating disorder becomes pregnant, conflicts about changes in body shape can result in a recrudescence or an exacerbation of the disorder. Even women who had "disordered eating habits" before pregnancy are at increased risk for complications of pregnancy (26). Because anorectic and bulimic behaviors during pregnancy can jeopardize maternal and fetal health, early diagnosis and treatment are essential. Consultation with a physician who has expertise in the medical complications of eating disorders is imperative.

REFERENCES

1. **Pryor T.** Diagnostic criteria for eating disorders: DSM-IV revisions. Psychiatr Annals. 1995;25:40-9.

2. **Mehler PS, Gray MC, Schulte M.** Medical complications of anorexia nervosa. J Womens Health. 1997;6:533-41.

3. **Batal H, Johnson M, Lehman D, Steele A, Mehler PS.** Bulimia: a primary care approach. J Womens Health. 1998;7:211-9.

4. **de Simone G.** Cardiac abnormalities in young women with anorexia nervosa. Br Heart J. 1994;71:287-91.

5. **Cooke RA, Chamber JB, Singh R.** QT interval in anorexia nervosa. Br Heart J. 1994;72:69-73.

6. **Mehler PS, Weiner KC.** Anorexia nervosa and total parenteral nutrition. Int J Eat Disord. 1993;14:297-309.

7. **Siemers B, Lhakmakijan Z, Gench B.** Bone density patterns in women with anorexia nervosa. Int J Eat Disord. 1996;19:179.

8. **Klibanski A.** The effects of estrogen administration on trabecular bone loss in young women. J Clin Endocrinol Metab. 1995;80:898-903.

9. **Rydall AC, Rodin GM, Olmsted MP.** Disordered eating behavior and microvascular complications in young women with IDDM. N Engl J Med. 1997;336:1849-54.

10. **Chami TN, Andersen AE, Crowell MD.** Gastrointestinal symptoms in bulimia nervosa. Am J Gastroenterol. 1995:90:88-93.

11. **Greenfield D.** Hypokalemia in outpatients with eating disorders. Am J Psychiatry. 1995;152:60-5.

12. **Mehler PS.** Pseudo-Bartter's. Eating Disorders: The Journal of Prevention and Treatment. 1998;6:65-8.

13. **Devnyst O, Lambert N, Rodhain J.** Hematological changes in anorexia nervosa. QJM. 1993;86:791-5.

14. **Stewart DE, Raskin J, Garfinkel PE.** Anorexia nervosa, bulimia and pregnancy. Am J Obstet Gynecol. 1987;157:1194-8.

15. **Mitchell JE, Seim HC, Glotter D.** A retrospective study of pregnancy in bulimia nervosa. Int J Eat Disord. 1991;10:209-14.

16. **Conti J, Abraham S, Taylor A.** Eating behaviors and pregnancy outcome. J Psychosom Res. 1998;44:465-77.

17. **Franko DL, Walton BE.** Pregnancy and eating disorders. Int J Eat Disord. 1993;13:41-8.

18. **Lingham R, McCluskey S.** Eating disorders associated with hyperemesis gravidarum. J Psychosom Res. 1996;40:231-4.

19. **Namir S, Melman K, Yager J.** Pregnancy in anorexia nervosa. Int J Eat Disord. 1986;5:837-45.

20. **Lacey JH, Smith G.** Bulimia nervosa: the impact of pregnancy on mother and baby. Br J Psychiatry. 1987;150:777-81.

21. **Lenberg R, Phillips J.** The impact of pregnancy on anorexia nervosa and bulimia. Int J Eat Disord. 1989;8:285-95.

22. **Fairburn CG, Stein A, Jones R.** Eating habits and eating disorders during pregnancy. Psychosom Med. 1992;54:665-72.

23. **Fahy TA.** Eating disorders in pregnancy. Psychol Med. 1991;21:577-80.
24. **Stein A, Fairburn CG.** Eating habits and attitudes in the postpartum period. Psychosom Med. 1996;58:321-5.
25. **Bonne OB, Rubinoff B, Berry EM.** Delayed detection of pregnancy in patients with anorexia nervosa. Int J Eat Disord. 1996;20:423-5.
26. **Abraham S, King W, Jones D.** Attitudes to body weight, weight gain and eating behavior in pregnancy. J Psychosom Obstet Gynecol. 1994;15:189-95.

IV. Illicit Drug Use
Ellen D. Mason

Over the past decade, illicit drug use during pregnancy has been recognized as a major public health problem, the ultimate economic and social ramifications of which have yet to be determined. The epidemic use of crack cocaine in the 1980s segueing into the widespread use of inhaled opiates in the 1990s dramatically expanded the population of chemically dependent women while simultaneously heightening concern about the effect of maternal drug use on fetuses, infants, and children exposed to drugs in utero. Public concern has stimulated intensive study of the prevalence of use and the obstetric, perinatal, neonatal, and long-term developmental consequences of drug use during pregnancy. The results of many of these investigations are now becoming available. Familiarity with recent findings in perinatal drug research is important for any clinician who cares for women with reproductive potential. This knowledge can and should be incorporated into the routine medical and obstetric care of women.

Epidemiology

Reliable prevalence data on the use of illicit drugs during pregnancy is difficult to obtain. Fear of the consequences of disclosure limits the accuracy of responses to large-scale telephone surveys and drug history screening questionnaires. Nonetheless, in a recent anonymous national U.S. survey, 1.8% of pregnant women admitted to having used an illicit drug in the preceding month and 6.7% of nonpregnant women 15 to 44 years of age admitted to recent illicit drug use (1). When data are collected directly from pregnant women, the incidence of drug use as documented by self-report or urine toxicology screening ranges from 4% to 32% (2, 3).

The long-term health consequences of maternal substance abuse can be very costly. It is estimated that the initial cost of medical care for children born to mothers who used illicit drugs during pregnancy is $1100 to $4100 higher than the cost for unexposed infants (4). The additional costs of health care and special education projected out to age 18 years may be as much as $750,000 per child (5).

Identification of Pregnant Women Who Use Illicit Substances

Illicit drug use occurs in all ethnic and socioeconomic groups. Thus, it is mandatory that clinicians screen for the problem in a systematic and effective way. Despite the limitations of drug history screening tools, these tools are a vital part of perinatal drug use assessment because toxicology testing can generally only identify *recent* drug use. Many practitioners use standardized instruments, such as the CAGE (6) or MAST (*M*ichigan *A*lcohol *S*creening *T*est) (7) questionnaires, but these instruments are not appropriate for obtaining information about illicit drug use.

All pregnant women should be asked, in a nonjudgmental but specific way, about use of illicit drugs. If a patient has medical problems or behavioral issues that are associated with illicit drug use, such as preterm labor or noncompliance with prenatal visits, a more detailed history should be taken. The interviewer should emphasize that the drug history is asked of all pregnant women and is being taken for the purpose of understanding the patient's personal health and pregnancy issues as fully as possible. The history should include types of drugs used, frequency of use, duration of use, and route of use. The patient should be assured of the confidentiality of the interview at its onset.

Toxicology testing complements the drug history because self-report misses at least one fourth to one half of maternal substance users (8). Because urine toxicology testing is the most common testing method, clinicians should understand the methods and limitations of this testing. Thin-layer chromatography and high-performance liquid chromatography, which are used in most clinical laboratories, may not be sensitive enough to detect low concentrations of drugs in the urine of pregnant women because they are designed to screen specimens from patients with suspected drug overdoses (9). If an appropriately sensitive assay, such as the nonisotopic enzyme immunoassay, is used, it is still important to remember that the metabolites of many abused drugs, such as cocaine, heroin, and amphetamines, are present in urine for no more than 48 to 72 hours after ingestion. A negative result on urine toxicology screening does not rule out the use of drugs earlier in pregnancy. In addition, clinicians should be aware that false-positive results are possible because immunoassay and gas chromatography–mass spectrometry can yield positive results for drugs of abuse when patients have used certain prescription or over-the-counter medications (e.g., combination decongestant–antihistamine–antitussive preparations).

Investigation into the toxicologic testing of other biosubstances, such as neonatal meconium and maternal or neonatal hair, continues. Reliable drug screening of meconium and hair is potentially useful because the results reflect maternal drug ingestion as early as the first trimester. However, these tests are currently expensive, unstandardized, and largely experimental.

Treatment of Chemically Dependent Pregnant Women

Medical and Obstetric Management

When illicit drug use during pregnancy is suspected or diagnosed, more intensive prenatal and medical evaluation and care are required. Maternal drug abuse in combination with a drug-abusing lifestyle is associated with adverse outcomes, such as increased rates of maternal HIV infection (10), tuberculosis, sexually transmitted diseases, and vaginosis. Untreated infections, poor nutrition, and use of vasoactive substances, such as cocaine or amphetamines, are associated with intrauterine growth restriction (11, 12), preterm rupture of membranes (13, 14), LBW, and abruptio placenta (15, 16). Chemically dependent pregnant women should have more frequent obstetric visits than lower-risk women. The visits should include intensive surveillance for HIV infection and other sexually transmitted diseases as well as serial obstetric ultrasonography to assess fetal growth (17).

Treatment of Chemical Dependency

The diagnosis of illicit drug use during pregnancy should stimulate intervention by a clinician. Ideally, the intervention should consist of an estimate of addiction severity and an assessment of the patient's motivation to accept a treatment referral. When referring a woman for treatment, the clinician should nonjudgmentally give the woman information about the potential adverse effects of drug use in pregnancy. The patient should also be made aware of the various treatment options and behavioral modification strategies available to her (18). Consideration should be given to the patient's psychosocial situation, employment situation, child care issues, and comorbid disorders such as depression. Many pregnant drug users initially refuse treatment or deny their need for treatment because feelings of guilt or denial put them in the "pre-contemplation" state described by Prochaska and colleagues (19). It is important that clinicians continue to try to move such patients from a "precontemplation" to an "action" state with respect to treatment.

Since the 1980s, many women's treatment demonstration projects have been funded by the National Institute on Drug Abuse and the National Institute on Alcohol Abuse and Alcoholism. In 1988, the U.S. Congress passed the Anti-Drug Abuse Act (20), which provided funding to increase the number of treatment slots for women and children and to rigorously evaluate innovative treatment methods. Meta-analysis of pregnancy outcomes in some research demonstration programs shows that participants had better outcomes as measured by infant birthweight and other variables (21).

Busy clinicians can obtain information on drug treatment programs from state or county departments of alcohol and substance abuse. These agencies can be readily contacted by telephone or mail. They maintain and distribute up-to-date listings of comprehensive, sex-specific programs. Unfortunately, despite a U.S. federal law that gives pregnant women priority in admission to publicly funded treatment programs, there are still too few treatment slots available, especially for low-income pregnant women. It is estimated that fewer than one fourth of persons who need treatment receive it (22).

Medicolegal Issues Associated with Substance-Using Pregnant Women

Mandated Reporting

In the United States, the legal status of the fetus remains ambiguous. Attempts to criminalize maternal drug use in pregnancy continue, although they have been largely unsuccessful. Most authorities believe that, ultimately, such sanctions drive pregnant drug users away from vital care and resources (23). Several states mandate the reporting to local child protective services of any infant who has a positive result on a urine toxicologic test at the time of birth (24). It is prudent for clinicians who treat women of reproductive age to keep abreast of local and federal statutes pertaining to drug use in pregnancy.

Confidentiality of Drug Abuse Treatment Information

It is essential that clinicians work collaboratively with the drug treatment programs that their patients enter, but they must be aware that federal confidentiality regulations on drug and alcohol treatment are stricter than most other confidentiality rules (25). Except in cases of medical emergency, treatment programs may not disclose any information about a patient unless a valid consent form is signed. Clinicians should be proactive about arranging for an appropriate exchange of information so that they can effectively follow and encourage patients who enter treatment.

Cocaine

The recreational use of cocaine by women of reproductive age became widespread in the past decade and continues to be a common cause of complications in pregnancy. Although recent data indicate that numbers of casual or "recreational" and adolescent users seem to be decreasing, "hard-core" use in older women seems unabated (26). Cocaine use in pregnancy is strongly associated with adverse obstetric outcomes. These outcomes, in turn, have been shown to increase health care costs in both urban and rural settings (27, 28).

Cocaine is an ester of benzoic acid that is derived from the leaves of the coca plant, *Erythroxylum coca*. Application of hydrochloric acid to raw coca paste yields cocaine hydrochloride, which can be snorted or injected. Treatment of the hydrochloric cocaine salt with a base, followed by solvent extraction, produces alkaloidal cocaine, or *crack*, which is heat stable and therefore can be inhaled (29). Cocaine readily crosses the placenta, although placental passage may be limited by cocaine-induced vasoconstriction of uterine arteries (30). Cocaine inhibits the re-uptake and metabolism of norepinephrine and epinephrine at neural junctions, activating the adrenergic nervous system peripherally and centrally. The primary physiologic manifestations of cocaine are central nervous system (CNS) stimulation, peripheral vasoconstriction, and hypertension. Studies in animal models suggest that the hormonal milieu of pregnancy enhances cocaine toxicity, particularly in the heart and peripheral circulation (31, 32). In addition, cocaine has been shown to directly augment the contractility of the pregnant human uterus by adrenergic and nonadrenergic mechanisms (33).

Maternal Effects

Complications of cocaine use result primarily from the sympathomimetic actions of the drug. A large body of literature documents many adverse consequences of cocaine use in pregnancy, including cardiovascular events, such as transient malignant hypertension, myocardial ischemia and infarction, cardiac arrhythmia, cardiomyopathy, and aortic rupture (34–37). Catastrophic CNS complications associated with cocaine use include seizures (38) and cerebrovascular accidents in pregnant and postpartum women (39, 40). Pulmonary, metabolic, and psychiatric problems are also common in the setting of acute or chronic cocaine use (41, 42).

Obstetric and Fetal Effects

Epidemiologic studies of cocaine use in pregnancy are limited by confounding factors, such as polysubstance abuse, tobacco smoking, poor nutrition, lack of prenatal care, and poverty. Nonetheless, strong associations have been seen between maternal cocaine use and placental abruption (43), preterm premature rupture of membranes (44, 45), pregnancy-induced hypertension (46), a preeclampsia–like syndrome (47), and uterine rupture (48, 49). These outcomes are presumed to be a consequence of cocaine-induced elevations of circulating catecholamine levels, maternal blood pressure, uterine contraction intensity, and body temperature and decreased uterine artery blood flow.

Cocaine-medicated vasoconstriction of uterine arteries, with subsequent decrements in placental perfusion, is presumed to be responsible for the increased rates of fetal growth restriction and LBW seen in the offspring of pregnant cocaine users (50, 51). The pattern of growth restriction is usually symmetrical and is presumed to be due to reductions in fetal nutrient delivery associated with decreased uterine artery perfusion. Some investigators have reported a "reversal" in the usual pattern of growth restriction, with larger reductions in head circumference than in other somatic variables (52).

The spectrum of congenital anomalies associated with maternal cocaine use is still incompletely defined. Unlike alcohol, cocaine is not highly or predictably teratogenic. The teratogenicity of cocaine is presumed to be largely due to the vasoconstrictive effects of the drug in the fetal circulation. Animal and human data indicate an increased incidence of genitourinary malformations, cardiac defects, structural ophthalmic anomalies, cerebral infarctions, and hydroencephaly in cocaine-exposed fetuses (53–55). Cerebral infarctions and hydroencephaly may be direct effects of cocaine or may occur in premature births precipitated by antepartum cocaine use (56).

Neurobehavioral Effects on Newborn and Child

Although neurobehavioral abnormalities, such as tremulousness and increased startle response, have been seen in some cocaine-exposed neonates (57), evidence is insufficient to support the routine diagnosis of a distinctive neonatal cocaine abstinence syndrome in exposed infants (58). Enormous interest and concern about potential cognitive and behavioral abnormalities in cocaine-exposed children has launched longitudinal studies of these children that are still underway. A few preliminary results indicate that attention deficit disorders may be more common in prenatally exposed school-age children (59). Prominent authorities in child development stress that, although these findings are of great concern, the extent to which they can be modified by subsequent environmental factors and care is unknown (60, 61).

Narcotics

Epidemiology

The recreational use of narcotics by pregnant women has been a persistent problem since the 1950s. Recent prevalence studies indicate that the use of opiates, particularly inhalational heroin, is on the rise. The National Household Survey on Drug Abuse reported a fourfold increase in heroin use between 1990 and 1995, and the Drug Abuse Warning Network documented a significant increase in heroin-related emergency department visits between 1993 and 1995 (62). Increased use of heroin by both low-income and middle-class women (attributed to the fact that the available drug is now both purer and cheaper) can be expected to lead to a substantial increase in the number of children exposed to heroin in utero.

Maternal Effects

Information on the adverse health effects of heroin has largely been drawn from data gathered on parenteral drug users. Recognized complications in this group include increased rates of HIV infection, bacterial endocarditis, viral hepatitis, and cellulitis. Most of these complications are due in part to the parenteral injection of unsterile particulate matter or a drug-using lifestyle and are not direct effects of heroin itself. Regardless of the route of use, opiate overdose is a potential complication in any heroin user and should be suspected in pregnant women who present with coma, miotic pupils, and respiratory depression. Judicious use of narcotic antagonists, such as naloxone, in resuscitation is appropriate because overuse may precipitate withdrawal symptoms in both mother and fetus.

Obstetric and Fetal Effects

The obstetric complications associated with opiate use during pregnancy are engendered by a complex interaction between the effects of the drugs themselves and the effects of a drug-using lifestyle, which generally includes poor nutrition and inadequate prenatal care.

Diagnosis of pregnancy may be delayed in the setting of opiate addiction because menstrual abnormalities are seen in as many as 60% to 90% of heroin-dependent women (63, 64).

Nausea, vomiting, and fatigue, which are common in early pregnancy, may be misinterpreted by addicted women as signs of withdrawal. This may lead to increased drug consumption and a concomitant delay in the diagnosis of pregnancy.

Fetal and Neonatal Effects

Use of heroin during pregnancy is associated with an increased incidence of LBW resulting from premature delivery and symmetric growth restriction (65). Intrauterine fetal demise is increased in opiate-exposed fetuses (66). Nonstress tests should be initiated in the third trimester for opiate-using women, although the reactivity of the test has been shown to be decreased in women receiving methadone maintenance therapy (67).

The neonatal abstinence syndrome is common in infants antenatally exposed to opiates, and it contributes to the increase in overall neonatal mortality seen in pregnancies that involve opiate exposure (68). Symptoms characteristic of this syndrome include hyperirritability, tremor, gastrointestinal dysfunction, and autonomic symptoms, such as yawning, sneezing, and fever. Severe symptoms, such as seizures, may necessitate the short-term use of depressant medications, such as barbiturates. A scoring system has been devised to evaluate children with neonatal abstinence syndrome and help predict their need for specialized neonatal care (69). The syndrome usually occurs within 72 hours after birth, although it may appear at any time until 2 weeks after delivery.

Treatment of Opiate Dependency in Pregnancy

Maternal narcotic withdrawal during pregnancy jeopardizes fetal well-being and may be associated with spontaneous abortion (70) and intrauterine fetal stress (71). Methadone treatment during pregnancy prevents fluctuating narcotic levels in the fetus as well as intrauterine fetal withdrawal. In addition, methadone, given in conjunction with comprehensive care (including prenatal care and drug rehabilitation), reduces obstetric complications and neonatal morbidity and mortality rates (72, 73).

Ongoing controversy about the association of higher-dose methadone and the neonatal abstinence syndrome during pregnancy precludes consensus recommendations on dosing. In general, given the marked intravariation and intervariation of plasma methadone levels seen in pregnant women, individualization of dose is the only sensible strategy. A reasonable objective is to abolish all maternal withdrawal symptoms (74).

Pregnant candidates for methadone therapy should be given an initial dose of 10 to 20 mg/d, depending on their drug histories. Five milligrams should be given every 4 to 6 hours over 24 to 48 hours until all narcotic withdrawal symptoms are extinguished (75). Establishing the correct dose for a given patient may require brief hospitalization because few outpatient treatment programs are able to dispense multiple doses in a single day. Patients receiving methadone who become pregnant may maintain their prepregnancy dosage. Intrapartum analgesia for labor should not be withheld from women receiving methadone therapy because long-term use of methadone will not lessen the pain experienced during labor. Postpartum, women who continue to receive methadone therapy may require downward adjustment of their usual doses. The AAP considers methadone to be compatible with breastfeeding. No adverse effects have been reported in nursing infants with a maternal dosage of 20 mg/24 hours or less (76).

Marijuana

Marijuana is one of the illicit drugs most commonly used by women of child-bearing age, but relatively little is known about its effects in human pregnancy. The 1995 National Pregnancy and Health Survey indicated that of the 4 million women who gave birth in 1992, 2.9% reported having used marijuana during their pregnancy (77). Despite the high prevalence of use, marijuana is arguably the least-studied illicit drug used in pregnancy.

Marijuana is prepared from the plant *Cannabis sativa*. The principal active ingredient is delta-9-tetrahydrocannabinol (delta-9-THC). Inhalation of marijuana is associated with rapid absorption of THC into the bloodstream. Physical effects include increased heart rate, decreased blood pressure, and CNS effects such as drowsiness and impaired concentration. Few chronic adverse health effects are associated with marijuana use, although acute and chronic bronchitis and alterations in pituitary, ovarian, and adrenal hormone levels have been reported (78, 79).

Effects in Pregnancy

The antiemetic effect of delta-9-THC may diminish the nausea often experienced early in pregnancy. Human and animal data suggest that the placenta is a partial barrier to the transport of delta-9-THC (80, 81). Several prospective studies have found no association between marijuana use and an increased incidence of congenital anomalies in human pregnancy. Animal data show that crude marijuana extract is teratogenic in some species, depending on dose and route of administration (82, 83).

Studies of the effect of marijuana on birthweight have had somewhat equivocal results, and no effect has been reported when birthweights are corrected for gestational age (84, 85). Overall, given the sparseness of the data on the effects of marijuana use in pregnancy and the common occurrence of this use, it is clear that further study in this area is greatly needed if clinicians are to properly advise women of reproductive age.

REFERENCES

1. **Coleman F, Kay J.** Biology of addiction. Obstet Gynecol Clin North Am. 1998;25:1.
2. **Gillogley KM, Evens AT, Hansen RL, et al.** The impact of cocaine, amphetamine and opiate use detected by universal intrapartum screening. Am J Obstet Gynecol. 1990;163:1535-42.
3. Statewide prevalence of illicit drug use by pregnancy women—Rhode Island. MMWR Morb Mortal Wkly Rep. 1990;39:354-5.
4. **Chasnoff IJ.** Drugs, alcohol, pregnancy and the neonate. JAMA. 1991;266:1567-8.

5. Drug Exposed Infants: A Generation at Risk. Report to the Chairman Committee on Finance, U.S. Senate, June 1990. U.S.General Accounting Office.

6. **Mayfield D, Mcleod G, Hall P.** The CAGE questionnaire: validation of a new alcoholism screening instrument. Am J Psychiatry. 1974;131:1121-3.

7. **Selzer ML.** The Michigan Alcoholism Screening Test: the quest for a new diagnostic instrument. Am J Psychiatry. 1971;127:89-95.

8. Drug Exposed Infants: A Generation at Risk. Report to the Chairman Committee on Finance, U.S. Senate, June 1990. U.S.General Accounting Office.

9. **Kwong TC, Shearer D.** Detection of drug use during pregnancy. Obstet Gynecol Clin North Am. 1998;25:43-64.

10. **Ward JW, Karon J, Fleming P, et al.** Trends in AIDS incidence in the United States, 1990-1994 [abstract]. Presented at the Eleventh International Conference on AIDS, Vancouver; July 7-12, 1996; p36.

11. **Sprauve ME, Lindsay MK, Herbert S, et al.** Adverse perinatal outcome in parturient who use crack cocaine. Obstet Gynecol. 1997;89:674-8.

12. **Oro AS, Dixon SD.** Perinatal cocaine and methamphetamine mphetamine exposure: maternal and neonatal correlates. J Pediatr. 1987;111:571-8.

13. **Dinsmoor MJ, Irons SJ, Christmas JT.** Preterm rupture of the membranes associated with recent cocaine use. Am J Obstet Gynecol. 1994;171:305-9.

14. **Delaney DB, Larrabee KD, Monga M.** Preterm rupture of the membranes associated with recent cocaine use. Am J Perinatol. 1997;14:285-8.

15. **Shiono P, Klebanof M, Nugent R, et al.** The impact of cocaine and marijuana use on low birth weight and preterm birth: a multicenter study. Am J Obstet Gynecol. 1995;172:19-27.

16. **Little BB, Snell LM, Gilstrap LC 3d.** Methamphetamine abuse during pregnancy: outcome and fetal effects. Obstet Gynecol. 1988;72:541-4.

17. **Mitchell JL.** Treatment Improvement Protocol Series (TIPS): Pregnant, Substance Using Women. Rockville, MD: U.S. Dept of Health and Human Services; 1993.

18. **Rosen RK, Dube CE, Lewis DC, et al., eds.** March of Dimes Substance Abuse Curriculum for Obstetricians and Gynecologists. White Plains, NY: March of Dimes Birth Defects Foundation; 1995.

19. **Prochaska JO, DiClemente CC, Norcross JC.** In search of how people change: applications to addictive behaviors. Am Psychol. 1992;1102-13.

20. **Rahdert E, ed.** Treatment for Drug-Exposed Women and Their Children: Advances in Research Methodology. National Institute for Drug Abuse Research Monograph 166. Rockville, MD: National Institute on Drug Abuse; 1996.

21. Final Report: Evaluation of the Demonstrations To Improve Access to Care for Pregnant Substance Abusers. Washington, DC: Mathematic Policy Research, Inc.; 1997.

22. Substance Abuse: The Nation's Number One Health Problem—Key Indicators for Policy. Institute for Health Policy, Brandeis University, for The Robert Wood Johnson Foundation, Princeton, New Jersey; 1993:60-3.

23. **Chavkin W.** Mandatory treatment for drug use during pregnancy. JAMA. 1991;266: 1556-62.

24. Epidemiological Study of the Prevalence of Alcohol and Other Drug Use among Pregnant and Parturient Women in Illinois. Chicago: National Association for Perinatal Research and Education; 1992.

25. **Lopez F, ed.** Treatment Improvement Protocol Series (TIPS) #13: Confidentiality of Patients' Records for Alcohol and Other Drug Treatment. Rockville, MD: U.S. Dept of Health and Human Services, Public Health Service, Center for Substance Abuse Treatment;.

26. **Jones J.** The rise of the modern addict. Am J Public Health. 1995;85:1157-62.

27. **Benke M, Eyler FD, Conlon M, et al.** How fetal cocaine exposure increase neonatal hospital costs. Pediatrics. 1997;99:204-8.

28. **Calhoun BC, Watson PT.** The cost of maternal cocaine abuse. I. Perinatal cost. Obstet Gynecol. 1991;78:731-4.

29. **Farrar HC, Kearns GL.** Cocaine: clinical pharmacology and toxicology. J Pediatr. 1989;115:665.

30. **Mittelman RE, Corofino JC, Hearn WL.** Tissue distribution of cocaine in a pregnant woman. J Forensic Sci. 1989;34:481-6.

31. **Kurtzman JT, Thorp JM, Spielman FJ, et al.** Estrogen mediates the pregnancy-enhanced cardiotoxicity of cocaine in the isolated perfused rat heart. Obstet Gynecol. 1994;83:613-5.

32. **Woods JR, Scott KJ, Plessinger MA.** Pregnancy enhances cocaine's actions on the heart and within the peripheral circulation. Am J Obstet Gynecol. 1994;170:1027-35.

33. **Hurd WW, Betz AL Dombrowski MP, Fomin VP.** Cocaine augments contractility of the pregnant human uterus by both adrenergic and non-adrenergic mechanisms. Am J Obstet Gynecol. 1998;178:1077-81.

34. **Isner JM, Estes M, Thompson PD, et al.** Acute cardiac events temporally related to cocaine abuse. N Engl J Med. 1986;315:1438-43.

35. **Nanjii AA, Filpenko JD.** Asystole and ventricular fibrillation associated with cocaine intoxication. Chest. 1984;85:132-3.

36. **Weiner RS, Lockhart JT, Schwartz RG.** Dilated cardiomyopathy associated with maternal cocaine abuse. Am J Med. 1986;81:519-20.

37. **Mendelson MA, Chandler J.** Postpartum cardiomyopathy associated with maternal cocaine abuse. Am J Cardiol. 1992;70:1092-4.

38. **Myers JA, Earnest MP.** Generalized seizures and cocaine abuse. Neurology. 1984;34:675-6.

39. **Mecado A, Johnson F, Calver D, et al.** Cocaine, pregnancy and postpartum intracerebral hemorrhage. Obstet Gynecol. 1989;73:467-78.

40. **Iriye B, Asrat T, Adashek J.** Intraventricular hemorrhage and maternal brain death associated with antepartum cocaine abuse. Br J Obstet Gynecol. 1995;102:68-9.

41. **Gawin FH, Ellenwood EE.** Cocaine and other stimulants: actions, abuse and treatment. N Engl J Med. 1988;3188:1173-82.

42. **Brody SL, Slovis CM, Wrenn KD.** Cocaine-related medical problems: consecutive series of 233 patients. Am J Med. 1990;88:325-31.

43. **Bateman DA, Ng SK, Hansen CA, et al.** The effects of intrauterine cocaine exposure in newborns. Am J Public Health. 1993;83:190-3.

44. **Delaney DB, Larabee KD, Monga M.** Preterm premature rupture of the membranes associated with recent cocaine use. Am J Perinatol. 1997;14:285-8.

45. **Dinsmoor MJ, Irons SJ, Christmas JT.** Preterm rupture of the membranes associated with recent cocaine use. Am J Obstet Gynecol. 1994;171:305-9.

46. **Little BB, Snell LM, Klein VR, et al.** Cocaine abuse during pregnancy: maternal and fetal implications. Obstet Gynecol. 1989;73:157-60.

47. **Towers CV, Pircon RA, Nageotte MP, et al.** Cocaine intoxication presenting as preeclampsia and eclampsia. Obstet Gynecol. 1993;81:545-7.

48. **Gonsoulin W, Borge D, Moise KJ Jr.** Rupture of unscarred uterus in primigravid women in association with cocaine use. Am J Obstet Gynecol. 1990;163:526-7.

49. **Iriye BK, Bristow RE, Hsu CD, et al.** Uterine rupture associated with recent antepartum cocaine abuse. Obstet Gynecol. 1994;83:340-1.

50. **Spruave ME, Lindsay MK, Herbert S, Graves W.** Adverse perinatal outcome in parturient who use crack cocaine. Obstet Gynecol. 1997;89(5 pt 1):674-8.

51. **Eyler FD, Behnke M, Conlon NS, Wobie K.** Birth outcome from a prospective, matched study of prenatal crack/cocaine use: I. Interactive and dose effects on health and growth. Pediatrics. 1998;101:229-37.

52. **Little BB, Snell LM.** Brain growth among fetuses exposed to cocaine in utero: asymmetrical growth retardation. Obstet Gynecol. 1991;77:361-4.

53. **Chasnoff IJ, Chisum GM, Kaplan WE.** Maternal cocaine use and genitourinary tract malformations. Teratology. 1988;37:201-4.

54. **Lipshultz SE, Frassica JJ, Orav EJ.** Cardiovascular abnormalities in infants prenatally exposed to cocaine. J Pediatr. 1991;118:44-51.

55. **Sliva-Arujo A, Tavares MA.** Development of the eye after gestation exposure to cocaine: vascular development in the retina of rats and humans. Ann N Y Acad Sci. 1996;801:274-88.

56. **Singer LT, Yamshita TS, Hawkins S, et al.** Increased incidence of intraventricular hemorrhage and developmental delay in cocaine-exposed very low birth weight infants. J Pediatr. 1994;124:765-71.

57. **Chasnoff IJ, Burn W, Schnoll S, et al.** Cocaine use in pregnancy. N Engl J Med. 1985; 313:666-9.

58. **Little B, Wilson GN, Jackson G.** Is there a cocaine syndrome? Dysmorphic and anthropometric assessment of infants exposed to cocaine. Teratology. 1996;54:145-9.

59. **Richardson GA, Conroy ML, Day NL.** Prenatal cocaine exposure: effects on the development of school-age children. Neurotoxicol Teratol. 1996;18:727-634.

60. **Mayes L, Granger R, Bornstein M, et al.** The problem of prenatal cocaine exposure: a rush to judgement. JAMA. 1992;3:406-8.

61. **Zuckerman B, Frank D.** "Crack kids": not broken. Pediatrics. 1992;89:337-9.

62. **Kaltenbach K, Berghella V, Finnegan L.** Opioid dependence during pregnancy: effects and management. Obstet Gynecol Clin North Am. 1998;25:139-51.

63. **Gaulden EC, Littlefield DC, Putoff OE, et al.** Menstrual abnormalities associated with heroin addiction. Am J Obstet Gynecol. 1964;90:155-60.

64. **Santen RJ, Sofsky J, Bilie N, et al.** Mechanisms of action of narcotics in the production of menstrual dysfunction in women. Fertil Steril. 1975;26:538-48.

65. **Kandall SR, Albin S, Lowinson J, et al.** Differential effects of maternal heroin and methadone use on birth weight. Pediatrics. 1976;58:681-5.

66. **Fricker H, Segal S.** Narcotic addiction, pregnancy and the newborn. Am J Dis Child. 1978;132:360-6.

67. **Levine AB, Rebarber A.** Methadone maintenance treatment and the non-stress test. J Perinatol. 1995;15:229-31.

68. **Stimmel B, Goldberg J, Reisman A, et al.** Fetal outcome in narcotic-dependent women: the importance of the type of maternal narcotic used. Am J Drug Alcohol Abuse. 1982;9:383-95.

69. **Green M, Suffet F.** The neonatal narcotic withdrawal index: a device for the improvement of care in the abstinence syndrome. Am J Drug Alcohol Abuse. 1981;8:203-13.

70. **Remnteria JL, Nuang NN.** Narcotic withdrawal in pregnancy: stillbirth incidence with a case report. Am J Obstet Gynecol. 1973;116:1152-6.

71. **Naeye RL, Blanc W, Beblance W, et al.** Fetal complications of maternal heroin addiction: abnormal growth, infections and episodes of stress. J Pediatr. 1973;83:1055-61.

72. **Jarvis MA, Schnoll S.** Methadone treatment during pregnancy. J Psychoactive Drugs. 1994;26:155-61.

73. **Suffet F, Brotman R.** A comprehensive care program for pregnant addicts: obstetrical, neonatal and child development outcomes. Int J Addict. 1984;19:199-219.

74. **Mitchell JL.** Treatment Improvement Protocol Series (TIPS): Pregnant, Substance Using Women. Rockville, MD: US Dept of Health and Human Services; 1993.

75. **Kaltenbach K, Silverman N, Wapner RJ.** Methadone maintenance during pregnancy. In: State Methadone Treatment Guidelines, Center for Substance Abuse Treatment. Rockville, MD: US Dept of Health and Human Services; 1992.

76. **Briggs GG, Freeman RK, Yaffe SJ.** In: Mitchell CW, ed. Drugs in Pregnancy and Lactation. Baltimore: Williams & Wilkins; 1994:556-8.

77. **National Institute of Drug and Alcohol Abuse.** National pregnancy and health survey—drug use among women delivering live births. Rockville, MD: NCADI; 1992: publication no. BKD192.

78. **Institute of Medicine.** Marijuana and Health. Washington, DC: National Academy Press; 1982.

79. **Harclerode J.** The effect of marijuana on reproduction and development. In: Peterson, ed. Marijuana Research Findings: 1980. Rockville, MD: National Institute of Drug Abuse; 1980:137-66.

80. **Abrams R, Cook C, Davids K, et al.** Plasma delta-9-tetrahydrocannabinol in pregnant sheep and fetus after inhalation of smoke from a marijuana cigarette. Alcohol Drug Res. 1986;6:361-9.

81. **Harbison RD, Mantilla-Plata B.** Placental toxicity, maternal distribution and placental transfer to tetrahydrocannabinol. J Pharmacol Exp Ther. 1972;180:446.

82. **Linn S, Schoenbaum SC, Manson RR, et al.** The association of marijuana with outcome of pregnancy. Am J Public Health. 1983;73:1161-4.

83. **Abel E.** Prenatal exposure to cannabis: a critical review of effect on growth, development and behavior. Behav Neural Biol. 1980;29:137-56.

84. **Fried PA, Watkinson B, Wilan A.** Marijuana use during pregnancy and decreased length of gestation. Am J Obstet Gynecol. 1984;150:23-7.

85. **Gibson GT, Baghurst PA, Colley DP.** Maternal alcohol, tobacco and cannabis consumption and the outcome of pregnancy. Aust N Z J Obstet Gynaecol, 1983;23:15-9.

V. Tobacco and Alcohol Use
Lisa M. Latts

Of all the medical complications of pregnancy, those that are often most difficult for a clinician to address are those that are self-inflicted as a result of a pregnant woman's personal habits. The harms to the fetus of maternal smoking, alcohol use, and drug use are becoming better understood, but our ability to treat and prevent these problems is still limited. The actions taken towards a woman who drinks or uses drugs in pregnancy may now come from the courts instead of the physician's office. The presence of the courtroom in prenatal care raises a myriad of issues, including the rights of the fetus versus the rights of the mother and the right to privacy. Punitive actions toward substance-abusing pregnant women raise the concern that women will be frightened away from prenatal care.

This section describes the epidemiology surrounding commonly used substances in pregnancy, the fetal effects of these substances, and possible ways to encourage cessation of and abstinence from smoking, alcohol use, and drug use in pregnant women.

Smoking and Pregnancy

Epidemiology

In 1973, the U.S. Surgeon General issued a warning about the dangers of smoking in pregnancy, yet tobacco is still the substance most commonly used in pregnancy. The situation is improving. In 1965, 40% of women of reproductive age smoked cigarettes (1). Birth certificate data from the National Center for Health Statistics show that the prevalence of smoking in pregnancy was 13.6% in 1996, down from 20% in 1989 (2). Smoking is increasing among teenagers, however. Of teenagers 15 to 17 years of age, 15.7% smoked in 1996, 5% more than in 1989 (2). Women with 9 to 11 years of education were much more likely than women who had graduated from college to smoke during pregnancy (29% compared with 3%) (3). Smoking during pregnancy was also significantly more likely in women receiving Medicaid than in non–Medicaid-funded women (44% compared with 16.3%) (4) and in unmarried than in married women (5).

Fetal Effects

Tobacco smoke consists of nicotine, carbon monoxide, and approximately 500 other chemicals. The harmful effects of nicotine on the fetus were first discovered in 1957 (6). Nicotine readily crosses the placenta and is 15% more concentrated in the fetal circulation than in the maternal circulation. Nicotine causes vasoconstriction of the uterine and placental blood vessels. Much of the harm of smoking in pregnancy may be related to fetal hypoxia resulting from carbon monoxide. Fetal hemoglobin has a much greater affinity for oxygen than adult hemoglobin does. Carbon monoxide from tobacco smoke is transmitted to the fetus and binds to fetal hemoglobin, creating carboxyhemoglobin. The greater oxygen affinity of fetal hemoglobin facilitates the bond. The fetal carboxyhemoglobin level can be 10% to 15% higher than the maternal level, effecting a 60% reduction in fetal blood flow (7).

Smoking is the leading cause of LBW in the United States. It has been estimated that 21% to 39% of all cases of LBW are due to maternal smoking, and smoking thus accounts for more than 4600 infant deaths per year (8). On average, women who smoke cigarettes during pregnancy have infants that are 150 to 250 g lighter than the infants of women who do not smoke (9). Women who smoke more than one pack per day increase the risk for a LBW infant by 130% (5). The growth restriction seen with smoking in pregnancy is symmetrical, developing early in pregnancy and manifesting as decreased biparietal diameter, decreased crown-to-heel length, and decreased chest and shoulder circumference (1). Smoking cessation during pregnancy can decrease the risk for LBW. If a woman successfully quits smoking during the first trimester or early in the second trimester, her risk for a LBW infant approaches that of a nonsmoker (10, 11).

Smoking during pregnancy is also linked to increased perinatal and neonatal mortality rates. Smoking increases risk for spontaneous abortion, premature delivery, and placental abruption. The relative risk of spontaneous abortion in a smoker compared with a nonsmoker is 1.2 to 1.8 (8, 12). Infants exposed to smoke in utero and in the home after birth are at increased risk for the sudden infant death syndrome (SIDS). The child of a woman who smoked during pregnancy is three times more likely than the child of a nonsmoker to die of SIDS. In addition, a child exposed to environmental tobacco smoke in the home has relative risk for death from SIDS of 2.2 to 2.4 compared with a child in a smoke-free environment (13). Twenty-two percent of annual deaths from SIDS—1178 deaths in 1990—can be attributed to smoking (12).

Children exposed to smoke in utero are more likely to have cognitive and behavioral problems. Mounting evidence indicates an increased risk for mental retardation, lower IQ, and attention deficit with hyperactivity disorder (ADHD) in the offspring of pregnant smokers (14–16). These effects persist after parental IQ and socioeconomic status are controlled for. Naeye and colleagues (16) compared siblings for cognitive ability and attention deficit disorder and found that test scores in the sibling exposed to tobacco smoke in utero were an average of 2% to 4% lower than those in the unexposed sibling. Exposed siblings were also more likely to have ADHD (16).

Additional risks from smoking during pregnancy are being discovered regularly. Some evidence indicates that HIV-positive women who smoke are more likely than nonsmokers to transmit HIV to the fetus (relative risk, 1.45 [95% CI, 1.07 to 1.96]) (17). Preterm infants born to smoking mothers have impaired respiratory function compared with non–tobacco-exposed infants

(18). Infants of mothers who smoke are at increased risk for neonatal respiratory infections and asthma (19).

Cessation Methods

The motivation to quit smoking during pregnancy is strong; 25% to 40% of smokers quit on their own when they become pregnant (1, 20). This quit rate is higher than that at any other point in life. Of women who quit, 21% to 35% have relapse before the end of the pregnancy; 50% resume smoking within 3 months of giving birth; and 70% have relapse within 1 year of delivery. Those who continue to smoke usually smoke fewer cigarettes per day during pregnancy (21).

The clinician plays an important role in encouraging smoking cessation among women who continue to smoke. Smoking cessation early in pregnancy provides the most benefit to the fetus, but cessation at any time will decrease the chances of LBW and SIDS. Even decreasing the number of cigarettes smoked per day is beneficial. One study found that an average decrease of nine cigarettes per day was associated with a 100-g increase in birthweight (22). In 1996, the Agency for Health Care Policy and Research released smoking cessation guidelines that included recommendations for pregnancy (Box 3-4). On the basis of a comprehensive review of the literature, the guideline task force recommends that clinicians strongly encourage all pregnant

---

Box 3-4 Smoking Cessation Guidelines

Recommendation: Pregnant smokers should be strongly encouraged to quit throughout pregnancy. Because of the serious risks of smoking to the pregnant smoker and fetus, pregnant smokers should be offered intensive counseling treatment. (Strength of evidence = A)

Recommendation: Minimal interventions should be used if more intensive interventions are not feasible. (Strength of Evidence = C)

Recommendation: Motivational messages on the impact of smoking on both the pregnant smoker and fetus should be given. (Strength of Evidence = C)

Recommendation: Nicotine replacement should be used during pregnancy only if the increased likelihood of smoking cessation with its potential benefits outweighs the risk of nicotine replacement and potential concomitant smoking. (Strength of Evidence = C)

From Fiore MC, et al. Smoking Cessation. Clinical Practice Guideline No 18. Rockville, MD: US Dept of Health and Human Services, Public Health Service, Agency for Health Care Policy and Research; 1996: AHCPR publication no. 96-0692.

women to quit smoking and refer women to an intensive counseling program if possible (23).

Multiple behavioral interventions to improve rates of smoking cessation in pregnancy have been developed and studied. Greater motivation to quit increases the success of smoking cessation programs in pregnant women compared with programs in the nonpregnant population. Study sites have included public clinics that treat mostly low-income women, private clinics, and health maintenance organization settings. The typical intervention is a 10- to 20-minute counseling session with a health care provider trained in smoking cessation. Most programs include educational materials specific to smoking cessation in pregnancy. Cessation rates in the treatment group range from 4.9% to 31.9%; risk ratios for smoking cessation range from 0.9 to 7.1. Dolan-Mullen and co-workers (11) did a meta-analysis that calculated a combined risk ratio for all studies. The combined risk ratio was 1.50 (95% CI, 1.22 to 1.86), suggesting that intensive counseling can increase the rate of smoking cessation 50% from baseline. Generally, the more intensive and interventional the program, the higher the rate of smoking cessation.

The Centers for Disease Control and Prevention sponsored the Smoking Cessation in Pregnancy project, which was conducted in partnership with state health departments. The elements of the intervention used by this project are outlined in Box 3-5. The critical first step to a successful intervention is identification. A detailed smoking history should be taken at the initial prenatal visit, and follow-up inquiries should be made at subsequent visits. Many

---

Box 3-5 Elements of Smoking Intervention Used by Smoking Cessation in Pregnancy Project

1. Assess smoking status—elicit a smoking history at the prenatal visit and reassess at each visit by using smoking as a "vital sign."
2. Counsel on harms of smoking.
3. Set a quit date, if possible, and, together with the pregnant patient, develop a smoking cessation plan.
4. Teach the necessary smoking cessation skills—provide information on withdrawal, evaluation of smoking patterns and triggers, behavior modification, and coping skills.
5. Provide reinforcement.
6. Prevent relapse.

Adapted from Floyd RL et al. Smoking during pregnancy: prevalence, effects, and intervention strategies. Birth. 1991;18:48-53.

women quit smoking initially as a result of first-trimester morning sickness. These women should receive encouragement and positive reinforcement so that they do not resume smoking after resolution of the morning sickness (5).

The Agency for Health Care Policy and Research guidelines recommend nicotine replacement therapy during pregnancy only if the benefits can be shown to outweigh the risks. The FDA classifies the nicotine patch as a category C drug. In 1991, Benowitz (7) called for the study of the nicotine patch in pregnancy, arguing that the benefits would probably outweigh the risks in certain pregnant smokers, especially those who smoked many cigarettes per day. Few studies have evaluated the use of the nicotine patch in pregnancy. Wright and associates (24) studied the patch in pregnant women over a 6-hour application period and noted no adverse effects. Oncken and colleagues (25) examined a 5-day course of nicotine gum in 19 pregnant smokers. All but two women tolerated the gum without difficulties, and 15 of the 19 were able to refrain from smoking during the trial. There have been no studies of bupropion (Wellbutrin, Zyban) for smoking cessation in pregnancy. Bupropion is a class B drug (i.e., there are no adverse animal data and no human data). Burroughs-Welcome has established a registry for pregnant women exposed to bupropion. Despite the lack of clinical trials and objective data, some practitioners treat heavy smokers with nicotine replacement (26).

Postpartum Period

Many women who successfully quit smoking during pregnancy have relapse after giving birth. Infants exposed to environmental tobacco smoke are at increased risk for SIDS, respiratory infections, asthma, ear infections, and many other problems (27). A few studies extend smoking cessation interventions into the postpartum period to prevent relapse (28). One unique solution is to introduce a counseling intervention into a well-child visit at the pediatrician's office. Severson and co-workers (29) found improved quit rates and lower relapse rates among counseled women compared with controls at 6 months, but no significant difference was seen at 1 year.

Economic Impact

Smoking in pregnancy is associated with significant costs. The Centers for Disease Control and Prevention estimate that costs attributable to prenatal smoking were $1.4 billion in 1995 (30). Break-even points for smoking cessation programs in pregnancy have been estimated at $32 to $80 per patient (31, 32). The estimated ratio of cost to benefit for smoking cessation in pregnancy is 1:3 to 1:6 for short-term benefits and as much as 1:17 for long-term benefits (1).

Alcohol and Pregnancy

Drinking during pregnancy leads to the fetal alcohol syndrome (FAS), a specific pattern of birth defects that includes mental retardation, prenatal and postnatal growth restriction, craniofacial abnormalities, and CNS disorders. A milder form of the condition, fetal alcohol effects (FAE), consists of prenatal or postnatal growth deficiency, mental deficits, and mild facial dysmorphology. The diagnosis of FAS or FAE is made clinically; no genetic or biological markers can help identify children with these disorders. Because of the cognitive component of FAS, this diagnosis is very difficult to make at birth, especially if the history of alcohol use during pregnancy is not known. Occasionally, the diagnosis is not made until a child is enrolled in school. This makes estimates of the true incidence of FAS difficult to determine. Advisories warning of the dangers of alcohol use during pregnancy were released in 1981, 1990, and 1995, yet women continue to drink during pregnancy.

Epidemiology

The use of alcohol during pregnancy may be increasing. Twelve percent of pregnant women surveyed for the Behavioral Risk Factor Surveillance Survey in 1991 reported having drunk alcohol during the preceding month. In 1995, this figure was 16%. The rate of frequent drinking (defined as consumption of an average of seven or more drinks per week or five or more drinks on at least one occasion) also increased significantly, from 0.8% in 1991 to 12.6% in 1995 (33).

The incidence of FAS in the literature varies greatly, depending on whether data were obtained from a passive data source (such as birth certificate or vital statistics data), from a hospital or clinic, or from population-based ascertainment studies. The Centers for Disease Control and Prevention's Birth Defects Monitoring Program reported an incidence of FAS of 6.7 per 10,000 live births in 1993. Using a combination of sources, Abel (34) identified the incidence of FAS in the United States as 2 per 1000—20 times greater than the incidence in Europe. Among children born to heavy drinkers, 4% will have FAS (34). The syndrome is much more common in Native Americans and Alaska natives, possibly because of a genetic predisposition as well as greater use of alcohol in pregnancy (35).

Mothers who deliver children with FAS or FAE tend to be older (>30 years of age), of African-American or Native American ethnicity, and long-term heavy drinkers (36). Having one child with FAS greatly increases the risk for having another. Women who drink alcohol during pregnancy are far more likely to smoke or use other drugs. Cigarettes, when combined with alcohol use, act as a permissive factor for FAS (37).

The estimated annual economic cost of FAS is $74.6 million (38). The major cost associated with the syndrome is the cost of care for mentally retarded persons who require residential care. The figure of $74.6 million does not take into account the costs of other sequelae of prenatal alcohol exposure.

Clinical Characteristics of the Fetal Alcohol Syndrome

Jones and colleagues (39) first described the clinical syndrome of FAS in mothers with chronic alcoholism in 1973. Exposure to alcohol in utero causes a spectrum of abnormalities, with FAS at one extreme and FAE at the other. Children with FAS may have mild or no evidence of facial dysmorphology while showing typical behavioral characteristics or mental retardation (36). No safe threshold has been established for drinking during pregnancy. The likelihood of delivering a child with FAS depends on the timing (the critical period) and the dosage of alcohol use. Binge drinking, which is associated with higher blood alcohol levels, increases the chance that a fetus will have FAS (37). However, even a small daily dose of alcohol can lead to learning impairment (40).

Growth deficiency in FAS is usually moderate to severe. Children with FAS do not exhibit catch-up growth and remain below the 10th percentile for height, weight, and head circumference (36). They may require hospitalization for failure to thrive as infants and may have short stature as adults.

The CNS dysfunction manifests in newborns as irritability and tremulousness (41). As the infants grow, they exhibit IQ deficits; the average IQ is in the range of mild retardation, 60 to 75. If significant facial dysmorphology exists, severe cognitive impairment is more likely (36). Children with FAS also have characteristics of ADHD, especially impulse-control problems and difficulty in school.

Facial dysmorphology is the most noted feature of FAS (Figures 3-2 and 3-3). Children have a flat midface, a flat or absent philtrum, a thin upper-lip vermilion border, a short, upturned nose, epicanthal folds, and short palpebral fissures. These features may become more distinct and recognizable as the child ages (42).

Children with heavy exposure to alcohol in utero are more likely to have major congenital abnormalities, such as cleft palate, intraocular defects, atrial and ventricular septal defects, congenital hip dislocation, vertebral anomalies, and urinary tract abnormalities. They are at risk for certain brain abnormalities, the most common of which are hydrocephalus, cerebral dysgenesis, and cerebellar hypoplasia (41).

In addition to creating the risk for FAS, drinking during pregnancy increases the risk for spontaneous abortion. Women who drink 1 oz of alcohol twice weekly double their chance of a miscarriage (41). The estimated perinatal mortality rate in women with heavy alcohol intake is 17% (43).

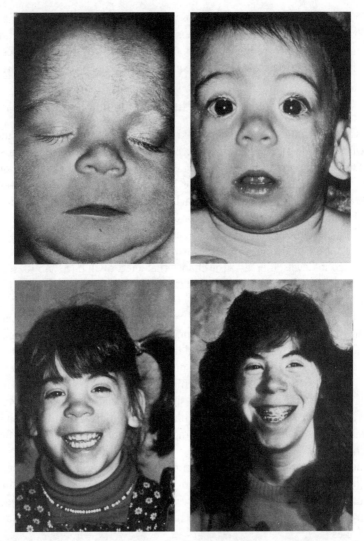

Figure 3-2 Adolescent girl with diagnosis of fetal alcohol syndrome, photographed at birth, at 9 months of age, at 5 years of age, and at 14 years of age. While facial features are gradually maturing, small palpebral fissures, relatively long, smooth philtrum, and narrow upper vermilion persist. (From Streissguth AP, Aase JM, Clarren SK, et al. Fetal alcohol syndrome in adolescents and adults. JAMA. 1991;265:1963; with permission.)

Screening

Because alcohol use is self-reported, it is often difficult to identify patients with alcohol problems. The first barrier is asking the questions. Only 65% of women with a history of heavy alcohol and drug abuse report being asked by

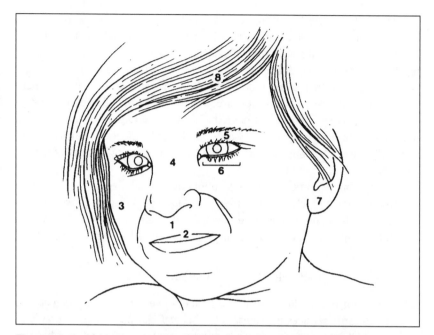

Figure 3-3 Facial features associated with fetal alcohol syndrome. 1. Absent philtrum. 2. Thinned upper vermilion. 3. Hypoplastic midface. 4. Low nasal bridge. 5. Epicanthal fold. 6. Shortened palebral fissure. 7. Low-set ears. 8. Microcephaly. (From Coles CD. Impact of prenatal alcohol exposure on the newborn and the child. Clin Obstet Gynecol. 1993;36: 255; with permission.)

their physicians whether they used drugs or alcohol during pregnancy (44). Of those who were asked, 43% told the truth and 13% lied. Important aspects of the history include concomitant drug and tobacco use and the drinking habits of the father as well as the mother (42).

Screening questionnaires can assist in the identification of persons at risk. Traditional questionnaires include the MAST and the CAGE. Newer questionnaires include the TWEAK (*T*olerance to alcohol, *W*orry (by spouse) about your drinking, have you ever had an *E*ye-opener, *A*mnesia, have you ever felt you needed to *C*ut down on you drinking) and the T-ACE (*T*olerance; do you get *A*nnoyed if someone criticizes your drinking; have you *C*ut down; do you ever have an *E*ye-opener) (45). All four of these questionnaires could greatly increase the identification of heavy drinkers if used aggressively.

Treatment for Alcohol Use

Once a woman is identified as an alcohol user, intervention may be required. In one survey of pregnant women who admitted their alcohol or drug use to a physician, 5% were referred to a drug or alcohol program, 5% were referred to child protective services, and 59% were given no information at all (44).

The Center for Substance Abuse Treatment has called for pregnant women to be given priority at alcohol and drug treatment centers (46). All centers that receive substance abuse block grant funds must treat pregnant women. Nonetheless, few treatment centers are prepared or equipped to care for pregnant women. They often do not have the day care, nutrition, or medical care that may be necessary to care for these complicated patients. Treatment is behaviorally based; Antabuse should be avoided in pregnancy because of teratogenicity (42).

Many pregnant women who use alcohol have a dual diagnosis of the alcohol problem and a psychiatric disorder (47). These dual diagnoses are difficult to treat and often go unrecognized. Specialized treatment centers for women with these diagnoses have only recently been developed and very few exist.

Treatment for Fetal Alcohol Syndrome

It is important that children with FAS be identified early so that they can be directed towards services appropriate to their special needs (48). Behavioral problems and, occasionally, failure to thrive, must be addressed. Cardiac defects often close spontaneously and rarely require surgery. Children with FAS have increased risk for otitis and dental caries, so good hygiene and dental visits are important (42).

It is also important that families with children who have FAS be identified to social services. Women who are heavy alcohol users during pregnancy are likely to continue drinking in the postpartum period. Early intervention may allow for treatment of the mother and may improve the home environment.

REFERENCES

1. **Floyd RL, Rimer BK, Giovino GA, Mullen PD, Sullican SE.** A review of smoking in pregnancy: effects on pregnancy outcomes and cessation efforts. Annu Rev Public Health. 1993;14:379-411.
2. **Ventura SJ, Martin JA, Curtin SC, Mathews TJ.** Report of final natality statistics, 1996. Monthly Vital Statistics Report. 1998;46(11 suppl):1-100.
3. National Center for Health Statistics, Public Health Service. Health, United States, 1995-1996; Hyattsville, MD: PHS 96-1232-1; 89 pp.
4. **Frost FJ, Cawthon ML, Tollestrup K, Kenny FW, Schrager LS, Nordlund DJ.** Smoking prevalence during pregnancy for women who are and women who are not Medicaid-funded. Am J Prev Med. 1994;10:91-6.
5. **Floyd RL, Zahniser SC, Gunter EP, Kendrick JS.** Smoking during pregnancy: prevalence, effects, and intervention strategies. Birth. 1991;18:48-53.
6. **Lambers GS, Clark KE.** The maternal and fetal physiologic effects of nicotine. Semin Perinatol. 1996;20:115-26.

7. **Benowitz NL.** Nicotine replacement therapy during pregnancy. JAMA. 1991;266:3174-7.

8. **U.S. Surgeon General.** The Health Consequences of Smoking for Women: A Report of the Surgeon General, 1983. Washington, DC: U.S. Government Printing Office, U.S. Dept of Health and Human Services; 1983.

9. **Bardy AH, Seppala T, Lillsunde P, Kataja JM, Koskela P, Pikkarainen J, et al.** Objectively measured tobacco exposure during pregnancy: neonatal effects and relation to maternal smoking. Br J Obstet Gynaecol. 1993;100:721-6.

10. **Li CQ, Windsor RA, Perkins LL, Goldenberg R, Lowe JB.** The impact on infant birth weight and gestational age of cotinine-validated smoking reduction during pregnancy. JAMA. 1993;269:1519-24.

11. **Dolan-Mullen P, Ramirez G, Groff JY.** A meta-analysis of randomized trials of prenatal smoking cessation interventions. Am J Obstet Gynecol. 1994;171:1328-34.

12. **DiFranza JR, Lew RA.** Effect of maternal cigarette smoking on pregnancy complications and sudden infant death syndrome. J Fam Pract. 1995;40:385-94.

13. **Schoendorf KC, Keily JL.** Relationship of sudden infant death syndrome to maternal smoking during and after pregnancy. Pediatrics. 1992;90:905-8.

14. **Drews CD, Murphy CC, Yeargin-Allsopp M, Decoufle P.** The relationship between idiopathic mental retardation and maternal smoking during pregnancy. Pediatrics. 1996;97:547-53.

15. **Milberger S, Biederman J, Faraone SV, Chen L, Jones J.** Is maternal smoking during pregnancy a risk factor for attention deficit hyperactivity disorder in children? Am J Psychiatry. 1996;153:1138-42.

16. **Naeye RL, Peters EC.** Mental development of children whose mothers smoked during pregnancy. Obstet Gynecol 1984;64:601-7.

17. **Turner BJ, Hauck WW, Fanning TR, Markson LE.** Cigarette smoking and maternal-child HIV transmission. J Acquir Immune Defic Syndr Hum Retrovirol. 1997;14:327-37.

18. **Hoo A, Henschen M, Dezateax C, Costeloe K, Stocks J.** Respiratory function among preterm infants whose mothers smoked during pregnancy. Am J Respir Crit Care Med. 1998;158:700-5.

19. **American College of Obstetrics and Gynecology.** Smoking and reproductive health. ACOG Technical Bulletin. 1993;180.

20. **Fingerhut LA, Kleinman JC, Kendrick JS.** Smoking before, during and after pregnancy. Am J Public Health. 1990;80:541-4.

21. **Hebel JR, Fox NL, Sexton M.** Dose-response of birth weight to various measures of maternal smoking during pregnancy. J Clin Epidemiol. 1988;41:483-9.

22. **Secker-Walker RH, Vacek PM, Flynn BS, Mead AM.** Smoking in pregnancy, exhaled carbon monoxide, and birth weight. Obstet Gynecol. 1997;89:648-53.

23. **Agency for Health Care Policy and Research.** Clinical Guideline No. 18: Smoking Cessation. Washington, DC: Agency for Health Care Policy and Research; 1996.

24. **Wright LN, Thorp JM, Kuller JA, Shrewsbury RP, Anath CV, Hartmann KE.** Transdermal nicotine replacement in pregnancy: maternal pharmacokinetics and fetal effects. Am J Obstet Gynecol. 1997;176:1090-4.

25. **Oncken CA, Hatsukami DK, Lupo VR, Lando HA, Gibeau LM, Hansen RJ.** Effects of short-term use of nicotine gum in pregnant smokers. Clin Pharmacol Ther. 1996;59:654-61.

26. **Hickner J, Cousineau A, Messimer S.** Smoking cessation during pregnancy: strategies used by Michigan family physicians. J Am Board Fam Pract. 1990;3:39-42.

27. **DiFranza JR, Lew RA.** Morbidity and mortality in children associated with the use of tobacco products by other people. Pediatrics. 1996;97:560-8.

28. **Lowe JB, Windsor RA, Balanda KP, Woodby L.** Smoking relapse prevention methods for pregnant women: a formative evaluation. American Journal of Health Promotion. 1997;11:244-6.

29. **Severson HH, Andrews JA, Lichtenstein E, Wall M, Akers L.** Reducing maternal smoking and relapse: long-term evaluation of a pediatric intervention. Prev Med. 1997;26:120-30.

30. Medical-care expenditures attributable to smoking during pregnancy—United States, 1995. MMWR Morb Mortal Wkly Rep. 1997;46:1048-50.

31. **Shipp M, Croughan-Minihane MS, Petitti DB, Washington AE.** Estimation of the break-even point for smoking cessation programs in pregnancy. Am J Public Health. 1992;82:383-90.

32. **Hueston WJ, Mainous AGI, Farrell JB.** A cost-benefit analysis of smoking cessation programs during the first trimester of pregnancy for the prevention of low birthweight. J Fam Pract. 1994;39:353-7.

33. **Wagner CL, Katikaneni LD, Cox TH.** Alcohol consumption among pregnancy and childbearing-aged women—United States, 1991 and 1995. MMWR Morb Mortal Wkly Rep. 1997;46:346-50.

34. **Abel EL.** An update on incidence of FAS: FAS is not an equal opportunity birth defect. Neurotoxicol Teratol. 1995;17:437-43.

35. **Burd L, Moffatt MEK.** Epidemiology of fetal alcohol syndrome in American Indians, Alaskan Natives, and Canadian Aboriginal Peoples: a review of the literature. Public Health Rep. 1994;109:688-93.

36. **Wekselman K, Spiering K, Hetteberg C, Kenner C, Flandermeyer A.** Fetal alcohol syndrome from infancy through childhood: a review of the literature. J Pediatr Nurs. 1995;10:296-303.

37. **Abel EL, Hannigan JH.** Maternal risk factors in fetal alcohol syndrome: provocative and permissive influences. Neurotoxicol Teratol. 1995;17:445-62.

38. **Stockbauer JW, Land GH.** Changes in characteristics of women who smoke during pregnancy: Missouri, 1978-88. Public Health Rep. 1991;106:52-8.

39. **Jones KL, Smith DW, Ulleland CH, Streissguth AP.** Pattern of malformation in offspring of chronic alcohol mothers. Lancet. 1973;1:1267-71.

40. Surgeon General's Advisory on Alcohol and Pregnancy. FDA Drug Bulletin. 1981;2:10.

41. **Clarren SK.** Recognition of fetal alcohol syndrome. JAMA. 1981;245:2436-9.

42. **Lewis DD, Woods SE.** Fetal alcohol syndrome. Am Fam Physician. 1994;50:1025-32.

43. **Hanson JW, Jones KL, Smith DW.** Fetal alcohol syndrome: experience with 41 patients. JAMA. 1976;235:1458-60.

44. **Gehshan S.** Missed opportunities for intervening in the lives of pregnant women addicted to alcohol or other drugs. J Am Med Wom Assoc. 1995;50:160-3.

45. **Russel M, Martier SS, Sokol RJ, Mudar P, Jacobson SW, Jacobson JL.** Detecting risk drinking during pregnancy: a comparison of four screening questionnaires. Am J Public Health. 1996;86:1435-9.

46. **Nagy PG.** Intensive outpatient treatment for alcohol and other drug abuse. Rockville, MD: US Dept of Health and Human Services; 1994.

47. **Grella CE.** Background and overview of mental health and substance abuse treatment systems: meeting the needs of women who are pregnant or parenting. J Psychoactive Drugs. 1996;28:319-43.

48. **Wagner CL, Katikaneni LD, Cox TH, Ryan RM.** The impact of prenatal drug exposure on the neonate. Obstet Gynecol Clin North Am. 1998;25:169-94.

VI. Violence and Pregnancy
Mary Hepburn

Background

Violence against women is prevalent, takes many forms, and is most often inflicted by men. Moreover, the perpetrator is most often the woman's partner or ex-partner, and the violence is most often experienced at home. Although the term *domestic violence* can imply abuse or violence by either partner in a relationship that may be heterosexual or homosexual, as recognized by a 1995 United Nations report (1), the most common manifestation of domestic violence is violence against women by male partners. In the 1992 British Crime Survey, domestic violence constituted the single largest category of assaults, and 80% of this violence was directed against women (2). In the United States, it is estimated that 95% of battered partners are women (3). Domestic violence can be difficult to define, but a definition such as "the psychological, emotional and economic as well as physical and sexual abuse of women by male partners or ex-partners" (4) indicates the wide range of ways in which women can be abused and the likely circumstances of such abuse.

Although statistics confirm that partners pose the biggest threat of violence and that violence most often occurs in the home, women can be at risk for violence from men in any sexual relationship or in any encounter with men in which sex is a factor. Consequently, women with a particularly high risk for violence are those who engage in prostitution. Like domestic violence, the violence associated with prostitution can be physical, sexual, or psychological. However, it can be inflicted by sexual partners (i.e., those buying the woman's services) or by those who control her activities. In some situations, the violence associated with prostitution overlaps considerably with domestic violence.

Pregnancy affords no protection from either domestic or prostitution-associated violence. Research shows that domestic violence often begins or escalates during pregnancy (5, 6), and women whose financial circumstances necessitate prostitution usually must continue to work during pregnancy. Regardless of the form it takes, violence against women has implications for the health of the woman and any children she may have. Violence against pregnant women also has major implications for the health of the unborn child. This violence is therefore the concern of all those involved in providing care for pregnant women.

Although domestic violence and prostitution-related violence may seem to be disparate problems, they overlap considerably, not only in practical terms but also in cause. In pregnancy, many consequences for mother and baby are common to both types of violence. However, they occur in different circumstances and evoke contrasting national, institutional, professional, and individual responses. As two examples of violence against pregnant women. they provide an interesting contrast.

Domestic Violence

Prevalence

It is difficult to estimate the prevalence of domestic violence against women because many victims are unwilling to involve authorities such as the police or law courts. Moreover, authorities have historically been reluctant to recognize violence between partners as within their remit. Indeed, in the United Kingdom until 1829, a husband had a legal right to chastise his wife, provided that he used a stick "no thicker than a man's thumb." When the violence is sexual, it is even less likely to be recognized as an assault, and the existence of rape within marriage has only been legally recognized in Scotland since 1989 and in England and Wales since 1991. As a result, most reports of domestic violence are gross underestimates. However, in the United States, an estimated 2 to 4 million women are battered each year (1) and 2000 women (30% of female homicide victims) are murdered each year in association with battering (3). Surgeon General Koop, in 1985 (7), declared that domestic violence is a public health epidemic that affects the lives of millions. In the United Kingdom, the Home Affairs Select Committee Report on Domestic Violence (1993) (8) concluded that domestic violence is "common," and the 1992 British Crime Survey (2) stated that 11% of women reported physical violence in their relationships. However, a 1993 crime survey (9) in Islington, London, found that 1 in 4 women reported an experience of domestic violence in their lifetime. The Canadian national survey done in 1993 (10), the most comprehensive survey to date, interviewed 12,300 women older than 18 years of age. It found that at least 3 in 10 women had a history of at least one episode of abuse from a marital partner.

Reported estimates for domestic violence during pregnancy vary from 1/50 (11) to 1/6 (12) pregnant women. During pregnancy, changes are seen in the pattern of violence. The frequency of violence increases. Battered women typically suffer violence at multiple sites and, in pregnancy, the breasts and the pregnant abdomen are particular targets (5).

Characteristics of Abusers and Abused

In the common image of domestic violence, a man from a low social class is beating up his wife while affected by alcohol, drugs, or mental illness. This picture is far from accurate. Although men who abuse their female partners undoubtedly have a range of personality disorders, domestic violence is a world-wide problem that occurs throughout the social spectrum. No consistent relation has been found between domestic violence and employment status or income (13). Although social factors (e.g., unemployment, stress from overwork, drugs, alcohol) are sometimes identified as triggers for abuse and although violence may occur in association with some of these factors, no evidence indicates that it is caused by them. The 1996 British Crime Survey found that offenders were under the influence of alcohol less often in domestic violence situations than in stranger and acquaintance violence situations (14).

Conversely, battering may cause women to develop mental illness; problem drug or alcohol use; or social problems, including homelessness. Poverty and poor social circumstances may limit the ability to escape from the abuse. Women assaulted during pregnancy are more likely to have had psychiatric problems, to have attempted suicide, to smoke or drink alcohol more heavily (13), and to have problem drug use (15). Domestic violence is also more common among separated or divorced women, women of greater parity, teenagers, women with unintended pregnancies, and women who present late for antenatal care (13, 15, 16). However, the important point is that there is no typical abuser and no typical abused woman. Health care providers should be aware that any woman who presents for maternity care is a potential victim of domestic violence. It has been estimated that this violence may be experienced by up to 20% of women seen at antenatal clinics (17).

Health Effects in Pregnancy

Women who experience domestic violence are more likely to present late or irregularly for antenatal care, and they have a higher rate of pregnancy complications, including miscarriage, preterm labor, LBW, and fetal death (18). They are also more likely to have poor health, depression (including suicide attempts), and addiction (5, 13), which add to the risks for their pregnancies. The injuries seen in abused women include bruises, cuts, fractured bones, and internal injuries (19); reported injuries during pregnancy include maternal rupture of the uterus, spleen, or liver, placental abruption, premature spontaneous rupture of membranes, miscarriage, and fetal death (20).

Identification

Most battered women, pregnant or not, are unlikely to volunteer a history of abuse unless they are asked. Unfortunately, they are rarely asked. In one study of 290 pregnant women (21), 23% of women reported battering in the past or present, yet none had been asked about violence by any of the health care providers that they had seen (22). Patients are often more ready for inquiry than providers are. In one U.S. primary care survey, 75% of women favored routine inquiry about physical abuse and 97% of female and male respondents said that they would answer truthfully if asked directly (23). Only 7% reported ever being asked directly by a clinician.

There are many reasons why health care providers may not directly inquire about abuse (22). Many have not been trained to consider the possibility of abuse or to know what to do when it occurs. Some providers fear offending the patient. Furthermore, if violence is identified, advice is too often limited to a recommendation to leave the batterer, frustrating both physician and the patient when the advice is not followed. It is worthwhile for physicians to address their personal barriers to dealing effectively with this common problem. Respectful support for the victim not only reinforces what is often poor self-esteem but also opens the door to discussions with more limited but realistic goals.

Given the possible consequences of domestic violence during pregnancy, identification of this violence is important. It is easy to suspect violence in the presence of injuries, but many professionals do not make the connection. The presence of injuries at various sites and of various ages should ring alarm bells. Other features, such as the woman's age, parity, or marital status, may be associated with an increased relative risk for domestic violence, but many abused women do not have these features, and many women who have not been abused do. The factors associated with increased risk are therefore not specific enough to allow effective screening for domestic violence. Because we have no reliable markers for identification, it seems sensible to ask women directly; consequently, routine inquiry has been recommended by the U.S. Surgeon General (24) and in guidelines issued by the American Medical Association in 1992 (25).

Management

All pregnant women should be asked about violence, and the circumstances of the interview must be conducive to disclosure. All pregnant women should be seen alone at some point during their initial visit. It is vital that a woman who gives a history of abuse is reassured that her story is believed and that confidentiality will be maintained. A woman may deny assault because it did not occur, but denial does not preclude violence, with or without the presence of injuries. Nevertheless, if a woman does not give a history of domestic violence, the caregiver must respect this choice, even if he or she believes that violence has occurred. Maternity care involves relatively lengthy contact between patient and physician and, in time, with development of trust, the woman may feel able to disclose the violence. Even if she does not, the caregiver may find ways to help even without a history of violence ever being made explicit. Awareness should be maintained, especially if subsequent evidence of new or continued injury is seen.

Physical injuries and acute complications of pregnancy require treatment, and the circumstances in which the injuries were sustained should be explored. Careful and detailed documentation of the history and of any injuries is vital because it may be required later as legal evidence. However, the physician's responsibility does not end with medical management.

Whether or not the woman requires admission to hospital, the immediate level of risk to her and her existing children should be ascertained, and appropriate assistance should be offered. The caregiver may think that the woman's best and only course of action is to leave her abusive partner, but most abused women know that this may increase the risk for violence (26). Women who are advised to leave but are unable to do so may feel ashamed of their "weakness" and may therefore not keep subsequent appointments. It is essential to avoid giving such directive advice.

Even if the woman does not want to leave or is unable to leave immediately, she may appreciate help in devising a contingency plan in case she feels able to leave or has to leave urgently at some time in the future. Information, including addresses and contact telephone numbers of relevant agencies for use in such an eventuality, will be helpful and welcome even if the woman does not use it immediately.

Implications for Physicians and Health Care Workers

Those who care for pregnant women must be aware of the true prevalence and distribution of domestic violence, must recognize their responsibility to identify and deal with the violence appropriately, and must possess the necessary knowledge and skills to do this. This requires training at the undergraduate as well as the postgraduate level, and this training should be an integral part of the curriculum for relevant health care workers. Until this is achieved, however, progress can still be made by concentrating on those professionals already providing care who, even if they are aware of the problem of domestic violence, believe that they do not have the skills to deal with it.

Although it is essential that those who ask the questions know how to deal with the answers, all professionals should (and most do) possess the necessary basic skills and already use them in their day-to-day work with pregnant women. Appropriate training is essential, but just as important are an awareness of the problem, the confidence to ask the questions, and the factual knowledge required to provide appropriate management. Organizations in the United States, including the American Medical Association and the College of Obstetricians and Gynecologists (ACOG), were at the forefront of an increasing international response to the issue of domestic violence. Their publications provide detailed information and guidelines for appropriate management of the problem, and educational materials are available through the ACOG resource center.

Prostitution

Prevalence and Predisposing Factors

Like domestic violence, prostitution is hard to define and can take many forms. The legal status of selling and buying physical sexual services varies in different countries, but it is often associated with other illegal activities and is, in one way or another, considered immoral. Because many persons are therefore reluctant to admit their involvement in prostitution, there is a dearth of accurate prevalence data. Both males and females provide sexual services for money, but more females than males provide these services and far more males than females purchase them. Like domestic violence, prostitution occurs throughout the social spectrum. However, at the lower end of the spectrum, financial pressures are greater and options for income generation are fewer. Moreover, problem drug use is more prevalent in association with socioeconomic deprivation, and many women sell sexual services to finance a drug habit. At the lower end of the market, the financial rewards are less and the working environment is more dangerous. Such women, particularly those working on the street, therefore have greater exposure to the various risks—including risk for violence—associated with their work.

Women in the sex industry are usually viewed as willingly engaging in sexual activities, but their willingness is often more apparent than real. Their financial need prevents genuine freedom of choice; moreover, many women are forced to work as prostitutes to provide money for a partner or another man (often, to finance his drug habit). The sex industry is market driven, and women continue to work as prostitutes because there is an enormous and continued demand for their services. Nevertheless, because they are perceived to be willing participants, they are also perceived to be willingly exposing themselves to the risks associated with prostitution. Consequently, the sexual activities that occur are not considered abusive, and violence that occurs in the course of these activities, although recognized as assault, is often perceived as partly the fault of the woman who invited it by engaging in prostitution. However, prostitution's place in the continuum of violence against women was recognized in the United Nations 1995 report (1).

Prostitution in Pregnancy

Women who provide physical sexual services for money often continue to do so during pregnancy. They continue because the circumstances that first brought them to prostitution do not disappear when they become pregnant. In addition, the activities of these women are demand led, and a definite demand for pregnant prostitutes exists. Consequently, women with the greatest financial need often have little choice but to continue to expose themselves to not only the usual risks of prostitution but also to additional risks to their own health and the health of their unborn baby that result from prostitution during pregnancy.

Prostitution during pregnancy carries many risks and causes many problems. Women who engaged in commercial sex around the time of conception are often uncertain about paternity. Although these women may not acknowledge the possibility that their regular partner is not the father—claiming that they use condoms with clients but not with partners—the increased rates that are often paid for unprotected sex make this possibility very real. Partners aware of or involved in the prostitution often collude with the women in this self-deception. Nevertheless, despite this denial, women sometimes admit that the possibility causes them anxiety, especially if there is a risk that it may be confirmed (for example, by the birth of a baby whose ethnicity is obviously not compatible with those of the woman and her partner). Such uncertainty can also lead to violence from the partner during pregnancy. The pregnancy may have been unintended, and this may lead to violence from the partner or a person controlling the woman's activities who perceives that the woman's earning potential will be reduced or interrupted.

Violence from an abusive partner who may or may not be involved in the woman's activities is common and incurs all of the hazards incurred in domestic violence. Violence from clients is also common. For women who work as prostitutes, violent death is an ever-present risk. As discussed above, women who work at the lower end of the market (particularly on the streets) have poorer social circumstances; are more likely to have other problems, such as drug use, that compromise their ability to protect themselves; and work in more dangerous circumstances. These women are especially vulnerable to all of the risks of prostitution, but the potential consequences are greater for those who are pregnant.

Unprotected intercourse with multiple partners carries the risk for sexually transmitted diseases, including HIV infection. During pregnancy, such diseases not only are harmful to the mother but can compromise fetal well-being. They may be transmitted to the baby in utero and can affect development or growth as well as causing both short- and long-term morbidity for the baby from the disease itself. They can also cause complications in pregnancy, including early rupture of the membranes or early delivery. These effects often occur in addition to those resulting from co-existing drug or alcohol abuse and other social factors, such as smoking, poor diet, housing problems, and stress due to lifestyle and general circumstances. All of these effects are frequently compounded by inadequate or absent antenatal care. These women therefore have the potential for very high-risk pregnancies.

Identification

Given the legal and moral status of prostitution, it is not surprising that few women volunteer a history of involvement in it. Unlike the identification of domestic violence, identification of prostitution by routine inquiry is not appropriate. However, it is important that clinicians be constantly aware of the possibility of social problems and be receptive to any markers revealed by a good social history. Problem drug or alcohol use, financial difficulties, or a history of violence should prompt further questioning. Any indication that the woman is unhappy with the estimated gestation or concerned about paternity or the diagnosis of a sexually transmitted disease should lead to a full sexual history. Establishing the situation may take some time and many visits, and more detailed inquiry may not lead to either a direct question about or an admission of involvement in prostitution. As with domestic violence, a woman may not volunteer the information for two reasons: either because it is not true or because she chooses not to tell. Her choice must be respected. However, a high index of suspicion may allow more appropriate and sensitive management, even in the absence of an explicit admission.

Management

Medical management depends on the particular problems identified. If a sexually transmitted disease is considered likely or possible, appropriate screening should be done and treatment should be given if needed. Contact tracing and treatment of sexual partners should also be done if possible and appropriate. Acute obstetric complications should be dealt with in the routine manner, and fetal well-being should be monitored, if necessary, as in any high-risk pregnancy. Conflict between estimated gestation and professed paternity should be handled sensitively and sympathetically. Inappropriate management would obviously not be justified, but a small discrepancy might be resolved by judiciously timed delivery.

Maternal or fetal medical problems due to violence should receive appropriate treatment, and a history of violence in the absence of current injury should prompt assessment of risk. The woman should be helped to escape immediately or to make contingency plans for the future. She should also receive a referral to or information about relevant agencies.

Social management is not the responsibility of health care professionals. However, these professionals should be aware of possible social problems and try to identify them. Underlying problems, such as problem drug or alcohol use, should be addressed, and the woman with the problem should be offered treatment and help from appropriate agencies. In the absence of a specific problem, she will still need assistance from social services, but this should be offered supportively and should, as far as possible, be negotiated with her cooperation. Imposition against her wishes may discourage her from further attendance. Social problems, including drug or alcohol use, should not necessarily be regarded as incompatible with adequate child care. Their effect on the woman's lifestyle should be assessed, and appropriate help should be given to address the problems and minimize their destabilizing effect.

Legal management is currently ineffective and counterproductive. As British barrister Helena Kennedy has observed, "Selling sex as a commodity is perceived as depraved, but it is the seller, not the buyer, who bears the responsibility. The purchaser is seen as the victim of his own sexual needs; again the law promotes the myth that men are ruled by their libido. Prostitution is tolerated because of an acceptance of male promiscuity which is not afforded women" (27). Legislation aims to protect society from the nuisance of prostitution; public health initiatives aim to protect clients from risks, such as risk for HIV infection. There is less emphasis on protecting prostitutes; instead, these persons are punished by legislation that is considered an effective way to eliminate prostitution. However, prosecution of prostitutes is ineffective in reducing prostitution because it does not remove the woman's need to earn money. Indeed, it is often counterproductive because it leads to a fine that simply increases the woman's need to work.

The law gives women little opportunity to protect themselves. The legal view is that prostitutes are "bad" women, and any legal action that they take is unlikely to succeed (27). The police response to the murder of a prostitute contrasts with that to the murder of an "innocent" or "respectable" woman; the latter is seen as a much graver offense indicating mental derangement (27). It is interesting that during a recent series of murders of prostitutes in Glasgow suggestions that a serial killer might be responsible caused great public alarm. Apparently, it is much less disturbing to think that several men rather than one single deranged person might be killing prostitutes.

Summary

Women are at risk for violence in a variety of circumstances and, often, in association with or as a result of other problems. Both the violence and the problems associated with it can affect the physical, psychological, and emotional well-being of the woman and any children she may have. The predisposing circumstances and the consequent violence also occur during pregnancy, when the health of an unborn child is also at risk. Health care professionals often believe that their responsibility is limited to the treatment of injuries and acute medical or obstetric problems that are a direct result of physical violence. However, both the violence and the associated social problems can affect the health of mother and baby in other ways. Consequently, even in the absence of injuries, they are a legitimate concern of health care professionals and, during pregnancy, of persons providing maternity care.

Health care professionals should possess the skills needed to identify these problems and the knowledge necessary to give women relevant information and to involve appropriate agencies. Despite the differing attitudes of society and the law to the different circumstances and types of violence that occur, these professionals should be able to give appropriate care in a nonjudgmental way.

The management of violence against women is merely one example of the need to recognize the link between social problems and health and to adopt a social model of health. Although this concept is gaining increasing recognition, acceptance of it is far from universal. An interagency response, coupled with national recognition that this is an important issue for both health services and those responsible for training health care professionals, is necessary.

REFERENCES

1. Violence Against Women: A World-wide Report. New York: United Nations; 1995.
2. Mayhew P, Maung NF, Mirrlees-Black C. The 1992 British Crime Survey. London: HMSO; 1993.
3. Jones RF. Domestic violence—a physician's perspective. In: Bewley S, Friend J, Mezey G, eds. Violence Against Women. London: Royal College of Obstetricians and Gynaecologists; 1997:76-82.
4. Scottish Needs Assessment Programme. SNAP Report. Glasgow: Scottish Forum for Public Health Medicine; 1997.
5. Stark E, Flitcraft A, Frazier W. Medicine and patriarchal violence. The social construction of a private event. Int J Health Serv. 1979;9:41-93.
6. Bowker LH. Beating Wife Beating. Lexington, MA: Lexington; 1983.
7. Report of the Surgeon General's Workshop on Violence and Public Health. Washington, DC: U.S. Dept of Health and Human Services; 1985.
8. Home Affairs Select Committee. Domestic Violence. London: HMSO; 1993.

9. **Mooney J.** The Hidden Figure: Domestic Violence in North London. London: Islington Council; 1994.

10. **Statistics Canada.** Wife assault: the findings of a national survey. Juristat Service Bulletin. 1994;14:.

11. **Campbell J.** Nursing assessment for risk of homicide, with battered women. Am J Nurs. 1986;86:910-3.

12. **McFarlane J.** Assessing for abuse during pregnancy. JAMA. 1992;267:3176-8.

13. **Hillard PJA.** Physical abuse in pregnancy. Obstet Gynecol. 1985;66:185-90.

14. **Mirrlees-Black C, Mayhew P, Percy A.** The 1996 British Crime Survey: England and Wales. London: The Stationary Office; 1996.

15. **Plichta S.** The effects of woman abuse on health care utilisation and health status: a literature review. Womens Health Issues. 1992;2:154-63.

16. **Gazmararian JA, Adams MM, Saltzman LE, et al.** The relationship between pregnancy intendedness and physical violence in mothers of newborns. Obstet Gynecol. 1995;85:1031-8.

17. **Mezey G.** Domestic violence in pregnancy. In: Violence Against Women. London: Royal College of Obstetricians and Gynaecologists; 1997:191-8.

18. **Bullock L, McFarlane J.** The birthweight/battering connection. Am J Nurs. 1989;98: 1153-5.

19. **Dobash RE, Dobash RP.** Violence against wives. London: Open Books; 1980.

20. **James-Hanman D, Long L.** Crime prevention: an issue for midwives? B J Midwif. 1994;2:29-32.

21. **Helton AS, McFarlane J, Anderson ET.** Battered and pregnant: a prevalence study. Am J Public Health. 1987;77:1337-9.

22. **Sugg NK, Inui T.** Primary care physicians' response to domestic violence: opening Pandora's box. JAMA. 1992;267:3194-5.

23. **Friedman LS, Samet JH, Roberts MS, Hudlin M, Hans P.** Inquiry about victimization experiences: a survey of patient preferences and physician practices. Arch Intern Med. 1992;152:1186-90.

24. **Young A, McFarlane J.** Preventing abuse during pregnancy: a national educational model for health providers. J Nurs Educ. 1991;30:202-6.

25. **American Medical Association.** American Medical Association diagnostic and treatment guidelines on domestic violence. Arch Fam Med. 1992;1:39-47.

26. **Geberth VJ.** Stalkers. Law and Order. 1992;October:138-43.

27. **Kennedy H.** Naughty but nice. In: Eve Was Framed: Women and British Justice. London: Chatto & Windus; 1992.

CHAPTER 4

Hypertension and Renal Disease

I. Hypertension and Preeclampsia
Raymond O. Powrie, MD, and Karen Rosene-Montella, MD

II. Acute Renal Failure
John M. Davison, MD

III. Chronic Renal Disease
John P. Hayslett, MD

I. Hypertension and Preeclampsia
Raymond O. Powrie and Karen Rosene-Montella

Hypertension is the most common chronic medical condition encountered in women of childbearing age. Its estimated incidence among women 20 to 45 years of age varies with race but ranges from 20% to 50%. The management of hypertension in pregnancy is complicated by three factors: the effects of normal pregnancy on blood pressure, the potential effects of antihypertensive agents on the fetus, and the relationship between chronic hypertension and preeclampsia.

Key Values and Normal Physiologic Changes for Hypertension and Renal Disease

	Direction of Change	Percentage Change or Normal Range for Pregnancy
24-hour urinary protein excretion	↑	≤300 mg
Albumin level	↓	3.0 to 3.2 g/dL
Blood pressure	↓	Gradually returns to prepregnancy levels by term
Blood urea nitrogen level	↓	8 to 12 mg/dL
Creatinine clearance rate	↑	120 to 160 mL/min (50% increase)
Creatinine level	↓	0.4 to 0.7 mg/dL
HCO_3	↓	18 to 22 mq/L
Oncotic pressure	↓	10% to 15% decrease
pH	↑	7.44
Renal plasma flow	↑	60% to 80% increase
Renal ultrasonogram	↑	Renal size increased by 1 cm; hydronephrosis
Renin/angiotensin level	↑	2× to 4× increase
Ureteral peristalsis	↓	Ureteral dilatation common
Uric acid level	↓	2.4 to 4.0 mg/dL
Urinary glucose test	↑	2 to 4+

↑ Increase
↓ Decrease
↔ No change

Treatment guidelines for chronic hypertension are based on the role of this condition as a risk factor for cardiovascular illness and death, outcomes that, for the most part, develop over decades rather than in weeks or months. Treatment guidelines for chronic hypertension during pregnancy should focus on fetal and maternal well-being. Chronic severe hypertension in pregnancy has been associated with intrauterine growth restriction (IUGR) and, possibly, placental abruption. However, this is not because of the effects of chronic hypertension per se but rather because of hypertension's role as a risk factor for, and manifestation of, preeclampsia, a condition that can have significant short-term effects on both mother and fetus. Most hypertensive women have excellent pregnancy outcomes. Currently, we have no practical or effective way to predict which women with chronic hypertension will develop preeclampsia or to prevent preeclampsia from occurring in those at risk. In particular, it has been repeatedly shown that good control of blood pressure in the pregnant woman with chronic hypertension does not decrease risk for preeclampsia.

Chronic Hypertension

Proper Measurement of Blood Pressure

Patient Position

Blood pressure in pregnancy should be measured while the patient is in the sitting position. Inferior vena caval compression by the gravid uterus while the patient is supine can alter readings substantially, and measurement of blood pressure in the supine position during pregnancy should therefore be avoided. Up to 10% of pregnant women will have a decrease in systolic blood pressure of more than 30% when supine during the third trimester (the supine hypotensive syndrome) (1). Other women may have aortic compression when supine in the third trimester, and this can lead to a minor degree of aortic coarctation that elevates blood pressures in the arm out of proportion to those in the leg. The common practice of measuring blood pressure while the pregnant patient is lying on her left side should be avoided. If it is necessary to measure blood pressure while the patient is in this position, care should be taken to ensure that the blood pressure cuff and brachial artery are kept at the level of the heart to avoid falsely lowering the blood pressure measurement.

Technique

Use of an automatic blood pressure cuff should be avoided because some evidence indicates that the machines lack validity in the setting of preeclampsia. The diastolic blood pressure should be determined by using Korotkoff sound phase V (extinction of sounds) rather than phase IV (muffling) to maintain consistency with practice in nonpregnant persons. However, data suggest that the disparity between phase IV and phase V is increased in pregnancy and may exceed 10 mm Hg in up to 5% of women. Therefore, some experts have advocated that both phase IV and phase V measurements be obtained and recorded in pregnancy (2).

Role of 24-Hour Blood Pressure Monitors

Despite initial concerns that ambulatory blood pressure monitoring might give inaccurate results in patients with vasospastic conditions, such as preeclampsia, the existing data seem to suggest that 24-hour blood pressure monitors are reliable in assessing blood pressure control in pregnant women (3). The exact role of 24-hour ambulatory blood pressure monitoring in pregnancy has not yet been determined. Some evidence suggests that "white coat hypertension" may be more common and more pronounced in pregnant women. If this is true, ambulatory blood pressure monitoring may help avoid unnecessary hospitalization and treatment in pregnant women. The finding that the normal nocturnal decrease in systolic and diastolic blood pressure is dampened in pregnant women who later develop preeclampsia provides some hope that 24-hour blood pressure monitoring may help in the early identification of pregnant women who will later develop preeclampsia (4).

Normal Changes in Blood Pressure

Systemic arterial blood pressure decreases 10 to 15 mm Hg during pregnancy, with a greater decrease in the diastolic than in the systolic pressure. This decrease begins in the first trimester and reaches a nadir toward the end of the second trimester. During the third trimester, blood pressure returns to baseline. The decrease may be exaggerated in some women with chronic hypertension. The mechanism of this is not clear, but it may be related to the decrease in sensitivity to exogenous angiotensin II noted in pregnant women. In the first few days postpartum, blood pressures often increase above baseline values.

The second-trimester decrease in blood pressure is important because it may mask mild to moderate chronic hypertension during the first two trimesters. Many young women never have their blood pressure measured before they become pregnant, and the new development of blood pressure greater than 140/90 mm Hg in the third trimester can be due either to the development of preeclampsia or to chronic hypertension that was previously masked.

Definition of Hypertension

The definition of hypertension in pregnancy is the same as the definition of hypertension in the nonpregnant population: Blood pressures greater than 140/90 mm Hg are arbitrarily considered "hypertensive." Severe hypertension in pregnancy is defined as a systolic blood pressure greater than 160 mm Hg or a diastolic blood pressure greater than 110 mm Hg. However, it is important to emphasize that most pregnant women have diastolic blood pressures less than 70 mm Hg at 20 weeks of gestation and that a diastolic blood pressure of 85 mm Hg at the end of the second trimester is not particularly "normal" and may indicate underlying chronic hypertension or evolving preeclampsia.

Classification of Hypertension

It is common practice to view any hypertension seen before 20 weeks of gestation as evidence of chronic hypertension. Patients with hypertension that presents for the first time after 20 weeks of gestation should be carefully and frequently evaluated for evidence of preeclampsia and may need to be hospitalized for close observation.

Because of the confusing and overlapping nature of the diagnoses of chronic hypertension and preeclampsia or pregnancy-induced hypertension (PIH), the American College of Obstetrics and Gynecology (ACOG) recommends using a four-category classification when discussing hypertension that occurs during pregnancy. This classification system is shown in Table 4-1.

Table 4-1 American College of Obstetrics and Gynecology Classification of Hypertension in Pregnancy

Class	Description	Comments
I	Disorders unique to pregnancy (preeclampsia, eclampsia)	Significant risk for fetal and maternal morbidity. Almost never occurs before 20 weeks of gestation and usually occurs close to term.
II	Disorders unrelated to pregnancy (chronic hypertension of any cause)	Chronic hypertension not associated with preeclampsia carries minimal risk to the pregnant woman. Risk for intrauterine growth restriction and placental abruption is probably present in less than 1% of women with chronic hypertension without superimposed preeclampsia. Secondary causes of hypertension, such as pheochromocytoma and moderate-to-severe renal disease, can present significant risk to both mother and fetus.
II	Preeclampsia or eclampsia superimposed on chronic hypertension	Because of normal increase in blood pressure that occurs in the third trimester, diagnosis of this entity should never be based solely on increases in blood pressure. Criteria for this diagnosis should include such things as new-onset proteinuria, hyperuricemia, and thrombocytopenia. Substantial increased risk to mother and fetus.
IV	Transient or late hypertension of pregnancy	Isolated blood pressures >140/90 mm Hg toward term. The blood pressure elevation rapidly resolves postpartum. Documentation of normal blood pressures both before and after pregnancy is required. May be a harbinger of chronic hypertension.

Management of Chronic Hypertension

Three Approaches

Although the most important aspect of management in the woman who has chronic hypertension during pregnancy is watching for the onset of signs and symptoms of preeclampsia, the hypertension itself is also a concern. The first management option is for the patient to continue using her current antihypertensive medication, if it is one that has been shown in research and clinical experience to be reasonable for use in pregnancy. Blood pressure should be checked regularly, and the antihypertensive dose should be adjusted as necessary. The need for dosing adjustments during pregnancy is due to the effects of pregnancy on both blood pressure and drug pharmacokinetics. Hepatic metabolism, renal clearance, and volume of distribution of medications are all increased in pregnancy.

The second option is for the patient to take advantage of the physiologic decrease in blood pressure associated with pregnancy and stop using her antihypertensive medication. In this case, the U.S. National High Blood Pressure Education Program (5) advises that medication use be resumed only if the blood pressure exceeds 160/100 mm Hg. The Canadian Consensus recommendations are more conservative and recommend treatment of all persons with blood pressure greater than 140/90 mm Hg (6–8). However, no evidence suggests that control of blood pressure to below 160/100 mm Hg during the 9 months of gestation provides any specific benefits to mother or fetus (9). Surprisingly, despite the simplicity of this management choice, many women who have accepted the diagnosis of chronic hypertension find the idea of discontinuing their medication use for 9 months difficult to accept.

The third option is to switch the patient from a medication that lacks good pregnancy data (either because the medication has a known ill effect on the fetus or because clinical or research experience with the medication in pregnancy is nonexistent) to one for which there is good pregnancy data and to check the blood pressure regularly, adjusting antihypertensive drug dosing as needed.

Specific Antihypertensive Agents

Those medications that are best tolerated and are favored by clinicians who care for patients with hypertension in pregnancy are alpha-methyldopa and labetalol (see Drugs for Chronic Hypertension table at the end of this chapter) (10, 11). Hydralazine, the beta-blockers with intrinsic sympathomimetic activity (pindolol, oxprenolol, and acebutolol), and the calcium-channel blocker nifedipine should be considered second-line agents. All of these agents have been used and studied extensively for the control of hypertension in pregnancy, and their use seems to be relatively free of fetal or maternal complications. Drugs that should be considered third-line agents include other beta-blockers (atenolol and propranolol), clonidine, diltiazem, verapamil, and thiazide diuretics. Use of these agents, however, is limited by either an increased incidence of adverse fetal effects or a relative lack of experience with the drugs in pregnancy.

The only antihypertensive agents that are absolutely contraindicated in pregnancy are the angiotensin-converting enzyme (ACE) inhibitors; their use should be discontinued as soon as pregnancy is diagnosed. Although little evidence of teratogenesis exists with the ACE inhibitors, multiple case reports of fetal anuric renal failure, fetal renal dysplasia, and fetal loss associated with ACE inhibitors have led to their placement in the U.S. Food and Drug Administration's pregnancy classification category X. Some investigators believe that fetal renal perfusion is highly angiotensin II–dependent, and this theory is substantiated by the similarities between ACE inhibitor–induced fetal renal complications and renal complications described in fetuses that received a hypotensive injury in utero (such as that seen in the donor twin in twin–twin transfusion syndrome) (12). The newer angiotensin-receptor antagonists losartan and valsartan are also contraindicated in pregnancy.

Methyldopa is the only antihypertensive agent for which there has been long-term follow-up of children exposed in utero (13). Data clearly show that children exposed to methyldopa in utero had normal physical and mental development similar to that in a control group of children born to mothers who did not use aldomet during pregnancy. Unfortunately, methyldopa is only a moderately effective antihypertensive drug and often leaves women feeling fatigued and mentally "slowed down." Labetalol is, in our opinion, a much better tolerated and more effective antihypertensive agent, although it lacks the long-term follow-up data that makes methyldopa unique.

The second-line antihypertensive agents pindolol, oxprenolol, and acebutolol are as effective as labetalol in controlling blood pressure but are considered second-line agents because of concerns about possible effects on the fetus. The β-blockers propranolol and atenolol have been associated with small-for-gestational-age fetuses when used beginning early in gestation and with neonatal complications such as hypoglycemia and tremor. However, these complications were infrequent with the ISA β-blockers pindolol, oxprenolol, and acebutol.

Dosing of Antihypertensive Agents in Pregnancy

Many antihypertensive agents are cleared more rapidly from the systemic circulation during pregnancy because of a pregnancy-associated increase in hepatic and renal clearance (14). Therefore, hypertension that recurs toward the end of a standard dosing interval should not necessarily be viewed as a treatment failure and can often be managed by shortening the interval. A classic example of this would be the use of atenolol every 12 hours in pregnancy despite the standard use of once-daily dosing in nonpregnant persons. Pharmacokinetic studies of oral labetalol and short-acting nifedipine in pregnancy also suggest a need for dosing intervals shorter than in the nonpregnant patient.

Antihypertensive Agents in the Postpartum Period and in Breastfeeding
All antihypertensive agents, including the ACE inhibitors, are compatible with breastfeeding. It is important to remember that postpartum blood pressure changes may necessitate closer follow-up. In particular, if antihypertensive doses have been increased during pregnancy, patients will probably need to be switched back to their pre-pregnancy dosing in the days after delivery.

Preeclampsia and Pregnancy-Induced Hypertension

Definition

Preeclampsia, toxemia, preeclampsia toxemia, and *PIH gestosis* are often used as interchangeable terms, but the term *preeclampsia* is preferred. This term should be used only to refer to the syndrome in which pregnant women develop manifestations of a multisystem disorder that affects the endothelium; produces diffuse vasospasm; and has a variety of features that can include hypertension, proteinuria, edema, hyperuricemia, renal dysfunction, elevated liver enzyme levels, and thrombocytopenia.

Preeclampsia has no one pathognomonic feature. Although PIH (defined as hypertension occurring in the setting of pregnancy) is one of the main manifestations of preeclampsia, it is not sufficient for the diagnosis. Proteinuria and hypertension are considered to be the key manifestations of this syndrome, but neither is absolutely essential to the diagnosis. The manifestations of preeclampsia should be thought of like the diagnostic criteria for systemic lupus erythematosus: The presence of each manifestation increases the likelihood of the eventual diagnosis. It is important to realize that the clinical and laboratory features of preeclampsia are not the disease itself but are reflections of an underlying process that we are only beginning to understand.

Incidence

Preeclampsia is common and complicates at least 5% to 10% of pregnancies. It is very rare before 20 weeks of gestation, and the vast majority of cases occur close to term (near 38 to 40 weeks of gestation).

Risk Factors

The risk factors for preeclampsia are listed in Box 4-1. Chronic hypertension and nulliparity are the most common important risk factors in the general

---

Box 4-1 Risk Factors for Preeclampsia

Maternal factors
  First pregnancy
  New partner, previous use of barrier contraception, donor sperm
  Age <18 or >35 years
  History of preeclampsia
  Family history of preeclampsia in mother or sister
  Heavy lifting, forced work pace
  Daily consumption of more than four cups of coffee
  Black race
Medical factors
  Chronic hypertension
  Type 1 diabetes, type 2 diabetes, or gestational diabetes; further increase with
    retinopathy, nephropathy, or vasculopathy
  Renal disease
  Systemic lupus erythematosus
  Obesity
  Thrombophilia
Placental or fetal factors
  Multiple gestation
  Hydrops fetalis
  Gestational trophoblastic disease
  Triploidy

---

population; the other factors offer intriguing clues about the possible causes of preeclampsia. The diverse nature of the many risk factors suggests that preeclampsia may be an end point common to a variety of processes.

Pathophysiology

On a pathophysiologic level, preeclampsia is characterized by diffuse endothelial damage and vasospasm. Pathologic examination of affected organs shows areas of endothelial swelling, edema, microinfarctions, and microhemorrhages. The main target organs for preeclampsia are the brain, kidney, liver, lungs, and heart.

Etiology

The etiology of preeclampsia is one of medicine's greatest mysteries, and, in fact, we have a remarkably poor understanding of preeclampsia as a whole. What we do know about the causes of preeclampsia is that the process probably begins early in gestation and is a failure of normal placentation. It has been shown that trophoblastic invasion of the maternal endometrium does not occur normally in women who develop preeclampsia (15). In particular, the interface between the maternal and fetal circulatory systems is less extensive in women who develop preeclampsia than in women who do not. Many manifestations of preeclampsia are therefore thought to be related to a relative ischemia of the placenta. That preeclampsia is a disease of first pregnancies and that its incidence seems to be decreased by a woman's exposure to her partner's semen suggests that at least some of the failure of the placenta to establish adequate circulation within the uterus may be due to an immune response in the mother to foreign antigens that can be at least partly modulated by recurrent exposure to paternal antigens. Associations between preeclampsia and conditions such as diabetes and the thrombophilias suggest that causes of placental ischemia other than inadequate trophoblastic invasion may be involved in some cases of preeclampsia. We still have much to learn about why and how preeclampsia occurs. If, in fact, placental ischemia is important in causing preeclampsia, the mechanisms by which this results in diffuse endothelial damage in the mother remain unclear.

Manifestations

The manifestations of preeclampsia are outlined in Table 4-2.

Table 4-2 Manifestations of Preeclampsia

System	Manifestations of Preeclampsia or Eclampsia
Neurologic	Headache, visual scotoma, scintillations, hyperreflexia, clonus, seizures, cerebral hemorrhage, cerebral ischemia, retinal vasospasm, cortical blindness, exudative retinal detachment
Renal	Proteinuria, hyperuricemia, renal insufficiency, acute tubular necrosis, renal cortical necrosis
Cardiac	Hypertension, generalized edema (including ascites), excessive weight gain, diastolic or systolic cardiac dysfunction
Respiratory	Pulmonary edema
Hepatic	Elevated transaminase levels, hepatic tenderness, hepatic rupture, hepatic infarction, hepatic hemorrhage
Hematologic	Hemoconcentration (elevated hemoglobin concentration), microangiopathic hemolytic anemia, thrombocytopenia, decreased haptoglobin concentration, elevated lactate dehydrogenase and bilirubin levels
Coagulation	Decreased fibrinogen levels, increased fibrin degradation products, elevated INR, and PTT, DIC
Fetal/placental	Oligohydramnios (decreased amniotic fluid), intrauterine growth restriction, evidence of intrauterine hypoxemia on fetal testing, placental infarction, placental abruption, fetal demise

Symptoms

The main symptoms of preeclampsia are visual disturbance, headache, epigastric discomfort, swelling (edema), and rapid weight gain.

Visual Disturbances

The visual disturbances that characterize preeclampsia are scintillations or scotomas and are presumed to be due to cerebral vasospasm. Transient blindness is reported in 1% to 5% of patients who have eclamptic seizure. Serous retinal detachments can also occur and are related to retinal edema.

Headache

The headache that characterizes preeclampsia is usually frontal in location and throbbing in quality. In many ways, it resembles a migraine headache. This is not surprising, given that the mechanism of both migraine headaches and preeclamptic headaches is cerebral vasospasm.

Epigastric Pain

The epigastric discomfort that occurs in preeclampsia can be marked and may be out of proportion to the degree of liver enzyme abnormalities. It is believed to be caused by edema in the liver that stretches the hepatic capsule. In rare cases, it may actually be caused by hepatic infarction. The associated hepatic tenderness can be dramatic. We emphasize the importance of a gentle examination of the liver in patients in whom preeclampsia is suspected because the edematous liver of the preeclamptic patient is at risk for the rare but disastrous complication of hepatic hemorrhage and rupture.

Edema

Edema is present in more than 30% of pregnant women and is therefore not a reliable sign of preeclampsia. Rapid weight gain or edema in the hands or facial area (nondependent edema) is more suggestive of preeclampsia but is still seen in normal pregnancies. Thus, edema is best viewed as a sign that should lead the clinician to consider the possibility of preeclampsia. It is not an essential diagnostic feature of the disorder.

Signs

Signs of preeclampsia include hypertension, retinal vasospasm, right upper quadrant (hepatic) tenderness, and clonus.

Hypertension

Hypertension is an important manifestation of preeclampsia but is not seen in all cases. It is defined as a sustained increase in blood pressure to more than

140 mm Hg (systolic) or 90 mm Hg (diastolic). In the past, a documented increase of more than 30 mm Hg (systolic) and 15 mm Hg (diastolic) from baseline during the course of pregnancy was also viewed as an acceptable criterion for the diagnosis of preeclampsia, but this is no longer thought to be a reliable diagnostic feature of preeclampsia. In fact, evidence from 24-hour ambulatory blood pressure monitoring in pregnancy suggests that normotensive women without preeclampsia may have variations in blood pressure that approach a change of 30/15 mm Hg in the course of 24 hours.

Retinal Disease

Retinal vasospasm can be seen on fundoscopic examination as segmental narrowing of arterial vessels. Retinal edema (in the form of soft exudates), hemorrhage, and exudative retinal detachment can also be seen, but papilledema is remarkably rare. Although many patients using magnesium sulfate report some visual blurring or diploplia, careful testing of visual acuity and fundoscopic examination allows detection of preeclampsia-related cortical or retinal visual alterations. Data suggest that preeclampsia is a potent risk factor for deterioration of retinopathy during pregnancy in patients with type 1 diabetes (16).

Clonus

Clonus is an important sign of preeclampsia but should not be overdiagnosed. Pregnant women often have very brisk reflexes and are not considered to have abnormal deep tendon reflexes until three beats of clonus have been demonstrated.

Laboratory Findings

The laboratory findings in preeclampsia reflect the many systems involved in the process (Table 4-3).

Life-Threatening Manifestations

The life-threatening manifestations of preeclampsia include seizures, cerebral hemorrhage, pulmonary edema, disseminated intravascular coagulopathy (DIC), acute renal failure (ARF), and hepatic rupture.

Seizures

Seizures are the most well-known manifestation of preeclampsia. In fact, the term *preeclampsia* literally means "pre-seizure." Once a seizure has occurred, the diagnosis is changed from preeclampsia to eclampsia. It is estimated that eclampsia is associated with a maternal mortality rate of 5% and a perinatal mortality rate of 130 to 300 per 1000. Fortunately, eclampsia is

Table 4-3 Laboratory Findings in Preeclampsia

	Findings Suggestive of Preeclampsia
Complete blood count	Hemoconcentration evidenced by hemoglobin concentration >12 g/dL (normally near 10 g/dL in gravid women late in pregnancy); thrombocytopenia <150 or sequential decreases within normal range; microangiopathic hemolytic anemia may occur
Urinalysis	Useful only as a screening test for proteinuria; if preeclampsia is suspected, a 24-hour urine study should be collected
24-hour urine collection for measurement of creatinine clearance and total protein	Creatinine clearance <150 or a 24-hour urinary protein level >300 mg should be considered abnormal
Creatinine level	>0.8 mg/dL (70 mmol/L); intravascular volume depletion, renal artery vasospasm, and glomerular endotheliosis all probably contribute
Uric acid level	>5 mg/dL (0.3 mmol/L); renal tubular dysfunction can be an early feature of preeclampsia that precedes proteinuria and is manifested by hyperuricemia (11,12)
AST level	Elevated hepatic transaminase levels are an important manifestation of preeclampsia; even in cases of preeclampsia without epigastric pain or tenderness, elevations in transaminase levels may be seen
INR, PTT	Not routinely necessary unless transaminase levels are elevated, platelet count is low, or patient is set for surgical delivery; a coagulopathy can occur in preeclampsia because of a consumptive coagulopathy; thrombocytopenia and microangiopathic hemolytic anemia may also be present
D-dimer, fibrinogen, FDP levels	Decreased levels of fibrinogen with increased levels of D-dimer and FDP are suggestive of preeclampsia-related intravascular coagulation, but tests for this should not be routinely ordered in the absence of elevated AST, INR, and PTT
Lactate dehydrogenase, bilirubin, and hepatoglobin levels; blood smear to look for fragmented erythrocytes	Findings may suggest preeclampsia-related microangiopathic hemolytic anemia, but tests for this should not be routinely ordered in the absence of a decreasing hemoglobin concentration; lactate dehydrogenase may also increase secondary to liver involvement

currently rare in the developed world (estimates range from 1 in 1000 to 1 in 20,000), presumably because of the aggressive approach taken to early identification of and delivery in preeclamptic patients. Eclamptic seizures are typically *grand mal* with classic clonic–tonic muscular activity followed by a postictal period. However, focal and Jacksonian-type seizures have been described. Classically, seizures are preceded by evidence of neuromuscular irritability with tremulousness, agitation, nausea, vomiting, and clonus, but some patients may have seizure as the initial presentation of preeclampsia. Most eclamptic seizures occur in the context of established preeclampsia with hypertension and proteinuria. However, they have been reported in the absence of proteinuria and hypertension and may occur as late as 7 days postpartum. There have been case reports of eclamptic convulsions occurring as late as 23 days postpartum. The cause of the eclamptic seizure is unclear and is not the same as that of seizures seen with hypertensive encephalopathy because eclampsia can occur with only mild elevations in blood pressure. Autopsies in women who died with eclampsia show varying degrees of cerebral edema, microinfarction, petechial hemorrhage, and fibrinoid necrosis of the cerebral arterioles that are not typical of hypertensive encephalopathy. Electroencephalograms may show epileptiform abnormalities but usually show only a nonspecific diffuse slowing that may persist for weeks after delivery. Computed tomography (CT) and magnetic resonance imaging (MRI) of the eclamptic patient can be normal or can show a wide variety of findings ranging from diffuse edema to focal areas of hemorrhage or infarction. The MRI seems to be more sensitive in detecting abnormalities in eclamptic patients, but both CT and MRI of the brain can be normal in patients who have had eclamptic convulsions. This is particularly true if the imaging study is done in the first 24 hours after the seizure (17).

Cerebral Hemorrhage
Cerebral hemorrhages account for 50% to 65% of deaths from preeclampsia. They can be unpredictable. They are not necessarily due to severe elevations in blood pressure and do not always occur in association with eclamptic convulsions (18).

Pulmonary Edema
Pulmonary edema occurs in about 2.9% of cases of preeclampsia and causes significant maternal morbidity. It is usually seen in the postpartum period, when mobilization of fluid from the third space begins. It occurs as a result of the interplay of decreased preeclampsia-related ventricular function and pulmonary endothelium damage with low plasma oncotic pressure associated with pregnancy, preeclampsia, and the postpartum period. Ventricular dysfunction is seen in up to one third of severe cases of preeclampsia, and echocardiographic studies suggest that both systolic and diastolic dysfunction may occur. Both are believed to be manifestations of vasospastic coronary ischemia and usually resolve rapidly with resolution of preeclampsia. Pulmonary edema may be severe enough to warrant mechanical ventilation.

Disseminated Intravascular Coagulopathy

Disseminated intravascular coagulation can occur as a late and severe complication of preeclampsia or eclampsia. Because most patients with DIC have low platelet counts or elevated transaminase levels, DIC screening in the absence of these abnormalities is generally not necessary (19).

Acute Renal Failure

Although acute preeclampsia is often associated with some degree of renal impairment, ARF in preeclampsia is, fortunately, rare. In addition to the previously described glomerular lesions seen with preeclampsia, acute tubular necrosis (ATN) and partial or total cortical necrosis have been described in preeclampsia and are thought to be related to vasospasm-induced renal ischemia. A full discussion of other causes of ARF in pregnancy is found in the next section of this chapter.

HELLP Syndrome

A particular clustering of the manifestations of preeclampsia is the HELLP syndrome (*H*emolysis, *E*levated *L*iver enzymes, and *L*ow *P*latelet counts). This constellation of symptoms represents a particularly severe form of preeclampsia with significant risk for maternal illness and fetal illness and death (20). Hemolytic anemia may be prominent, and large numbers of schistocytes (fragmented erythrocytes) are seen on peripheral smears of the blood. Haptoglobin levels are usually decreased, and lactate dehydrogenase levels are usually increased.

Hepatic Infarction, Hemorrhage, and Rupture

Hepatic failure may be related to preeclampsia, and when it occurs, a diagnosis of acute fatty liver of pregnancy (AFLP) should be seriously considered. Hepatic infarction, hemorrhage, and rupture have all been reported in preeclampsia and usually present with severe epigastric or right upper quadrant pain. If transaminase levels are 3 to 4 times higher than normal, these vascular injuries should be sought on ultrasonography or CT of the liver.

Fetal Effects

In addition to having maternal manifestations, preeclampsia has significant adverse fetal effects, including decreased amniotic fluid volume, IUGR, placental abruption, and intrauterine death. Often, these complications precede the maternal clinical manifestations of preeclampsia. Placental abruption in preeclampsia usually occurs in the setting of moderate to severe hypertension and is associated with significant fetal morbidity and mortality rates.

Management

In-Patient Monitoring

The unpredictable clinical course and frequent rapid deterioration seen in preeclampsia necessitates hospitalization when the diagnosis of preeclampsia is suspected. Although some studies point to a role for closely monitored outpatient management of mild gestational hypertension remote from term, this management approach can be supported only when a patient is very reliable and a clinician remains very involved in the patient's care (21). Currently, there is no way to predict in whom and when the serious complications of preeclampsia will develop. Thus, close monitoring is required so that a rapid response can address any change in status.

Once in the hospital, the patient should be placed on bedrest, and preeclampsia laboratory screening tests should be done (complete blood count; measurement of creatinine, uric acid, lactate dehydrogenase, and AST; and urinalysis) if they have not already been undertaken. A 24-hour urine sample should be collected for measurement of protein level, creatinine clearance, and creatinine level (to ensure adequacy of collection).

If there is clear evidence of the diagnosis of preeclampsia and the patient is nearing or past 37 weeks of gestation with well-established pregnancy dating, continuing the pregnancy has no benefit. Delivery is always the best treatment for the mother. However, there may be a fetal reason to continue the pregnancy if no maternal life-threatening complications of preeclampsia are present. If there is evidence of fetal compromise, delivery is necessary. Bedrest will decrease blood pressure and edema in preeclamptic patients, but no evidence suggests that it will change outcome. In fact, the treatment of hypertension may mask ongoing multisystem disease and fetal compromise and is appropriate only to prevent malignant hypertension in the mother. Any delay in delivery must be because of uncertainty about the diagnosis or because of fetal immaturity. Guidelines from the ACOG on when it is no longer advisable to delay delivery in a preeclamptic woman at less than 37 weeks of gestation are reviewed in Box 4-2.

Laboratory Tests

If delivery is delayed, laboratory values such as complete blood count, platelet count, AST level, and creatinine level should be monitored closely because they can deteriorate precipitously. It is standard practice to check these tests every 1 to 2 days in a stable, hospitalized preeclamptic patient and with any deterioration or change in the patient's clinical status. In the setting of severe preeclampsia, it is not unreasonable to obtain these values and a coagulation profile every 6 to 8 hours.

Box 4-2 Severe Manifestations of Preeclampsia That Warrant Delivery Before 37 Weeks of Gestation

---

Persistent or frequent blood pressure >160 to 180 mm Hg (systolic) or >110 mm Hg (diastolic) despite treatment

Grand mal seizure

Acute-onset renal failure (serum creatinine level elevated 1 mg/dL above baseline or oliguria <500 mL/24 hours)

Platelet count <100,000/L

Evidence of microangiopathic hemolysis

Elevated alanine aminotransferase or aspartase aminotransferase level to greater than two times normal

Symptoms suggestive of end-organ damage: headache, visual disturbances, epigastric or right upper quadrant pain

Retinal hemorrhage, retinal exudates, papilledema

Pulmonary edema

Fetal compromise suggested by nonstress test or biphysical profile, amniotic fluid index <2, estimated fetal weight less than fifth percentile, reverse umbilical artery end-diastolic flow, abnormal contraction stress test

---

Delivery

When severe preeclampsia is diagnosed, it is always in the mother's interest to deliver the baby. Once delivery has occurred, the manifestations of pre-eclampsia generally resolve rapidly, although preeclampsia can present de novo after delivery. In general, vaginal deliveries can be safely and successfully induced even in patients with severe preeclampsia, and Cesarean section is usually reserved for obstetric indications, such as failure to progress, malpresentation, and fetal distress.

Seizure Prophylaxis and Treatment

Aside from delivery, the most important supportive measure for the preeclamptic woman is the use of an anticonvulsant to prevent seizures. Anticonvulsant therapy is usually started prophylactically once the diagnosis of preeclampsia is firmly established and the manifestations are severe enough to warrant a plan for immediate delivery (Table 4-4). Magnesium sulfate has proven to be the drug of choice for this purpose (22). It is usually given as an intravenous bolus of 4 to 6 g followed by a continuous intravenous infusion of 1 to 4 g/hour to attain a therapeutic plasma concentration of 4 to 7 mmol/L. Alternatively, it can be given in a series of regular intramuscular injections.

Table 4-4   Regimens for Administering Anticonvulsants Used to Prevent Seizures in Patient with Preeclampsia

Agent and Method of Administration	Precautions
Magnesium 4 to 6 g IV load (4 g over 5 to 10 min or 6 g over 30 min) followed by 2 to 3 g IV per hour (40 g in 1 L D5/Ringer lactate at 50 mL/hour)	Therapeutic level for seizure prophylaxis is 4 to 8 mg/dL. Levels of 8 to 12 mg/dL can cause loss of patellar reflexes, diploplia, slurring of speech, flushing, and somnolence. Levels >12 mg/dL can lead to muscular paralysis, hypoventilatory respiratory failure, and cardiac collapse. Antidote for magnesium toxicity is 10 mL of 10% calcium gluconate administered as slow IV push.
IM magnesium 10 g (of a 50% magnesium solution) followed by 5 g IM q4h	Same precautions as above.
Phenytoin 1000 mg IV (in 250 mL normal saline) over 1 hour followed by 500 mg PO 10 hours later (11)	Less effective than magnesium in preventing seizures in preeclampsia but can be used if magnesium fails, acute renal failure is present, or the fluid administration necessary for magnesium infusion is contraindicated and the IM route cannot be used because of thrombocytopenia or coagulopathy.

The only role of magnesium in preeclampsia is that of an anticonvulsant. Despite the possibility of a transient decrease in blood pressure with its initial administration, magnesium has no significant sustained effect on blood pressure. Its mechanism of action remains unclear, but it does not seem to have any intrinsic anticonvulsant effect and may actually prevent seizures through its action as a cerebral vasodilator. If the woman is seizing (Box 4-3), an intravenous benzodiazepine (lorazepam is an excellent choice) is indicated. If an eclamptic convulsion occurs while a patient is receiving magnesium, most clinicians add phenytoin to the regimen. Anticonvulsant therapy can generally be stopped once postpartum diuresis has begun and the manifestations of preeclampsia have started to improve. Although hypertension is usually seen in women with eclampsia, it is not essential to the diagnosis, and control of blood pressure in the setting of preeclampsia has never been shown to decrease a person's risk for seizure.

Treatment of Hypertension

The level at which elevated blood pressure should be treated in the setting of preeclampsia is controversial. It is agreed that blood pressures greater than 180 mm Hg (systolic) and 110 mm Hg (diastolic) should always be treated acutely. In the setting of obvious hypertensive end-organ damage (retinal he-

---

Box 4-3 Acute Management of Eclamptic Seizure

---

1. Ensure that airway is protected and maternal oxygenation is maintained.
2. Give intravenous lorazepam or diazepam to stop seizure acutely.
3. Initiate fetal monitoring.
4. Administer anticonvulsant (*see* Table 4-4).
5. Keep blood pressure <170/110 mm Hg (or <160/100 mm Hg in some recommendations).
6. Check "preeclampsia labs" (especially CBC, creatinine level, AST ± INR, PTT) if they have not been measured recently, and follow closely.
7. Initiate plans for imminent delivery (route to be determined on basis of obstetric indications).

---

morrhage, papilledema, pulmonary edema, severe headache, or renal failure), it is advisable to decrease the blood pressure to no more than 160/100 mm Hg. Beyond this consensus, opinions vary considerably. Although no evidence suggests that blood pressures less than 180/110 mm Hg improve maternal or fetal outcomes in the setting of preeclampsia (23), many persons believe that the risks for seizure, placental abruption, and cerebral hemorrhage are decreased by bringing blood pressures down into the normal or mildly hypertensive range. The alternative position is that because preeclampsia is a dynamic vasospastic disorder with associated target-organ ischemia, it is safest to let blood pressures run in a moderately severe range to avoid worsening ischemia in areas of regional vasospasm. Severe, sudden decreases in maternal blood pressure should be avoided because they may adversely affect uteroplacental and cerebral perfusion. In the absence of direct evidence of end–target-organ damage from severe hypertension, blood pressures should be kept below 170/110 mm Hg.

If urgent or emergent blood pressure reduction is required, intravenous labetalol or intravenous hydralazine can be used. Some evidence indicates that labetalol may be a better choice, although both agents are acceptable (24). Calcium-channel blockers like nifedipine, although previously used by many persons in this setting, should be avoided if the patient is using magnesium because the combination has been associated with severe hypotension and cardiovascular collapse in several case reports. Diuretics should not be used unless pulmonary edema is present. Once the patient has delivered, any antihypertensive agent can be used for blood pressure control. At that point, nitroprusside and nitroglycerin are excellent choices because of their very short half-lives. The doses of the various agents are listed in Table 4-5.

Table 4-5 Drugs Used to Treat Acute Severe Hypertension in Pregnancy

Agent	Bolus Treatment	Infusion	Comments
Intravenous Agents			
Hydralazine	5–10 mg IV every 20–30 min to a total bolus dose of 40 mg	0.5–10 mg/h	Generally considered the first-line parenteral agent for acute control of BP in pregnancy Flushing, tachycardia, nausea, and headache are common maternal side effects Fetal distress and neonatal thrombocytopenia reported
Labetalol	Start with 5–10 mg IV bolus and use a progressively increasing dose (20, 40, 80 mg) every 10 min as needed to control BP up to a total bolus dose of 300 mg	1–2 mg/min	Generally considered a second-line agent after hydralazine IV infusion should be monitored carefully for evidence of cumulative effect (and infusion rate often needs to be decreased with prolonged use)
Nitroprusside	Always should be given as infusion due to extremely short half life	50 mg in 250 mL D5W; start at 0.3 µg/kg/min Titrate to maximum of 10 µg/kg per min Watch thiocyanate levels	Not a first-line agent antepartum because of theoretical possibility of increased fetal sensitivity to thiocyanate
Nitroglycerin	Should always be given as infusion because of extremely short half life	50 mg in 250 mL D5W (i.e., 200 µg/mL), start at 5 µg/min (2 mL/h) and titrate upwards as needed by doubling dose every 5 min	Less widely used in this setting despite theoretical advantages
Oral Agents			
Clonidine	0.1 mg PO load; repeat every hour until desired BP is obtained or maximum of 0.7 mg is given	0.1 mg PO bid; titrate up to maximum of 2.4 mg/d	Risk for rebound hypertension if discontinued suddenly
Methyldopa	1000 mg load PO	500 to 1000 mg PO bid increased by 250 mg per dose until desired effect is obtained or dose of 4 g/d is reached	Effect not usually seen before 4 to 6 h
Labetalol	100 mg PO	100 mg PO bid; titrate to maximum dose of 2400 mg/d	May need to dose tid
Nifedipine	10 mg PO every 3–4 hours	30 mg of long-acting formulation once daily; titrate to maximum of 120 mg/d	Interaction with magnesium sulfate reported to cause severe precipitous hypotension Associated with decreased uteroplacental flow, fetal hypoxia, and acidosis in monkeys

Prevention and Treatment of Pulmonary Edema

It is important to minimize intravenous fluids in the patient with preeclampsia because of the propensity for pulmonary edema. Regular auscultation of the lungs and use of transcutaneous pulse oximetry is critical to identifying pulmonary edema early in patients with severe preeclampsia. This careful observation should be continued in the postpartum period because pulmonary edema often occurs as late as 2 to 3 days after delivery. Acute treatment of pulmonary edema should involve supplemental oxygen, furosemide, and if needed, morphine. An effective dose of furosemide in this setting is often as low as 10 to 20 mg intravenously. If severe hypertension is present, control of blood pressure is very important because increased afterload can be an important contributor to pulmonary edema. Intubation and mechanical ventilation may become necessary if the above measures do not improve the patient's oxygenation.

Acute Renal Failure

Most renal failure in the setting of preeclampsia is rapidly reversible, but if significant hypotension has occurred (as may happen with placental abruption or DIC-related hemorrhage), ATN or renal cortical necrosis may result and necessitate dialysis. In persons with sustained oliguria in the setting of preeclampsia, use of a maximum of two small intravenous fluid boluses (250 cc) to try to improve urinary output is useful. These boluses should be given under close monitoring because of the risk for pulmonary edema. Diuretics should be avoided in the absence of pulmonary edema because of the intravascular volume depletion present in most patients with preeclampsia. If the patient is unresponsive to small fluid boluses, the use of central hemodynamic monitoring to guide appropriate therapy should be considered. However, sustained oliguria in preeclampsia is unusual and therefore significant, and rapid peripartum renal deterioration should also lead to consideration of the differential diagnoses of the hemolytic uremic syndrome (HUS), thrombotic thrombocytopenic purpura, and an entity known as *postpartum renal failure*. Careful microscopic examination of urinary sediment should be done to search for casts and a peripheral smear reviewed for hemolysis.

Postpartum Manifestations

Preeclampsia, like eclampsia, can worsen or even initially present postpartum. Why this is so is difficult to explain. Blood pressure may remain elevated from preeclampsia for 6 weeks to 3 months postpartum, even in the absence of a history of underlying chronic hypertension. However, if laboratory abnormalities, such as thrombocytopenia, elevated creatinine level, or LFT abnormalities persist, further investigation may be warranted. Therefore, careful postpartum follow-up and adjustment of antihypertensive dosing may be necessary in the first several weeks postpartum.

Prevention

Despite considerable research, we have no proven way to prevent preeclampsia. Dietary salt restriction, calcium supplementation, and low-dose acetylsalicylic acid (ASA) have all failed to show a significant effect on the incidence of preeclampsia among women at risk. Calcium supplementation was advocated as a potential preventive intervention because of studies showing that women who developed preeclampsia had decreased urinary calcium levels during pregnancy that may have been due to deficient calcium intake. The use of ASA was advocated because of favorable results in many small trials and the fact that low-dose ASA causes a decrease in thromboxane relative to prostacyclin that was thought to be important in preventing preeclampsia. Unfortunately, the results of major trials with calcium or ASA have been disappointing, and the use of these agents to decrease the incidence of preeclampsia is not supported (25). However, a tantalizing study published in 1997 suggests that the timing of ASA administration during the day may influence ASA's effects, and we may yet hear more about the role of ASA in the prevention of preeclampsia (26). We remain frustratingly ignorant about preeclampsia, and our inability to prevent it in those at risk is a reflection of our lack of understanding of the basic physiologic process that underlies it.

Counseling Women Who Have Had
Preeclampsia about Subsequent Pregnancies

The overall recurrence rate of preeclampsia in subsequent pregnancies seems to be about 18%. Although we would hardly discourage a woman from becoming pregnant again after a pregnancy complicated by preeclampsia, it is important to inform a patient of the risk for recurrence. Women who have severe, early (before 27 weeks of gestation) preeclampsia seem to have an especially high incidence of recurrence of preeclampsia in subsequent pregnancies (66%) and, in particular, a high rate of recurrence of preeclampsia before 27 weeks of gestation (21%) (27). Such women also seem to have a very high incidence of underlying medical disease, including chronic hypertension, renal disease (particularly IgA nephropathy), and thrombophilias. It is therefore recommended that physicians evaluate all patients with early preeclampsia several months after delivery for the presence of these conditions. Women who have atypical and severe manifestations of preeclampsia should be evaluated for underlying hypertension or renal disease several months after delivery to ensure that an underlying chronic medical condition has not been misdiagnosed as preeclampsia (28).

REFERENCES

1. Incidence of supine hypotensive syndrome in late pregnancy. J Obstet Gynecol British Empire. 1960;67:254-8.

2. **Perry IJ, Stewart BA, Brockwell J, et al.** Recording diastolic blood pressure in pregnancy. BMJ. 1990;301:1198.

3. **Biswas A, Choolami MA, Anandakumar C, Arulkumaran S.** Ambulatory blood pressure monitoring in pregnancy induced hypertension. Acta Obstet Gynecol Scand. 1997;76:829-33.

4. **Ayala DE, Hermida RC, Mojon A, Fernanadez JR, Silva I, Ucieda R, Iglesias M.** Blood pressure variability during gestation in healthy and complicated pregnancies. Hypertension. 1997;30:611-8.

5. **National High Blood Pressure Education Program.** National high blood pressure education program working group report on high blood pressure in pregnancy. Am J Obstet Gynecol. 1990;163:1691-712.

6. **Helewa ME, Burrows RF, Smith J, Williams K, Brain P, Rabkin SW.** Report of the Canadian Hypertension Society Consensus Conference: definitions, evaluation and classification of hypertensive disorders in pregnancy. Can Med Assoc J. 1997;157:715-25.

7. **Moutquin J, Garner PR, Burrows RF, Rey E, Helewa ME, Lange IR, Rabkin SW.** Report of the Canadian Hypertension Society Consensus Conference: nonpharmacologic management and prevention of hypertensive disorders in pregnancy. Can Med Assoc J. 1997;157:907-19.

8. Report of the Canadian Hypertension Society Consensus Conference: pharmacologic management of hypertensive disorders in pregnancy. Can Med Assoc J. 1997;157:907-19.

9. **Sibai BM, Mabie WC, Shansa F, Villar MA, Anderson GD.** A comparison of no medication versus methyldopa or labetalol in chronic hypertension during pregnancy. Am J Obstet Gynecol. 1990;162:960-7.

10. **Khedun SM, Moodley J, Naicker T, Maharaj B.** Drug management of hypertensive disorders of pregnancy. Pharmacol Ther. 1997;74:221-58.

11. **Henriksen T.** Hypertension in pregnancy: use of antihypertensive drugs. Acta Obstet Gynecol Scand. 1997;76:96-106.

12. **Pryde PG, Sedman AB, Nugent CE, Barr M.** Angiotensin-converting enzyme fetopathy. J Am Soc Nephrol. 1993;3:1575-82.

13. **Cockburn J, Moar VA, Ounsted M, Redman CWG.** Final report of study on hypertension during pregnancy: the effects of specific treatment on the growth and development of the children. Lancet. 1982;i:647-9.

14. **Loebstein R, Lalkin A, Koren G.** Pharmacokinetic changes during pregnancy and their clinical relevance. Clin Pharmacokinet. 1997;33:328-43.

15. **Khong TY, De Wolf F, Robertson WB, Brosens I.** Inadequate maternal vascular response to placentation in pregnancies complicated by preeclampsia and by small for gestation-al age infants. Br J Obstet Gynecol. 1986;93:1049-59.

16. **Lovestam-Adrian M, Agardh CD, Aberg A, Agardh E.** Preeclampsia is a potent risk factor for deterioration of retinopathy during pregnancy in type 1 diabetics. Diabet Med. 1997;14:1059-65.

17. **Royburt M, Seidman DS, Serr DM, Mashiach S.** Neurologic involvement in hypertensive disease of pregnancy. Obstet Gynecol Surv. 1991;46:656-63.

18. **Sanders TG, Calyman DA, Sanchez, Ramos L, Vines FS, Russo L.** Brain in eclampsia: MRI imaging with clinical correlation. Radiology. 1991;180:475-8.

19. **Kramer RL, Izquierdo LA, Gilson GJ, Curet LB, Qualls CR.** Preeclamptic labs for evaluating hypertension in pregnancy. J Reprod Med. 1997;42:223-8.

20. **Dotsch J, Hohmann M, Kuhl PG.** Neonatal morbidity and mortality associated with maternal hemolysis elevated liver enzymes and low platelets syndrome. Eur J Pediatr. 1997;156:389-91.

21. **Baron JR, Stanziano GJ, Sibai BM.** Monitored outpatient management of mild gestational hypertension remote from term. Am J Obstet Gynecol. 1994;170:765-9.

22. **Lucas MJ, Leveno KJ, Cunningham FG.** A comparison of magnesium sulfate with phenytoin for the prevention of eclampsia. N Engl J Med. 1995;333:201-5.

23. **Witlin AG, Sibai BM.** Hypertension in pregnancy: current concepts of preeclampsia. Annu Rev Med. 1997;48:115-27.

24. **Mabie WC, Gonzalez AR, Sibai BM.** A comparative trial of labetalol and hydralazine in the acute management of severe hypertension complicating pregnancy. Obstet Gynecol. 1987;70:328.

25. **Collaborative Low Dose Aspirin Study in Pregnancy Collaborative Group.** CLASP: a randomized trial of low dose aspirin for the prevention and treatment of preeclampsia among 9364 pregnant women. Lancet. 1994;343:619-29.

26. **Hermida RC, Ayala DE, Iglesias M, Mojon A, Siolva I, Ucieda R, Fernanadez JR.** Time-dependent effects of low dose aspirin administration on blood pressure in pregnant women. Hypertension. 1997;30:589-95.

27. **Sibai BM, Mercer B, Sarinoglu C.** Severe preeclampsia in the second trimester: recurrence risk and long term prognosis. Am J Obstet Gynecol. 1991;165:1408-12.

28. **Goodlin RC.** Preeclampsia as the great impostor. Am J Obstet Gynecol. 1991;164:1577-81.

II. Acute Renal Failure
John M. Davison

Acute renal failure is a clinical syndrome characterized by a sudden and marked decrease in the glomerular filtration rate (GFR), increasing serum creatinine and urea levels, and, usually, urinary output decreased to less than 400 mL/24 hours. Thus, the definition of ARF describes the functional state of the renal tract without defining pathology (1). For the most part, obstetric ARF, whether it occurs during or after pregnancy, occurs in women with previously healthy kidneys. Such patients require multidisciplinary evaluation and treatment, the principles of which resemble those for the nonpregnant patient. However, there are also specific diagnostic and management points that physicians must bear in mind when considering ARF in pregnancy (2). This section focuses on the clinical pathology of ARF and the presentations of ARF that can arise in obstetric practice.

Pathology and Clinical Evolution

Alterations in Renal Morphology and Function

There are three common patterns of ARF that are probably all versions, varying in severity, of one pathologic process: preglomerular vasoconstriction causing renal hypoperfusion with preferential cortical ischemia.

Prerenal Failure or Vasomotor Nephropathy
Vasomotor nephropathy is a relatively mild form of ARF that is caused by moderate degrees of renal ischemia. No changes in renal morphology are seen. The condition is reversible if renal perfusion is promptly improved.

Acute Tubular Necrosis
Acute tubular necrosis occurs if renal ischemia is more severe or persistent. Damage is limited to the most metabolically active tubular cells. Blood vessels and glomeruli do not show significant alteration. This condition is reversible after a variable period of renal shutdown.

Acute Cortical Necrosis
Acute cortical necrosis (ACN) occurs if renal ischemia is very severe or protracted or if intense intravascular coagulation is present. Complete disintegration of glomeruli and tubules throughout the entire cortex of both kidneys may occur, usually with an irreversible clinical course. In pregnancy, however, renal involvement may be patchy; thus, some reversibility may be seen.

Clinical Phases

The three sequential consecutive phases of ARF have important management implications. *Oliguria* is defined as a urine volume less than 400 mL/24 hours for a few days to several weeks. Complete anuria is uncommon in ATN and is usually a manifestation of massive ACN or complete obstruction. Nonoliguric forms of ACN, in which urine volumes seem adequate but renal function is severely impaired, are occasionally seen.

In *polyuria*, urine volumes increase markedly and can be as high as 10 L/24 hours for several days to 2 weeks. Urine is dilute and, despite the large volumes excreted, metabolic waste products are not eliminated efficiently.

Thus, serum urea and creatinine levels continue to increase for several days parallel to increased urinary output. Profound fluid and electrolyte losses endanger survival if not adequately replaced.

In *recovery*, urine volumes decrease toward normal. Renal function gradually improves, nearing the level seen before ARF developed.

Significance

In the 1950s and 1960s, the incidence of ARF in pregnancy was 0.02% to 0.05% and ARF represented about 2% of all cases of renal failure (2, 3). At that time, ARF was a substantial cause of maternal death; at least 20% of women with this complication died.

At the beginning of this new century, ARF still has a bimodal distribution that corresponds to septic abortion early in gestation and bleeding problems and preeclampsia late in pregnancy, but a marked decline overall in obstetric ARF has been seen. This is largely because of the liberalization of abortion laws and to improvements in perinatal care that have reduced the incidence of complications such as sepsis, hypovolemia, severe hemorrhage, and eclampsia (3). The current incidence of ARF in pregnancy is less than 0.005%, but complications with transient mild-to-moderate decrements in the GFR occur in 1 in 8000 deliveries.

Guidelines for Assessment of Obstetric Acute Renal Failure

Before anuria or oliguria is ascribed to ARF, prerenal failure (vasomotor nephropathy) caused by dehydration or hypotension, as well as blockage of the urinary tract (obstructive uropathy), must be excluded. These exclusions are particularly important in obstetric practice. It is all too easy to forget about volume depletion or unwitting damage to the urinary tract when dealing with obstetric emergencies, even though these may cause ARF later (4) (Table 4-6).

It is also crucial to review the history and reappraise all findings and events in conjunction with a nephrologist (2). This review may reveal a background of hemorrhage, obstetric trauma, severe hyperemesis, abortion, chronic renal disease, preeclampsia, sensitization to drugs, inadequate intravascular replacement, or incompatible blood transfusion. It is also important to think of the rare causes of sudden renal dysfunction: sarcoidosis, lymphoma, the Goodpasture syndrome, systemic illnesses (such as endocarditis), ingestion of nephrotoxins, and structural infiltration of the kidneys secondary to extrarenal disease.

Table 4-6 Causes of Acute Renal Failure in Pregnancy

Urinary tract obstruction	Damage to ureters during cesarean section and repair of cervical or vaginal lacerations
	Pelvic hematoma
	Broad ligament hematoma
	Marked polyhydramnios or multiple gestation
Volume contraction/ hypotension	Antepartum hemorrhage (placenta previa)
	Postpartum hemorrhage from uterus or extensive soft tissue trauma
	Abortion
	Hyperemesis gravidarum
	Adrenocortical failure; usually, failure to augment steroids to cover delivery in patient receiving long-term therapy
Volume contraction/ hypotension and coagulopathy	Antepartum hemorrhage (abruptio placentae)
	Preeclampsia or eclampsia
	Amniotic fluid embolism
	Incompatible blood transfusion
	Drug reaction(s)
	Acute fatty liver of pregnancy
	Hemolytic-uremic syndrome
Volume contraction/ hypotension, coag- ulopathy, and infection	Septic abortion
	Chorioamnionitis
	Pyelonephritis
	Puerperal sepsis

Diagnosis and Investigation

Blood should be drawn for complete blood count; measurement of serum urea, creatinine, electrolyte, glucose, amylase, and protein (especially albumin) levels; and measurement of osmolality. Liver function tests should be done, and coagulation indices and acid-base status should be determined in an arterial blood sample. Urine specimens should be tested for specific gravity, osmolality, and electrolyte and protein levels. Determination of the ratio of urine osmolality to plasma osmolality is valuable; the ratio is greater than 1.5 in vasomotor nephropathy and is closer to unity in ATN or ACN. Table 4-7 outlines other relevant tests.

Blood cultures (aerobic and anaerobic), vaginal swabs, and midstream urine should undergo bacteriologic assessment. Abnormalities on the electrocardiogram do not necessarily correlate with the degree of hyperkalemia or hypokalemia. Initially in hyperkalemia, there are peaked T waves with QRS prolongation and then disappearance of P waves with deformation of the QRS complex. Fluid balance must be assessed. Total anuria or alternating periods of anuria and polyuria strongly suggest obstruction, but normal volumes do

Table 4-7 Differential Diagnosis of Oliguria

	Prerenal Failure (Vasomotor Nephropathy)	Acute Tubular Necrosis
History	Vomiting, diarrhea, other causes of dehydration	Dehydration, ischemic insult, nephrotoxin ingestion but no specific history in 50% of cases
Physical examination	Decreased blood pressure, increased pulse rate, poor skin tugor	May have signs of dehydration, but physical examination often normal
Urinalysis	Concentrated urine; few formed elements on sediment but many hyaline cases	Isothenuria; sediment contains renal tubular cells and pigmented casts but may be normal
Urinary sodium	<20 mEq/L; most <10 mEq/L	≥25; usually >60 mEq/L
Urine-to-plasma osmolality ratio	High (often ≥1.5)	Low (<1.1)
Urea	≥20	≤3
Creatinine	>40	<1
Fractional sodium excretion $(U/P_{Na}/U/P_{creatinine})$	<1%	>1%
Renal failure index $(U/P_{Na}/U/P_{creatinine})$	<1	>1

not exclude obstruction. The bladder should be catheterized with continuous drainage so that volumes can be recorded hourly. Central hemodynamic monitoring may be necessary if anuria persists. A separate intravenous-therapy line, preferably in a central vein, should be established. Exact therapy depends on the biochemical disturbances and central venous pressure, renal artery pressure, or wedge pressure readings.

Administration of large amounts of fluid in ATN is both useless and fraught with danger. Blood loss must be taken into account and is frequently underestimated, especially if an antepartum hemorrhage (which is often concealed) has occurred.

Increments in urine flow produced by "loop diuretics," such as furosemide, may represent conversion of oliguric renal failure to a polyuric form rather than reversal of prerenal failure. Furthermore, no evidence shows that loop diuretics have beneficial effects on periods of oliguria, immediate prognosis, or the incidence of death. Proper fluid management should reduce volume overload, but diuretics may be necessary on occasion.

A decision on the timing and route of delivery may need to be made. Ureteric obstruction by the enlarging uterus is very uncommon but does occur, especially in women with a solitary kidney, polyhydramnios, or multiple gestation. Such hydronephrosis might progress to ARF, but the situation usually resolves after amniotomy. If delivery is inappropriate, ultrasonography-guided percutaneous nephrostomy is safe and reliable (1).

To allow assessment of prognosis, biopsy is indicated in patients with protracted oliguria or anuria who fail to improve. Diagnosing ACN early, however, is not mandatory, because the management of the acute stage is no different from the management of ATN.

Pregnancy Complications Associated with Acute Renal Failure

Septic Abortion

Acute renal failure is associated with septic abortion for many reasons (3). Dehydration and hypotension can lead to considerable renal ischemia. Soap and Lysol, common abortifacients, may have specific nephrotoxic effects. The marked hemolysis (with severe anemia) caused by some bacteria and chemical abortifacients is, in itself, enough to provoke renal shutdown. Most sepsis in pregnancy is due to gram-negative bacteria, and clostridia are responsible for only 0.5% of cases in which patients develop shock. Clostridia are also responsible for one of the most devastating syndromes complicating pregnancy.

Presentation can be dramatic, with an abrupt increase in body temperature (to 40 °C) that is often associated with myalgias, vomiting, and diarrhea that is occasionally bloody (2, 3). Once symptoms begin, hypotension, tachypnea, and progression to frank shock occur within hours. The patient is usually jaundiced and has a bronzelike color in association with cutaneous vasodilation, cyanosis, and pallor. Despite fever, the extremities are often cold, and purplish areas that may be precursors of small patches of necrosis are often seen on the toes, fingers, and nose. The clinician may be misled by an asymptomatic patient admitted with an incomplete abortion who rapidly develops shock. Myalgia, often most intense in the thorax and abdomen, may lead to a misdiagnosis of intra-abdominal inflammatory processes. This is especially true when a history of provoked abortion is denied or is not sought because heavy vaginal bleeding is not prominent. Abdominal radiography, however, may show air in the uterus or abdomen as a result of gas-forming organisms or perforation of the uterus.

Knowledge of recent treatment with antibiotics or other drugs is important if bacterial resistance, suppressed infection, and drug-modified physiology are to be diagnosed. Diabetes must be excluded, but blood from a finger prick should not be used if skin perfusion is poor. Leukocytosis (25,000/mm^3) with marked shifts to the left is usual, as is thrombocytopenia (platelet count

<50,000/mm^3). Hypercalcemia severe enough to provoke tetany can occur. The patient may be hypoxic through ventilation-perfusion inequality. The severity of DIC correlates with poor peripheral oxygenation and severity of shock. An increasing and irreversible metabolic acidosis is also a bad prognostic sign.

High doses of antibiotics are essential, but use of clostridia antitoxin, steroids, and surgical intervention is controversial (3). Some favor the radical surgical approach and perform abdominal hysterectomy if the woman responds poorly to resuscitation. On the other hand, modern antibiotics can usually contain infection in the pelvis and eventually eradicate it from the uterus. This may be preferable because many women with a septic abortion may want a pregnancy in the future. In an appreciable number of cases, anuria may persist for 3 weeks or more. Often, the polyuric phase begins just when the patient is thought to have ACN rather than ATN. However, some women with septic abortion do develop ACN, perhaps because of the severity of the ischemic insult or massive DIC.

Pyelonephritis

In the absence of complicating features, such as obstruction, calculi, papillary necrosis, and analgesic nephropathy, it is rare for acute pyelonephritis to cause ARF in nonpregnant persons. However, this association seems to be more common in pregnant women (5). It is known that acute pyelonephritis in pregnancy, in contrast to acute pyelonephritis in nonpregnant patients, is accompanied by decrements in the GFR. It has been suggested that the vasculature in pregnancy may be more sensitive to the vasoactive effect of bacterial endotoxins or cytokines. Pyelonephritis can be a common cause of the adult respiratory distress syndrome in pregnancy.

Preeclampsia, Eclampsia, and HELLP Syndrome

The characteristic renal lesion of preeclampsia is glomerular endotheliosis, in which the glomeruli are enlarged and ischemic as a result of swelling of the intracapillary cells. Significant decreases in the GFR are seen (6). Oliguria is not uncommon and may be a normal response to short-lived prerenal causes. Reduced intravascular volume, poor fluid intake, vasospasm, and decreased arterial pressure secondary to antihypertensive treatment can all predispose to decreased urinary output. Of greater concern is prerenal failure presenting as oliguria after acute blood loss from abruptio placentae or postpartum hemorrhage. This is particularly dangerous if DIC supervenes.

In preeclampsia, ARF preeclampsia is usually due to ATN, but ACN may also occur. It is possible that ATN is the obligatory outcome of glomerular cell swelling, loss of anionic charge, and complete obliteration of the capillary lumen. If the ARF is related solely to preeclampsia without chronic hypertension or renal disease before pregnancy, long-term renal function is normal in about 80% of cases. Underlying chronic problems reduce this figure to 20%; all other patients need long-term dialysis.

The HELLP syndrome was originally thought to be a rare complication of severe preeclampsia, but as more attention has been paid to liver and hematologic function in gravidas, it has been diagnosed more often (6). It is not clear, however, whether ARF is a specific component of the HELLP syndrome itself or a complication of a particularly severe multisystem condition. It may occur, without evidence of hemolysis, as the HELLP syndrome (7).

Acute Renal Failure Specific to Pregnancy

Acute Fatty Liver

Acute fatty liver of pregnancy (AFLP), or obstetric pseudoacute yellow atrophy, is a rare complication of late pregnancy or the early postpartum period; it occurs in approximately 1/13,000 deliveries (3). It is characterized by jaundice; severe hepatic dysfunction, including coma; and varying degrees of renal failure. Reversible urea-cycle enzyme deficiencies (orthinine transcarbamylase and carbamyl phosphate synthetase) resembling those seen in Reye syndrome have been described.

The ARF seems to be due to hemodynamic factors, as it is in the hepatorenal syndrome, but some cases have been associated with DIC (2).

Hemolytic-Uremic Syndrome

The hemolytic-uremic syndrome (HUS), also called *idiopathic postpartum renal failure, postpartum malignant nephrosclerosis, and irreversible postpartum renal failure*, is a rare and often fatal entity characterized by onset of renal failure as late as 3 to 10 weeks postpartum. It usually follows an uneventful pregnancy and delivery (3, 4). The patient develops marked azotemia and severe hypertension, which is often associated with microangiopathic hemolytic anemia and platelet aggregation with formation of microthrombi in the terminal portions of the renal vasculature. It should be remembered that renal failure, microangiopathic hemolytic anemia, and thrombocytopenia may also be associated in gravidas with severe preeclampsia, the HELLP syndrome, AFLP, and thrombotic thrombocytopenic purpura (7, 8, 8a). Distinguishing between these antenatal disorders may be difficult (Table 4-8); close long-term follow-up is required.

Table 4-8 Conditions with Hematologic and Hepatic Involvement Linked to Acute Renal Failure

	Preeclampsia	AFLP	TTP	HUS	Viral or Drug-Induced Hepatitis
Symptoms					
Onset	>20 wk	>28 wk	Any time	Any time	Any time
Nausea and vomiting	− or +	+++	+	+ to ++	+++
Abdominal pain	+ to +++	++	+	−	+/++
Signs					
Hypertension	+ to +++	−/+	+	+ to +++	−
Fever	−	−/+	+	−/+	−/+
Abnormal mental status	− to +++	− to +++	− to +++	−/+	−/+
Liver function tests					
Bilirubin level	NL to 5× ↑	SL to 30× ↑	↑ indirect	↑ indirect	5 to 40× ↑
ALT (SGPT) level	SL to 100× ↑	SL to 30× ↑	NL to SL ↑	NL to SL ↑	SL to >100× ↑
Glucose level	NL	SL to 20× ↑	NL	NL	NL or ↓
Ammonia level	NL	NL or ↓	NL	NL	NL or ↑
Hematologic studies					
White blood cell count	NL to ↑	↑↑	NL or ↑	NL or ↑	NL or ↑
Schistocyte count	+/+++	+/+++	+++	+++	−
Normoblast count	−	+++	+++	+++	−
Platelet count	30K to NL	20 to 150L	5 to 100K	5 to 100K	NL
Prothrombin time	NL or SL ↑	NL to ↑↑↑	NL	NL	NL to ↑↑↑
Fibrinogen level	NL or SL ↓	NL or ↓	NL	NL or SL ↓	↑, NL or ↓
Fibrin degradation products level	NL or SL ↑	NL or ↓	NL	NL or SL ↑	NL
Antithrombin III level	↓	↓	NL	NL	↓
Renal factors					
Creatinine level	NL to 5× ↑	NL to 10× ↑	NL to 5× ↑	Rapid or marked	NL
Proteinuria	1+ to 4++	1+ to 4+	0 to 4+	0 to 4+	NL
Uric acid level	↑	↑	NL or ↑	↑	NL

NL = normal; SL = slight; AFLP = acute fatty liver of pregnancy; TTP = thrombotic thrombocytopenia purpura; HUS = hemolytic-uremic syndrome.

Many patients die despite dialysis, plasmapheresis, exchange transfusion, immunosuppression, and use of heparin, streptokinase, dipyridamole, aspirin, or corticosteroids, alone or in combination. Others survive but require long-term dialysis or transplantation with a risk for recurrence of the HUS lesion in the graft. One etiologic theory implicates lack of prostacyclin, a powerful vasodilator and potent endogenous inhibitor of platelet aggregation. Attempts at management have included exchange transfusion, plasma infusion, plasmapheresis, and prolonged prostacyclin infusion. None of these treatments has proven beneficial (2).

Cortical Necrosis

The incidence of cortical necrosis of pregnancy has decreased over the years to less than 1/80,000 (3). Although cortical necrosis may involve the entire renal cortex, resulting in irreversible renal failure, the "patchy" variety occurs more often in pregnancy. It is more prevalent in multigravidas older than 30 years of age and may be associated with overwhelming septicemia, placental abruption, unrecognized longstanding intrauterine death, and, occasionally, diabetes or preeclampsia. Most cases present in the third trimester or the puerperium.

An initial episode of severe oliguria, which lasts much longer than the episode seen in uncomplicated ATN, is followed by a variable return of function and a stable period of moderate renal insufficiency. Years later, for reasons that are still obscure, renal function may decrease again, often leading to end-stage renal failure.

Management of Obstetric Acute Renal Failure

Treatment of ARF in pregnancy resembles the treatment of ARF in nonpregnant populations and aims to prevent the appearance of uremic symptoms, acid-base and electrolyte disturbances, and volume problems (e.g., overhydration when the patient is oliguric or dehydration in the polyuric phase). There must also be awareness of the propensity of patients with ARF to develop infection, which can be serious in pregnant women (3, 9). Many cases respond to judicious conservative management, but if such an approach is unsuccessful, dialysis is necessary.

Dialysis in patients with ARF can be prescribed "prophylactically"; that is, before the appearance of electrolyte imbalance, acidemia, or uremic symptoms. Such prophylactic dialysis seems even more necessary in pregnant patients who have an immature fetus and in whom temporization is desired (4, 10). Metabolic and biochemical guidelines are given elsewhere (2, 9).

Peritoneal dialysis is effective and safe as long as the catheter is inserted high in the abdomen under direct visualization through a small incision. In fact, there is no difference in outcome factors between hemodialysis and peritoneal dialysis (11, 12). Volume shifts during hemodialysis should be minimized to avoid impairment of uteroplacental blood flow (13). Shorter, more frequent dialysis may be helpful. Controlled anticoagulation with heparin (including monitoring to verify that activated clotting time is maintained between 150 and 180 seconds) is desirable during hemodialysis. Vigilance for vaginal bleeding is also important. Premature contractions or onset of labor often occurs during or immediately after dialysis, and progesterone may be dialyzed, resulting in reduced levels (1, 9). The fetus should be monitored after 28 weeks of gestation during and shortly after dialysis.

In patients with ARF, early delivery (as dictated by fetal maturity) should be done if possible. Blood lost should be replaced quickly to the point of slight overtransfusion because in pregnant patients, uterine bleeding may be concealed and thus underestimated (13, 14).

When delivery is imminent, nursery personnel should be advised that the neonate may be subject to rapid dehydration as a result of increased levels of urea and other solutes in the fetal circulation that precipitate osmotic diuresis.

REFERENCES

1. **Baylis C, Davison JM.** The urinary system. In: Chamberlain G, Broughton-Pipkin F, eds. Clinical Physiology in Obstetrics. Oxford: Blackwell; 1998:263-307.

2. **Lindheimer MD, Katz AI, Ganeval D, Grunfeld JP.** Renal failure in pregnancy. In: Brenner BM, Lazarus JH, eds. Acute Renal Failure, 3d ed. New York: Churchill-Livingstone; 1993:417-39.

3. **Pertuiset N, Grunfeld JP.** Acute renal failure in pregnancy. Baillieres Clin Obstet Gynaecol. 1994;8:333-51.

4. **Krane K, Cucuzzella A.** Acute renal insufficiency in pregnancy: a review of 30 cases. J Mat Fet Med. 1995;4:12-8.

5. **Cunningham FG, Lucas MJ.** Urinary tract infections complicating pregnancy. Baillieres Clin Obstet Gynaecol. 1994;8:353-73.

6. **Gaber LW, Spargo BH, Lindheimer MD.** Renal pathology in preeclampsia. Baillieres Clin Obstet Gynaecol. 1994;8:443-68.

7. **Sibai BM, Ramadan M.** Acute renal failure in pregnancies complicated by hemolysis, elevated liver enzymes and low platelets. Am J Obstet Gynecol. 1993;168:1682-90.

8. **Sibai BM, Kustermann L, Velasco J.** Current understanding of severe preeclampsia pregnancy-associated hemolytic uremic syndrome, thrombotic thrombocytopenic purpura, hemolysis, elevated liver enzymes and low platelet syndrome and postpartum acute renal failure: different clinical syndromes or just different names? Curr Opin Nephrol Hypertens. 1994;3:436-45.

8a. **Kahra K, Draganov B, Sund S, Hovig T.** Postpartum renal failure: a complex case with probable coexistence of hemolysis, elevated liver enzymes, low platelet count, and hemolytic uremic syndrome. Obstet Gynecol. 1998;92:698-700.

9. **Okundaye IB, Abrinko P, Hou SH.** Registry of pregnancy in dialysis patients. Am J Kidney Dis. 1998;31:766-73.

10. **Jones DC, Hayslett JP.** Outcome of pregnancy in women with moderate or severe renal insufficiency. N Engl J Med. 1996;336:226-32.

11. **Jungers P, Chauveau D, Choukronn G, et al.** Pregnancy in women with impaired renal function. Clin Nephrol. 1997;47:281.

12. **Jungers P, Chauveau D.** Pregnancy in renal disease. Kidney Int. 1997;52:871.

13. **Hou SH, Firanek C.** Management of the pregnant dialysis patient. Adv Renal Rep Ther. 1998;5:24-30.

14. **Oosterhof H, Navis CJ, Go JG, et al.** Pregnancy in a patient on haemodialysis: fetal monitoring by Doppler velocimetry of the umbilical artery. Br J Obstet Gynaecol. 1993;100:1140-1.

III. Chronic Renal Disease
John P. Hayslett

Renal disease during pregnancy, whether it results from primary renal disease or systemic disorders, may threaten fetal development as well as the health of the mother. Because assessment of renal function in pregnancy must consider the significant and unique functional changes that occur in normal gestation, these changes are reviewed before the maternal and fetal complications associated with the more common renal disorders are discussed.

Renal Function and Volume Homeostasis

Normal pregnancy is characterized by the gradual cumulative retention of 500 to 900 mmol (mEq/L) of sodium and 6 to 8 L of water, which are distributed between the maternal extracellular fluid and the products of conception. Maternal plasma volume increases 30% to 45%. The incremental increase is most marked in the second trimester and is sustained until term. Renal plasma flow increases by 80% between conception and the second trimester and then, towards term, decreases to a level about 60% greater than the nonpregnant level. The glomerular filtration rate (Figure 4-1) incrementally achieves an increase of 30% to 50% by the ninth week of gestation and is sustained until term, after which it rapidly decreases to nongravid levels (1). The mechanism responsible for this remarkable alteration in renal function is probably caused by the generalized and profound vasodilation that characterizes pregnancy. Observations in normotensive women show that hyperfiltration is caused by plasma flow increments, with only a minor contribution from reduction in capillary oncotic pressure (2).

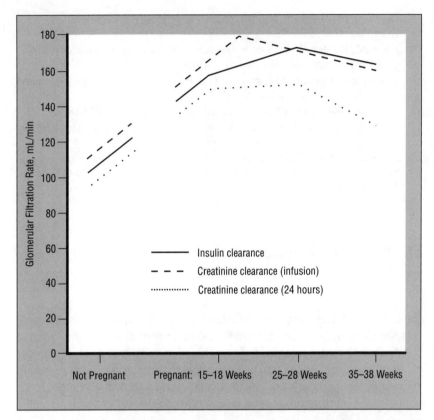

Figure 4-1 Mean glomerular filtration rate by three methods in ten healthy women at 15 to 18, 25 to 28, and 35 to 38 weeks of pregnancy, and again at 8 to 12 weeks postpartum (nonpregnant). (From Davison JM, Hytten FE. Glomerular filtration during and after pregnancy. J Obstet Gynaecol Br Commonwealth. 1974;81:588–95; with permission.)

In clinical practice, simple screening techniques for estimating the GFR usually rely on measurements of serum levels of urea nitrogen and creatinine. Because of the expansion of extracellular fluid and the increase in the GFR, levels of these substances are substantially lower during gestation than in nongravid women. Compared with nongravid values of 13 ± 3 mg/dL (4.7 ± 1 mmol/L) (mean ± SD) of serum urea nitrogen and 0.67 ± 0.14 mg/dL (59 ± 12 µmol/L) of plasma creatinine, levels fall to 8.7 ± 1.5 mg/dL (3.1 ± 0.5 mmol/L) and 0.46 ± 0.13 mg/dL (41 ± 11 µmol/L), respectively, in pregnancy. Concentrations that exceed 13 mg/dL (4.7 mmol/L) of urea nitrogen and 0.8 mg/dL (70 mmol/L) of creatinine suggest the possibility of renal insufficiency. In patients with known or suspected renal insufficiency, formal estimates of GFR are required. In early pregnancy, the GFR can be estimated from the cre-

Table 4-9 Normal Renal Values in Pregnancy by the Second Trimester

Blood urea nitrogen	4–13 mg/dL
Creatinine	0.2–0.8 mg/dL
Glomerular filtration rate	125–200 mL/min
Protein excretion in 24 hours	100–300 mg
Serum albumin	2.8–3.6 g/dL
Uric acid	2.0–4.5 mg/dL

atinine clearance rate, which is obtained from 24-hour urine collections. In the second half of pregnancy, however, the 24-hour estimate of creatinine clearance rate underestimates the maximal capacity for filtration because of pooling of fluid in the lower extremities (see Figure 4-1). Therefore, the creatinine clearance rate should be measured in later pregnancy with the woman lying on her side after hydration with water in such a manner that urine flow exceeds 5 to 6 mL/min.

Mean protein and albumin excretion in pregnancy are also increased. In a series of 270 healthy pregnant women without underlying renal disease, mean protein excretion was approximately 117 mg/24 hours (upper 95% confidence limit, 260 mg/24 hours) and mean albumin excretion was approximately 12 mg/24 hours (upper 95% confidence limit, 29 mg/24 hours) (3). Therefore, protein excretion exceeding 300 mg/24 hours and albumin excretion exceeding 30 mg/24 hours are abnormal in pregnancy. Patients with asymptomatic protein excretion early in pregnancy often develop nephrotic range proteinuria in the third trimester

Table 4-9 gives the normal renal values in pregnancy by the second trimester.

Effect of Intrinsic Renal Disease on Pregnancy

Chronic renal disease may be caused by many types of tissue injury. Regardless of the type of injury, the functional consequences that result in morbidity usually take one of two nonexclusive forms: the nephrotic syndrome and renal insufficiency. This discussion is oriented toward these common clinical expressions of renal disease.

Nephrotic Syndrome

The nephrotic syndrome is defined as proteinuria of at least 3.0 g/d and a serum albumin level of less than 3 g/dL. Patients with this syndrome inevitably have a reduced capacity to excrete sodium and will retain salt and water if sodium intake exceeds the maximum excretory rate. In addition, and apparently as a consequence of hypoalbuminemia, these patients usually have elevated cholesterol and triglyceride levels due to increased lipid production or decreased metabolic clearance. The GFR may be normal or reduced, depending on the severity of the renal injury. It should be emphasized that the nephrotic syndrome always results from an injury reaction that affects the glomerulus (whether due to primary renal disease or systemic disease), which increases the rate of filtration of plasma proteins. Lesser rates of proteinuria can result from either glomerular or tubulointerstitial injury.

The nephrotic syndrome in pregnancy may be caused by pre-existing renal disease, renal disease that develops de novo during pregnancy, or preeclampsia. The distinction between intrinsic renal disease and preeclampsia has important clinical implications because patient management for these conditions differs. In intrinsic renal disease, the goal is usually full-term delivery; in preeclampsia, the aim is delivery when fetal maturity is reached. In patients who have established renal disease before pregnancy or who have proteinuria documented before 20 weeks of gestation, the diagnosis of renal disease is readily made. The onset of proteinuria in the latter part of pregnancy, however, presents diagnostic uncertainty because of the similar clinical features of intrinsic renal disease and preeclampsia. In this case, it may not be possible to confirm a diagnosis of preeclampsia in the absence of coagulation and/or liver function disturbances and/or hemolytic anemia that may suggest preeclampsia. Whenever the distinction between intrinsic renal disease and preeclampsia cannot be made with confidence, it is recommended that the physician make preeclampsia the working diagnosis to reduce the risk of intrauterine death or other fetal complications of preeclampsia that may occur if delivery is delayed (4).

The difficulty in distinguishing between intrinsic renal disease and preeclampsia is highlighted by a report that analyzed 176 patients with proteinuria and hypertension in whom the underlying renal injury was documented by renal biopsy within 6 days of delivery (5). Among primigravidas, the incidence rates of preeclampsia, intrinsic renal disease, and hypertensive glomerulosclerosis were 83%, 12%, and 5%, respectively. Although the nephrotic syndrome is not a common complication of preeclampsia, preeclampsia was the most common cause of de novo nephrotic syndrome in this series. In contrast, in multiparous patients, only 38% had preeclampsia, 26% had renal disease, and 24% had hypertensive renal disease. Because a clinical diagnosis of preeclampsia was made in almost all of these patients during pregnancy, this study shows that primary renal disease can present clinically with the same features as preeclampsia.

Although a complications rate of 4.5% from renal biopsy during pregnancy was reported not to exceed the incidence in nonpregnant patients in one large series from Australia (6), we agree with Lindheimer and Davison (7) that renal biopsy is rarely indicated during pregnancy. The major risk of concern is excessive perirenal bleeding that may compromise the fetus. In cases where fetal survival is unlikely because of severe progressive renal failure in the early stage of gestation, that potential complication may not be an important consideration. However, when the continuation of pregnancy is possible, therapy can usually be introduced based on the apparent clinical diagnosis whereas the histopathological diagnosis is delayed until after delivery.

Three important practical questions arise when pregnancy and renal disease coexist:

1. Does pregnancy adversely affect the course of the underlying renal disease?
2. Are the odds of a successful outcome of pregnancy lowered?
3. What are the maternal complications?

In patients in whom the nephrotic syndrome is caused by intrinsic renal disease, pregnancy is reported to not affect the natural course of the underlying renal disease in the absence of severe hypertension or renal insufficiency (8). In like manner isolated severe preeclampsia is not associated with long-term complications of either hypertension or renal dysfunction (9). In an analysis of a published series of patients who had nephrotic syndrome due to intrinsic renal disease and had preserved renal function, fetal survival was usually normal. Fetal outcome may be worse in patients with nephrotic syndrome due to preeclampsia compared with patients with lesser amounts of proteinuria, probably because high rates of proteinuria represent a more severe form of preeclampsia (5).

With respect to maternal morbidity, the progressive expansion of extracellular fluid can cause massive edema, especially near term, that increases risk for thromboembolic disease, aggravates or causes hypertension, and has been reported to complicate vaginal delivery because of vulvar edema. A recent report (10) also shows that women with preeclampsia-induced nephrotic syndrome may develop dilutional hyponatremia. The impairment in water excretion was ascribed to the nonosmotic mechanism for release of vasopressin, which was activated by a reduction in plasma volume.

The clinical management of patients with nephrotic syndrome should aim to reduce the severity of edema formation. Because proteinuria in patients with asymptomatic levels of proteinuria usually increases during pregnancy to nephrotic levels, we recommend initiating a low sodium intake (1.5 g) in early pregnancy to reduce the rate of edema formation. A low sodium diet is also indicated in all patients with nephrotic syndrome. Dietary sodium restriction is not associated with a reduction of fetal survival or birthweight but does reduce pregnancy-induced increases in plasma volume and cardiac output (11). In addition, frequent periods of bed rest with the woman lying on her side to promote a higher GFR, especially in late pregnancy, will enhance the rate of sodium excretion. In most patients, these conservative measures will suffice to prevent symptomatic edema formation. In cases of primary renal disease where dietary salt restriction does not prevent severe symptomatic edema formation, we recommend diuretics, such as furosemide, to reduce edema to a more tolerable level. To prevent reaccumulation of edema, a natriuretic dose of furosemide is readministered after a weight gain of several pounds but not more often than once every two to three days, while a low sodium intake is maintained. This regimen prevents resistance to the action of loop diuretics and electrolyte abnormalities. Diuretics, however, are not used in preeclamptic patients, where circulating volume is reduced, because of the risk of impairing placental blood flow.

In the absence of significant hypertension or renal insufficiency in patients with intrinsic renal disease, pregnancy is carried to term with the expectation of a vaginal delivery. In preeclamptic patients, the usual approach to this condition is employed. Most patients have spontaneous diuresis, associated with a gradual decrease in urinary protein and an increase in serum albumin, within 2 to 4 weeks of delivery. In patients in whom the cause of nephrotic syndrome has not been established, renal biopsy can be done within 1 week of delivery to determine the type of underlying lesion.

Renal Disease with Normal or Near-Normal Renal Function

Even before the introduction of effective oral antihypertensive agents and modern techniques for monitoring fetal growth and development, some authors reported that the course of pregnancy was relatively uneventful in patients with renal disease who had preserved renal function. The first of several large series of patients with primary renal disease with normal or near-normal renal function was reported in 1980. That study (8) analyzed 121 pregnancies in 89 gravidae. Criteria for inclusion were continuation of pregnancy beyond the first trimester and sufficient data to evaluate the effect of the pregnancy on the underlying renal disease. In all patients, a histologic diagnosis was established. At the onset of pregnancy, the serum creatinine level was 1.4 mg/dL or less in all women, the nephrotic syndrome was present in one third of women, and hypertension was noted in 20% of women. During pregnancy, hypertension increased or occurred de novo in about one quarter of patients, renal function decreased in 16% (most often in women with diffuse glomerulonephritis), and protein excretion increased in 50% and exceeded 3 g/L/d in 39 of 57 pregnancies [68%]). These changes generally resolved after delivery, and the decline in renal function during long-term follow-up was found in this (8) and other studies (12) to be similar to that of the natural course seen with the underlying types of renal disease. The live birthrate was 93%, and the neonatal mortality rate was 5% (Table 4-10). The incidence rates of

Table 4-10 Obstetric Complications in Primary Renal Disease with Preserved and Moderately Reduced Renal Function

	Preserved Renal Function (Cr ≤ 1.4 mg/dL)*	Moderately Reduced Renal Function (Cr > 1.4 mg/dL)†	General U.S. Population‡
No. of pregnancies	121	82	–
Preterm deliveries (<37 weeks), %	20	59	11
Growth restriction (<10th percentile), %	24	37	10
Birthweight ± SD, g	2693 ± 878	2239 ± 839	2800
Stillbirths, %	5	5	0.7
Fetal deaths, %	2	7	0.7
Neonatal deaths, %	4.9	2	0.7
Infant survival rate, %	89	91	98.6

* Data from Katz et al. (8). Cr = creatinine level.
† Data from Jones and Hayslett (18).
‡ Data from Williams' Obstetrics. 20th ed. Stamford, CT: Appleton & Lange, 1997, Chapter 1.

preterm delivery (20%) and small-for-gestational-age infants (24%) were substantially greater than corresponding rates in normal pregnancies (11% and 10%, respectively). These results, which indicate a moderate incidence of reversible maternal complications and a moderate decrease in fetal survival, have been confirmed in other large series that also conclude that pregnancy does not seem to affect the course of the underlying disease. It should be noted that because hypertension was present in a large fraction of patients, it is difficult to determine whether the high incidence of fetal growth restriction and preterm delivery was due to hypertension or another factor related to renal disease. In patients with preserved renal function, however, an analysis of 360 patients with various types of glomerular disease showed that hypertension was associated with a lower rate of renal survival (12).

Reflux nephropathy has been shown to carry a significant risk for prematurity and progression in patients with hypertension, active infection, and abnormal renal function. Patients with adult autosomal dominant polycystic kidney disease tend to do well unless they are hypertensive or have advanced disease; however, they have an increased risk for pyelonephritis and complications from liver cysts (although this is rare) (13). No adverse influence of gestation on the natural course of IgA nephropathy was noted in a series of 36 pregnant patients with preserved renal function compared with 35 controls (14). Diabetic nephropathy and lupus nephropathy have been studied as distinct entities and are discussed in Chapters 5 and 9, respectively.

The use of antihypertensive agents in pregnancy is uncertain and controversial because of the lack of prospective studies involving sufficiently large numbers of patients and the absence of long-term evaluation of these drugs on the physical and mental development of offspring, especially with the newer classes of agents. The Consensus Report of the National Institutes of Health (4) indicates that women with renal disease are at increased risk for superimposed preeclampsia, perinatal morbidity and death, and the possibility of deterioration of renal function, and suggests the use of antihypertension agents if the diastolic blood pressure ≥100 mm Hg. Subsequent studies, however, demonstrate that control of hypertension significantly reduces the rate of decline of renal function in patients with chronic renal disease (15). Based on this information we recommend treatment when the diastolic blood pressure is ≥90 mm Hg. The action and safety of antihypertensive agents in pregnancy are discussed elsewhere (4, 16).

Renal Disease with Moderate or Severe Renal Insufficiency

In contrast to gravidae with preserved renal function, gravidae with moderate (serum creatinine level >1.4 mg/dL [124 μmol/L] and <2.5 mg/dL [222 μmol/L]) or severe (serum creatinine level >2.5 mg/dL [222 μmol/L]) renal insufficiency have been reported to have accelerated underlying disease and markedly reduced fetal survival (50% or less) (17).

The risks for maternal and obstetric complications in pregnancies with pre-existing primary renal disease and a serum creatinine level greater than 1.4 mg/dL (124 μmol/L) at the onset of gestation were recently reported in a series of 82 pregnancies in 67 women (18). These women were equally divided in their type of renal disease; half had chronic glomerulonephritis and half had tubulointerstitial disease. Follow-up in almost all women 12 months after delivery permitted an assessment of the long-term effects of pregnancy on the natural course of renal disease. Maternal complications included a doubling in the incidence of hypertension in the third trimester compared with the first antepartum visit (48% compared with 28%) and the rate of high-grade proteinuria (41% compared with 28%). In addition, a pregnancy-related loss of renal function (occurring during pregnancy or within 6 weeks of delivery) was seen in almost half of all cases. In 23% of this subgroup (10% of the total series), there was rapid progression to end-stage renal failure within 6 months after delivery. The risk for accelerated progression was highest when serum creatinine levels exceeded 2.0 mg/dL (177 μmol/L) at the beginning of pregnancy. Obstetric complications were also more common than in pregnancies associated with preserved renal function and included preterm delivery (59%) and small-for-gestational-age infants (37%). Despite these complications, the overall fetal survival rate was 91% (see Table 4-10).

These findings corroborate several smaller recent studies of 19 to 37 pregnancies that reported fetal survival rates of 76% to 80% (19–21). In these studies 16% to 50% of women had a gestational loss of renal function. The better obstetrical outcomes in recent studies than in older reports probably reflect improved medical and perinatal care and the increased availability of intensive care nurseries for perterm infants.

The effect of hypertension on pregnancy outcome has been examined in women with moderate or severe hypertension. In smaller series a higher incidence of superimposed preeclampsia, preterm deliveries, fetal growth restriction, and fetal loss was observed in women with moderate or severe hypertension than in normotensive gravidae (20, 21). In the large study of 82 pregnancies (18), however, hypertension at onset of gestation did not correlate with fetal survival, preterm delivery, or fetal growth restriction. When present in the third trimester, hypertension was associated with a higher rate of preterm delivery (72% vs. 46%) but not with increased intrauterine growth restriciton (36% vs. 38%) or reduced fetal survival. The presence of high-grade proteinuria at any time during pregnancy had no effect on its outcome.

Dialysis

Dialytic treatment has been employed during gestation when renal failure occurs in women who conceived before the development of severe renal insufficiency and in women receiving chronic dialysis. In the latter case, pregnancy is usually diagnosed in the second trimester because menstrual irregularities are common in renal failure and the typical symptoms of pregnancy are usually attributed to other causes. Ultrasonography is useful for diagnosis as well as for assessment of gestational age because HCG levels are elevated in severe renal insufficiency as a result of a reduction in metabolic clearance.

Information on maternal complications and pregnancy outcome in gravidae supported by dialysis is available only from case reports and small series that probably favor pregnancies with better outcomes. The scarcity of data reflects, at least in part, the fact that dialysis is not commonly used in pregnancy. For example, in 1980 the European Dialysis and Transplant Association (22) reported 16 successful pregnancies in more than 13,000 women of reproductive age receiving chronic dialysis. A recent report from Saudi Arabia (23), however, suggests that the prevalence of fertility in women receiving chronic dialysis may be higher than published reports suggest. In a survey of the incidence of pregnancy in 50% of all women in the country younger than 50 years of age who were receiving long-term hemodialysis between 1985 and 1990, 27 pregnancies were reported in 380 women (incidence, 7%). Ten pregnancies, including the eight that continued for at least 34 weeks, were successful (survival rate, 37%). This result highlights the importance of counseling women of reproductive age on the need for birth control if they wish to avoid pregnancy.

Fetal death is most often related to preterm delivery due to premature labor, although abruptio placenta, fetal distress, and maternal bleeding are also common causes of early delivery. Both hemodialysis and chronic ambulatory peritoneal dialysis have been used, with about equal rates of successful outcome (20% to 50%) (24). Peritoneal dialysis may have theoretical advantages because it avoids dramatic changes in fluid volume and the absence of heparin and allows greater ease in continuing an unrestrictive diet. Redrow and associates (25) reported a consecutive series of eight pregnancies in which peritoneal dialysis was used as therapy for end-stage renal disease. They showed that it was feasible to implant Tenckhoff catheters intraoperatively during pregnancy and that enough space was available in the peritoneal cavity to accommodate adequate volumes of dialysate.

It is common practice to perform hemodialysis daily or every other day (rather than the usual three times per week) to maintain the urea nitrogen level at less than 50 mg/dL and to reduce the likelihood of large changes in fluid volume and electrolytes. The prescription for dialysis, largely based on theoretical considerations, is detailed elsewhere (26). It proposes using a bicarbonate dialysate, rather than one containing acetate, maintaining plasma levels of ionized calcium within a normal range by administering oral calcium and 1,25-vitamin D, and making appropriate adjustments in the dialysate level of calcium. Only minimum doses of heparin are used to reduce risk for bleeding. In addition, control of hypertension to blood pressures no greater than 140/90 mm Hg is recommended. Although there is no significant experience in the use of recombinant erythropoietin in pregnancy, it seems reasonable to use this agent to maintain hematocrit levels above 30% (27, 28).

Renal Transplantation and Pregnancy

Because successful renal transplantation restores fertility as well as renal function, it is not surprising that some women become pregnant or wish to become pregnant after transplantation. The report by Davison (29) on 34 pregnancies in 18 renal allograft recipients managed at a single center provides important insights into pregnancy outcome and the effect of pregnancy on long-term graft function. Of 24 pregnancies in 17 women that went beyond early pregnancy, 11 had adverse prenatal outcomes: five growth-restricted babies, five stillbirths, and one neonatal death. Preterm delivery was common (46%), and five pregnancies ended at or before 32 weeks of gestation. Pregnancy outcome correlated with maternal complications, which included uncontrolled hypertension, renal function deterioration, and graft rejection. A successful obstetric outcome was seen in 73% of women who had complications before 28 weeks of gestation and 92% of women who did not have early complications.

With respect to the effect of pregnancy on graft function, a case-control study done in the same series compared renal function in 18 renal allograft recipients who became pregnant with renal function in 18 matched controls who did not become pregnant (29). No significant difference in graft function was seen during 15 years of follow-up (30).

Lindheimer and Katz (31) stress that counseling at the time of transplantation is important because women who were previously infertile may not be aware of the possible change in their fertility status. In addition, they suggest that women be advised to avoid pregnancy for at least 24 months after surgery because of the higher incidence of rejection, infection, and permanent loss of graft function in the early postoperative period. Recommended guidelines for transplant recipients considering pregnancy are listed in Box 4-4.

A National Transplantation Registry was established in 1991 to study pregnancy outcomes in transplant recipients. Results from the survey of transplantation centers in the United States, published in 1995, are shown in Table 4-11 according to whether patients were immunosuppressed with or without cyclosporine (32). These data show that the incidence rates of live births were 88% in the group without cyclosporine and 70% in the group with cyclosporine. The incidence of low birthweight (<2500 g) was high, from 37% to 50%, primarily because of premature delivery. Table 4-11 also shows that the rate of graft rejection during pregnancy was about 6% to 11% and that the rate of graft loss within 2 years of delivery was about 5% to 10%. Rates of maternal complications, including hypertension, preeclampsia, and infection, were high. Multivariate analysis showed that low birthweight correlated with

---

Box 4-4 Recommended Guidelines for Transplant Recipients Considering Pregnancy

General good health for ≥2 years post-transplant
No (or minimal) proteinuria
No hypertension
No evidence of graft rejection
No pelvic caliceal distention on recent IVP
Stable renal function
On maintenance immunosuppression

Adapted from Lindheimer MD, Katz AI. Pregnancy in the renal transplant patient. Am J Kidney Dis. 1992;19:173-6.

Table 4-11 Obstetric and Maternal Complications in 500 Pregnancies in Transplant Recipients

Variable	Non-CsA	CsA
No. of pregnancies	252	197
Obstetric complications, %		
Premature (<37 wks)	52	54
Low birthweight (<2500 g)	37	40
Live births	88	70
Maternal complications, %		
Hypertension	21	56
Preeclampsia	20	29
Infection	18	22
Rejection	6.5	11.1
Graft loss (2 years after delivery)	4.5	8.9

Adapted from Radomski JS et al. Outcomes of 500 pregnancies in 335 female kidney, liver and heart transplant patients. Transplant Proc. 1995;27:1089-90. CSA = cyclosporine administration.

hypertension, a plasma creatinine level greater than 1.5 mg/dL, and pregnancy within 2 years of surgery.

The Registry data therefore confirm earlier experience in female renal transplant recipients that showed fetal survival in about 75% of pregnancies, a rate associated with a high incidence of obstetric and maternal complications, including a 5% to 10% chance of loss of graft function. These data also provide information on the introduction of cyclosporin A in graft management and show that the incidence of low-birthweight infants and maternal hypertension is higher than in the azathioprine era.

REFERENCES

1. **Davison JM, Baylis C.** Pregnancy in patients with underlying renal disease. In: Davison JM, Cameron JC, Grunfeld J-P, Kerr DNS, Ritz E, Winearls CG, eds. Oxford Textbook of Nephrology, 2d ed. Oxford: Oxford Univ Press; 1998:2327-48.

3. **Roberts M, Lindheimer MD, Davison JM.** Altered glomerular permselectivity to neutral dextrans and heteroporous membrane modeling in human pregnancy. Am J Physiol. 1996;270:338-43.

3. **Higby KM, Suiter CR, Phelps JY, Siler-Khodr T, Langer O.** Normal values of urinary albumin and total protein excretion during pregnancy. Am J Obstet Gynecol. 1994; 171:984-9.

4. National High Blood Pressure Education Program Working Group Report on High Blood Pressure in Pregnancy. Am J Obstet Gynecol. 1990;163:1691-712.

5. **Fisher KA, Luger A, Spargo BH, Lindheimer MD.** Hypertension in pregnancy: clinical-pathological correlations and remote prognosis. Medicine (Baltimore). 1981;60: 267-76.

6. **Packham DK, Fairley KF.** Renal biopsy: indications and complications in pregnancy. Br J Obstet Gynaecol. 1987;94:935-9.

7. **Lindheimer MD, Davison JM.** Renal biopsy in pregnancy. "To b...or not to b...?" Br J Obstet Gynaecol. 1987;94:932-4.

8. **Katz AI, Davison JM, Hayslett JP, Singson E, Lindheimer MD.** Pregnancy in women with kidney disease. Kidney Int. 1980;18:192-206.

9. **Chesley LC.** Remote prognosis. In: Chesley LC, ed. Hypertensive Disorders of Pregnancy. New York: Appleton-Century-Crofts; 1978:421.

10. **Hayslett JP, Katz DL, Knudson JM.** Dilutional hyponatremia in preeclampsia. Am J Obstet Gynecol. 1998;179:1312-6.

11. **Steegers EAP, van Lakwijk HPJM, Jongsma HW, Fast JH, deBoo T, Eskes TKAB, Hein PR.** (Patho)physiological implications of chronic dietary sodium restriction during pregnancy: a longitudinal prospective randomized study. Br J Obstet Gynecol. 1991;98:980-7.

12. **Jungers P, Houillier P, Forget D, Labrunie M, Skhiri H, Giatras I, Descamps-Latsscha B.** Influence of pregnancy on the course of primary chronic glomerulonephritis. Lancet. 1995;346:1122-4.

13. **Gabow P, Johnson A, Kaehny WD, et al.** Factors affecting the progression of renal disease in autosomal dominant polycystic kidney disease. Kidney Int. 1992;41:1311-9.

14. **Abe S.** The influence of pregnancy on the long-term renal prognosis of IgA nephropathy. Clin Nephrol. 1994;41:61-4.

15. **Zucchelli P, Zuccala A, Borghi M, Fusaroli M, Sardelli M, Stallone C, Sanna G, Gaggi R.** Long-term comparison between captopril and nifedipine in the progression of renal insufficiency. Kidney Int. 1992;42:452-8.

16. **Sibai BM.** Treatment of hypertension in pregnant women. N Engl J Med. 1966;335:257-65.

17. **Lindheimer MD, Katz AI.** Gestation in women with kidney disease: prognosis and management. Baillieres Clin Obstet Gynecol. 1994;8:387-404.

18. **Jones DC, Hayslett JP.** Outcome of pregnancy in women with moderate or severe renal insufficiency. N Engl J Med. 1996;335:226-32.

19. **Hou SH, Grossman SD, Madias N.** Pregnancy in women with renal disease and moderate renal insufficiency. Am J Med. 1985;78:185-94.

20. **Imbasciati E, Pardi G, Capetta P, Ambroso G, Bozzetti P, Pagliari B, Ponticelli C.** Pregnancy in women with chronic renal failure. Am J Nephrol. 1986;6:193-8.

21. **Cunningham FG, Cox SM, Harstad TW, Mason RA, Pritchard JA.** Chronic renal disease and pregnancy outcome. Am J Obstet Gynecol. 1990;163:453-9.

22. **The Registration Committee of the European Dialysis and Transplant Association.** Successful pregnancies in women treated by dialysis and kidney transplantation. Br J Obstet Gynaecol. 1980;87:839-45.

23. **Souqiyyeh MZ, Huraib SO, Saleh AGM, Aswad S.** Pregnancy in chronic hemodialysis patients in the Kingdom of Saudi Arabia. Am J Kidney Dis. 1992;19:235-8.

24. **Hou S.** Peritoneal dialysis and hemodialysis in pregnancy. Baillieres Clin Obstet Gynaecol. 1987;1:1009-25.

25. **Redrow M, Cherem L, Elliot J, et al.** Dialysis in the management of pregnant patients with renal insufficiency. Medicine (Baltimore). 1988;67:199-208.

26. **Hou SH, Grossman SD.** Pregnancy in chronic dialysis patients. Semin Dial. 1990;3:224-9.

27. **Yankowitz J, Piraino B, Laifer SA, Frassetto L, Gavin L, Kitzmiller JL, Cromble-holme W.** Erythropoietin in pregnancies complicated by severe anemia of renal failure. Obstet Gynecol. 1992;80:485-8.

28. **Scott LL, Ramin SM, Richey M, Hanson J, Gilstrap LC 3d.** Erythropoietin use in pregnancy: two cases and a review of the literature. Am J Perinatol. 1995;12:22-4.

29. **Davison JM.** Pregnancy in renal allograft recipients: prognosis and management. Baillieres Clin Obstet Gynaecol. 1987;1:1027-1045.

30. **Sturgiss SN, Davison JM.** Effect of pregnancy on the long-term function of renal allografts: an update. Am J Kidney Dis. 1995;26:54-6.

31. **Lindheimer MD, Katz IK.** Pregnancy in the renal transplant patient. Am J Kidney Dis. 1992;19:173-6.

32. **Radomski JS, Ahlswede BA, Jarrell BE, Mannion J, Cater J, Moritz MJ, Armenti VT.** Outcomes of 500 pregnancies in 335 female kidney, liver, and heart transplant recipients. Transplant Proc. 1995;27:1089-90.

APPENDIX: DRUGS FOR CHRONIC HYPERTENSION

The drug table on page 233 is for reference when there is a clinical indication for treatment with one of the medications listed. Decisions about medication use in pregnancy should be made on the basis of a benefit-to-risk ratio, avoiding unnecessary treatment of symptoms but with consideration of the fact that fetal well-being depends on maternal well-being. Because the U.S. Food and Drug Administration is working on a new classification system of medications used in pregnancy, we have classified medications as follows:

Data Suggest Drug Use May be Justified When Indicated
When data and/or experience supports the safety of the drug.

Data Suggest Drug Use May Be Justified in Some Circumstances
When less extensive or desirable data are reported, but the drug is reasonable as a second-line therapy or may be used on the basis of the severity of maternal illness.

Data Suggest Drug Use Is Rarely Justified
Use drug only when alternatives supported by more experience and/or a better safety profile are not available.

Pregnancy pharmacokinetics may necessitate a significant increase in dose or dosing frequency, and dosing recommendations may require modification according to individual circumstances.

Drugs for Chronic Hypertension

Drug	Use May Be Justified When Indicated	Use May Be Justified in Some Circumstances	Use Is Rarely Justified	Comments/Dose Adjustments
ACE inhibitors Captopril Enalapril Lisinopril			√	Cause fetal renal failure; only use is for scleroderma renal crisis
Acebutolol		√		Preferred in class
Alpha-Methyldopa	√			
Atenolol		√		Other beta-blockers may be preferred because of IUGR
Clonidine			√	Causes somnambulance and night terrors
Diltiazem			√	Limited data for use as an antihypertensive agent
Hydralazine	√			
Hydrochloro-thiazide			√	Rarely used for treatment of hypertension; prevents normal expansion of blood volume
Labetalol	√			May need to increase dose or dosing frequency
Metoprolol		√		
Nifedipine		√		Synergistic with $MgSO_4$; may cause hypotension; useful for hyperaldosteronism
Oxprenolol		√		
Pindolol		√		Preferred beta-blocker
Prazosin		√		Useful for alpha-blockade in presence of pheochromo-cytoma
Propranolol			√	Other beta-blockers pre-ferred because of IUGR
Verapamil			√	Limited data for use as an antihypertensive agent

CHAPTER 5

Endocrine Problems

I. Overview of Gestational Diabetes
Jami Star and Donald R. Coustan

Gestational diabetes mellitus (GDM), as defined by the Third International Workshop Conference on Gestational Diabetes Mellitus (1), is "carbohydrate intolerance of variable severity with onset or first recognition during preg-

Key Values and Normal Physiologic Changes for Endocrine Problems

	Direction of Change	Percentage Change or Normal Range for Pregnancy
Adrenocorticotropic hormone	↑	5.2 ± 2.8 pmol/L Unchanged reposne to corticotropin-releasing hormone Blunted response to metyrapone*
Aldosterone	↑	3× increase early, up to 10× by term
Angiotensin	↑	2× to 4× increase
Calcium (ionized)	↔	
Calcium (total)	↓ (due to ↓ albumin)	<10.0 mg/dL
Catecholamines	↔	
Cortisol	Plasma ↑ Urinary ↑	Plasma >80 μg/dL (4× increase) Urinary 10× to 20 × increase/24 hours
Corticoropin-releasing hormone (CRH)	↑↑	10× increase by term
Free T$_4$, free T$_3$	↑ then ↔	
FSH/LH	↓	Suppressed, may be undetectable Flat response to gonadotropin-releasing hormone
Growth hormone	↔ then ↑	Blunted response to hypoglycemia Nl response to CRH
Glucose	↓	Fasting, <100 mg/dL
Hb A$_{1c}$	↔	3.8% to 6.4%
hPL	↑ (secreted by placenta)	Resembles growth hormone
Pituitary size	↑	35% increase
Prolactin	↑↑	Up to 10-fold increase
PTH (parathyroid hormone)	Slight ↑	
Renin activity (plasma)	↑	2× to 3× increase
TBG (thyroid-binding globulin)	↑	2× increase
Total T$_4$, total T$_3$	↑↑	> 10 μg/dL
T$_3$ resin uptake	↓	Inversely proportional to TBG
Thyroid antibodies	↔ or ↓	Increased response to TRH
TSH	Early ↓ then ↔	Increased response to TRH
Vasopressin	↔	Normal response to water deprivation*

↑ = Increase.
↓ = Decrease.
↔ = No change.
* Test not recommended in pregnancy.

nancy." By definition, this includes both cases of new-onset disease and cases of previously unrecognized glucose intolerance. Reclassification may be done at the time of postpartum testing by using standard criteria for the diagnosis of diabetes in the nonpregnant population (2). The U.S. national prevalence of GDM is approximately 4% but varies widely, ranging from 1% to 14% depending on the ethnicity of the population and the methods used for screening and diagnosis (3). Most U.S. obstetricians practice routine screening for GDM, but there is international debate over the importance of making this diagnosis. Despite the lack of controlled trials to support the benefit of widespread screening, data suggest that in the undiagnosed and untreated state, GDM has implications for both maternal and fetal morbidity (4).

Pathophysiology

Pregnancy is a hyperinsulinemic state characterized by a decrease in insulin sensitivity. This insulin resistance is at least partly explained by the presence of "diabetogenic" hormones, such as human placental lactogen, progesterone, cortisol, and prolactin. Fasting plasma glucose levels are generally lower in pregnancy than in the nonpregnant state, but postprandial values tend to be higher, particularly in persons who cannot adequately augment their insulin response. Late pregnancy may be described as a time of "accelerated starvation"; this implies an increased turnover of maternal metabolic fuels in the fasting state and the replacement of carbohydrate metabolism by fat use sooner than in the nonpregnant state (5, 6).

Patients with GDM may have a further decrease in insulin sensitivity, somewhat akin to that seen in type 2 diabetes, but they also have a relative deficit in insulin secretion (7). However, the pathophysiology of GDM is not completely understood. Even though all pregnant women are insulin resistant, less than 10% develop GDM. The severity of GDM may be influenced by several factors, including maternal age, body weight, and genetic predisposition (5).

Implications

Fetal Implications

One of the most significant manifestations of GDM is fetal macrosomia, which is defined by a birthweight greater than 4000 g or greater than the 90th percentile for gestational age. According to the Pedersen hypothesis (1954), maternal hyperglycemia results in fetal hyperinsulinemia, leading to excessive fetal growth. This hypothesis was expanded on by Freinkel and colleagues in 1979; they described the condition as "fuel-mediated teratogenesis," implicating the importance of other maternal metabolites. Clearly, maternal hyperglycemia alone does not completely account for the development of macrosomia, nor is its absence entirely preventive. As many as 25% of infants of mothers with GDM may have complications of this condition, despite relatively normal maternal fasting and postprandial glucose levels (8). Finally, macrosomia is not limited to the diabetic population.

An increased perinatal mortality rate has been reported in infants of mothers with poorly controlled GDM, but the evidence for this was collected in the 1960s and 1970s (before modern obstetric care was implemented) and without controlling for other maternal conditions. Recent evidence suggests an increase in congenital defects in GDM, including central nervous system and urinary tract abnormalities, but this may be due to the presence of undiagnosed diabetes around the time of conception and organogenesis (9). No such increases were found in a population whose prepregnancy diabetic status was well characterized (10).

Neonatal and Childhood Implications

Newborns of mothers with GDM are at risk for complications, such as hypoglycemia, hypocalcemia, hyperbilirubinemia, and polycythemia (11). Accumulating evidence also suggests that the offspring of mothers with GDM are at increased risk for obesity in childhood and for glucose intolerance in childhood and adulthood (12).

Maternal Implications

Because of concerns about fetal macrosomia and resultant birth trauma, mothers with GDM have an increased risk for intervention, including induction and cesarean section (13). They also have an increased risk for hypertensive disorders of pregnancy (e.g., preeclampsia). Beyond having implications for the pregnancy, GDM confers an increased lifetime risk for overt diabetes (generally type 2): Approximately 50% of mothers with GDM develop diabetes within 20 years of an affected pregnancy (14).

Screening

Historical risk factors are not sensitive enough to identify all patients at risk for GDM (15). The recommendations of the Fourth International Workshop Conference on Gestational Diabetes Mellitus (Box 5-1) suggest beginning with risk assessment at the first prenatal visit. In general, screening should be done in all patients with the exception of "low-risk" patients who meet *all* of the following criteria: age less than 25 years, normal weight before pregnancy, no known diabetes in a first-degree relative, no history of abnormal glucose metabolism, no previous poor obstetric outcome, and ethnicity associated with a low prevalence of GDM (high-prevalence groups include Hispanic-Americans, African-Americans, Native Americans, and Pacific Islanders). Screening for

---

Box 5-1 Indications for Screening for Gestational Diabetes at 24 to 28 Weeks of Gestation*

Screening should be done in all patients unless *all* of the following criteria are met:

Age <25 years

Normal weight

Ethnic background not associated with a high prevalence of diabetes

No first-degree relatives with diabetes

Previous poor obstetric history

No history of abnormal glucose metabolism

---

* Earlier screening is indicated in "high-risk" patients with any of the following characteristics: obesity, family history of type 2 diabetes, history of gestational diabetes or glucose intolerance, glucosuria, or treatment with medications that predispose to hyperglycemia. From Metzger BE, Coustan DR. Summary and recommendations of the Fourth International Workshop Conference on Gestational Diabetes Mellitus. Diabetes Care. 1998;21(Suppl 2):B161-7; with permission.

GDM is generally done between 24 and 28 weeks of gestation. Earlier testing may be considered in women with a history of the disease (whose risk for recurrence is as high as 50%), women in whom type 2 diabetes is strongly suspected, or women using medications that predispose to hyperglycemia.

The initial screening method most often used in the United States is a 1-hour, 50-g oral glucose load test; the patient does not need to be fasting (3). Occasionally, patients cannot tolerate this test, and alternatives are available. One alternative is the "jellybean test"; one study noted that the ingestion of 18 Brach's jellybeans, with a result at 1 hour of more than 120 mg/dL, had diagnostic sensitivity and specificity similar to those of oral glucose load testing (16). Another alternative is the "breakfast tolerance test," which uses a standard 600-kcal mixed-nutrient challenge in the fasting state and a 1-hour plasma glucose cutoff of 100 mg/dL (17). Outside of the United States, a 2-hour, 75-g oral glucose tolerance test is often used. This test should be done after 3 days of unrestricted intake (at least 150 g of carbohydrate) and an overnight fast of at least 8 hours (2). Efforts are currently underway to establish a worldwide consensus on methods and diagnostic criteria.

Diagnosis

The American Diabetes Association (ADA) recommends a cutoff of 140 mg/dL (7.8 mmol/L) or more for the 50-g glucose challenge test (3). Other authorities suggest a cutoff of 130 mg/dL because approximately 10% of patients with GDM have values of 130 to 140 mg/dL (18). Use of the lower value will increase the sensitivity of the test to almost 100%, but more women will undergo further testing. A normal test result early in pregnancy should be followed by repeated screening at 24 to 28 weeks of gestation.

A value below the selected cutoff necessitates no further testing. Patients whose value exceeds 130 to 140 mg/dL undergo the gold standard of testing: a 3-hour, 100-g oral glucose tolerance test done in the fasting state. Because of the changes in carbohydrate metabolism that accompany pregnancy, the cutoff values for a diagnosis of diabetes in pregnancy should not be identical to those used for diagnosis in nonpregnant persons but should be specifically derived for pregnancy (19).

The original criteria for diagnosis of GDM (O'Sullivan and Mahan, 1964) were based on the likelihood of subsequent development of diabetes in the mother, although these criteria were later correlated with an increased risk for perinatal death and illness. Because of changes in laboratory methods, the original values were converted by the National Diabetes Data Group. However, use of the glucose oxidase method required additional revision, resulting in the Carpenter and Coustan conversion of the original O'Sullivan criteria (20). These criteria are now recommended by the Fourth International Workshop Conference on Gestational Diabetes Mellitus (Table 5-1) (2). Two elevated values are required for diagnosis. Like the 75-g oral glucose tolerance test, the 3-hour test should be conducted after 3 days of unrestricted intake and an overnight fast. An abnormal value should be followed with a repeated 3-hour test 1 month later because one third of patients with one abnormal value will ultimately meet the diagnostic criteria and are at increased risk for fetal macrosomia (21). In patients who have an initial 50-g glucose challenge test result greater than 180 to 200 mg/dL, one alternative to the 100-g, 3-hour oral glucose tolerance test is to obtain fasting and postprandial plasma glucose levels. An abnormal fasting or postprandial value could be considered

Table 5-1 Criteria for Diagnosis of Gestational Diabetes*

Patient Status	Glucose Level on 3-hour, 100-g Oral Glucose Tolerance Test (NDDG)	Glucose Level on 3-hour, 100-g Oral Glucose Tolerance Test (Carpenter/Coustan)	Glucose Level on 2-hour, 75-g Oral Glucose Tolerance Test (CDA)
	◄——————————— (mg/dL) ———————————►		
Fasting	105	95	95
1 hour after eating	190	180	180
2 hours after eating	165	155	155
3 hours after eating	145	140	

NDDG = National Diabetes Data Group; CDA = Canadian Diabetes Association.

diagnostic, whereas a normal fasting value would require follow-up with the 3-hour oral glucose tolerance test.

Plasma Glucose Monitoring

The absolute cutoff for glycemic control necessary to prevent fetal morbidity has not been determined. According to evidence presented at the Fourth International Workshop Conference on Gestational Diabetes (2), the goals during pregnancy include maintenance of a fasting plasma glucose level less than 95 mg/dL (5.27 mmol/L) and postprandial plasma glucose levels less than 140 mg/dL (7.8 mmol/L) at 1 hour and less than 120 mg/dL (6.66 mmol/L) at 2 hours. In the presence of euglycemia, perinatal mortality rates should not be increased above those seen in the general population. Testing should be done at least weekly, although evidence suggests that four-times-daily monitoring of fasting and postprandial values may result in decreased perinatal morbidity rates. Capillary blood or venous plasma may be used, and postprandial circulating glucose measurements are preferred to preprandial measurements because they are more predictive of outcome (22). In general, self-monitoring of glucose should be encouraged because it has been associated with improved fetal outcome (i.e., a decreased incidence of macrosomia) (23) (Figure 5-1). Glucose is often found in the urine of pregnant patients and its measurement in urine is not useful. Serial measurements of glycosylated hemoglobin A_{1c} are not considered helpful in GDM because they have poor discriminatory value (23–25).

Treatment

Dietary Therapy

Once GDM is diagnosed, dietary therapy is begun in an effort to normalize the blood glucose level. Attention is also given to necessary weight gain and maternal nutritional status. For the woman of average weight and height, the American College of Obstetricians and Gynecologists (ACOG) recommends a total weight gain of 10 to 12 kg through the second and third trimesters at a rate of approximately 350 to 400 g/wk; this recommendation may be modified depending on the patient's body mass index (BMI). Nutritional counseling, preferably by a registered dietitian, is advised for guidance about caloric distribution. Generally, dietary recommendations are similar to those used in patients with type 1 and type 2 diabetes mellitus. With this approach, approximately 75% to 80% of women become euglycemic (25).

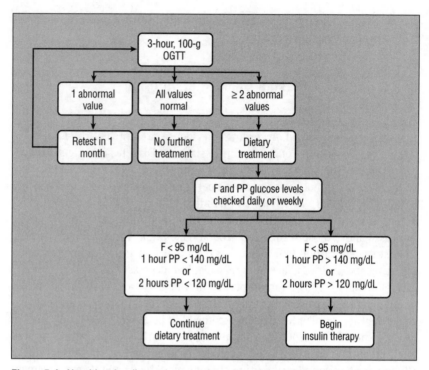

Figure 5-1 Algorithm for diagnosis and management of gestational diabetes. F = fasting; OGTT = oral glucose tolerance test; PP = postprandial.

The guidelines recommended by various organizations differ. The recommendations of the Fourth International Workshop Conference on Gestational Diabetes Mellitus (2) are in keeping with those of other groups (e.g., the ADA) in advising that optimal weight gain varies according to prepregnancy weight. For example, patients who are underweight (BMI <19.8 kg/m²) should gain up to 18 kg in pregnancy; in those who are overweight (BMI >29 kg/m²), overall weight gain should not exceed 7 kg. There is no consensus on the absolute minimum caloric intake for patients with GDM, although ketonuria should be avoided. It is not known how the distribution of carbohydrates throughout the day may influence adverse perinatal outcomes, such as macrosomia. One common approach divides total intake so that 25% of calories are consumed at breakfast, 30% are consumed at lunch, 30% are consumed at dinner, and 15% are reserved for a bedtime snack (24). Another approach, for patients receiving insulin, is to divide total intake into three meals and three or more snacks (6). Complex carbohydrates are preferred to simple sugars because they cause less-extreme blood glucose excursions. Recent evidence suggests that restricted carbohydrate intake (calories from carbohydrates accounting for <42% of calories) may reduce the incidence of macrosomia further and result in fewer requirements for insulin (26). As a general rule, persistent ketosis should be avoided, and dietary manipulation may be required if evidence of ketonuria is seen.

The usefulness of exercise in the treatment of GDM is not well studied, although one might expect exercise to enhance insulin sensitivity much as it does in patients with type 2 diabetes (25). One small randomized trial (27) comparing diet alone with diet and exercise (arm ergometers) found improved glycemic control in patients who exercised.

Insulin Therapy

If fasting or postprandial cutoff values (>95 mg/dL fasting; >140 mg/dL 1 hour after eating; and >120 mg/dL 2 hours after eating) are exceeded twice or more in a 2-week period, insulin therapy is advised (24). Approximately 15% to 20% of patients require insulin. Human insulin, which is less immunogenic than animal preparations, is preferred because it tends to be absorbed faster and to have a shorter duration of action and therefore results in fewer glucose excursions outside of the desired range (23). Insulin therapy may be started at a dose of 0.9 U/kg of ideal body weight divided into two administrations, with two thirds of the dose given in the a.m. hours and one third given in the p.m. hours. The a.m. dose should be two thirds NPH or intermediate-acting insulin and one third regular insulin. The p.m. dose should be half NPH and half regular insulin. Occasional patients may require separate injections of regular insulin before dinner and intermediate-acting insulin at bedtime. Patients maintained on insulin therapy are advised to check their glucose levels at least four times daily (while fasting and after each meal) (23). An alternative is a starting dose of 20 U of NPH and 10 U of regular insulin 15 to 30 minutes before breakfast, with subsequent titration based on plasma glucose values 2 hours after meals. If evening or fasting plasma glucose levels are elevated, a second dose of insulin (usually a 1:1 combination of intermediate and short-acting insulins) before dinner is prescribed .

It should be noted that the precise level of glucose control required to eliminate risk for macrosomia has not been determined. In fact, most large babies are born to nondiabetic mothers. However, there seems to be a continuum between degree of carbohydrate intolerance and adverse perinatal outcomes, such as macrosomia. A large multicenter trial in Toronto (28) assessed pregnancy outcomes in women with carbohydrate intolerance that was insufficient to meet the criteria for diagnosis of GDM. The risk for macrosomia increased in a graded manner with increasing degrees of carbohydrate intolerance on the glucose challenge test and the oral glucose tolerance test.

In patients with GDM, the risk for macrosomia persists to some degree despite therapy. Even with objective evidence of "good" glycemic control, other factors (i.e., maternal age, parity, and obesity) contribute to birthweight. The use of insulin therapy at lower fasting and postprandial values is occasionally recommended to further reduce the risk for fetal macrosomia.

Fetal Surveillance and Delivery

The necessity of weekly fetal surveillance in a normoglycemic patient who has diet-controlled GDM and no other risk factors (e.g., hypertension, previous poor obstetric outcome) is controversial (29). These patients are considered to have low risk for fetal death. Some authors recommend daily kick counts in this setting; others initiate formal testing between 34 and 40 weeks of gestation. In the presence of insulin therapy, poorly controlled diabetes, or other risk factors (e.g., hypertension, intrauterine growth restriction [IUGR], previous stillbirth), fetal well-being testing should be considered when the patient reaches 32 to 36 weeks of gestation or sooner, depending on the individual circumstances. The frequency, nature, and timing of testing may be influenced by the individual clinical situation. Options include nonstress testing, contraction stress testing, and biophysical profiles done weekly or twice weekly; fetal growth estimation should not be done more often than every 10 to 14 days (2, 24).

Because the risk for shoulder dystocia is approximately 3 times higher in patients with GDM, there is great concern about its prevention. However, there is no clear consensus on a birthweight cutoff at which cesarean section should be done. One of the biggest limitations in this regard is reliance on ultrasonography for fetal weight assessment; this procedure may under- or overestimate fetal weight. Previous obstetric history and pelvic assessment are taken into consideration in such a case. However, many practitioners offer or recommend cesarean section at an estimated fetal weight of 4250 to 4500 g in a GDM pregnancy (30). (There are no absolute fetal weight cutoffs in the absence of diabetes.) Given the inaccuracies of ultrasonography in fetal weight testing, it is advisable to combine clinical and sonographic assessment.

The timing of delivery may be individualized. No clear evidence shows that expectant management results in significant increases in perinatal morbidity or mortality rates. However, it may increase the risk for a large-for-gestational-age infant. One randomized trial (31) compared expectant management with induction of labor in insulin-treated patients with GDM at term. They found that those managed expectantly had an increased prevalence of macrosomia and shoulder dystocia but no increased risk for cesarean section. It is not unreasonable, therefore, to consider induction of labor at or after 38 weeks of gestation in insulin-treated patients with GDM in an effort to reduce the likelihood of macrosomia.

Some controversy surrounds the need for fetal lung maturity assessment by amniocentesis before delivery in patients with GDM. Patients at or beyond 38 weeks of gestation (with reliable pregnancy dating criteria) who have good glycemic control do not require amniocentesis before delivery because they have a very small risk for an infant with respiratory distress syndrome. If elective delivery is considered before 38 weeks of gestation, or if the patient has poor glycemic control or there is uncertain gestational dating, then amniocentesis to confirm fetal pulmonary maturity (i.e., a lecithin-to-sphingomyelin ratio greater than 2:1 or a positive phosphatidylglycerol test result) is recommended (2, 16).

Labor

Maternal hyperglycemia should be avoided during labor. Fetal hyperglycemia may increase the risk for acidemia (32), and fetal hyperinsulinemia may place the neonate at risk for hypoglycemia. During labor, maternal circulating glucose levels should be assessed every 1 to 2 hours, and continuous intravenous insulin should be given as needed to maintain a plasma glucose level less than 120 mg/dL. In the event of a planned cesarean section, insulin should be withheld on the morning of surgery if the fasting glucose level is normal. In general, glucose-containing intravenous fluids in amounts beyond the minimum required to maintain basal energy requirements (0.12 to 0.18 g/kg per hour) should be avoided. After delivery, treatment with insulin is rarely necessary (2).

Postpartum Follow-up

In the immediate postpartum period, it is not necessary to continue treatment or testing unless type 2 diabetes is very strongly suspected.

The diagnosis of GDM carries an increased risk for subsequent type 2 diabetes. This risk is modified by other factors, such as ethnic background, age, body weight, and family history. For example, more than 50% of Hispanic women in Los Angeles develop diabetes within 5 years of a pregnancy complicated by GDM (33).

In a patient with the diagnosis of GDM, testing is recommended within the first few months after delivery (i.e., 6 to 12 weeks postpartum) to rule out overt diabetes mellitus or impaired glucose tolerance (2, 24). According to the most recent ADA guidelines, a fasting plasma glucose level of 126 mg/dL or more on two or more occasions is diagnostic of diabetes, and a level between 110 to 125 mg/dL is diagnostic of impaired fasting glucose. If the fasting plasma glucose level is less than 126 mg/dL, a 2-hour, 75-g oral glucose tolerance test should be done. A 2-hour value of 200 mg/dL or more is diagnostic of diabetes, and a 2-hour value of 140 to 199 mg/dL is consistent with impaired glucose tolerance (34). Even with normal testing, patients should be encouraged to have annual plasma glucose sampling and should receive careful preconception evaluation before another pregnancy. In addition, for patients at high risk for diabetes, dietary and lifestyle recommendations (including weight loss, increased physical activity, and a low-fat, high-carbohydrate diet) should be made (35).

A diagnosis of GDM should not discourage the practice of breastfeeding; in fact, breastfeeding should be encouraged. Options for contraception are similar to those for patients without diabetes and include hormonal preparations as well as barrier methods. Some data suggest that breastfeeding women using a progestin-only oral contraceptive have an increased risk for type 2 diabetes. Low-dose combination oral contraceptives may be considered in the absence of other contraindications (2, 36).

Recurrence

Worldwide, the rate of recurrence of GDM in a subsequent pregnancy ranges from 30% to 60%. This risk may be modified by limitation of weight gain between pregnancies. The risk for type 2 diabetes is greatest in women with recurrent GDM, but the overall lifetime risk for type 2 diabetes is increased even in women who revert to normal glucose tolerance in a subsequent pregnancy (35).

REFERENCES

1. **Metzger BE.** Summary and recommendations of the Third International Workshop Conference on Gestational Diabetes Mellitus. Diabetes. 1991;40:197-201.

2. **Metzger BE, Coustan DR.** Summary and recommendations of the Fourth International Workshop Conference on Gestational Diabetes Mellitus. Diabetes Care. 1998; 21(Suppl 2):B61-7.

3. **American Diabetes Association.** Position statement: gestational diabetes mellitus. Diabetes Care. 1998;21(Suppl 1):S60-1.

4. **Adams KM, Li H, Nelson RL, Ogburn PL, Danilenko-Dixon DR.** Sequelae of unrecognized gestational diabetes. Am J Obstet Gynecol. 1998;178:1321-32.

5. **Boden G.** Fuel metabolism in pregnancy and gestational diabetes mellitus. Obstet Gynecol Clin North Am. 1996;23:1-10.

6. **Gunderson EP.** Intensive nutrition therapy for gestational diabetes. Diabetes Care. 1997;20:221-6.

7. **Kuhl C.** Etiology and pathogenesis of gestational diabetes. Diabetes Care. 1998;21 (Suppl 2):B19-26.

8. **Hod M, Langer O.** Fuel metabolism in deviant fetal growth in offspring of diabetic women. Obstet Gynecol Clin North Am. 1996;23:259-77.

9. **Martinez-Frias ML, Bermajo E, Rodriguez-Pinilla E, Prieto L, Frias JL.** Epidemiological analysis of outcomes of pregnancy in gestational diabetic mothers. Am J Med Genet. 1998;78:140-5.

10. **Pettitt DJ, Knowler WC, Baird R, Bennett PH.** Gestational diabetes: infant and maternal complications of pregnancy in relation to third-trimester glucose tolerance in Pima Indians. Diabetes Care. 1980;3:458-64.

11. **Persson B, Hanson U.** Neonatal morbidities in gestational diabetes mellitus. Diabetes Care. 1998;21(Suppl 2):B79-84.

12. **Vohr BR, McGarvey ST, Tucker R.** Effects of maternal gestational diabetes on offspring adiposity at 4-7 years of age. Diabetes Care. 1999;22:1284-91.

13. **Sermer M, Naylor CD, Farine D, Kenshole AB, Ritchie JWK, Fare DJ, et al.** The Toronto tri-hospital gestational diabetes project. Diabetes Care. 1998;21(Suppl 2):B33-42.

14. **O'Sullivan JB.** Body weight and subsequent diabetes mellitus. JAMA. 1982;248:949-52.

15. **Coustan DR, Nelson C, Carpenter MW, Carr SR, Rotondo L, Widness JA.** Maternal age and screening for gestational diabetes: a population-based study. Obstet Gynecol. 1989;73:557-61.

16. **Boyd KL, Ross EK, Sherman SJ.** Jelly beans as an alternative to a cola beverage containing 50 grams of glucose. Am J Obstet Gynecol. 1995;173:1889-92.

17. **Coustan DR, Widness JA, Carpenter MW, Rotondo L, Pratt DC.** The "breakfast tolerance test": screening for gestational diabetes with a standardized mixed nutrient meal. Am J Obstet Gynecol. 1987;157:1113-7.

18. **Carr SR.** Screening for gestational diabetes mellitus. Diabetes Care. 1998;21(Suppl 2):B14-8.

19. **Coustan DR.** Screening and diagnosis of gestational diabetes. Baillieres Clin Obstet Gynaecol. 1991;5:293-313.

20. **Carpenter MW, Coustan DR.** Criteria for screening tests for gestational diabetes. Am J Obstet Gynecol. 1982;144:768-73.

21. **Coustan DR.** Screening and testing for gestational diabetes. Obstet Gynecol Clin North Am. 1996;23:125-36.

22. **de Veciana M, Major CA, Morgan MA, Asrat T, Toohey JS, Lien JM, et al.** Postprandial versus preprandial blood glucose monitoring in women with gestational diabetes mellitus requiring insulin therapy. N Engl J Med. 1995;333:1237-41.

23. **Homko CJ, Khandelwal M.** Glucose monitoring and insulin therapy during pregnancy. Obstet Gynecol Clin North Am. 1996;23:47-74.

24. **American College of Obstetricians and Gynecologists.** Technical Bulletin 200: Diabetes in Pregnancy. Washington, DC: American College of Obstetricians and Gynecologists; 1994.

25. **Langer O, Hod M.** Management of gestational diabetes mellitus. Obstet Gynecol Clin North Am. 1996;23:137-59.

26. **Major CA, Henry J, De Veciana M, Morgan MA.** The effects of carbohydrate restriction in patients with diet controlled gestational diabetes. Obstet Gynecol. 1998;91:600-4.

27. **Jovanovic-Peterson L, Durak EP, Peterson CM.** Randomized trial of diet versus diet plus cardiovascular conditioning on glucose levels in gestational diabetes. Am J Obstet Gynecol. 1989:161:415-9.

28. **Sermer M, Naylor CD, Gare DJ, Kenshole AB, Ritchie JWK, Farine D, et al.** Impact of increasing carbohydrate intolerance on maternal-fetal outcomes in 3637 women without gestational diabetes: the Toronto tri-hospital gestation diabetes project. Am J Obstet Gynecol. 1995;173:146-56.

29. **Landon MB, Gabbe SG.** Antepartum fetal surveillance in gestational diabetes mellitus. Diabetes. 1985;34(Suppl 2):50-4.

30. **American College of Obstetricians and Gynecologists.** Technical Bulletin 159: Fetal Macrosomia. Washington, DC: American College of Obstetricians and Gynecologists; 1991.

31. **Kjos SL, Henry OA, Montoro M, Buchanan TA, Mestman JH.** Insulin-requiring diabetes in pregnancy: a randomized trial of active induction of labor and expectant management. Am J Obstet Gynecol. 1993;169:611-5.

32. **Lawrence GF, Brown VA, Parsons RJ, Cooke ID.** Feto-maternal consequences of high-dose glucose infusion during labour. Br J Obstet Gynecol. 1982;89:27-32.

33. **Kjos SL, Peters RK, Xiang A, Henry OA, Montoro M, Buchanan TA.** Predicting future diabetes in Latino women with gestational diabetes. Diabetes. 1995;44:586-91.

34. **American Diabetes Association.** Committee Report: Report of the Expert Committee on the Diagnosis and Classification of Diabetes Mellitus. Diabetes Care. 1998;21(Suppl 1):S5-19.

35. **Dornhorst A, Frost G.** The potential for dietary intervention postpartum in women with gestational diabetes. Diabetes Care. 1997;20:1635-7.

36. **Kjos SL, Peters RK, Xiang A, Schaefer U, Buchanen TA.** Hormonal choices after gestational diabetes. Diabetes Care. 1998;21(Suppl 2):B50-7.

II. Controversies in Gestational Diabetes
Erin Keely and Peter R. Garner

The practice of screening for and treating GDM is recommended in North America by most expert organizations, including the ADA (1), the ACOG (2), and the Canadian Diabetes Association (3). However, we still lack international consensus on the best diagnostic criteria, optimal screening strategies, and benefits of treatment with respect to fetal mortality and morbidity. The debate is fueled by a lack of properly randomized studies of sufficient power.

The goal of diagnosing and treating GDM is to reduce fetal morbidity and mortality rates. The main concern, as outlined in the preceding section, is macrosomia. However, most large babies are not born to diabetic mothers. Maternal characteristics other than GDM, such as obesity, advanced maternal age, increased parity, and postmaturity, are also strongly associated with macrosomia and may be more powerful predictors of macrosomia than is maternal hyperglycemia (4, 5). However, there seems to be a continuum between the degree of carbohydrate intolerance and adverse perinatal outcomes, such as macrosomia. A large multicenter trial in Toronto (6) assessed pregnancy outcomes in women who had carbohydrate intolerance that was not sufficient to meet the criteria for diagnosis of GDM. The risk for macrosomia increased in a gradual manner with increasing degrees of carbohydrate intolerance on the glucose challenge test and the oral glucose tolerance test.

It is the adverse events associated with increased birthweight, such as trauma, surgical delivery, perinatal asphyxia, shoulder dystocia, clavicular fractures, and brachial palsy lesion, that are clinically relevant. However, less than 2% of macrosomic infants have permanent sequelae, and most of these sequelae occur in infants weighing more than 4500 g (7). An increased perinatal mortality rate in women with GDM was first suggested by O'Sullivan and Mahan in the 1960s, before the advent of modern obstetric care and without controlling for other maternal conditions, such as obesity and hypertension. Improved obstetric care, resulting in an overall decrease in fetal mortality rates, makes it difficult to know the true effect of GDM on fetal mortality. Clinical trials to assess this are not feasible because of the sample size that would be required to show a difference in mortality. The offspring of mothers with GDM have an increased risk for obesity and type 2 diabetes (8). Excessive fetal insulin production, as assessed by amniotic fluid insulin levels, is correlated with both obesity and impaired glucose tolerance, but no prospective studies of the benefit of maternal glycemic control on these childhood outcomes have been done.

The diagnosis of GDM occurs in two steps: screening and definitive diagnosis. Most data suggest a continuum of risk for macrosomia with maternal hyperglycemia, making arbitrary cutoff values difficult to determine. Star and Coustan, in the preceding section, outline the diagnostic criteria proposed by the major U.S. organizations. However, the reader should know that there is much debate internationally about the best criteria. The Canadian Diabetes Association (CDA), in its recently published clinical practice guidelines (3), recommends a 2-hour, 75-g glucose tolerance test rather than the 3-hour, 100-g test because of its ease of administration and available normative data (grade D consensus recommendation). The CDA recognizes the lack of data on obstetric outcomes for all diagnostic criteria and thus proposes these criteria as an interim measure until further information is available.

Before starting a treatment program in the patient with GDM, the physician should remember that the potential maternal and fetal gains from therapy must be balanced against the potential harmful effects of therapy, including the risks to the mother from surgical delivery. In the Toronto tri-hospital study (9), the rate of cesarean section was 33% in GDM pregnancies and 20.2% in non-GDM pregnancies, despite normalization of birthweight by tight glycemic control. This suggests that the label *GDM* puts women at increased risk for surgical delivery and thus for infection, blood transfusion, and wound dehiscence.

The studies reported to date on benefits of treatment have been contradictory and methodologically flawed. In a large population-based study, Langer and colleagues (10) compared intensive therapy with more conventional glycemic control. Significant improvement in rates of macrosomia, cesarean section, shoulder dystocia, stillbirth, and neonatal metabolic complications was seen in the intensive therapy group. However, patients were not truly randomized, and this may have resulted in selection bias. The proportion of small-for-gestational-age infants was also increased in the intensive therapy group; this characteristic may result in an increase in neonatal morbidity and, ironically, in future type 2 diabetes (11). In contrast, other randomized controlled trials have found little difference in mean birthweight, incidence of macrosomia, or rate of cesarean section among women with GDM who received no treatment, dietary therapy alone, or dietary therapy plus insulin (12, 13).

Coustan and Lewis (14) assessed the incidence of macrosomia in the infants of 72 women with GDM. The incidence rates were 7% for women treated with diet and insulin, 30% for women treated with diet alone, and 50% in women who received no treatment. However, randomization in this trial was not strictly adhered to and, despite reduced rates of macrosomia, no reduction in the incidence of cesarean section or midforceps delivery was seen.

In a later study, Coustan and Imarah (15) showed reductions in the rates of both macrosomia and surgical intervention in women with GDM who were treated with diet and insulin compared with women with GDM who were treated with diet alone or who received no treatment. However, because this study was a retrospective, nonrandomized chart review of populations that differed in socioeconomic status, the potential for bias was present. Thompson and co-workers (16) found a significantly lower mean birthweight and incidence of macrosomia in women with GDM who were treated with diet and insulin compared with women with GDM who were treated with diet alone. However, no difference was seen in important clinical outcomes, such as surgical delivery, shoulder dystocia, or neonatal metabolic complications.

We completed a pilot project of 299 pregnant women with GDM who were randomly assigned to standard obstetric care or to usual care for GDM (17). We found no significant differences in birthweight, incidence of macrosomia, or poor obstetric outcome. Although this study was the largest prospective trial to date, the sample size was insufficient to definitively show whether treatment of GDM is beneficial. A true picture of maternal and fetal risks and benefits will require a large, multicenter trial of approximately 3000 deliveries if birth trauma, hypoglycemic seizures, and perinatal mortality are used as the clinically relevant sequelae. Until a trial shows a clear benefit of treatment for maternal or fetal outcome, the question of whether to screen patients for GDM will remain unanswered.

Because most women do not have serious sequelae even with mean blood glucose levels greater than 140 mg/dL, it is important to determine which women and infants are at risk and to target therapy to this high-risk group. We cannot rely solely on maternal glucose values. Two approaches for identifying fetuses at risk are to estimate fetal weight with ultrasonography (18) and to measure the insulin level in the amniotic fluid (19). Further studies into the benefits of targeting at-risk infants rather than all infants are needed.

Antepartum management of the patient with GDM uses a team approach and involves a diabetic nurse practitioner, a dietitian, and an obstetrician or another physician in association with an outpatient unit for maternal fetal assessment. Many different strategies are used; the major constituents of maintaining euglycemia are patient education, home glucose monitoring, initial dietary adjustment, and, if diet alone does not suffice, use of supplemental insulin. In our experience, approximately 15% of patients with GDM require insulin. Others suggest that up to 50% of women with GDM require insulin; this translates to about 2% of all pregnant women (20). Star and Coustan suggest using 0.9 U/kg divided into two injections. We prefer to assess the pattern of hyperglycemia and target the insulin for the time of day at which the highest blood glucose levels are seen. We begin with lower dosages (e.g., 0.3 U/kg) to avoid maternal hypoglycemia. Adjustments are made over the telephone by a diabetic nurse specialist every 2 to 3 days, as needed. If glucose control is too tight (fasting blood glucose levels <4.8 mmol/L), the risk for growth restriction increases. Thus, overzealous treatment should be avoided (21). Hypoglycemia must also be avoided during labor and delivery because of the risk for serious reactions, including hypoglycemic seizures. Intravenous insulin is rarely needed in the delivery room for women with GDM.

In summary, many issues in the diagnosis and management of GDM are still controversial. Further, properly designed studies are needed to clearly define the benefits of treatment on clinically relevant obstetric and childhood outcomes. Further work on defining those pregnancies at highest risk is needed to that we can target therapy to those who truly need it. In the meantime, we have only consensus guidelines based on few data to guide clinical practice.

REFERENCES

1. **American Diabetes Association.** Gestational diabetes mellitus: clinical practice recommendations—1999. Diabetes Care. 1999;22(Suppl 1):S74-6.

2. **American College of Obstetricians and Gynecologists.** ACOG Technical Bulletin: Diabetes and Pregnancy. Washington, DC: American College of Obstetricians and Gynecologists; 1994. (Available at www.acog.com/publications/educational bulletins/btb200.htm.)

3. **Meltzer S, Leiter L, Daneman D, Gerstein HC, Lau D, Luwig S, et al.** 1998 clinical practice guidelines for the management of diabetes in Canada. Can Med Assoc J. 1998;159(Suppl 8):S1-29.

4. **Jacobson VD, Cousins L.** A population-based study of maternal and perinatal outcome in patients with gestational diabetes. Am J Obstet Gynecol. 1989;161:981-6.

5. **Cnattingius S, Bergstrom R, Lipworth L, Kramer MS.** Prepregnancy weight and the risk of adverse pregnancy outcomes. N Engl J Med. 1998;338:147-52.

6. **Sermer M, Naylor CD, Farine D, Kenshole AB, Ritchie JWK, Fare DJ, et al.** The Toronto tri-hospital gestational diabetes project. Diabetes Care. 1998;21(Suppl 2):B33-42.

7. **Blank A, Grave G, Metzger B.** Effects of gestational diabetes on perinatal morbidity reassessed. Report on the international workshop on adverse perinatal outcomes of gestational diabetes mellitus, December 3–4 1992. Diabetes Care. 1995;18:127-9.

8. **Pettitt DJ, Knowler WC.** Long term effects of the intrauterine environment, birthweight, and breastfeeding in Pima Indians. Diabetes Care. 1998;21(Suppl 2):B138-41.

9. **Naylor CD, Sermer M, Chen E, Sykora K.** Cesarean delivery in relation to birth weight and gestational glucose tolerance: pathophysiology or practice style? JAMA. 1996;275:1165-70.

10. **Langer O, Rodriguez DA, Xenakis EMJ, McFarland MB, Berkus MD, Areendondo F.** Intensified versus conventional management of gestational diabetes. Am J Obstet Gynecol. 1994;170:1036-47.

11. **Phillips DIW.** Birthweight and the future development of diabetes. Diabetes Care. 1998;21(Suppl 2):B150-5.

12. **Li DFH, Wong VCW, O'Hoy KMKY, Yeung CY, Ma HK.** Is treatment needed for mild impairment of glucose tolerance in pregnancy? A randomized controlled trial. Br J Obstet Gynecol. 1987;94:851-4.

13. **Persson B, Stangenberg M, Hansson V, Norlander E.** Gestational diabetes mellitus comparative evaluation of two treatment regimens, diet versus insulin and diet. Diabetes. 1985;34(Suppl 2):101-5.

14. **Coustan DR, Lewis SB.** Insulin therapy for gestational diabetes. Obstet Gynecol. 1978;51:306-10.

15. **Coustan DR, Imarah J.** Prophylactic insulin treatment of gestational diabetes reduces the incidence of macrosomia, operative delivery and birth trauma. Am J Obstet Gynecol. 1984;150:836-42.

16. **Thompson DJ, Porter KB, Gunneils DJ, Wagner P, Spinnato JA.** Prophylactic insulin in the management of gestational diabetes. Obstet Gynecol. 1990;75:960-4.

17. **Garner P, Okun N, Keely E, Wells G, Perkins S, Sylvain J, Belcher J.** A randomized controlled trial of strict glycemic control and tertiary level obstetric care versus routine obstetric care in the management of gestational diabetes: a pilot study. Am J Obstet Gynecol. 1997;177:190-5.

18. **Buchanan TA, Kjos SL, Schafer U, Peters RK, Xiang A, Byrne J, et al.** Utility of fetal measurements in the management of gestational diabetes mellitus. Diabetes Care. 1998;21:(Suppl 2):B99-106.

19. **Hopp H, Vollert W, Rogosch V, Novak A, Weitzel HK, Glockner E, Besch W.** Indication and results of insulin therapy for gestational diabetes mellitus. J Perinat Med. 1996;25:521-30.

20. **Langer O.** Maternal glycemic criteria for insulin therapy in gestational diabetes mellitus. Diabetes Care. 1998;21(Suppl 2):B91-8.

21. **Langer O, Levy J, Brustman L, Anyaegbunam A, Merkatz R, Divon M.** Glycemic control in gestational diabetes mellitus. How tight is tight enough? Small for gestational age versus large for gestational age. Am J Obstet Gynecol. 1989;161:646-53.

III. Type 1 and Type 2 Diabetes
Anne Kenshole, Joel Ray, and Erin Keely

Women with existing diabetes are the group in whom internists have the greatest opportunity to affect fetal outcome. The benefits of prepregnancy glycemic control—a primary task of the internist and endocrinologist—on fetal outcome are unquestioned. This section provides practical management strategies for helping women with type 1 diabetes. A discussion of type 2 diabetes is included at the end of the section.

Pregnancy Risks for Women with Type 1 Diabetes

Metabolic Control

Pregnancy is associated with significant changes in fuel metabolism. Beginning in the first trimester, fasting blood glucose levels decrease as a result of accelerated starvation. Postprandial levels increase as a result of the insulin resistance caused by increased maternal cortisol and prolactin as well as placental production of human placental lactogen. These changes predispose to fasting hypoglycemia early in pregnancy and to postprandial hyperglycemia later in pregnancy. By term, overall insulin requirements are generally two to three times the prepregnancy amounts.

Hypoglycemia unawareness (lack of autonomic symptoms, such as tremors, palpitations, and diaphoresis) results in the inability to detect decreasing blood sugar until neuroglycopenic symptoms (decreased level of consciousness, seizures, and coma) occur. In pregnancy, severe hypoglycemia occurs in 30% to 40% of women in the first half of pregnancy, most often between midnight and 8:00 a.m. (1), because of intensified insulin management and a diminished counter-regulatory response to hypoglycemia. Women with severe hypoglycemia before pregnancy, hyperemesis, and gastroparesis are at greatest risk. Reinforcement of the importance of 1) a bedtime snack that includes starch, fat, and protein; 2) carrying a supply of fast-acting carbohydrates (e.g., juice, hard candies, dextrogel); 3) monitoring blood sugars overnight on a weekly basis; and 4) maintaining availability of a glucagon injection kit are vital. Intermittent maternal hypoglycemia seems to have no adverse effect on fetal or neonatal outcomes (2).

Pregnancy also predisposes to accelerated starvation, which can result in ketonuria after an overnight fast. Diabetic ketoacidosis (DKA) may develop more rapidly than usual in pregnancy and is associated with adverse fetal outcome. Tocolytics and corticosteroids may precipitate DKA, and it may occur at glucose levels lower than those seen in the nonpregnant state. DKA complicates about 1% of pregnancies and is associated with a 35% fetal mortality rate (3). The diagnosis and management of DKA in pregnancy are the same as for DKA in the nonpregnant state except that more aggressive management of acidosis with earlier bicarbonate replacement should be considered (3). The fetal heart rate must be monitored continuously until acidosis has ceased. Maternal acidosis should be corrected before surgery is done, because any emergency surgical delivery confers significant risk to the acidotic mother.

Deterioration of Chronic Complications

One of the biggest fears of both patients and health care providers is that pregnancy may hasten the progression of retinal damage or renal failure. It is difficult, at times, to distinguish the natural history of these events over a 9-month period from a pregnancy-hastened decline.

Diabetic Retinopathy

The presence and degree of diabetic retinopathy are associated with the duration of diabetes and glycemic control. Persons who have had diabetes for more than 15 years have a 90% incidence of retinopathy. This rate may be lower in the future as a result of improved glycemic control, which is now the goal of therapy. Diabetic retinopathy may be classified as nonproliferative diabetic retinopathy (microaneurysms, intraretinal hemorrhage, or exudates), in which visual loss is rare, or proliferative retinopathy (retinal neovascularization with the potential for vitreous hemorrhage, fibrosis, and retinal detachment), which seriously threatens vision.

Most studies have shown some worsening of retinopathy over the course of a pregnancy relative to a 40-week period in the nonpregnant state (7–11). Proliferative retinopathy was an indication for pregnancy termination 30 years ago because of the associated risk for blindness. With the advent of laser therapy, this risk has diminished. Diabetic retinopathy may worsen in pregnancy for several reasons, including suddenly tightened glycemic control (multiple studies have shown that this transiently worsens retinopathy), increased cardiac output, the hypercoagulable state of pregnancy, and the increased production of growth factors. Table 5-2 summarizes data on the progression of diabetic retinopathy during pregnancy. Women with severe nonproliferative diabetic retinopathy and proliferative diabetic retinopathy have an approximately 50% chance of worsening during pregnancy. Risk factors for progression include poor initial glycemic control, rapid normalization of blood sugar, chronic hypertension, pregnancy-induced hypertension, nephropathy, and degree of retinopathy at conception (4). Macular edema may also worsen, especially in the presence of proteinuria, and can cause permanent visual loss.

Table 5-2 Course and Prognosis of Diabetic Retinopathy in Pregnant Women

Type of DR at Conception	Characteristics	Percentage That May Worsen to Next Level of DR or More During Pregnancy	Percentage Whose Retinopathy Worsened to This Level During Pregnancy Who Will Return to Prepregancy Level of DR after Delivery
Absent	No DR present	10–18	Not applicable
Nonproliferative		18–36	Completely: 30
			Partially: 50
Mild/moderate	<10 microaneurysms or dot hemorrhages		
Severe	>10 microaneurysms with or without hemorrhage, hard exudates, cotton-wool spots, and intraretinal microvascular abnormalities	54.8	Completely: 17 Partially: 58
Proliferative	Retinal neovascularization, history of laser therapy, previous vitreous hemorrhage	58.5*	

* Indicates percentage with current or previous proliferative DR who require laser photocoagulation during pregnancy.

To avoid vision-threatening changes during pregnancy, it is essential that women be assessed by an ophthalmologist before conception and, if retinopathy is present, in each trimester. In women with severe disease, monthly follow-up is indicated. Ideally, photocoagulation should be completed before pregnancy with time to ensure regression of the peripheral diabetic retinopathy before conception. In preventing blindness, laser therapy is as effective in the pregnant woman as in the nonpregnant woman, and it can safely be used in pregnancy if needed. When active neovascularization is present, the risk for precipitating retinal bleeding by using the Valsalva maneuver during labor remains controversial, but cesarean section has not been shown to be advantageous (12).

Diabetic Nephropathy

Diabetic nephropathy represents a spectrum of disease ranging from an increased glomerular filtration rate (GFR) to microalbuminuria (microalbumin, 30 to 300 mg/d or a microalbumin-to-creatinine ratio >2 mg/mmol) to overt nephropathy (>300 mg of protein/24 hours) to end-stage renal failure. Nephropathy complicates approximately 4% of diabetic pregnancies and is associated with increased maternal and perinatal morbidity rates.

In the nonpregnant state, tight glycemic control, angiotensin-converting enzyme (ACE) inhibition, and, possibly, dietary protein restriction have been shown to slow the rate of progression of diabetic nephropathy. Thus, most women with nephropathy are using an ACE inhibitor at the time of conception. Exposure to ACE inhibitors in early pregnancy does not seem to be harmful, but ACE inhibition must be stopped upon confirmation of pregnancy to avoid later toxic effects on the fetus. Discontinuing use of the ACE inhibitor may unmask hypertension, which necessitates use of another antihypertensive agent known to be safe in pregnancy (see Chapter 4) (13). Ideally, use of the ACE inhibitor should be discontinued before patients actively try to conceive, but continuing ACE inhibition until conception is theoretically advantageous because pregnancy begins while the woman is at the lowest level of proteinuria and because the least amount of time elapses without the protective effect of ACE inhibitors.

Pregnancy is associated with a 50% increase in the GFR and a subsequent decrease in the serum creatinine level to less than 60 μmol/L. The normal excretion of protein also increases to as much as 300 mg/d. Women with diabetic nephropathy may not have normal physiologic responses to pregnancy. About one third show the expected increase in GFR, one third have no significant change in GFR, and one third show a decline in GFR (14).

Microalbuminuria usually increases but rarely to the level of overt nephropathy. An increased risk for preeclampsia is associated.

Most women with proteinuria have a significant, progressive increase in protein excretion, often into the nephrotic range (>3 g/24 hours). The mean increase in protein excretion is about 3 g/24 hours throughout gestation (15). This massive proteinuria may be associated with severe edema, hypertension, retinal edema, decreased mobility, and hypercoagulability. Nephrotic-range proteinuria or elevated serum creatinine levels are relative contraindications to pregnancy because fetal compromise and significant maternal morbidity are probable.

In one study of women with moderate or severe renal insufficiency from various causes, the incidence of urinary protein excretion greater than 3 g/L increased from 23% in the first trimester to 41% in the third trimester. Furthermore, of 70 pregnancies, 8 (10%) were associated with rapid progression of maternal renal insufficiency. Obstetric complications included a preterm delivery rate of 59%, an IUGR rate of 37%, and an infant survival rate of 93% (16). Although pregnancy may accelerate the progression of nephropathy for several theoretical reasons, including hyperfiltration and increased dietary protein levels, postpartum renal function will return to prepregnancy levels in most cases. No evidence suggests that pregnancy is an independent risk factor for the acceleration of nephropathy in most women (15). The exception is women with moderate-to-severe renal impairment (serum creatinine level >124 µmol/L), who have a 45% risk for pregnancy-related permanent decline in GFR (17). It seems that pregnancy shortens the time to end-stage renal failure by 36 months in women with moderate renal insufficiency. It may be prudent to recommend delaying pregnancy until after transplantation in women with severe renal impairment. In women who have no nephropathy at the time of pregnancy, poor glycemic control and transient proteinuria during pregnancy are associated with the subsequent development of nephropathy (4).

Hypertension is seen in 30% of women with diabetic nephropathy in the first trimester and in 75% by the third trimester (14). Women with nephropathy have an increased risk for superimposed preeclampsia (65%) compared with those without nephropathy (9%) (15). Other risk factors for preeclampsia in diabetic women include nulliparity and poor glycemic control. Deteriorating renal function and superimposed preeclampsia are responsible for the high rates of preterm delivery (>50%), low birthweight, and cesarean section. Despite the potential fetal and maternal complications, 90% of pregnancies in women with early nephropathy are successful.

It is important to note that pregnancies are less likely to be planned in women with renal disease than in women without nephropathy (30% compared with 70%). This may be because of irregular menses associated with renal disease or because of discouraging advice given by health care providers. Counseling of such women and their partners must include discussion of the multiple problems that develop as nephropathy progresses, the decline in fertility with chronic renal insufficiency, and the major disruption in lifestyle and the shortened life expectancy that follow the development of end-stage renal disease.

Neuropathy

Peripheral and cranial neuropathies do not usually cause problems in pregnancy. In fact, symptomatic peripheral neuropathy may be alleviated as a result of tightened glucose control. Autonomic neuropathy may lead to many disabling symptoms, including symptomatic postural hypotension, hypoglycemia unawareness, and worsening gastroparesis. Severe hyperemesis gravidarum exacerbates gastroparesis and often necessitates hospitalization for fluid, electrolyte, and nutritional management.

Coronary Artery Disease

Fortunately, coronary artery disease is uncommon in diabetic women of childbearing age. Before conception, any woman in whom angina is suspected on the basis of symptoms or evidence of atherosclerotic disease should undergo formal exercise stress testing. Maternal and fetal survival rates have improved significantly in recent years; the current maternal mortality rate is 13%, much lower than the previously reported 50% rate (18). Nevertheless, any woman with coronary artery disease who is considering pregnancy should be fully informed of the hazards associated with pregnancy and delivery and of her reduced life expectancy.

Infections

Infections are more common in women with type 1 diabetes than in nondiabetic persons and may precipitate DKA. Compared with nondiabetic controls, women with type 1 diabetes have an increased rate of antepartum infections (83% compared with 26%), including urinary, genital, and respiratory tract infections (19). *Candida albicans* is the most common isolate. The post–cesarean section infection rate is also higher in these women (24.6% compared with 4.6%), although it may be decreased by intraoperative antibiotic prophylaxis (20).

All prepregnant and antepartum patients should be screened for asymptomatic bacteriuria, which should be treated with oral antibiotics because successful eradication results in a reduction in maternal pyelonephritis, with its associated risks of preterm delivery and low birthweight (21).

Effect of Type 1 Diabetes on the Fetus and Neonate

Fetal and Neonatal Loss

The rate of first-trimester pregnancy loss has clearly been shown to be increased in women with poor glycemic control. However, it is not increased in women in good control (Figure 5-2) (22, 23). Late pregnancy loss may be due to congenital anomalies or "unexplained fetal death." The risk for stillbirth increases from 36 weeks of gestation (12). Fetal death may result from chronic fetal hypoxia, acidosis, intravascular thrombosis due to platelet aggregation and polycythemia, or severe fetal hypertrophic cardiomyopathy causing left-ventricular outflow obstruction. Poor glycemic control, fetal macrosomia, maternal vascular disease, renal disease, preeclampsia, and maternal ketoacidosis all increase risk for stillbirth. Fetal ventricular septal hypertrophy is thought to be due to fetal hyperinsulinemia and is diagnosed with fetal echocardiography in the third trimester or after birth. The effectiveness of tight glycemic control in late pregnancy in reversing this condition is unknown, but it generally regresses by 3 to 6 months of age (24). Despite improved fetal surveillance, maternal glycemic control, and intensive

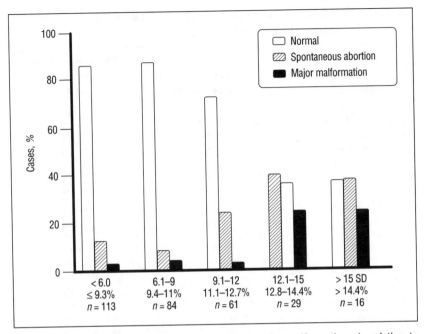

Figure 5-2 Incidence of spontaneous abortion and major malformations in relation to first-trimester hemoglobin A_{1c} level. (From Combs CA, Kitzmiller JL. Spontaneous abortion and congenital malformations in diabetes. Baillieres Clin Obstet Gynaecol. 1991;5:315–31; with permission.)

care treatment of neonates, the overall fetal and neonatal loss rate is 2% to 4%, five times the rate in the general population (25).

Congenital Anomalies

Major congenital anomalies now account for approximately 50% of neonatal deaths in infants born to women with type 1 diabetes (26). Such infants have a twofold to fourfold increase in risk for congenital anomalies compared with the general population (the risk is approximately 2% in healthy women), and this risk is directly related to the hemoglobin A_{1c} level at the time of conception. All organ systems are at risk, but risks for some defects, such as the caudal regression syndrome, are greatly increased in type 1 diabetes (Table 5-3). Because organogenesis occurs very early in fetal life (most major systems are established by 7 weeks after the first missed period), the insult to normal development occurs very early and often before the woman knows that she is pregnant (Figure 5-3).

Table 5-3 Major Congenital Anomalies in Infants of Diabetic Mothers Compared with Infants of Nondiabetic Mothers

Malformation	Relative Risk in Infants of Diabetic Mothers	Incidence in Infants of Diabetic Mothers per 1000 births
Cardiac	4	10
Central nervous system		7.2
Anencephaly	5	3.0
Spina bifida	3	1.7
Isolated hydrocephalus	3	1.7
Other	6	0.8
Skeletal		7.0
Talipes	2	1.7
Arthrogryposis	28	0.3
Urinary tract		3.2
Ureteral duplication	23	0.7
Cystic kidney	4	0.6
Agenesis	5	0.3
Gastrointestinal		3.2
Ureteral duplication	23	0.7
Cystic kidney	4	0.6
Agenesis	5	0.3
Cleft lip/palate	1.5	1.8
Caudal regression syndrome	212	1.3
Pseudohermaphroditism	11	0.6

From Combs CA, Kitzmiller JL. Spontaneous abortion and congenital malformations in diabetes. Baillieres Clin Obstet Gynaecol. 1991;5:315–31; with permission.

Risk factors for congenital anomalies include poor preconception glycemic control and maternal disease, especially nephropathy and hypertension. Most evidence points towards a direct effect of hyperglycemia on the developing embryo, but this has not been confirmed in all studies (12). There seems to be a direct correlation between first-trimester glycosylated hemoglobin levels and risk for congenital anomalies (see Figure 5-2). Several studies have confirmed that the rate of congenital anomalies is reduced in women who receive prepregnancy counseling that results in lower levels of hemoglobin A_{1c} (19). Folic acid supplementation has been shown to reduce neural tube defects in both the high-risk and the general population. Although no studies have been done specifically in diabetic women, it seems prudent to recommend folic acid supplementation for all women considering pregnancy. A dosage of 1 mg/d is probably adequate for these women. Investigations to determine the risk for and presence of congenital anomalies should include a first-trimester measurement of hemoglobin A_{1c}, estimation of maternal serum alpha-feto-

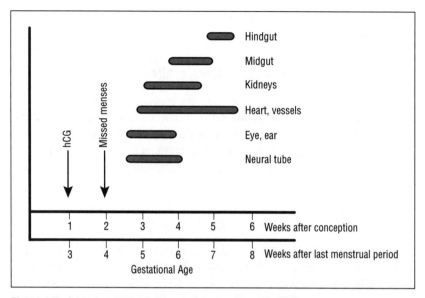

Figure 5-3 Critical periods of development for major body systems resulting in major malformations in infants of diabetic mothers. hCG = human chorionic gonadotropin. (From Combs CA, Kitzmiller JL. Spontaneous abortion and congenital malformations in diabetes. Baillieres Clin Obstet Gynaecol. 1991;5:315–31; with permission.)

protein level (as part of a maternal triple screening) at 15 to 18 weeks of gestation, fetal anatomic ultrasonography at 18 to 20 weeks, and, in high-risk situations, fetal echocardiography at 18 to 22 weeks.

Low or High Birthweight

Macrosomic (>4500 g) or large-for-gestational-age (>95% of normal for gestational age) babies are at increased risk for traumatic or surgical delivery, shoulder dystocia, brachial plexus lesions (Erb palsy), and neonatal metabolic complications. Excess fetal growth is believed to be due in part to fetal hyperinsulinemia in response to maternal hyperglycemia. However, other factors, such as maternal weight, maternal weight gain during pregnancy, parity, ethnicity, and other genetic factors, also affect birthweight. Potential prevention of macrosomia by intensive management of maternal glucose levels has been postulated, but rates of macrosomia continue to be 8% to 43% (12). Macrosomia may be an indication for delivery by vaginal induction at 38 weeks of gestation or for cesarean section.

Small-for-gestational-age babies are a complication in about 20% of these pregnancies. Cigarette smoking, placental insufficiency from vascular disease, hypertension, chronic renal failure, and preeclampsia are the most common causes of small-for-gestational-age babies (12).

Neonatal Metabolic Disturbances

In the final weeks of pregnancy, maintenance of maternal blood glucose levels between 3.5 and 7.5 mmol/L before delivery is important in lessening the risk for neonatal hypoglycemia (14). All neonates should have frequent capillary glucose measurements and, if the blood glucose level is less than 2 mmol/L (<36 mg/dL), early oral feeding or the use of intravenous dextrose, depending on severity, should be implemented.

Risk for Type 1 Diabetes

A common concern is whether the baby is at increased risk for diabetes. The overall risk is low but somewhat higher if the father has type 1 diabetes (risk to the child, 2.5% to 6%) than if the mother has it (1% to 3%); the risk in the general population is 0.3% (27). The question of increasing risk for childhood diabetes by early exposure to cow's milk when either parent has diabetes remains controversial (28).

Preconception Assessment and Counseling

Mounting evidence suggests that women with diabetes who plan and, if necessary, delay their pregnancies have better neonatal outcomes than do those whose pregnancies are unplanned (28, 29). Optimal glycemic control before conception reduces rates of first-trimester loss and congenital anomalies. If metabolic control is poor—especially if diabetic retinopathy is present—glucose levels should be decreased slowly. Ideally, pregnancy should be delayed until the hemoglobin A_{1c} level is less than 7.0%, but there is little increased risk for anomalies with a value less than 8.0%. Women should be warned that it may take several weeks or months to achieve optimal control and that effective contraception must be used in the interim.

Prepregnancy counseling must be provided by the primary caregiver together with any other health care professional who is involved with the woman's comprehensive management, ideally through a specialized pregnancy and diabetes center (30). This vital opportunity to affect fetal and maternal outcomes continues to be missed in women with unplanned pregnancies. In a retrospective study (31), less than 41% of women attempted to achieve optimal blood glucose control before becoming pregnant. Even after a community-based education program by health care providers to promote preconception counseling, only 34% of women actually received such counseling (32). Four times as many fetal and neonatal deaths and congenital anomalies occurred in the group that did not receive counseling. Women who fail to seek counseling generally include teenagers, smokers, those with lower income and education levels, those who lack marital support or are single, those who have poor relationships with health care providers, and those who perceive health care professionals as being unduly discouraging (32). However, in one study, about 50% of women with unplanned pregnancies were white, well educated, and married and had private insurance and an endocrinologist involved in their management.

Although prepregnancy clinics seem to be effective for the self-selected group of women who use them, "grassroots" counseling must occur at every opportunity from puberty on and must be documented in the medical record (30). Counseling must include assessment of fetal and maternal risk, quantitation of any maternal complications, setting of appropriate blood sugar goals to control hyperglycemia while minimizing hypoglycemia (especially hypoglycemia unawareness), and effective use of self-monitoring and dietary therapy (33). The emphasis should be on enlisting the woman's enthusiastic cooperation and promoting informed self-management whenever possible (Figure 5-4). Any choice to conceive should be an informed decision based on the risk assessment provided by the primary physician with the input of other health care providers.

Management During Pregnancy

Optimal care during pregnancy (Box 5-2) requires a multidisciplinary team of experts, including an obstetrician or perinatologist, an internist or endocrinologist, a dietitian, a nurse clinician, and an ophthalmologist.

Glycemic Control

The target values for capillary glucose measurement are a fasting (premeal) value of 4 to 6 mmol/L (72 to 108 mg/dL) and a 2-hour post-meal value of less than 8 mmol/L (144 mg/dL). Evidence suggests that targeting postprandial measurements may help prevent macrosomia in infants of mothers with GDM, but this has not been shown in pregestational diabetes (34). All prepregnant and pregnant women should, ideally, do four-times-daily home blood glucose monitoring, and more frequent testing may be required in persons whose glucose levels are particularly difficult to control. Overnight (3:00 A.M.) readings should be taken in any woman suspected of having overnight hypoglycemia. The glycosylated hemoglobin test reflects an average of the

1. Strongly Recommended Baseline Tests and Investigations

Tests/Investigations to Order	Optimal Test Result	Repeat Test in "X" Months	
		Before Pregnancy	During Pregnancy
Glycosylated hemoglobin level	Less than 4 SD of my control value (<7% most laboratories)	3 months	3 months
Compare venous and capillary (personal meter) values at same time	Personal meter value within 5% of venous value	6 months	3 months
Random urine microalbumin to creatinine ratio; if positive, 24 h urine for creatinine, protein, microalbumin	Ratio less than 1.5 (or random urine microalbumin less than 10 mg/L)	12 months	3 months
TSH (for type 1 only)	0.5 to 5.5 mU/L	12 months	If normal, no repeat
Serum creatinine	Less than 100 μmol/L (0.8 mg/dL)	12 months	If normal, no repeat
Ophthalmologic examination	Absent or minimal non-proliferative retinopathy Treated proliferative retinopathy	12 months, or more frequently if necessary	If no evidence of retinopathy, then repeat at 6 months

2. Strongly Recommended Patient Interventions

1. Use effective contraception until metabolic control is optimized.

2. Take folic acid 1 mg PO daily.

3. Assess and record capillary blood glucose testing qid.

4. Use insulin dosing bid to qid to achieve AC capillary glucose level of 4–6 mmol/L (72–108 mg/dL); self-adjust insulin.

5. Carry a nonperishable glucose source at all times, as well as keep a source in automobile and at bedside table, in order to deal with early hypoglycermia. Partner should be able to inject glucagon.

6. Visit diabetic nutritionist for dietary counseling.

3. Other Considerations

Other Conditions or Comorbidity	List of Medications	Should This Drug Be Stopped Once Pregnancy Is Confirmed? (Y/N)
Known hypertension?		
Known neuropathy?		
Known gastroparesis?		
Other endocrine disorder?		
Smoker?		
Known coronary, carotid, or peripheral arterial disease?		

Figure 5-4 Preconceptual care for women with type 1 and type 2 diabetes.

Box 5-2 Monitoring of Maternal and Fetal Well-Being Before and Throughout Pregnancy

Before pregnancy
Assessment of retinal, renal, and cardiovascular status
Discontinue ACE inhibitors
Optimization of glycemic control (Hb A_{1c} < 0.07)
Treat asymptomatic bactermia
Folic acid 1 mg PO

First trimester
Accurate dating of pregnancy by ultrasonography
(Re)examination of eyes by ophthalmologist
(Re)evaluate proteinuria
Evaluate glycemic control
  Hypoglycemia, especially overnight
  Hyperglycemia, Hb A_{1c}
  Dietary adjustment

Second trimester
Glycemic control
  Insulin requirements starting to increase
Complications
  Repeat eye examination and evaluation of urinary protein, depending on severity
Fetal
  Maternal serum screening
  Level 2 ultrasonography for anatomic survey
  Consider fetal cardiac ultrasonography

Third trimester
Glycemic control
  Rapid increase from 28 weeks of gestation onward
  Significant decrease in insulin requirements suggests placental insufficiency
Complications
  Monitor closely for hypertension, worsening nephropathy, and superimposed
    preeclampsia
Fetal
  Growth (macrosomia, IUGR)
  Well-being (biophysical profiles, nonstress test)
  Cardiac hypertrophy
Delivery plan

Postpartum period
Glycemic control
  Reduce dose to less than prepregnancy values
  Try to maintain patient's enthusiasm for tight control
Complications
  Maternal (infections)
  Neonatal (hypoglycemia, polycythemia, hyperbilirubinemia, hypocalcemia)
Lactation
  Dietary requirements
Follow-up for diabetes care and contraception, thyroiditis

past 120 days of erythrocyte hemoglobin exposure to blood glucose levels. Normal hemoglobin is defined as HbAA. If a patient has an ethnic predisposition to the sickle cell or thalassemia trait, she should have hemoglobin electrophoresis. The hemoglobin A_{1c} results for HbSS or HbSC for homozygotes are not interpretable, but for heterozygotes the test results may be interpretable in some laboratories (35, 36).

Frequent insulin adjustments will be needed and should be tailored to individual needs. Multiple doses of insulin (34) with self-adjustment for glucose values, exercise, and food intake are usually required to meet treatment goals. In general, premixed insulins are not recommended because they lack flexibility, but their use may simplify treatment in the few women who have difficulty with self-adjustment. Continuous-infusion insulin-pump therapy may be effective in pregnancy, but we do not usually initiate pump therapy in an already pregnant woman because of the time required to achieve an appropriate dosing regimen. Pump therapy has not been shown to be superior to multiple doses during pregnancy (12). Although published data on the use of lispro (Humalog) insulin in pregnancy are limited, this insulin is unlikely to be teratogenic. Thus, lispro insulin use can probably be maintained or initiated during pregnancy after discussion with the patient, particularly if it can facilitate tight glycemic control. There have been case reports of congenital anomalies in the infants of mothers who used lispro insulin, but there is no definite indication that the insulin caused the anomalies. The beneficial effects of less hypoglycemia and reduction of postprandial glycemic excursion may make lispro insulin ideal for use in pregnancy. This is especially true in women with hyperemesis because lispro insulin can be injected after successful food intake. Further studies are required.

Dietary therapy must be adjusted to accommodate the increased energy and calcium requirements of pregnancy. A daily 30 kcal/kg diet with 50% carbohydrates divided into three meals and three snacks is generally recommended. A weight gain of approximately 0.3 kg (0.7 lb) per week in the second and third trimesters is ideal. Hyperemesis and gastroparesis may necessitate changes in dietary management and the use of metoclopramide.

Monitoring for Worsening Microvascular Complications

All women with retinopathy must be followed by an ophthalmologist throughout pregnancy; the frequency of the visits will depend on the severity of the retinopathy. Laser photocoagulation can and should be used if needed.

Women with known microalbuminuria or overt proteinuria must be monitored for worsening renal function and hypertension as well as for superimposed preeclampsia, which may occur as early as 22 weeks of gestation. A 24-hour urine collection for creatinine clearance and protein excretion should be obtained in each trimester and more often if progression is seen. Hypertension should be treated with agents safe for use in pregnancy. Differentiating preeclampsia from worsening nephropathy can be difficult because proteinuria and increasing blood pressure occur in both conditions. A sudden worsening of proteinuria, a sudden increase in blood pressure, or the presence of the HELLP syndrome (*H*emolysis, *E*levated *L*iver function, *L*ow *P*latelet count), strongly suggests the presence of superimposed preeclampsia.

Fetal Monitoring

Monitoring for fetal well-being is usually the domain of the obstetrician. However, it is important that the internist understand the information provided by these tests. First-trimester ultrasonography is essential to ensure accurate dating of the pregnancy. This is important in assessing the risks of premature delivery. To assess risk for congenital anomalies, maternal serum screening and fetal anatomic ultrasonography (at 18 weeks of gestation) should be done. Fetal echocardiography with quality four-chamber cardiac views should be done at approximately 20 weeks of gestation in women with elevated first-trimester hemoglobin A_{1c} levels. Fetal biophysical and growth profiles, including assessment of intraventricular septal hypertrophy, are generally done every 2 weeks from 32 weeks of gestation until delivery. Daily fetal kick counts may also be reassuring.

Management During Labor and Delivery

The timing of delivery is a joint obstetric and medical decision. Preterm delivery is indicated if continuing the pregnancy will pose a risk to maternal or fetal well-being (e.g., a mother with preeclampsia, uncontrollable hypertension, or worsening renal function, or a fetus with severe macrosomia or progressive growth restriction). If delivery is expected to occur before 32 weeks of gestation, corticosteroids are usually given to accelerate fetal lung maturity. This temporarily increases maternal glucose levels and may necessitate the use of intravenous insulin for 48 hours to maintain satisfactory glucose control. Vaginal delivery is preferred unless obstetric reasons necessitate cesarean section. The role of cesarean section in preventing trauma and injury when macrosomia is present is controversial.

In early labor, subcutaneous insulin use should be continued while the woman is still eating. When the woman is in active labor and no longer eating, intravenous insulin and dextrose administration should be started. In general, women need 1 to 1.5 U of insulin per hour, depending on the total daily insulin requirement, to keep the glucose level in the desired range (4 to 8 mmol/L [72 to 144 mg/dL]). With delivery of the placenta, insulin requirements may rapidly decrease. The insulin infusion should be stopped and subcutaneous-only insulin should be re-introduced once the capillary blood sugar level exceeds 10 mmol/L (180 mg/dL). Ketosis is rare during this "honeymoon period."

Postpartum Care

Immediately after delivery, insulin requirements decrease to prepregnancy levels. In fact, there may be a period of 24 to 48 hours in which euglycemia can be maintained without exogenous insulin. However, because of short hospital stays, reinstituting insulin therapy before a woman becomes hyperglycemic seems prudent. The target range postpartum is 8 to 12 mmol/L (144 to 216 mg/dL); this averts hypoglycemia in a woman who must be responsible for the care of her newborn yet keeps blood sugar low enough to reduce risk for infection. When the new mother has established a reasonable schedule, these glycemic targets should be lowered. One half to two thirds of the prepregnancy insulin requirement is an approximate starting dose. Women who breastfeed need less insulin than those who do not. Many women will have changed to a more intensive insulin regimen during pregnancy, and the more frequent dosing should be continued if the woman agrees. This is in the interest of maintaining the recognized benefits of intensive diabetes management.

If ACE inhibitors were used before pregnancy, their use can be safely restarted during breastfeeding. Contraceptive choices should be discussed. Postpartum thyroiditis is more common in women with type 1 diabetes (37). The thyroid-stimulating hormone (TSH) level should be measured if a woman is unduly fatigued or develops symptoms suggestive of hypo- or hyperthyroidism. Treatment is generally recommended only for symptomatic persons; thus, screening is not recommended.

Type 2 Diabetes in Pregnancy

Unique issues for pregnant women with type 2 diabetes include 1) the safety of oral hypoglycemic agents in pregnancy and 2) the effect and management of the comorbid conditions associated with insulin resistance, including obesity, hypertension, and hyperlipidemia. The risk associated with microvascular and macrovascular complications is the same as that in the population with type 1 diabetes.

Oral Hypoglycemic Agents

Controversy surrounds the risk for congenital abnormalities with first-trimester use of oral hypoglycemic agents. One study of 332 pregnancies

(38) showed a 16.9% rate of anomalies (11.7% major anomalies) that were not related to type of treatment: diet, sulfonylureas, or insulin. In another study (39) in 25 women with type 2 diabetes (7 were using metformin, and 18 were using sulfonylurea), there were two stillbirths, 23 living children, and one congenital anomaly (4%). Poor maternal glucose control is the major risk factor for anomalies (38). No data are available on the insulin sensitizers.

Neonatal hypoglycemia was found in 27% of women who received glyburide in the third trimester (40). Lactic acidosis or neonatal hypoglycemia with the use of metformin has not been reported.

In most women, the use of oral agents should be discontinued before pregnancy and insulin therapy should be initiated. This allows glycemic control to be optimized before pregnancy instead of in the first trimester, when the critical stage of fetal development has already passed. However, if a woman conceives while using oral agents, these agents may simply be replaced by insulin. Insulin therapy should be adjusted as in type 1 diabetes. Because of underlying insulin resistance, obese women with type 2 diabetes may need 200 to 300 U of insulin per day by term.

Few data are available on which to base breastfeeding recommendations. It is likely that both metformin and sulfonylurea are secreted into milk. Because of the potential risk for neonatal hypoglycemia and the lack of data, we prefer to continue insulin therapy during lactation in women whose blood sugar cannot be controlled with diet alone.

Comorbid Conditions

Insulin resistance is associated with hypertension, hyperlipidemia, and android obesity. Pre-existing hypertension and obesity increase a woman's risk for superimposed preeclampsia and the morbidity and mortality associated with it. Antihypertensive drugs must be switched for agents known to be safe in pregnancy. Use of ACE inhibitors must be stopped when pregnancy is continued or, preferably, before conception. They can be replaced with a safe agent if the blood pressure remains elevated. Obesity results in an increased risk for several adverse obstetric outcomes, including preeclampsia and macrosomia. Hyperlipidemic agents are not recommended for use in pregnancy, although postmarketing surveillance studies have not shown these agents to have any teratogenic potential (41, 42). Although statins have not been shown to have teratogenic effects, their use should be discontinued before pregnancy or when pregnancy is confirmed. In older women who have coronary risk factors (e.g., hypertension, hyperlipidemia, smoking) in addition to diabetes, investigation for silent ischemic heart disease should be considered before pregnancy.

REFERENCES

1. **Rosenn B, Siddiqi TA, Miodovnik M.** Normalization of blood glucose in insulin-dependent diabetic pregnancies and the risks of hypoglycemia: a therapeutic dilemma. Obstet Gynecol Surv. 1994;50:56-6.

2. **Kimmerle R, Heinemann L, Delecki A, Berger M.** Severe hypoglycemia: incidence and predisposing factors in 85 pregnancies of type I diabetic women. Diabetes Care. 1992;15:1034-7.

3. **Hogay ZJ.** Diabetic ketoacidosis in pregnancy: etiology, pathophysiology, and management. Clin Obstet Gynecol. 1994;37:39-49.

4. **Van Dyk DJ, Axer-Siegel R, Erman E, Hod M.** Diabetic vascular complications and pregnancy. Diabetes Rev. 1995;3:632-42.

5. **Axer-Siegel R, Hod M, Fink-Cohen S, Kramer M, Weinberger D, Schindel B, Yassur Y.** Diabetic retinopathy during pregnancy. Ophthalmology. 1996;103:1815-9.

6. **Klein BEK, Moss SE, Klein R.** Effect of pregnancy on progression of diabetic retinopathy. Diabetes Care. 1990;13:34-40.

7. **Laatikainen L, Teramo K, Hieta-Heikurainen H, Koivisto V, Pelkonen R.** A controlled study of the influence of continuous subcutaneous insulin infusion treatment in diabetic retinopathy during pregnancy. Acta Med Scand. 1987;221:367-76.

8. **Chew EY, Mills JL, Metzger BE, Remaley NA, Jovanovic-Peterson L, Knopp RH, et al.** Metabolic control and progression of retinopathy. The Diabetes in Early Pregnancy Study. Diabetes Care. 1995;18:631-7.

9. **Rosenn B, Miodovnik M, Kranias G, Khourt J, Combs CA, Mimouni F, et al.** Progression of diabetic retinopathy in pregnancy: association with hypertension in pregnancy. Am J Obstet Gynecol. 1992;166:1214-8.

10. **Kaaja RK, Sjoberg L, Hellsted T, Immonen I, Sane T, Teramo K.** Long-term effects of pregnancy on diabetic complications. Diabetes Med. 1995;13:165-9.

11. **Reece EA, Lockwood CJ, Tuck S, Coulehan J, Homko C, Wiznitzer A, et al.** Retinal and pregnancy outcomes in the presence of diabetic proliferative retinopathy. J Reprod Med. 1994;39:799-804.

12. **Garner P.** Type I diabetes mellitus and pregnancy. Lancet. 1995;346:157-61.

13. **Burrows RF, Burrows EA.** Assessing the teratogenic potential of angiotensin-converting enzyme inhibitors in pregnancy. Aust N Z J Obstet Gynecol. 1998;38:306-11.

14. **Kitzmiller JL, Coombs CA.** Diabetic nephropathy and pregnancy. Obstet Gynecol Clin North Am. 1996;23:173-203.

15. **Gordon M, Landon MB, Samuels P, Hissrich S, Gabbe SG.** Perinatal outcome and long-term follow-up associated with modern management of diabetic nephropathy. Obstet Gynecol. 1996;87:401-9.

16. **Jones DC, Hayslett JP.** Outcome of pregnancy in women with moderate or severe renal insufficiency. N Engl J Med. 1996;335:226-32.

17. **Purdy LP, Hantsch CE, Molitch ME, Metzger BE, Phelps RL, Dooley SL, et al.** Effects of pregnancy on renal function in patients with moderate to severe diabetic renal insufficiency. Diabetes Care. 1996;19:1067-96.

18. **Reece EA.** Coronary artery disease. In: Gleicher N, ed. Principles and Practice of Medical Therapy in Women. New York: Appleton; 1998:968-73.

19. **Stamler EF, Cruz ML, Mimouni F, et al.** High infectious morbidity in pregnant women with insulin-dependent diabetes: an understated complication. Am J Obstet Gynecol. 1990;63:1217-21.

20. **Riley LE, Heeren T, Tuomala RE, Greene MF.** Low risk of post-cesarean section infection in insulin requiring diabetic women. Diabetes Care. 1996;19:597-600.

21. **Smaill FG.** Antibiotic versus no treatment for asymptomatic bacteriuria. In: Keirse MJNC, Renfrew JM, Neilson JP, Crowther C, eds. Pregnancy and Childbirth Module. In: the Cochrane Pregnancy and Childbirth Database. The Cochrane Collaboration, Issue 2, Oxford: Update Software; 1995.

22. **Mills JL, Simpson JL, Driscoll SG, et al.** Incidence of spontaneous abortion among normal women and insulin-dependent diabetic women whose pregnancies were identified within 21 days of conception. N Engl J Med. 1988;319:1617-23.

23. **Rosenn B, Miodovnik M, Combs CA, Khoury J, Siddiqi TA.** Glycemic thresholds for spontaneous abortion and congenital malformations in insulin-dependent diabetes mellitus. Obstet Gynecol. 1994;84:515-20.

24. **Veille JC, Sivakoff M, Hanson R, Fanaroff AA.** Intraventricular septal thickness in fetuses of diabetic mothers. Obstet Gynecol. 1992;79:51-4.

25. **Casson IF, Clarke CA, Howard CV, McKendrick O, Pennycook S, Pharoah POD, et al.** Outcomes of pregnancy in insulin dependent diabetic women: results of a five-year population cohort study. BMJ. 1997;315:275-8.

26. **Coombs CA, Kitzmiller JL.** Spontaneous abortion and congenital malformations in diabetes. Baillieres Clin Obstet Gynaecol. 1991;5:315-31.

27. **Warram JH, Krolewski AS, Gottlieb MS, Kahn CR.** Differences in risk of insulin-dependent diabetes in offspring of diabetic mothers and diabetic fathers. N Engl J Med. 1984;311:149-52.

28. **Ellis TM, Atkinson MA.** Early infant diets and insulin-dependent diabetes. Lancet. 1996;347:1464-5.

29. **The Diabetes Control and Complications Trial Research Group.** Pregnancy outcomes in the Diabetes Control and Complications Trial. Am J Obstet Gynecol. 1996;174:1343-53.

30. **Gregory R, Tattersall RB.** Are diabetic pre-pregnancy clinics worthwhile? Lancet. 1992;340:656-8.

31. **Holing EV, Beyer CS, Brown ZA, Connell FA.** Why don't women with diabetes plan their pregnancies? Diabetes Care. 1998;21:889-95.

32. **Willhoite, MB, Bennert HW, Palomaki GE, Zaremba MM, Herman WH, Williams JR, Spear NH.** The impact of preconception counseling on pregnancy outcomes: the experience of the Maine Diabetes in Pregnancy Program. Diabetes Care. 1993;16:450-5.

33. **Van Allen MI.** Folate up for healthy babies. Can Med Assoc J. 1994;151:151-4.

34. **De Veciana M, Marjor CA, Morgan MI, Asrat T, Toohey JS, Lien JM, Evans AT.** Postprandial versus preprandial blood glucose monitoring in women with gestational diabetes mellitus requiring insulin therapy. N Engl J Med. 1995;333:1237-41.

35. **Allen LC.** Effects of hemoglobin variants on Hb A1c determinations using Bio-Rad columns. Clin Biochem. 198;18:173-5.

36. **Weykamp CW, Martina WV, van der Dijs FP, Penders TJ, van der Slik W, Muskiet FA.** Hemoglobin S and C: reference values for glycohemoglobin in heterozygotes, double-heterozygotes and homozygous subjects, as established by 13 methods. Clin Chim Acta. 1994;231:161-71.

37. **Gerstein HC.** Incidence of postpartum thyroid dysfunction in patients with type I diabetes mellitus. Ann Intern Med. 1993;118:419-23.

38. **Towner D, Kjos SL, Leung B, Montoro MM, Xiang A, Mestman JH, et al.** Congenital malformations in pregnancies complicated by NIDDM. Diabetes Care. 1995;18:1446-51.

39. **Hellmuth E, et al.** Congenital malformations in offspring of diabetic women treated with oral hypoglycaemic agents during embryogenesis. Diabetes Med. 1994;11:471-4.
40. **Briggs GG, Freeman RK, Yaffe SJ, eds.** Drugs in Pregnancy and Lactation. Philadelphia: Lippincott, Williams & Wilkins; 1998.
41. **Freyssinges C, Ducrocq MB.** Simvastatin and pregnancy. Therapie. 1996;51:537-42.
42. **Manson JM, Fressinges C, Ducrocq MB, Stephenson WP.** Postmarketing surveillance of lovastatin and simvastatin exposure during pregnancy. Reprod Toxicol. 1996;10:439-46.

IV. Thyroid Disease
Kai Yang and Gerard N. Burrow

Thyroid disease is common in women, particularly during the childbearing years. In this section, we discuss the diagnosis and management of common thyroid disorders in pregnant women and in the postpartum period.

Normal Thyroid Function in Women

During pregnancy, maternal iodine levels decrease because of an increase in the GFR (1, 2). In addition, active transfer of iodide from mother to fetus occurs. The thyroid becomes hyperplastic and, in countries with low or marginal iodine intake, pregnant women may become iodine deficient and develop goiter (3). The prevalence rate of goiter is related to iodine intake. In an iodine-sufficient area, such as the United States, the thyroid may enlarge slightly (10% to 20%) on ultrasonography, but the increase is usually not enough to cause physically noticeable goiter (4, 5). Therefore, goiter in a pregnant woman from an iodine-sufficient area is usually not a normal physiologic finding.

The thyroid gland primarily makes thyroxine (T_4) and smaller amounts of triiodothyronine (T_3). These are transported on carrier proteins, such as thyroxine-binding globulin (TBG) and albumin. Free T_4 is the biologically active component. It feeds back on the pituitary gland, resulting in increased secretion of TSH if the patient is hypothyroid and decreased secretion if the patient is hyperthyroid.

Common thyroid function tests are

1. Measurement of bound and free T_4 (total T_4)
2. Measurement of free T_4 only
3. Measurement of thyroxine-binding capacity, a functional measure of thyroxine-binding globulin
4. Measurement of T_3 resin uptake, an inverse measure of thyroxine-binding capacity

5. Measurement of the free T_4 index, an estimate of the amount of free T_4 available
6. Measurement of the TSH level
7. Measurement of total or free T_3 in the setting of hyperthyroidism

After conception, TBG increases (see the Key Values table on page 236) approximately twofold because of the effect of estrogen on increased synthesis and decreased clearance by the liver (6). The TBG level peaks in the 12th to 14th week of gestation and then plateaus, resulting in high total T_4 and T_3 levels during pregnancy (5, 7, 8).

Free T_4 also increases in the first trimester and decreases in the third trimester (Table 5-4). The first-trimester change is due to a rapid increase in human chorionic gonadotropin (hCG) levels after fertilization; these levels reach a peak of 50,000 mIU/mL during the first trimester. At this level, hCG has some TSH-like activity (equivalent to a TSH level of 35 U/L), and it increases the T_4 level and decreases the TSH level (9). Up to 15% of normal patients have suppressed TSH levels in the first trimester (7, 8).

Because pregnancy causes immunosuppression, interpretation of thyroid antibody tests may be difficult. Commonly measured antibodies include antithyroglobulin, antimicrosomal, and antithyroid peroxidase antibodies, which are detectable in most cases of autoimmune thyroid disease (10). Thyroid-stimulating immunoglobulin (TSIg) is present in Graves disease. Because TSIg is an IgG that crosses the placenta, its titer may be predictive of the development of neonatal Graves disease and may be helpful in the differential diagnosis of first-trimester thyrotoxicosis. The antithyroid peroxidase antibody is the most specific antibody found in Hashimoto thyroiditis. Measurements of this antibody during pregnancy may be falsely low, especially after the first trimester, probably as a result of increasing cortisol levels.

Normal Thyroid Function in the Fetus

The fetal thyroid gland begins to form at 10 weeks of gestation, and the fetal hypothalamic-pituitary-thyroid axis begins to form at 12 weeks. The fetus is

Table 5-4 Changes in Thyroid Function by Trimester

	First Trimester	Second Trimester	Third Trimester
Free thyroxine (T_4) level	↑	Normal	Normal or ↓
TSH (thyroid-stimulating hormone) level	↓	Normal	Normal or ↑
hCG (human chorionic gonadotropin) level	↑↑	↑	↑

able to make some T_4 and TBG at 8 to 10 weeks of gestation; T_4 and TBG levels increase and then plateau at 35 to 37 weeks of gestation (11). The fetal hypothalamic-pituitary-thyroid axis is relatively immature, as shown by the high levels of TSH present in the baby relative to the level of T_4 produced (11).

Maternal free T_4 and T_3 cross the placenta poorly, although some transfer occurs if the fetus has congenital absence of the thyroid gland (Figure 5-5). In such fetuses, the T_4 level in the amniotic fluid is 50% lower than that in normal infants (11).

In contrast, antithyroid drugs (ATDs) easily cross the placenta. Therefore, the lowest possible dose of an ATD should be used to prevent hypothyroidism and goiter in the fetus (12).

Hypothyroidism

Maternal and Fetal Risks

Hypothyroidism, if untreated, is associated with 70% anovulation. In those patients able to conceive, there is increased risk for spontaneous abortion and preeclampsia. There is no increase in congenital anomalies or abnormal neurologic development. If thyroid-blocking antibodies are transferred to the fetus (this is rare), maternal T_4 would be a crucial source of fetal thyroid hormone (12).

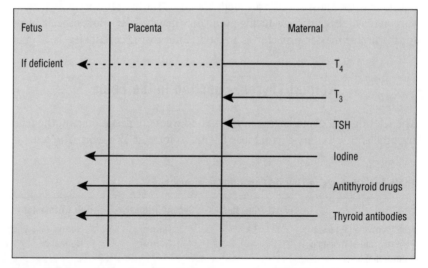

Figure 5-5 Placental transfer of thyroid hormones and antithyroid drugs.

Treatment

During pregnancy, the dose of thyroid hormone often must be increased (13, 14). The reasons for this are not clear and may involve

1) An increased extrathyroidal pool of T_4
2) The need to saturate large quantities of TBG
3) Increased deiodination or degradation of T_4 by placental, renal, or hepatic enzymes
4) Decreased gastrointestinal absorption of T_4 (especially if taken with iron supplement)
5) Increased transfer of T_4 from mother to fetus

Thus, pregnancy is associated with a relative thyroid hormone deficiency. In iodine-deficient areas, the decrease in maternal T_4 levels may lead to neonatal hypothyroidism and subsequent effects on IQ and neurologic function. In iodine-sufficient areas, the decrease causes normal pregnant women to increase iodine uptake and produce more T_4.

Because hypothyroid women cannot reliably increase their T_4 levels (12, 13), the T_4 dosage often needs to be adjusted. The TSH level is a sensitive indicator of the amount of thyroid hormone deficiency in a hypothyroid woman who is receiving inadequate replacement. An increase in the TSH level may occur as early as 4 to 8 weeks of gestation and as late as 6 months of gestation. Thirty percent of patients who have a normal TSH level on the first test subsequently have an elevated TSH level (15). Therefore, as soon as a hypothyroid woman is pregnant, TSH should be measured. If the level is clearly normal, the test should be repeated at 4 and 6 months of gestation. If the TSH level is high, the dose of thyroid hormone should be increased and the TSH should be checked again in 4 weeks. The TSH level should be checked every 4 to 6 weeks until it is stable.

In Kaplan's study (13), the amount of thyroid hormone needed to correct an elevated TSH level was estimated by using the TSH level. If the original TSH level was less than 10, the estimated increase in thyroid hormone was 41 ± 24 μg of T_4 per day; if the TSH level was between 10 and 20, the estimated increase was 65 ± 19 μg of T_4 per day; and if the TSH level was greater than 20, the estimated increase was 105 ± 32 μg of T_4 per day. The group with a history of thyroid ablation was more likely than the group with Hashimoto thyroiditis to show an increase in TSH (76% compared with 46%). Women with Hashimoto thyroiditis still have an intact thyroid that can respond by increasing thyroid hormone production, especially because autoimmune diseases often remits during pregnancy.

After the delivery, the dose should be decreased to the prepartum dose. The TSH level should be rechecked 6 to 12 weeks later.

Hyperthyroidism

Hyperthyroidism is the second most common endocrine problem (diabetes is first) in pregnant women (16). Clinical hyperthyroidism is seen in 0.1% to 0.2% of all pregnant women (2, 16, 17).

Maternal and Fetal Risks

Adverse fetal and maternal outcomes depend on whether the elevated T_4 levels are appropriately treated and on the cause of the underlying disorder. Most complications occur in patients who are undiagnosed or uncontrolled (18). These patients have greater risk for pregnancy-induced hypertension, premature delivery, congestive heart failure, thyroid storm, placenta abruptio, and infectious complications (2). It is not clear whether hyperthyroidism itself increases the miscarriage rate. Fetal or neonatal hyperthyroidism, IUGR leading to small-for-gestational-age babies, prematurity (19), and an increased incidence of stillbirths may affect the fetus (2). One study (20) also described an increased incidence of congenital malformations.

Is controlling hyperthyroidism during pregnancy important? In a study by Davis and associates (18), stillbirth was seen in 24% in patients with untreated hyperthyroidism and 5% to 7% of treated patients; premature delivery occurred in 53% of untreated patients and 9% to 11% of treated patients; and thyroid storm was seen in 21% of untreated patients and 5% of treated patients. Millar and colleagues (21) found that the relative risk for low-birthweight babies was 0.74 in mothers who were euthyroid throughout pregnancy. If hyperthyroidism occurred primarily during the first half of pregnancy, the relative risk for a low-birthweight baby was 2.36; if hyperthyroidism was seen throughout the pregnancy, the relative risk was 9.24 (21). Mitsuda and co-workers (22) noted that small-for-gestational age babies are more likely in mothers who were hyperthyroid for more than 30 weeks during pregnancy, had Graves disease for more than 10 years, had Graves disease beginning at an age less than 20 years, or had maternal TSIg or TSH-binding inhibitor IgG levels of more than 30%.

Diagnosis

Hyperthyroidism in pregnancy may be difficult to diagnose because many symptoms of normal pregnancy—including heat intolerance, fatigue, and increased basal metabolic rate—are similar to symptoms of hyperthyroidism. The more specific signs of hyperthyroidism include eye signs, weight loss, onycholysis, or heart rate that exceeds 100 beats/min and is unchanged with a Valsalva maneuver (17, 23).

The tests necessary to establish a diagnosis of hyperthyroidism include free T_4, TSH, total or free T_3, and antibody studies. Because T_4 levels can be high and TSH levels can be on the low side (they are even suppressed in 15% of normal patients), the diagnosis can be difficult to make in the first trimester. If the free T_4 level is very high and the TSH level is suppressed to less than 0.05 the patient is very likely to be truly hyperthyroid. Glinoer and associates (7) noted that a total T_4 level greater than 15 μg/dL or a T_3 level greater than 250 ng/dL is rare in normal pregnancy. Measurement of T_3RU may be useful. Typically, T_3RU levels are low during pregnancy, reflecting an increase in TBG. If the T_3RU level is high, there are fewer binding sites; this suggests the presence of hyperthyroidism (23). A level of thyroid-stimulating antibodies greater than 300% is highly suggestive of Graves disease, although TSIg may be normal in Graves disease.

A radioiodine scan is usually ordered in the work-up of hyperthyroidism in the nonpregnant patient. However, during pregnancy, radioiodine is *absolutely contraindicated* because it is taken up by the fetal thyroid and can cause fetal thyroid ablation.

Differential Diagnosis

Once the diagnosis of hyperthyroidism is secure, the causes of hyperthyroidism must be considered (Box 5-3). The causes of hyperthyroidism include hyperemesis gravidarum, Graves disease, toxic multinodular goiter, toxic

---

Box 5-3 Conditions Associated with Hyperthyroidism During Pregnancy

Excess secretion of hCG
  Hyperemesis gravidarum
  Trophoblastic disease
Graves disease
Thyroiditis
  Silent (lymphocytic)
  Subacute (granulomatous)
Solitary toxic nodule
Toxic multinodular goiter
Exogenous thyroid hormone
Struma ovarii
TSH-producing adenoma

Adapted from Inzucchi SE, Burrow GN. Hyperthyroidism in pregnancy. In: Bardin, ed. Current Therapy in Endocrinology and Metabolism, 6th ed. St. Louis, MO: Mosby; 1997:312-7.

adenoma, subacute thyroiditis, iatrogenic hyperthyroidism, TSH-secreting adenoma, ovarian struma, and hydatidiform mole (16).

Hyperemesis Gravidarum

Hyperemesis gravidarum, a poorly understood entity, occurs in 2 of every 1000 pregnancies (9). It is characterized by weight loss in excess of 5% of normal body weight, ketonuria, and vomiting in gestational weeks 6 to 9. Patients may have abnormal electrolyte and liver function test results (24). Two thirds of patients with hyperemesis gravidarum will have abnormal thyroid function tests, usually an elevated free T_4 level (59%), undetectable TSH (30%), or suppressed TSH (60%) (24). Patients usually have no stigmata of hyperthyroidism, including eye signs and goiter, and they usually test negative for antibodies (25). Most patients improve and have less vomiting by gestational weeks 16 to 20 without specific treatment of their biochemical hyperthyroidism (24, 25).

Although there is controversy over whether the hyperthyroidism causes the nausea and vomiting, most investigators believe that the symptoms are due to increased hCG production. The elevated hCG level also interacts with the TSH receptor to cause mild biochemical hyperthyroidism (26).

Hyperemesis gravidarum can be difficult to distinguish from true hyperthyroidism. If symptoms persist beyond 10 to 20 weeks, if the patient is positive for TSIg, or if signs and symptoms of hyperthyroidism antedate the pregnancy, it is more likely that the patient is truly hyperthyroid.

A more extreme case of inappropriate hCG secretion results from secretion by gestational trophoblastic neoplastic conditions, such as hydatidiform mole or choriocarcinoma (25). Trophoblastic disease occurs in 1 in 1500 pregnancies, although it is more common in Asian countries (1 in 300 to 500) (9, 27). Extreme levels of hCG (e.g., 1000 times normal levels) may cause hyperthyroidism in 50% of patients. These patients have biochemical hyperthyroidism, small goiter, and low TSH levels. Radioiodine uptake is high. Clinical symptoms range from none to severe thyrotoxicosis with thyroid storm (9, 27). Effective treatment involves surgical removal of the mole and the use of iodine, beta-blockers, and ATDs before surgery.

Graves Disease

Graves disease is an autoimmune disorder in which antibodies to the TSH receptor cause hyperthyroidism. Monitoring a patient with Graves disease during pregnancy involves two concerns: 1) controlling maternal hyperthyroidism without inducing fetal hypothyroidism and 2) evaluating for fetal hyperthyroidism (28).

The preconception management of patients with known Graves disease should establish an euthyroid state for at least 3 months before pregnancy.

Some investigators advocate radioactive iodine ablation of the thyroid in all young women with Graves disease (29) to avoid hyperthyroidism during pregnancy, although many clinicians do not recommend this. If a woman elects to have radioactive iodine treatment, she should wait several months after treatment before conceiving. If she continues to use ATDs, she should be euthyroid before conception.

In patients who have not been treated surgically or with radioactive iodine, Graves disease is usually worse in the first half of pregnancy and then remits because of the immunosuppressed state of pregnancy. Postpartum, Graves disease often flares because of the return to immunocompetence (16, 30).

Once the patient is pregnant, the ATD dose should be reduced with the goal of achieving thyroid function test results in the high normal to slightly hyperthyroid range (2, 31). The lowest possible ATD dose should be used because these drugs cross the placenta and can induce fetal hypothyroidism, goiter, and asphyxia (12, 29).

Thyroid function tests (free T_4, total T_3, and TSH) should be ordered frequently, at least every 4 weeks initially, until hyperthyroidism improves. The ATD dose should be decreased when the free T_4 level is in the near-normal range. The TSH level may remain in the suppressed range and should not be used to adjust antithyroid medication. Pregnant women tolerate mild hyperthyroidism well. Frequent monitoring is essential because 30% of patients can stop use of the ATD during the last weeks of gestation (16). However, ATD requirements often increase within 2 to 3 months after delivery.

All women with a history of Graves disease, including those who have been treated with radioactive iodine and who are either using no medications or are receiving T_4 replacement, are at risk for fetal hyperthyroidism. Although the mother is euthyroid because she has gone into remission or because her thyroid has been treated with radioactive iodine or surgically removed, she still carries autoantibodies to the thyroid. Fetal hyperthyroidism may occur when TSIg crosses the placenta and stimulates the fetal thyroid. Evidence of fetal tachycardia (heart rate >160 beats/min) or goiter, persistent hyperthyroidism or presence of a high antibody titer in the mother, or a previously affected sibling should alert the clinician to the possibility of fetal hyperthyroidism (10).

Neonatal hyperthyroidism is common, with an incidence rate of 1% to 5% (10). Babies with neonatal hyperthyroidism may have goiter, exophthalmos, tachycardia, failure to thrive, irritability, jaundice, heart failure, thrombocytopenia, advanced bone age, craniosynostosis, poor weight gain, and decreased feeding (10, 32). These symptoms should resolve within 3 months as maternal immunoglobulins are cleared, but some authors have noted persistence for as long as 7 months (32). If a mother is receiving ATDs, 5 to 10 days may pass before the appearance of hyperthyroid symptoms; this is due to the residual effect of ATDs. Very rarely, a patient may have both blocking and stimulatory antibodies and may manifest hypothyroidism alternating with hyperthyroidism or may manifest only transient hypothyroidism (1 in 220,000 births) (10, 28, 32).

Treatment

An asymptomatic woman with mild hyperthyroidism can probably be observed only. However, a pregnant woman with moderate to severe hyperthyroidism should be treated. In addition to the adverse effects to the mother and fetus, thyroid storm may be precipitated by cesarean section, labor and delivery, or preeclampsia.

Beta-blockers have been avoided because of early reports that the use of nonselective agents may cause IUGR, small placenta, postnatal hypoglycemia, bradycardia, increased fetal loss, and impaired response to anoxic stress (33–36). However, beta-blockers have not proved harmful for short-term use (until ATDs are effective) in a markedly symptomatic patient or as a preoperative regimen in patients with hyperthyroidism or in patients with thyroid storm. Propranolol 20 mg orally four times daily for 4 or 5 days before surgery or until the free T_4 level is reduced by medical therapy is useful.

The mainstay of therapy is the use of ATDs. There are two choices in the United States: propylthiouracil and methimazole (Tapazole). Both have side effects, such as rash, which occurs in 5% of patients. More serious side effects include hepatitis and agranulocytosis. Agranulocytosis occurs in 0.5% of patients. It is usually idiosyncratic with propylthiouracil and dose-related with methimazole (>40 mg/d) and may require hospitalization. Patients need to be counseled to hold the medication and have a leukocyte count checked in the presence of sore throat or fever. Hepatitis and agranulocytosis are serious side effects, and thionamides should not be given to the patient again.

The choice of an ATD depends on numerous factors (Table 5-5). Propylthiouracil and methimazole are equally effective in controlling hyperthyroidism and have similar adverse effects (37). Propylthiouracil probably crosses the placenta less well than methimazole does, although controversy surrounds this idea (25, 38, 39). Methimazole is used once or twice a day, and propylthiouracil is used three to four times daily; therefore, compliance may be better with methimazole. Methimazole concentrations in the mother's milk are 10 times higher than those of propylthiouracil; only 0.025% to 0.077% of a dose of propylthiouracil is excreted in milk (31, 40). Methimazole use has been reported in association with a congenital defect known as aplasia cutis congenita. In this disorder, localized patches of skin are absent at birth; 70% to 85% of these lesions occur on the scalp. The natural incidence rate of this defect is 0.03%. In other studies, however, methimazole did not cause such defects (20, 31). Propylthiouracil has not been associated with aplasia cutis.

Table 5-5 Comparison of Propylthiouricil and Methimazole

Variable	Propylthiouricil	Methimazole
Usual starting dose*	50–150 mg tid	10–15 mg bid
Half-life	1 hour	5 hours
Placental transfer	++	+++
Breast milk concentration	+	++

* Depends on severity of hyperthyroidism.

Overall, propylthiouracil and methimazole are equally effective in controlling hyperthyroidism. Propylthiouracil is probably the best choice, given the total absence of an association with aplasia cutis and the low concentrations of the drug in breastmilk. However, if a patient cannot tolerate propylthiouracil, methimazole is a viable alternative during pregnancy. The ATD dose should be kept as low as possible so that the mother's thyroid function test results are in the upper normal to mildly thyrotoxic range (31, 41).

Giving levothyroxine along with an ATD has no value because levothyroxine crosses the placenta poorly. Supplemental T_4 will prompt the use of higher doses of ATD, increasing the chance of fetal exposure to ATDs (19).

Lugol solution or iodine should be avoided because iodine may be taken up by the fetal thyroid and cause goiter. The only exceptions to this rule are during thyroid storm or before surgery (16).

Surgical excision of an overactive thyroid is an option for a patient who is noncompliant or intolerant of ATDs; excision is best done in the second trimester.

Postpartum Thyroiditis

Postpartum thyroid dysfunction can be caused by several distinct disorders, the most common of which are postpartum painless thyroiditis (PPT), postpartum Graves disease, postpartum Hashimoto thyroiditis, and postpartum toxic nodular goiter. The most common form of postpartum hyperthyroidism is PPT; it is six times more frequent than postpartum Graves disease.

Postpartum thyroiditis is seen in 3% to 6% of women in the 6 to 12 months after delivery (42). Classically, there is a destructive phase within the first 2 postpartum months during which release of preformed thyroid hormone causes hyperthyroidism. This is followed by hypothyroidism during the next 3 months. By 1 year postpartum, most patients are euthyroid. However, patients may develop symptoms of both hypothyroidism and hyperthyroidism, hyperthyroidism only, or hypothyroidism only. New mothers may not notice the symptoms of hyperthyroidism because weight loss, fatigue, and anxiety may be perceived as normal postpartum events. It is not until they develop hypothyroid features that many seek medical attention.

Seventy-five percent of patients with PPT are positive for antibodies, and this suggests an autoimmune pathogenesis (9, 43). Patients who have positive antibody studies in the first trimester have a threefold increased chance for PPT (6, 42). Patients who have type 1 diabetes also have an increased risk for PPT (44, 45).

Diagnosis in the hyperthyroid phase can be confirmed by a radioactive iodine uptake test unless the mother is breastfeeding. A low uptake distinguishes PPT from Graves disease. In patients who are not lactating and are not overly symptomatic, repeated thyroid function tests 1 month later are useful. They will show alleviation of the hyperthyroidism and, often, conversion to a hypothyroid phase that is not seen in Graves disease. Radioactive iodine uptake done in the hypothyroid phase is not helpful because the results are usually normal or slightly elevated.

Treatment involves observation during the thyrotoxic phase, with beta-blockers if needed for symptoms. Radioactive iodine and ATDs are not useful because the patient is releasing preformed thyroid hormone. Similarly, patients may receive observation only during the hypothyroid phase, with short-term T_4 therapy if symptoms are bothersome. Use of T_4 should be discontinued after 3 to 6 months, and the TSH level should be measured 6 weeks after discontinuation to determine whether the hypothyroidism has resolved. Twenty-three percent to 30% of these women develop permanent hypothyroidism and should have thyroid function tested yearly. Patients who have had PPT are also at risk for PPT with subsequent pregnancies (42).

In one interesting study (46), patients with Graves disease were predisposed to PPT and developed both Graves disease and PPT in the postpartum period. In patients who developed postpartum hyperthyroidism, uptake on radioactive scanning was low, normal, or high. Patients who had low or normal uptake also had increased urinary excretion of iodine consistent with iodine leakage from a damaged thyroid. Of these, most became euthyroid. However, 40% became hyperthyroid between months 4 and 9 postpartum and were then found to have high uptake consistent with Graves disease. Therefore, patients with Graves disease may have recurrence of their disease postpartum with or without associated PPT (46).

Thyroid Nodules and Thyroid Cancer

Thyroid nodules occur in 2% of pregnant women (9). As in nonpregnant patients, the optimal work-up includes fine-needle aspiration (47). Nodules are benign in 80% of cases, and the biopsy results may therefore reassure the patient (48). Only if the nodule is discovered after 20 weeks of gestation can fine-needle aspiration be delayed until after delivery. Patients with rapidly growing nodules, lesions associated with cervical adenopathy, or very large nodules should have immediate biopsy. Fine-needle aspiration may result in the following conclusions: insufficient material (<5%; the test should be repeated later); definitely benign (75%); definitely malignant (5%); or indeterminate (20%; these patients have follicular cells) (9). In patients who have follicular cells on biopsy, surgical excision of the lesion is recommended because it is only with full histologic evaluation that the lesion can be determined to be benign.

If fine-needle aspiration in a pregnant woman shows follicular cells, the surgical procedure can be delayed until the postpartum period (9). The question then arises as to whether the woman should have thyroid hormone suppression of the existing nodule. Pregnant women and their fetuses should tolerate the doses commonly used to treat thyroid nodules.

If the biopsy result indicates papillary cancer, the woman should have surgery regardless of the trimester, unless she is only weeks from term (49, 50). Surgery in the first trimester has been avoided because of the risk for spontaneous abortion, but there is no evidence of increased surgical risk during this time. The prognosis for patients with papillary thyroid cancer discovered before or during pregnancy or for patients with known papillary thyroid cancer who become pregnant is not worsened (50). Patients with papillary or follicular thyroid cancer often receive radioiodine therapy after surgery; this is inappropriate during pregnancy and breastfeeding and, if needed, can be scheduled in the postpartum period. After thyroidectomy, patients should be maintained on suppressive doses of levothyroxine (49, 50).

Previous treatment or scanning with radioiodine does not seem to increase the incidence of fetal malformations, infertility, or miscarriages unless a woman is in the first year after radioactive iodine treatment for thyroid cancer. In that case, the miscarriage rate is 40% compared with 20% (51).

REFERENCES

1. **Burrow GN, Fisher DA, Larsen PR.** Maternal and fetal function. N Engl J Med. 1985;313:1072.

2. **Inzucchi SE, Burrow GN.** Hyperthyroidism in pregnancy. In: Bardin CW, ed. Current Therapy in Endocrinology and Metabolism, 6th ed. St. Louis, MO: Mosby; 1997:312-7.

3. **Crooks J, Tulloch MI, Turnbull AC, Davidsson D, Skulason T, Snaedal G.** Comparative incidence of goiter in pregnancy in Iceland and Scotland. Lancet. 1967;2:625.

4. **Levy RP, Newman DM, Rejali LS, Barford DAG.** The myth of goiter in pregnancy. Am J Obstet Gynecol. 1980;137:701.

5. **Berghout A, Endert E, Ross A, Hogerzeil HV, Smits NJ, Wiersinga WM.** Thyroid function and thyroid size in normal pregnant women living in an iodine replete area. Clin Endocrinol. 1994;41:375-9.

6. **Brent GA.** Maternal thyroid function: interpretation of thyroid function tests in pregnancy. Clin Obstet Gynecol. 1997;40:3-15.

7. **Glinoer D, DeNayer P, Bourdoux P, Lemone M, Robyn C, Van Steirteghem A, et al.** Regulation of maternal thyroid during pregnancy. J Clin Endocrinol Metab. 1990;71:276-87.

8. **Weeke J, Dybkjaer L, Granlie K, Jensen SE, Kjaerulff E, Laurberg P, Magnusson B.** A longitudinal study of serum TSH, and total and free iodothyronines during normal pregnancy. Acta Endocrinol. 1982;101:531-7.

9. **Mazzaferri EL.** Evaluation and management of common thyroid disorders in women. Am J Obstet Gynecol. 1997;176:507-14.

10. **Brown RS.** Autoimmune thyroid disease in pregnant women and their offspring. Endocr Pract. 1996A;2:53-61.

11. **Fisher DA, Klein AH.** Thyroid development and disorder of thyroid function in the newborn. N Engl J Med. 1981;304:702-12.

12. **Burrow GN.** Neonatal goiter after maternal propylthiouracil therapy. J Clin Endocr. 1965;25:403-8.

13. **Kaplan MM.** Monitoring thyroxine treatment during pregnancy. Thyroid. 1992;2:147-52.

14. **Mandel SJ, Larsen PR, Seely EW, Brent GA.** Increased need for thyroxine during pregnancy in women with primary hypothyroidism. N Engl J Med. 1990;323:91-6.

15. **Larsen PR.** Monitoring thyroxine treatment during pregnancy. Thyroid. 1992;2:153-4.

16. **Mestman JH.** Hyperthyroidism in pregnancy. Endocrinol Metab Clin North Am. 1998;27:127-49.

17. **Burrow GN.** The management of thyrotoxicosis in pregnancy. N Engl J Med. 1985;313:562-5.

18. **Davis LE, Lucas MJ, Hankins GDV, Roark ML, Cunningham FG.** Thyrotoxicosis complicating pregnancy. Am J Obstet Gynecol. 1989;160:63-70.

19. **Mestman JH, Manning PR, Hodgman J.** Hyperthyroidism and pregnancy. Arch Intern Med. 1974;134:434-9.

20. **Momotani N, Ito K, Hamada N, BanY, Nishikawa Y, Mimura T.** Maternal hyperthyroidism and congenital malformations in the offspring. Clin Endocrinol (Oxf). 1984;20:695-700.

21. **Millar LK, Wing DA, Leung AS, et al.** Low birthweight and pre-eclampsia in pregnancies complicated by hyperthyroidism. Am J Obstet Gynecol. 1994, 84:946-9.

22. **Mitsuda N, Tamaki H, Amino N, et al.** Risk factors for developmental disorders in infants born to women with Graves Disease. Obstet Gynecol. 1992;80:359-64.

23. **Seely BL, Burrow GN.** Thyrotoxicosis in pregnancy. Endocrinologist. 1991;1:409-17.

24. **Goodwin TM, Montoro M, Mestman JH.** Transient hyperthyroidism and hyperemesis gravidarum: clinical aspects. Am J Obstet Gynecol. 1992A;167:648-52.

25. **Burrow GN.** Thyroid function and hyperfunction during gestation. Endocr Rev. 1993;14:194-202.

26. **Goodwin TM, Montoro M, Mestman JH, Pekary AE, Hershman JM.** The role of chorionic gonadotropin in transient hyperthyroidism of hyperemesis gravidarum. J Clin Endocrinol Metab. 1992B;75:1333-7.

27. **Rajatanavin R, Chailurkit L, Srisupandit S, Tungtrakul S, Bunyaratvey S.** Trophoblastic hyperthyroidism: clinical and biochemical features of five cases. Am J Med. 1988;85:237-41.

28. **Brown RS, Bellisario RL, Botero D, Fournier L, Abrams CAL, Cowger ML, et al.** Incidence of transient congenital hypothyroidism due to maternal thyrotropin receptor-blocking antibodies in over one million babies. J Clin Endocrinol Metab. 1996B; 81:1147-51.

29. **Hamburger JI.** Diagnosis and management of Graves' disease in pregnancy. Thyroid. 1992A;2:219-24.

30. **Amino N, Tanizawa O, Mori H, Iwatani Y, Yamada T, Kurachi K, et al.** Aggravation of thyrotoxicosis in early pregnancy and after delivery in Graves' disease. J Clin Endocrinol Metab. 1982;55:108-12.

31. **Mandel SJ, Brent GA, Larsen PR.** Review of antithyroid drug use during pregnancy and report of a case of aplasia cutis. Thyroid. 1994;4:129-33.

32. **McKenzie JM, Zakarija M.** Fetal and neonatal hyperthyroidism and hypothyroidism due to maternal TSH receptor antibodies. Thyroid. 1992;2:155-9.

33. **Sherif IH, Oyan WT, Bosairi S, Carrascal SM.** Treatment of hyperthyroidism in pregnancy. Acta Obstet Gynecol Scand. 1991;70:461-3.

34. **Pruyn SC, Phelan JP, Buchanan GC.** Longterm propranolol therapy in pregnancy: maternal and fetal outcome. Am J Obstet Gynecol. 1979;135:485-9.

35. **Habib A, McCarthy JS.** Effects on the neonate of propranolol administered during pregnancy. J Pediatr. 1977;91:808-11.

36. **Gladstone GR, Hordof A, Gersony WM.** Propanolol administration during pregnancy: effects on the fetus. J Pediatr. 1975;86:962-4.

37. **Wing DA, Millar LK, Koonings PP, Montoro MN, Mestman JH.** A comparison of PTU vs. methimazole in the treatment of hyperthyroidism in pregnancy. Am J Obstet Gynecol. 1994;170:90-5.

38. **Mortimer RH, Cannell GR, Addison RS, Johnson LP, Roberts MS, Bernus I.** Methimazole and propylthiouracil equally cross the perfused human term placental lobule. J Clin Endocrinol Metab. 1997;82:3099-102.

39. **Gardner DF, Cruikshank DP, Hays PM, Cooper DS.** Pharmacology of propylthiouracil (PTU) in pregnant hyperthyroid women: correlation of maternal PTU concentrations with cord serum thyroid function tests. J Clin Endocrinol Metab. 1986;62:217-20.

40. **Kampman JP, Hansen JM, Johansen K, Helweg J.** Propylthiouricil in human milk: revision of a dogma. Lancet. 1980;736-8.

41. **Mestman JH.** A comparison of propylthiouracil versus methimazole in the treatment of hyperthyroidism in pregnancy. Am J Obstet Gynecol. 1994;170:90-5.

42. **Browne-Martin K, Emerson CH.** Postpartum thyroid dysfunction. Clin Obstet Gynecol. 1997;40:90-101.

43. **Stagnaro-Green A.** Postpartum thyroiditis: prevalence, etiology, and clinical implications. Thyroid Today. 1993;16:1-9.

44. **Gerstein HC.** Incidence of postpartum thyroid dysfunction in patients with type I diabetes mellitus. Ann Intern Med. 1993;118:419-23.

45. **Alvarez-Marfany M, Roman SH, Drexler AJ, Robertson C, Stagnaro-Green A.** Long-term prospective study of post-partum thyroid dysfunction in women with insulin-dependent diabetes mellitus. J Clin Endocrinol Metab. 1994;79:10-6.

46. **Momotani N, Noh J, Ishikawa N, Ito K.** Relationship between silent thyroiditis and recurrent Graves' Disease in the postpartum period. J Clin Endocrinol Metab. 1994;79:285-9.

47. **Koutras DA.** Thyroid nodules in pregnancy. Thyroid. 1992;2:169-70.

48. **Hamburger JI.** Thyroid nodules in pregnancy. Thyroid. 1992B;2:165-8.
49. **Rosen IB, Korman K, Walfish PG.** Thyroid nodular disease in pregnancy: current diagnosis and management. Clin Obstet Gynecol. 1997;40:81-9.
50. **Choe W, McDougall IR.** Thyroid cancer in pregnant women: diagnostic and therapeutic management. Thyroid. 1994;4:433-5.
51. **Schlumberger M, DeVathaire F, Ceccarelli C, Delisle MJ, Francese C, Couette JE, et al.** Exposure to radioactive iodine-131 for scintigraphy or therapy does not preclude pregnancy in thyroid cancer patients. J Nucl Med. 1996;37:606-12.

V. Pituitary Disorders
Peter R. Garner and Erin Keely

Unassisted pregnancy is unusual in women with pituitary disease because normal pituitary function is necessary for both conception and maintenance of early pregnancy. It is interesting that a pregnant hypophysectomized woman will have normal gestation and spontaneous labor if she receives adequate replacement with corticosteroids, T_4, and vasopressin alone.

Physiologic and Anatomic Changes of the Pituitary

In pregnancy, the normal pituitary gland enlarges from 660 mg in the non-pregnant state to 760 mg by term. This is mainly due to an increase in the number and size of the lactotrophic cells. This increase in pituitary size does not result in visual-field changes if the woman has a normal pituitary gland before pregnancy. Visual-field changes that occur for the first time in pregnancy should therefore be fully investigated. Serial magnetic resonance imaging (MRI) of the pituitary done in the first and third trimesters by Gonzales and colleagues (1) showed an increased pituitary volume of about 136% overall and an increase in vertical and AP diameter of 2.6 mm, on average. They also found that MRI signal intensity was increased relative to that in the non-pregnant state. Physicians and radiologists should be aware of these normal changes—particularly the increased signal intensity, because this may lead to misinterpretation (1).

Anterior Pituitary Gland

The changes in pituitary hormone concentrations in pregnancy are listed in the Key Values table on page 236. These normal physiologic changes mean that it is very difficult to diagnose pituitary hypersecretion or hyposecretion during pregnancy and that confirmation often has to wait until the postpartum period.

The results of dynamic pituitary function testing (e.g., triple bolus testing) in pregnancy are also vulnerable to misinterpretation.

Lactotroph secretion of prolactin increases during the first trimester because of estrogen and progesterone stimulation of the lactotrophic cells. In the second and third trimesters, the decidua is a source of much-increased prolactin production. Decidual prolactin secretion is not suppressible by dopamine agonists. Prolactin response to thyrotropin-releasing hormone (TRH) infusion is similar in all three trimesters but is probably less than the nonpregnant response (2).

Maternal serum growth hormone (GH) levels are similar during early gestation and the nonpregnant state, but they increase in late gestation as a result of increasing levels of human placental GH, although maternal pituitary GH levels decrease. During pregnancy, placental GH levels increase progressively, but the regulation of placental GH secretion remains unknown. Insulin-like growth factor-1 is produced in response to GH and is elevated in pregnancy.

If it is necessary to measure GH levels during pregnancy, one must be sure that the assay used is specific for GH. Many older assays are nonspecific and measure human placental lactogen as GH; this leads to falsely elevated values in pregnancy. Growth hormone release and response to hypoglycemia is suppressed during pregnancy and up to 1 week postpartum, but testing for this during pregnancy is not advised. Growth hormone–releasing hormone stimulation testing in pregnancy is safe, and the response is unaltered (3).

Levels of TSH decrease in the first trimester with a reciprocal relationship to beta-hCG (4) (see Section IV). They then become slightly elevated by the third trimester but usually remain in the upper normal range (5). The higher the beta-hCG levels in the first trimester, the lower the TSH levels, and this may lead to erroneous diagnosis of hyperthyroidism in the first trimester, particularly in conditions associated with high first-trimester hCG levels, such as hyperemesis gravidarum.

Maternal adrenocorticotropic hormone (ACTH) levels increase progressively throughout pregnancy with a further increase during labor. The progressive increase is a response to elevated corticotropin-releasing hormone (CRH) concentrations in pregnancy, which increase several hundredfold by term. The elevated CRH levels in pregnancy are of placental origin (6). Of medical and practical importance is that placental ACTH is not suppressible after dexamethasone administration; this leads to difficulties in the interpretation of dexamethasone suppressive tests during pregnancy (see Section VI) (7).

Posterior Pituitary Function

Vasopressin release by the hypothalamus is controlled by alterations in plasma osmolarity, blood volume, and several other stress factors, both in pregnancy and in the nonpregnant state. In pregnancy, plasma osmolarity decreases from 285 to 275 mosm/kg (8). The mechanisms of osmoregulatory changes in pregnancy are controversial. Plasma levels of vasopressin are lower in healthy pregnant women than in nonpregnant controls. Release of vasopressin after dehydration or water loading remains unchanged in pregnancy. Pregnancy is characterized by incremental increases in intravascular volume. The volume-sensing vasopressin-release mechanisms seem to adjust as gestation progresses so that each new volume status is sensed as normal.

The metabolic turnover of vasopressin increases fourfold during pregnancy; the increase parallels that of circulating vasopressinase. This enzyme, which degrades vasopressin, is produced by the placenta in increasing amounts during pregnancy. This physiologic change has important medical consequences in the control of established diabetes insipidus during pregnancy.

The other hormone secreted by the posterior pituitary is oxytocin. Plasma oxytocin levels progressively increase during pregnancy, and a dramatic increase is seen at term. The hormone only facilitates human labor; although peaks occur in plasma oxytocin levels during labor, the onset of labor is not altered by hypophysectomy. Oxytocin levels increase during breastfeeding, with levels of 10 pg/mL at the initiation of feeding increasing to 55 pg/mL after 10 minutes.

Diagnostic Testing

Dynamic Pituitary Function Testing (Triple Bolus Test)

A normal triple bolus test consists of GnRH and TRH stimulation with added hypoglycemia induced by insulin for release of ACTH and GH. To avoid hypoglycemia, CRH and GHRH may be used in place of insulin. Although TRH, GnRH, and CRH seem to be safe in pregnancy, no standardized response range has been obtained in pregnant patients. Hypoglycemia can be dangerous and should not be used. Triple bolus testing in a case of suspected hypopituitarism (e.g., the Sheehan syndrome) should therefore be delayed until the postpartum period and should preferably be done at least 6 weeks after delivery.

Imaging of the Pituitary

It is safe to use MRI in pregnancy, and thin-section (2.5 to 3.0 mm) MRI is superior to computed tomography (CT) in pregnancy (9). To date, there is no evidence of embryo sensitivity to magnetic or radio frequency at the intensities encountered during MRI. The National Radiological Protection Board, however, suggests avoiding MRI in the first trimester if possible. High-resolution

CT of the pituitary produces a radiation dose to the pelvis of less than 10 mGy (1 Gy = 100 rads). The upper range of radiation acceptable to the pelvis is 25 mGy, but if CT is done during pregnancy, proper abdominal shielding measures are required.

Pituitary Tumors in Pregnancy

Although several distinct types of tumors can occur in the pituitary gland, pituitary adenomas derived from adenohypophyseal cells are the most common in pregnancy and represent 15% of all intracranial tumors (10). Pituitary adenomas are usually classified on the basis of immuno-electromicroscopic features or on the basis of size (microadenomas are <10 mm in diameter; macroadenomas are >10 mm in diameter). Classification on the basis of size has a practical application with respect to management in pregnancy.

The incidence of prolactinoma (lactotrophadenoma) is approximately 1/1000 women. Because estrogens stimulate lactotroph function, the effects of both pregnancy and estrogen therapy, including oral contraceptive use, have been intensively studied. The Pituitary Adenoma Study Group (10) suggests that no increase in risk for prolactinoma formation occurs as a result of oral contraceptive use. The benign course of pituitary adenoma in pregnancy has been emphasized by the results of large series by Gemzell and Wang (11) and Ruiz-Velasco and Tolis (12).

Prolactin-Secreting Pituitary Microadenomas

Ruiz-Velasco and Tolis (12) reviewed 2000 pregnancies in women with hyperprolactinemia. In particular, women whose pregnancies were induced by bromocriptine usually had an uneventful course, and less than 1% had an incidence of symptomatic complications, such as headache or visual-field defects. Serial MRI studies of women with microadenoma in pregnancy have shown that most microadenomas enlarge slightly during pregnancy but do not become symptomatic (1). Molitch (13), in a survey of 16 prolactinomas in pregnancy, illustrated the difference between prolactin-secreting microadenoma and macroadenoma responses to gestation. The survey also provides a rational approach to management.

Fertility in women who have hyperprolactinemia due to a microadenoma can be restored by use of a dopamine agonist, such as bromocriptine, pergolide, or cabergoline. For women who have adverse effects from or are resistant to dopamine agonist therapy for hyperprolactinemia, options include GnRH pulsatile therapy, human menopausal gonadotropin induction of ovulation, and trans-sphenoidal surgery. Bromocriptine is the treatment of choice because it produces a higher ovulation induction rate (80% to 90%) and a low risk for adenoma enlargement (Table 5-6). For women intolerant or resistant to bromocriptine, cabergoline is a useful alternative. Trans-sphenoidal surgery carries a higher morbidity rate and induces ovulation in only 60% of treated women with a rate of recurrence of hyperprolactinemia of 25% to 50% over 5 years of follow-up (14).

If ovulation induction is achieved with a dopamine agonist, microadenomas have a low risk (<1%) for complications related to pituitary expansion during pregnancy. In view of this low risk, use of the dopamine agonist can be discontinued upon confirmation of pregnancy. Because of the low risk for prolactinoma enlargement, routine periodic visual-field testing is not cost effective. In addition, because prolactin production is both combined pituitary and decidual in pregnancy, serum prolactin levels are variable and monitoring of microadenoma activity by serial estimations of prolactin has little value. Visual-field testing or MRI should be reserved for the rare woman who develops symptoms of tumor enlargement (i.e., headaches or visual-field changes).

After delivery, spontaneous remission of hyperprolactinemia have been noted in 40% to 65% of women with microadenoma, particularly if their prepregnancy levels were less than 60 µg/L. It is ironic that for many women with a microadenoma, pregnancy may be more of a treatment than a hazard. Breastfeeding should be encouraged because postpartum tumor regression has been seen on radiology in lactating women (15).

Prolactin-Secreting Macroadenoma

The management of macroadenoma differs from the management of microadenoma during pregnancy. This is because symptomatic tumor enlargement is greater in women with macroadenoma (16%) (see Table 5-6), but the risk is still low in women who were treated before conception with either irra-

Table 5-6 Effects of Pregnancy on Previously Treated versus Untreated Prolactin-Secreting Microadenomas and Macroadenomas

Type of Prolactinoma	No. of Tumors with Enlargement	Tumors with Symptomatic Enlargement (%)	Tumors with Asymptomatic Enlargement (%)
Untreated microadenoma	246	1.6	4.5
Treated macroadenoma	46	4.4	0
Untreated macroadenoma	45	15.5	8.9

Adapted from Molitch ME. Pregnancy and the hyperprolactinemic woman. N Engl J Med. 1985;312:1364-70.

diation or surgery (4%). Untreated women with macroadenoma greater than 1.1 cm often have visual-field defects during pregnancy (16).

The Bromocriptine Study Group has suggested that bromocriptine or another dopamine agonist be the initial choice for the management of women with macroadenoma who wish to conceive. Surgery or irradiation should be reserved for cases in which bromocriptine failed to reduce tumor size or caused excessive adverse effects or for cases of sudden visual deterioration. Response to therapy should be documented by repeated imaging before conception. Although it may be safe to discontinue bromocriptine therapy for the first trimester, the risk for tumor enlargement and the safety record of the medication may make it more desirable to continue therapy throughout the pregnancy or at least restart it in the second or third trimester. De Wit and Coelingh Bennink (17) showed that bromocriptine prophylaxis during pregnancy in women with macroadenoma prevents symptomatic enlargement. If bromocriptine prophylaxis is not used during gestation, women with macroadenoma require careful monitoring, including monthly Goldmann perimetric visual-field assessment and MRI confirmation in cases of suspected macroadenoma enlargement.

Because dopamine agonists are often used to induce ovulation in hyperprolactinemic women and are often used prophylactically during pregnancy to prevent adenoma enlargement, there has been great interest in the safety of bromocriptine in pregnancy. Bromocriptine freely crosses the placenta, and reports on fetal and neonatal outcome have been published by Krupp and Turkalj from the bromocriptine registry (18). The rates of spontaneous abortion (11.2%), multiple pregnancies (1.8%), and congenital malformations (major, 1%; minor, 2.5%) were similar to the rates seen in unexposed pregnancies (19). Longer-term follow-up studies have confirmed these initial findings, and postnatal development of children up to 5 years of age seems normal (18). Fewer data are available on the safety of cabergoline, quinagolide, and pergolide, but initial studies have shown no adverse effect of these agents on fetal or neonatal outcome.

Clinically, macroadenoma enlargement in pregnancy presents as headache; visual-field defects; diabetes insipidus; or, rarely, pituitary apoplexy. This can occur at any time during pregnancy but is more likely in the third trimester. If proven symptomatic macroadenoma growth occurs during pregnancy, bromocriptine should be the initial treatment of choice. Other therapeutic possibilities include dexamethasone treatment, trans-sphenoidal pituitary surgery, and delivery if deterioration occurs late in the third trimester.

Labor and delivery are usually uneventful, although it has been suggested that women with evidence of macroadenoma expansion should be delivered electively by forceps because intracerebral pressure may be markedly increased by maternal pushing. Postpartum breastfeeding does not cause macroadenomas to enlarge and should be encouraged.

Acromegaly

Acromegaly complicating pregnancy is rare; the prevalence is 5 cases per 100,000 persons. Disturbances of ovulation occur in 85% of women with acromegaly and are due primarily to associated hyperprolactinemia and impaired gonadotropin secretion. Excess GH may also result in maternal diabetes, hypertension, and left ventricular hypertrophy.

Acromegaly is usually due to a GH-secreting pituitary adenoma. Rarely, it may be due to a GH-releasing hormone–secreting tumor of the pancreas or a carcinoid tumor that leads to somatotrophic hyperplasia of the pituitary. Two large series of GH-secreting adenomas in pregnancy have been reported (19, 20). Expansion of GH-secreting adenomas has been reported in pregnancy but is unusual (20). Visual-field impairment is the usual presenting feature, and it often resolves spontaneously after delivery (20).

Before pregnancy is considered, active acromegaly should be treated by surgical removal of the adenoma followed by adjunct radiation or medical therapy if complete surgical ablation is not possible. Bromocriptine therapy normalizes GH levels in only 50% of acromegalic women, and it has little effect on tumor size. Long-acting somatostatin analogues are the medical treatment of choice in acromegaly, and successful pregnancies after treatment with the analogue Octreotide have been reported. Currently, the safety of Octreotide use throughout pregnancy or during lactation is not known.

Maternal GH does not cross the placenta, and elevated maternal GH levels have little effect on fetal growth and development. Macrosomic infants have been reported in mothers with active acromegaly because acromegaly is associated with elevated maternal glucose levels.

Adrenocorticotropic Hormone–Secreting Pituitary Tumor

Cushing disease due to a pituitary ACTH–secreting pituitary adenoma is discussed in Section VI.

Thyrotropin-Secreting Pituitary Adenomas

A successful pregnancy in an infertile woman with a thryotropin-secreting pituitary macroadenoma has been reported (21). Before the pregnancy, the woman was treated with Octreotide, which resulted in euthyroid status and reduced the size of the macroadenoma. Octreotide therapy was discontinued with pregnancy, but symptomatic adenoma enlargement occurred in the second trimester and the therapy was restarted. It thus seems that Octreotide is effective in controlling thyrotropin-secreting macroadenoma during pregnancy and, despite transplacental passage of Octreotide, no abnormalities in neonatal thyroid variables were found.

Gonadotropin-Secreting Pituitary Adenomas

Pregnancy was reported in a woman with a combined follicle-stimulating hormone (FSH) and prolactin-secreting pituitary macroadenoma after cabergoline treatment (22). Before pregnancy, the woman had presented with enlargement of both ovaries with hemorrhagic and serous cysts, which suggested that FSH was biologically active. After cabergoline treatment, both FSH and prolactin hypersecretion were restored to normal and the resulting pregnancy was uneventful.

Pregnancy was also reported in an infertile woman presenting with isolated luteinizing hormone (LH) hypersecretion. No evidence of a pituitary adenoma was seen on imaging, but the LH had normal bioactivity and normal molecular weight. The woman conceived twice after treatment with hCG.

Empty Sella Syndrome

Empty sella syndrome is a radiographic diagnosis made when incompetence of the diaphragma sella allows cerebrospinal fluid to enter the sella and flatten the pituitary gland. The incompetence of the diaphragma may be congenital or may follow tumor erosion, increased intracranial pressure, surgery, or even irradiation. Before pregnancy, pituitary function is usually normal. In the empty sella syndrome, varying degrees of hypopituitarism and hyperprolactinemia have been reported. Pregnancy in a woman with the empty sella syndrome is usually uneventful (23).

Diabetes Insipidus

Diabetes insipidus is caused by an abnormality of vasopressin secretion, action, or degradation. The presenting features are polydipsia, polyuria, and dehydration. Three types of diabetes insipidus are found in pregnancy: central, nephrogenic, and transient vasopressin-resistant (Table 5-7).

Central Diabetes Insipidus

Central diabetes insipidus is caused by decreased production of vasopressin by the paraventricular nuclei of the hypothalamus. It complicates 1/15,000 deliveries (24). Most often, a woman has known central diabetes insipidus before

Table 5-7 Causes of Diabetes Insipidus in Pregnancy

Type of Diabetes Insipidus	Cause
Central	Pregnancy DI worsening
	CNS tumor (e.g., prolactinoma)
	Granuloma (e.g., sarcoid)
	Histiocytosis X
	Leukemia, aneurysm
	Lymphocytic hypophysitis
	Sheehan syndrome
Nephrogenic	X-linked abnormality of vasopressin V_2 receptor
Transient vasopressin-resistant	Increased vasopressinase activity usually due to decreased degradation of vasopressinase in hepatic disease (e.g., acute fatty liver of pregnancy)
	Preeclampsia (particularly HELLP syndrome)
	Hepatitis

gestation because of tumor or another invasive disease, such as histiocytosis X. However, onset during pregnancy has been reported in the setting of the Sheehan syndrome and as a result of enlargement of a prolactinoma, histiocytosis X (25), and lymphocytic hypophysitis. It has also been reported as a complication of ventriculoperitoneal shunt during pregnancy (26).

Central diabetes insipidus often worsens in pregnancy because of increased clearance of endogenous vasopressin by vasopressinase (27). Vasopressinase (cystine aminopeptidase) is produced by the placenta, and its concentration dramatically increases during pregnancy in proportion to placental weight. It is metabolized in the liver; thus its activity is increased in liver disease. Subclinical central diabetes insipidus may be unmasked for the first time during pregnancy because of the need for vasopressin release at a lower serum osmolality and because of increased clearance of vasopressinase. During pregnancy, 60% of established cases of central diabetes insipidus worsen, but 25% improve and 15% remain the same (24).

Although central diabetes insipidus may appear for the first time during pregnancy, the diagnosis may be missed because many of the symptoms, such as polyuria, polydipsia, and dehydration, may be symptoms of pregnancy itself. In addition to these symptoms, profound electrolyte abnormalities, such as hypernatremia and severe oligohydramnios, have been reported and resolved with treatment (28).

Diagnosis of central diabetes insipidus occurring for the first time during pregnancy requires modification of the standard water deprivation test. Persons are normally required to lose up to 5% of their total body weight before dehydration adequately stimulates vasopressin release. Such dehydration can be dangerous in pregnancy and should not be used. The use of DDAVP as a test of urinary concentrating ability is preferred (29). Maximal urine osmolality over the next 11 hours is assessed. Any value greater than 700 mosmol/kg is considered normal (29).

Treatment of central diabetes insipidus in pregnancy is best achieved by using DDAVP 2 to 20 µg intranasally twice daily. This treatment can be given parenterally after cesarean section, but intravenous dosing is 5- to 20-fold more potent than the intranasal spray. Because it is not degraded by vasopressinase, DDAVP is the optimal treatment. Although it has mild oxytocic activity, the risk for premature labor is only theoretical. Transfer of DDAVP to breastmilk is minimal, and breastfeeding is not contraindicated. The largest material published on DDAVP and diabetes insipidus in pregnancy is by Kallen and colleagues (30). Their results suggest that maternal diabetes insipidus and treatment with DDAVP throughout pregnancy does not pose a major risk to the infant.

Labor proceeds normally in women with central diabetes insipidus, and surges of oxytocin can be detected during labor and the puerperium. This suggests that women with central diabetes insipidus, although they are vasopressin deficient, still secrete oxytocin normally. Lactation is not impaired.

Nephrogenic Diabetes Insipidus

The second type of diabetes insipidus seen in pregnancy is the nephrogenic type. Nephrogenic diabetes insipidus is a rare, X-linked disorder caused by mutation in the vasopressin V_2 receptor gene. At least six mutations in this gene have been identified, and direct mutational analysis can now be used for carrier detection and early prenatal diagnosis (31). Nonpregnant women are usually treated with thiazide diuretics or chlorpropamide. Chlorpropamide stimulates vasopressin release and enhances its action on the renal tubule, but it may cause fetal hypoglycemia and neonatal diabetes insipidus and therefore should not be used in pregnancy. Thiazide diuretics are a treatment of choice in nephrogenic diabetes insipidus in pregnancy (32).

Transient Vasopressin-Resistant Diabetes Insipidus of Pregnancy

Transient vasopressin-resistant diabetes insipidus in pregnancy is caused by increased vasopressinase activity due either to increased placental production of vasopressinase or to decreased hepatic vasopressinase metabolism from liver damage (33). The latter is the most common type and usually occurs in the third trimester in the setting of transient disturbances of liver function (e.g., acute fatty liver of pregnancy, preeclampsia, the HELLP syndrome, hepatitis) (34).

Treatment of transient vasopressin-resistant diabetes insipidus in pregnancy requires DDAVP because DDAVP is not degraded by vasopressinase. Close attention to electrolyte and fluid balance is important in the postpartum period, but the symptoms of transient vasopressin-resistant diabetes insipidus resolve a few days to a few weeks after delivery.

Hypopituitarism

After induction of ovulation, a hypophysectomized woman will have normal gestation and spontaneous labor if she receives adequate replacement with corticosteroids, T_4, and vasopressin alone (35). Women whose hypopituitarism is diagnosed before conception generally have good pregnancy outcome. Undiagnosed or poorly treated hypopituitarism carries an increased risk for spontaneous abortion, stillbirth, and maternal morbidity from hypotension and hypoglycemia (36). Hypopituitarism may result from a legion of disorders (Box 5-4), but it may present for the first time during pregnancy, particularly in the third trimester. The most likely causes of hypopituitarism in pregnancy are shown in Box 5-5.

The clinical diagnosis of hypopituitarism occurring for the first time in pregnancy is very difficult to make because the symptoms of nausea, vomiting, and fatigue are common in normal pregnancy. Presenting clinical features are often severe central frontal headache, visual-field changes, or diabetes insipidus. Dynamic testing of pituitary function during pregnancy is very difficult to interpret, but the pituitary-adrenal and pituitary-thyroidal

---

Box 5-4 Causes of Hypopituitarism Before Pregnancy

Congenital or acquired isolated hormone deficiences
Pituitary adenoma
Hypothalmic tumors, craniopharyngioma, germinoma, meningioma, glioma
Granulomatous disease, sarcoidosis, tuberculosis, syphilis, eosinophilic
  granuloma
Vascular diabetes, carotid aneurysm
Destructive or surgical causes
Pituitary surgery
Pituitary stalk section
Infiltration: hemochromatosis, amyloidosis

axes can be tested by a CRH/TRH combined challenge test. The physiologic changes that occur in ACTH and TSH levels during normal pregnancy should be considered when the test results are interpreted (5, 37, 38). Magnetic resonance imaging can be useful in distinguishing a pituitary adenoma from lymphocytic hypophysitis.

Treatment of hypopituitarism during pregnancy consists of hormone replacement therapy. Secondary hypoadrenalism requires maintenance doses of a corticosteroid such as cortisone acetate 25 mg in the A.M. hours and 12.5 mg in the P.M. hours. Parenteral corticosteroids are required to cover the stress of labor, intercurrent illness, infection, and emesis. An added mineralocorticoid is usually not required because the renin-angiotensin system is intact. Normal thyroid function is maintained by thyroxin replacement. Management of diabetes insipidus requires DDAVP.

Sheehan Syndrome

Severe hemorrhage, shock, or hypotension at delivery may lead to postpartum pituitary necrosis, or the Sheehan syndrome (39). The syndrome is now uncommon, and Sheehan himself estimated the incidence at less than 1/10,000 deliveries (40).

The pathogenesis of Sheehan syndrome is still not clear. Sheehan believed that the primary vascular disturbance was spasm of the arterial supply to the anterior lobe of the pituitary gland, resulting in pituitary gland ischemia and variable cellular damage. The hyperplastic pituitary gland of pregnancy is particularly vulnerable to ischemia and the edema that follows it, which further compromises circulation, leading to cellular necrosis and thrombosis in the portal sinuses and capillaries. Several of the patients whom Sheehan originally described were documented to have lymphocytic infiltration and other features found in lymphocytic hypophysitis (39).

Usually, only anterior pituitary function is affected because the posterior pituitary and hypothalamus are supplied by the inferior hypophyseal artery and the circle of Willis, making them less vulnerable to ischemic necrosis.

Box 5-5 Likely Causes of Hypopituitarism During Pregnancy

Diabetic peripartum necrosis
Enlarging prolactin-secreting macroadenoma
Lymphocytic hypophysitis
Histiocytosis X

However, some women with Sheehan syndrome have an impairment of ADH secretion that may lead to partial or overt diabetes insipidus (41).

The clinical presentation of Sheehan syndrome is variable; it may have an acute course or a chronic, slowly evolving one over many months, appearing for the first time again in a subsequent pregnancy. The acute syndrome has a high morbidity and mortality rate due to hypoglycemia and hypotension. There are usually no electrolyte imbalances because mineralocorticoid activity is not impaired, but hyponatremia can result from associated inappropriate ADH secretion and hypocortisolemia. Less-extensive pituitary destruction may produce a slower-evolving picture with loss of one or more of the tropic hormones. The pattern of loss of the tropic hormones is variable, but one of the first signs may be a failure to lactate.

In acute Sheehan syndrome, appropriate hormone replacement therapy with parenteral corticosteroids and hydration should be started immediately after baseline pituitary function tests (of TSH, free T_4, cortisol, GH, prolactin, LH, and FSH) are done. Free T_4 levels may not yet be decreased because of the long half life (7 days) of T_4. After stabilization and in the more chronic presentations, the definitive diagnosis of Sheehan syndrome, with dynamic pituitary function testing, can be made, preferably at 6 weeks postpartum.

Spontaneous recovery from hypopituitarism due to Sheehan syndrome with a normal subsequent pregnancy has been reported (42).

Lymphocytic Hypophysitis

Lymphocytic hypophysitis is a very uncommon autoimmune disorder that usually affects young women in late pregnancy or the postpartum period (43). It can occur in the presence of other autoimmune diseases, such as thyroid disorders and adrenalitis. Pathologically, the pituitary is enlarged secondary to inflammatory infiltrative lymphocytes and plasma cells. The ACTH- and TSH-producing cells seem to be the most affected. Circulating antihypophyseal antibodies have been detected. Most autoimmune diseases go into remission during pregnancy. It is unusual for this lesion to occur in the third trimester. One possible mechanism is that induction of the autoimmune process is initiated by an increased amount of antigen being produced by hyperplastic lactotrophic cells, and prolactin cell antibodies can be detected.

Clinically, the disorder presents with signs of an expanding intracellular mass (i.e., rapid visual-field changes in the third trimester or other neurologic signs) or hypopituitarism, including diabetes insipidus. The diagnosis should be considered in postpartum women with general malaise and persistent amenorrhea as well as hypothyroidism. The disorder can progress to chronic panhypopituitarism but, in some cases, it is reversible with a subsequent spontaneous pregnancy. Lymphocytic hypophysitis before a pregnancy does not adversely affect a future pregnancy, and pregnancy-related relapse of the disease does not seem to occur in the subsequent pregnancy (44).

The differential diagnosis includes an enlarging pituitary adenoma and the Sheehan syndrome, although there is no history of obstetric complication. Absolute differentiation from pituitary adenoma requires pituitary biopsy, but measurements of antithyroid antibodies and ANA suggest an autoimmune cause. In most cases, CT shows uniform contrast enhancement. Because of the preferential destruction of some cells, early striking diffuse homogeneous contrast enhancement on MRI has been noted, so MRI seems to be more helpful than CT in differentiating between this disorder and pituitary adenoma (45).

Treatment of lymphocytic hypophysitis, once it is diagnosed, requires correction of the hypopituitarism. A short course of high-dose corticosteroids produces dramatic resolution of visual-field defects in some women, but the response is not always obtained (46). In women who do not respond to corticosteroids, surgical decompression by partial hypophysectomy may be required.

Pituitary Surgery

Trans-sphenoidal surgery has become the treatment of choice for microadenomas and macroadenomas that are not responsive to medical treatment or that are producing signs or symptoms of enlargement. Trans-sphenoidal surgery done during pregnancy has been reported at least ten times (in five patients with Cushing disease, one patient with the Nelson syndrome, one patient with acromegaly, and three patients with enlarging prolactinoma) without increased maternal or fetal morbidity (14, 30, 47).

REFERENCES

1. **Gonzalez JG, Elizondo G, Galdivar D, Nanez H, Todd LE, Villa Real JZ.** Pituitary gland growth during normal pregnancy, an in vivo study using magnetic resonance imaging. Am J Med. 1988;85:217-20.

2. **Ylikorkald O, Kivinen S, Reinila U.** Serial prolactin and thyrotropin responses to thyrotropin-releasing hormone throughout normal pregnancy. J Clin Endocrinol Metab. 1979;48:288.

3. **Von Werder K, Muller OA, Harth R, et al.** Growth hormone releasing factor-stimulation test in normal controls and acromegalic patients. J Endocrinol Invest. 1984;7:185.

4. **Glinoer D, de Nager P, Bourdoux P, et al.** Regulation of maternal thyroid during pregnancy. J Clin Endocrinol Metab. 1990;71:276.

5. **Kotarba DD, Garner PR, Perkins S.** Changes in serum free thyroxine and free triiodothyronine and thyroid stimulating hormone reference intervals in normal term pregnant women. J Obstet Gynecol. 1995;15:5.

6. **Rees LH, Burke CW, Chard T, et al.** Possible placental origin of ACTH in normal human pregnancy. Nature. 1975;254:620.

7. **Garner PR.** Pituitary disorders in pregnancy. Curr Obstet Med. 1991;1:143.

8. **Thaper K, Kovacs K, Laws ER, et al.** Pituitary adenomas, current concepts in classif cation, histopathology and molecular biology. Endocrinologist. 1993;3:39.

9. **Stein AL, Levenick MN, Kletzky AA.** Computed tomography versus magnetic resonance imaging for the evaluation of suspected pituitary adenomas. Obstet Gynecol. 1989;73:996.

10. **Pituitary Adenoma Study Group.** Pituitary adenomas and oral contraceptives. A multicentre case-control study. Fertil Steril. 1983;39:753.

11. **Gemzell C, Wang CF.** Outcome of pregnancy in women with pituitary adenoma. Fertil Steril. 1979;31:3263.

12. **Ruiz-Velasco V, Tolis G.** Pregnancy in hyperprolactinemic women. Fertil Steril. 1984;41:793.

13. **Molitch ME.** Evaluation and management of pituitary tumors during pregnancy. Endocrinol Pract. 1996;2:287.

14. **Zervas NT.** Surgical results for pituitary adenomas: results of an international survey. In: Black PM, Zervas NT, Ridgway EC, Martiz JB, eds. Secretory Tumors of the Pituitary Gland. New York: Raven Press; 1984:377.

15. **Bergh T, Nillius SJ.** Prolactinomas: follow-up of medical treatment. In: Moliatti GM, ed. A Clinical Problem: Microadenoma. Oxford Excerpta Medica; 1982:115.

16. **Kupersmith MJ, Rosenberg C, Kleinberg D.** Visual loss in pregnant women with pituitary adenoma. Am Intern Med. 1994;121:473.

17. **de Wit W, Coelingh Bennink HJT.** Prophylactic bromocriptine treatment during pregnancy in women with macroadenoma: a report of 13 pregnancies. Br J Obstet Gynaecol. 1989;91:1059.

18. **Krupp P, Turkalj I.** Surveillance of bromocriptine in pregnancy and offspring. In: Jacobs HS, ed. Prolactinomas in Pregnancy. Lancaster: MTP Press; 1984:45-50.

19. **Abelove WA, Rupp JJ, Paschkis KE.** Acromegaly and pregnancy. J Clin Endocrinol Metab. 1954;14:32.

20. **Herman-Bonert, Seliverstov M, Melmed S.** Pregnancy in acromegaly, successful therapeutic outcome. J Clin Endocrinol Metab. 1998;83:727-31.

21. **Caron P, Gerbeau C, Pradayrol L, et al.** Successful pregnancy in an infertile woman with a TSH-secreting macroadenoma treated with Octreotide. J Clin Endocrinol Metab. 1996;81:1164.

22. **Paoletti AM, Depan GF, Meis V, et al.** Effectiveness of cabergoline in reducing follicle-stimulating hormone and prolactin hypersecretion from a pituitary macroadenoma in an infertile woman. Fertil Steril. 1994;62:882.

23. **Georgiev DB, Dokumov SI.** Continuous bromocriptine treatment of empty sella syndrome aggravating pregnancy. Gynecol Obstet Invest. 1991;32:243.

24. **Hime MC, Williams DJ.** Osmoregulatory adaptation in pregnancy and its disorders. J Endocrinol. 1992;132:7.

25. **DiMaggio LA, Lippes HA, Lee RV.** Histiocytosis X and pregnancy. Obstet Gynecol. 1995;85:806-9.

26. **Godsby L, Harlase F.** Central diabetes mellitus: a complication of ventriculoperitoneal shunt malfunction during pregnancy. J Obstet Gynecol. 1996;174:1655-7.

27. **Ryden G.** Cystine aminopeptidase activity in pregnancy. Acta Obstet Gynecol Scand. 1971;50:253.

28. **Hanson RG, Powrie RO, Lawson L.** Diabetes insipidus in pregnancy: a treatable cause of oligohydramnios. Obstet Gynecol. 1997;89:816.

29. **Hutchon DJR, Van Zijl JAWM, Campbell-Brown MB, et al.** Desmopressin as a test of urinary concentrating ability in pregnancy. J Obstet Gynecol. 1982;2:206.

30. **Kallen BA, Carlsson SS, Bergen BK.** Diabetes insipidus and the use of desmopressin during pregnancy. Eur J Endocrinol. 1995;132:144-6.

31. **Cheong HI, Park HW, Ha IS, et al.** Six novel mutations in the vasopressin V_2 receptor gene causing nephrogenic diabetes insipidus. Nephron. 1997;75:431.

32. **Uhrig JD, Hurley RM.** Chlorpropamide in pregnancy and transient neonatal diabetes insipidus. Can Med Assoc J. 1983;128:368.

33. **Durr JA, Hoggard JG, Hunt JM, et al.** Diabetes insipidus in pregnancy associated with abnormally high circulating vasopressinase activity. N Engl J Med. 1982;316:1070.

34. **Usta IM, Barton JR, Amon EA, et al.** Acute fatty liver of pregnancy: an experience in the diagnosis and management of fourteen cases. Am J Obstet Gynecol. 1994; 171:1342.

35. **Kaplan NM.** Successful pregnancy following hypophysectomy during the twelfth week of gestation. J Clin Endocrinol Metab. 1962;21:1139.

36. **Israel SL, Cornstain AS.** Unrecognized pituitary necrosis: a cause of sudden death. JAMA. 1952;148:189.

37. **Burrow GN, Polackwich R, Domabedian R.** The hypothalamic-pituitary-thyroid axis in normal pregnancy. In: Fisher DA, Burrow GN, eds. Perinatal Thyroid Physiology and Disease. New York: Raven Press; 1975:1-10.

38. **Fajardo MC, Florido J, Villaverde C, et al.** Plasma levels of beta-endorphin and ACTH during labor and immediate puerperium. Eur J Obstet Gynecol. 1994;55:105.

39. **Sheehan HL.** Postpartum necrosis of the anterior pituitary. J Pathol Bacteriol. 1937;45:189.

40. **Sheehan HL.** The recognition of chronic hypopituitarism resulting from postpartum pituitary necrosis. Am J Obstet Gynecol. 1971;111:852.

41. **Sheehan HL, Stornfield JP.** The pathogenesis of the anterior lobe of the pituitary gland. Acta Endocrinol. 1961;37:479.

42. **Grimes HG, Brooks MH.** Pregnancy in Sheehan's syndrome: report of a case and a review. Obstet Gynecol Surv. 1980;35:481.

43. **Pestell RG, Best JD, Alfard FP.** Lymphocytic hypophysitis: the clinical spectrum of the disorder and evidence for an autoimmune pathogenesis. Clin Endocrinol. 1990;33:457.

44. **Martin Caballero C, Garcia Lopez G, Cueto MJ.** Ovulation induction and normal pregnancy after panhypopituitarism due to lymphocytic hypophysitis. Obstet Gynecol. 1998;91:850-2.

45. **Powrie JK, Powell M, Ayers AB, Lowy C, Somksen PH.** Lymphocytic adenohypophysitis MRI features of two new cases and a review of the literature. Clin Endocrinol. 1995;42:315.

46. **Reusch JE, Kleinschmidt-De Masters BU, Lillehei KO, et al.** Preoperative diagnosis of lymphocytic hypophysitis unresponsive to short course dexamethasone. Neurosurgery. 1992;30:268.

47. **Freeman R, Wezenter B, Silverstein M, Ku D, Weiss KL, Kantrowitz AB.** Pregnancy associated subacute hemorrhage into a prolactinoma resulting in diabetes insipidus. Fertil Steril. 1992;58:427-9.

VI. Adrenal Disorders
Erin Keely and Peter R. Garner

Adrenal Cortex

During pregnancy, increased steroid hormone production is essential to meet both the maternal demand for increased estrogens and cortisol and the fetal demand for reproductive and somatic growth and development. In addition, alterations in the renin-angiotensin-aldosterone cascade are required to allow for a 50% increase in maternal blood volume without resulting in hypertension. These changes occur through a complex interaction among the maternal and fetal endocrine systems and the placenta.

Control of the Adrenal Cortex

Hypothalamic-Pituitary-Adrenal Axis
Corticotropin-releasing hormone is secreted from the hypothalamus as well as from the lungs, liver, gastrointestinal tract, adrenal glands, and placenta (1). It releases pro-opiomelanocortin and its breakdown products, including ACTH, from the anterior pituitary gland. Release of CRH from the hypothalamus is stimulated by stress, volume contraction, and other factors and is inhibited by glucocorticoids (cortisol) and ACTH.

During pregnancy, maternal CRH levels increase, predominately as a result of placental production (2). Placental CRH production is stimulated by circulating glucocorticoids, which, in contrast, exert negative feedback on hypothalamic production of CRH. Placental CRH enters both the maternal and fetal circulation. In the fetus, it may stimulate the fetal pituitary-adrenal axis. This, in turn, may play a role in fetal organ maturation and parturition (3).

During pregnancy, ACTH levels increase approximately twofold after the first trimester (see the Key Values table on page 236). This increase is, in part, placental in origin and may be a local paracrine effect of placental CRH production. Like placental CRH production, placental ACTH is not suppressible by glucocorticoids. The normal circadian rhythm of high morning and low evening ACTH and cortisol levels continues during pregnancy. The stress of labor causes ACTH levels to increase rapidly and then decrease within 2 days postpartum.

Cortisol circulates both bound (primarily to cortisol-binding globulin) and free. Both total (as measured by serum cortisol) and free (as measured by 24-hour urine free cortisol), cortisol levels increase twofold to threefold during pregnancy.

Exogenous corticosteroids are variably affected by placental enzymatic activity and thus have different rates of placental transfer (Table 5-8). This is important to consider when these preparations are prescribed because maternal and fetal availability will differ.

The adrenal cortex synthesizes three main androgens: androstenedione, dehydroepiandrosterone (DHEA), and DHEA sulfate. The levels of specific androgens during pregnancy are dependent on changes in both production rates and metabolic clearance. Androstenedione and total testosterone levels increase; DHEA and free testosterone levels decrease.

Renin-Angiotensin-Aldosterone System

The renin-angiotensin-aldosterone system is a cascade of events that regulates blood pressure, circulating volume, and sodium–potassium homeostasis. Renin production from the juxtaglomerulus apparatus in the kidney is controlled by renal arteriolar blood pressure, sodium concentration in the distal tubule, and beta-adrenergic receptors. The production of renin is the rate-limiting step in the pathway.

Aldosterone, the major circulating mineralocorticoid, promotes sodium reabsorption and potassium and bicarbonate excretion in the distal renal tubule. Its secretion is primarily controlled by angiotensin II, but hyperkalemia, ACTH, and vasopressin are also stimulants (4).

In pregnancy, the woman must increase plasma volume (and, thus, sodium reabsorption) without increasing blood pressure. Despite the increase in extracellular fluid volume, plasma renin activity levels increase fourfold between 8 and 20 weeks of gestation, after which they plateau (see the Key Values table) (5).

Angiotensin II levels are increased threefold as a result of increased renin and angiotensinogen. Paradoxically, marked resistance to the pressor effect of angiotensin II develops by 7 weeks of gestation, reaching a maximum at 28 weeks. After 30 weeks, there is some return of sensitivity but this does not

Table 5-8 Ratios of Maternal to Fetal Distribution of Synthetic Steroids

Compound	Maternal Concentration:Fetal Concentration
Prednisone	10:1
Hydrocortisone	6:1
Betamethasone	3:1
Dexamethasone	2:1

Adapted from Garner PG. Disorders of the Adrenal Cortex in Current Obstetric Medicine, v. 2. Lee R, ed. 1993:183-220.

reach the values seen in the nonpregnant state (6). The increase in prostaglandin E_2 production known to occur in pregnancy may account for this resistance (7).

Aldosterone levels, in response to increased renin and angiotensin II levels, increase fourfold by 8 weeks and continue to increase, reaching a 10-fold increase by term. However, urine sodium and potassium excretion do not change because of competitive inhibition by progesterone on mineralocorticoid receptors in the distal tubule.

Disorders of Adrenal Cortex

Cushing Syndrome

Cushing syndrome is caused by excess glucocorticoid production of any cause. It may be due to excess ACTH stimulation to the adrenal cortex (ACTH-dependent Cushing syndrome) from the pituitary gland (Cushing disease) or ectopic sources, or it may be independent of ACTH, as in adrenal adenoma or carcinoma and exogenous glucocorticoid therapy (Table 5-9). Hypercortisolism is rare in pregnancy because affected women (especially those with ACTH-dependent cases) have a 75% to 95% incidence of menstrual irregularities or anovulation (8). Adrenal causes of Cushing syndrome are overrepresented relative to ACTH-dependent causes in women who conceive compared with the nonpregnant population with Cushing syndrome (9).

Clinical Presentation

Several features of hypercortisolemia, such as moon facies, abdominal striae, and glucose intolerance, are common during pregnancy. Other features must therefore be present before investigation is warranted. In Cushing syndrome, the striae tend to be wider (>1 cm) and darker and to occur in sites other than the abdominal wall. The presence of proximal myopathy, hypertension, neu-

Table 5-9 Causes of Cushing Syndrome in Nonpregnant versus Pregnant Persons

Cause of Cushing Syndrome	Nonpregnant Persons (%)	Pregnant Persons (%)
ACTH-dependent causes		
Ectopic (lung cancer, carcinoid, islet-cell carcinoma)	16	2
Pituitary adenoma	59	33
ACTH-independent causes		
Adrenal adenoma	16	50
Adrenal carcinoma	9	10
Unknown		5

Adapted from Buescher MA et al. Cushing's syndrome in pregnancy. Obstet Gynecol. 1992:79:130-7.

ropsychiatric disturbances, hirsutism, acne, spontaneous bruising, and poor wound healing are more suggestive of a true hypercortisolemic state.

Pregnancy Outcome

Both maternal and fetal outcomes are compromised in hypercortisolemic states. Increased maternal morbidity is due to hypertension (67%), superimposed preeclampsia (10%), GDM (33%), and hypertension-induced congestive heart failure (10%). Maternal deaths from gastrointestinal bleeding, pulmonary edema, cardiac failure, and sepsis have been reported. Fetal morbidity is primarily due to preterm delivery (33% to 50%). Increased risk for spontaneous abortion and stillbirth (17% to 22%) is also seen (10–12).

Diagnosis

Cushing syndrome is one of the most difficult endocrine diagnoses to make in the nonpregnant state, and its diagnosis is even more challenging during pregnancy because of the altered hypothalamic-pituitary-adrenal axis and placental production of CRH and ACTH. As in the nonpregnant patient, investigation occurs in three stages: 1) a screening test for hypercortisolemia, 2) definitive biochemical diagnosis, and 3) determination of cause.

The best screening test is a 24-hour urine collection for free cortisol. The normal increase in 24-hour urinary cortisol excretion in pregnancy necessitates use of a higher reference range (229 to 680 nmol/24 hours). The diurnal variation of plasma cortisol may also be used because it is unaffected by pregnancy and is usually diminished in hypercortisolemic states. The serum cortisol level at 10:00 P.M. should be less than 50% of the serum cortisol level at 8:00 A.M. The 1.0-mg overnight dexamethasone suppression test is not accurate in patients with estrogen excess states due to the reliance on serum (total) cortisol measurements and resistance to glucocorticoid suppression during pregnancy.

If the screening tests suggest hypercortisolemia, a 2-day low-dosage (0.5 mg every 6 hours) dexamethasone test should be used. During pregnancy, urinary cortisol should suppress to less than 55 nmol/24 hours (10).

After hypercortisolemia is confirmed, its cause must be established. Measurement of ACTH is done to differentiate ACTH-dependent from ACTH-independent causes. Levels of ACTH are increased in pregnancy, but a value greater than 8 pmol/L suggests an ACTH-dependent cause and a value less than 1.1 pmol/L suggests an ACTH-independent cause (8).

Stimulation of CRH with or without inferior petrosal sinus sampling may be useful in the differential diagnosis of the Cushing syndrome. An increase of more than 50% in ACTH level or more than 20% in cortisol level after 1 μg/kg of ovine CRH suggests a pituitary source. Comparison of plasma ACTH levels in the venous drainage of the pituitary gland (inferior petrosal sinuses) with peripheral values allows localization to and lateralization within the pituitary gland (13). A modified approach through brachial rather than femoral veins, to reduce radiation exposure, has been reported in pregnancy (14). The specificity of CRH stimulation tests in pregnancy is unknown and may be altered by the downregulation of the anterior pituitary gland to exogenous CRH from placenta-derived CRH.

Imaging should be directed toward the appropriate area on the basis of biochemical investigations. There is a 10% to 20% chance of incidental pituitary or adrenal lesions in the normal population; thus, positivity on radiography without biochemical confirmation may be misleading. Magnetic resonance imaging is preferred for both pituitary and adrenal lesions because of its specificity and lack of ionizing radiation.

Treatment

Treatment should be aimed at the source of the cortisol excess. Although most case reports of the Cushing syndrome in pregnancy do not report the benefits of treatment during pregnancy, poor fetal and maternal outcomes seem to be improved when the hypercortisolemic state is treated.

Pituitary lesions can be selectively removed by the trans-sphenoidal route (cure rate, 80% to 90%). In three case reports, trans-sphenoidal surgery done at 16, 18, and 22 weeks of gestation resulted in two preterm deliveries (at 30 and 37 weeks of gestation) and one fetal death 17 weeks after surgery (15). For adrenal lesions, unilateral adrenalectomy during pregnancy decreases neonatal complications. This should be done unless the diagnosis is made late in the pregnancy (16). Cortisol replacement is required after both adrenal and pituitary surgery and should be continued until the hypothalamic-pituitary-axis has had time to recover.

If surgical therapy is contraindicated, medical therapy may be instituted. Metyrapone and ketoconazole have both been used in pregnancy in a very few persons. The fetal risks of these agents are unknown.

Hyperaldosteronism

Hyperaldosteronism is the excess production of aldosterone from the adrenal cortex causing hypertension, hypokalemia, and bicarbonate retention (metabolic alkalosis). It is a rare cause of secondary hypertension, accounting for approximately 0.5% to 2% of all hypertensive patients in the general population. Between 60% and 70% of cases are due to unilateral benign adrenal adenoma (17).

Clinical Presentation

Hypertension with hypokalemia is the classic presentation, but 7% to 38% of patients have normal potassium levels. The hypokalemia may be spontaneous or may appear after diuretic use, vomiting, or diarrhea. Markedly low potassium levels may cause headache, muscle weakness, muscle cramps, and fatigue.

Serum sodium levels are high normal, and metabolic alkalosis is present. In normal pregnancy, there is mild respiratory alkalosis with a compensatory decrease in bicarbonate of 4 mEq/L. Thus, one must compare bicarbonate levels in pregnancy to the reference range of 18 to 22 mEq/L.

Course in Pregnancy

During pregnancy, potassium retention is required to meet the needs of the fetus, placenta, breasts, and uterus. This retention occurs, despite elevated aldosterone levels in normal pregnancy, because of the antagonizing effect of progesterone on mineralocorticoid receptors. Thus, it seems that some of the clinical symptoms may be lessened during pregnancy. However, of the reported cases, some worsened during pregnancy (18–20) or postpartum.

Diagnosis

In the setting of hypokalemia, urinary potassium levels greater than 30 mmol/24 hours are required to confirm renal potassium wasting (the patient must not be receiving diuretics). Before further biochemical testing is done, it is necessary to correct the hypokalemia and to discontinue use of medications that suppress renin (such as beta-blockers and calcium-channel blockers) and spironolactone. Aldomet use may be continued during investigations.

The normal increase in aldosterone into the hyperaldosteronism range during pregnancy makes baseline plasma aldosterone levels difficult to interpret. Plasma renin levels should be decreased in primary hyperaldosteronism and are increased during pregnancy. In pregnant patients with primary hyperaldosteronism, renin levels are suppressed and are therefore helpful in diagnosis.

To confirm autonomous mineralocorticoid secretion, salt-loading studies may be done. In pregnancy, risk for volume overload, worsening hypokalemia, and lack of established diagnostic criteria limit the usefulness of this test. The response to upright posture is maintained in pregnancy, but normal values for renin stimulation during pregnancy have not been established.

Radiographic tests may be done after biochemical confirmation. Magnetic resonance imaging is preferred in pregnancy.

Treatment

The use of medical therapy to reduce the production or inhibit the action of mineralocorticoids is difficult because of the risk for adverse fetal effects. Spironolactone has been used, but there is concern about risk for feminization of a male fetus. The ACE inhibitors are helpful in nonpregnant persons without complete renin suppression, but they are contraindicated in pregnancy. Calcium-channel blockers have some reducing effect on aldosterone synthesis and release and are more effective than aldomet and beta-blockers (17).

Surgical removal of an identified adrenal adenoma is the treatment of choice in the nonpregnant state. In two cases of adrenalectomy at 15 and 17 weeks of gestation, blood pressure normalized and a healthy, term infant was delivered (19, 20). Thus, if hypertension or hypokalemia cannot be controlled medically, surgery during the second trimester is warranted.

Androgen Excess

Adrenal virilizing tumors are rare in pregnancy; only five cases have been reported to date. Maternal signs of virilization may be misinterpreted as changes of pregnancy. Definitive diagnosis of all cases occurred only after a virilized infant was delivered. Surgical therapy at the time of diagnosis is the treatment of choice.

Congenital Adrenal Hyperplasia

Congenital adrenal hyperplasia (CAH) is a group of autosomal-recessive inherited disorders of reduced or absent enzymatic activity of one of the stages of adrenal steroid biosynthesis resulting in reduced production of cortisol + mineralocorticoids (salt losers), increased release of ACTH due to the lack of negative feedback from cortisol, which in turn stimulates production of steroids not affected by the enzyme deficiency (i.e., androgens).

Three types of CAH may complicate a pregnancy: 21-hydroxylase deficiency, 11-hydroxylase deficiency, and 3-beta-dehydrogenase deficiency. The chromosomal sites of all of these types have been identified (21). All other forms are incompatible with reproduction. 21-Hydroxylase deficiency accounts for more than 90% of cases and is the focus of this discussion. In pregnancy, two issues are important: 1) appropriate treatment for mothers with CAH and 2) prevention of virilization of female fetuses affected by CAH.

Clinical Presentation of 21-Hydroxylase Deficiency

The clinical presentation of CAH depends on the enzyme defect and the severity of the enzyme deficiency. The severe, classic forms of CAH cause excess adrenal androgen production in early fetal life, resulting in virilization of female genitalia. In male fetuses, this excess androgen is of little clinical consequence. Postnatally, infants with the salt-losing form of CAH show classic aldosterone deficiency, including hyponatremia, hyperkalemia, and hypotension. Male infants who are not salt losers may have adrenal crisis due to glucocorticoid deficiency or may develop precocious puberty due to excess adrenal androgen production. Infants with the milder forms of 21-hydroxylase deficiency have no salt-wasting features and normal female external genitalia at birth. They generally present as premature adrenarche, accelerated growth, hirsutism, acne, menstrual irregularities, and infertility.

Women Known To Have Congenital Adrenal Hyperplasia Due to 21-Hydroxylase Deficiency

Fertility rates in women with classic 21-hydroxylase deficiency are often reduced because of oligo-ovulation, inadequate vaginal introitus despite surgical resection, and low marriage rates (22). In addition, an increase in first-trimester loss is seen (23). Successful conception requires good therapeutic compliance (to reduce androgen levels) and careful biochemical monitoring. There is an increased risk for cesarean section because these women tend to have android pelvis and, thus, cephalopelvic disproportion.

Women with CAH will be receiving glucocorticoid (usually, hydrocortisone or prednisone) and mineralocorticoid (if salt-losing) replacement. In the nonpregnant state, 17-OH progesterone levels are measured to assess the effectiveness of this treatment in lowering ACTH levels and, thus, stimulation to the adrenal cortex (24). However, during pregnancy, 17-OH progesterone measurement is not reliable because 17-OH progesterone normally increases throughout pregnancy. Free testosterone levels do not change and may be used as a marker of adequate suppression. Blood pressure, edema, and electrolytes should be monitored for adequacy of mineralocorticoid replacement. Most women do not require any change in either mineralocorticoid or glucocorticoid therapy, except at times of stress when parenteral stress doses are required (e.g., hyperemesis, labor, delivery) (see section on Adrenocortical Insufficiency below).

The woman with CAH will want to know her unborn child's risk for this disease. For the fetus to have CAH, the woman's partner must be a heterozygote carrier or a homozygote for the same enzyme defect. When the mother is affected and the father is a carrier, the fetus has a one in two chance of being affected and a one in four chance of being an affected female. The carrier incidence is approximately 1.2% to 6% and is higher among Yupik Eskimos, Ashkenazi Jews, and Hispanics. The partner may have ACTH stimulation tests with measurement of 17-OH progesterone or DNA testing to determine carrier status (25).

Prevention of Virilization in Affected Fetus

In most situations, fetuses at risk for virilization are discovered when a sibling is diagnosed at infancy or in childhood. This diagnosis confirms that both parents are carriers of the enzymatic defect of which they were previously unaware. Each subsequent pregnancy carries a one in four risk for an affected child and a one in eight risk for an affected female child.

Prenatal Treatment—The purpose of prenatal treatment is to prevent virilization in female fetuses; thus, one in eight fetuses may benefit from in utero intervention. The adrenal glands synthesize and secrete enough testosterone from 6 to 12 weeks of gestation on to masculinize female genitalia. If one can decrease the excess androgen by reducing ACTH stimulation to the fetal adrenal glands, the need for genital corrective surgery, the potential masculinization of the female brain, incorrect sex assignment at birth, and the psychological trauma of ambiguous genitalia for the parents and child may be avoided. Because of the early development of the external genitalia, treatment must be initiated before anyone knows whether the child is affected and what sex the child is. Thus, eight fetuses will be treated to prevent virilization in one (Figure 5-6).

To suppress fetal ACTH, glucocorticoids are given to the mother. They cross the placenta and provide negative feedback to the fetal hypothalamic-pituitary axis. Dexamethasone is the agent of choice because it has the greatest transplacental passage. Dosages of 0.5 mg three times daily or 20 µg/kg per day in two to three doses are recommended. To obtain the best results, treat-

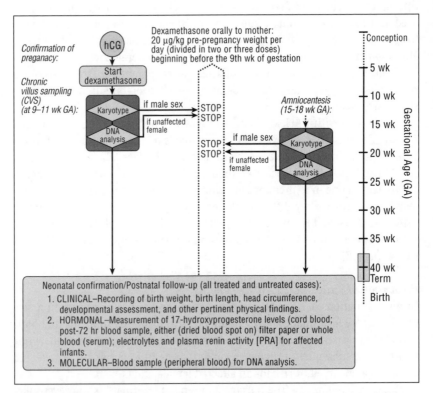

Figure 5-6 Alogrithm for prenatal diagnosis and treatment of 21-hydroxylase deficiency. (From Mercado AB, Wilson RC, Cheng KC, Wei J, New M. Prenatal treatment and diagnosis of congenital adrenal hyperplasia owing to steroid 21-hydroxylase deficiency. J Clin Endocrinol Metab. 1995;80:2014; with permission.)

ment must be started before 10 weeks of gestation and continued throughout pregnancy.

The fetal response to prenatal treatment is variable. Masculinization may be reduced but not necessarily eliminated. In one clinical series of 44 affected females treated from before 10 weeks of gestation to the end of pregnancy (24), 34% had normal genitalia, 52% had mild virilization not requiring surgery, and 14% required surgical correction. Of those in whom treatment was stopped before delivery (*n* = 7) or initiated after 10 weeks of gestation (*n* = 7), all required surgical intervention. Compared with their affected siblings, infants treated in utero before 10 weeks of gestation had significantly less virilization (26) (Figure 5-7).

The potential adverse effects of prenatal treatment to the fetus must be considered. No documented increase in congenital anomalies, long-term effects on psychomotor development, or intrauterine death has been seen. However, there have been reports of low birthweight, reduction of central nervous system DNA content in animal studies, white matter abnormalities on MRI, and impaired fine motor coordination (24). The consequences may not yet be apparent, given the small numbers and early ages of infants ex-

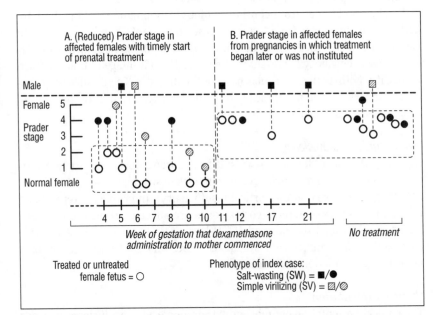

Figure 5-7 Effect of early dexamethasone on Prader stage of affected female infants compared with untreated affected siblings. (From Mercado AB, Wilson RC, Cheng KC, Wei J, New M. Prenatal treatment and diagnosis of congenital adrenal hyperplasia owing to steroid 21-hydroxylase deficiency. J Clin Endocrinol Metab. 1995;80:2014; with permission.)

posed to date. Parents must be informed that the risk-to-benefit ratio has not been clearly established and that controversy over the effectiveness of treatment continues (27).

Maternal adverse effects include Cushingoid features, excessive weight gain, hypertension, diabetes, emotional lability, and excessive striae (28). If they occur, it may be beneficial to reduce the dose of dexamethasone in the second or third trimester when critical external genitalia formation is complete. Risks known to occur in other settings of glucocorticoid replacement (e.g., osteoporosis and avascular necrosis) have not been studied.

Prenatal Diagnosis—The purposes of diagnosing CAH in utero include 1) to continue prenatal treatment in affected female fetuses, 2) to discontinue treatment in unaffected female fetuses and all male fetuses and thus reduce potential complications, and 3) to provide ongoing treatment in affected neonates to avoid complications of delayed diagnosis in infancy (e.g., adrenal crisis).

The gene for 21-hydroxylase lies in close approximately to the HLAB and DR locus and thus is usually inherited together. This is not the case for other causes of CAH. Comparison of HLA types among parents, affected sibling, and fetus has been used to predict whether the fetus is affected, but this form of testing has largely been replaced by genetic testing.

Fetal cells obtained from chorionic villous sampling or amniotic fluid, together with leukocytes from the index case and parents, can be studied with various molecular methods to determine whether the genetic defect for 21-hydroxylase deficiency is present in the fetus. The advantage of this approach is that it identifies the molecular basis of the disorder. The disadvantages include higher cost and a technically more difficult test. Details of the types of genetic testing are available (24).

Adrenocortical Insufficiency

Adrenocortical insufficiency may result from adrenal cortex destruction (primary adrenocortical insufficiency) or from lack of stimulation—that is, ACTH deficiency (secondary adrenocortical insufficiency). In primary adrenal gland destruction, all three adrenal cortex zones are affected. Thus, there is deficiency of all adrenal steroids and ACTH levels are elevated. With ACTH deficiency, the renin-angiotensin system is intact and continues to stimulate aldosterone production and release.

Clinical Presentation

The clinical presentation of undiagnosed adrenocortical insufficiency depends on the cause and acuity of presentation. Features of chronic adrenocortical insufficiency appearing for the first time in pregnancy may be identical to normal symptoms of pregnancy: nausea, vomiting, fatigue, orthostatic hypotension, and hyperpigmentation. Clues that may help differentiate the normal from the pathologic include excessive nausea, anorexia, and vomiting after the first trimester; weakness; and pigmentation early in pregnancy in the mucous membranes, extensor surfaces, and scars as compared to chloasma. The hyperpigmentation is due to elevations in ACTH precursor molecules that have melanocyte-stimulating activity and thus is present only in primary adrenocortical insufficiency. In addition, salt-wasting, decreased extracellular volume and electrolyte disturbances (hyponatremia and hyperkalemia) are associated with aldosterone deficiency.

Acute adrenal insufficiency (Addisonian crisis) can occur in undiagnosed or undertreated patients with chronic insufficiency in times of stress as well as in situations of sudden adrenal disturbance, such as preeclampsia, postpartum hemorrhage, anticoagulation, gram-negative bacteremia, and florid meningococcemia. It generally presents with fever, vomiting, confusion, hypotension, hypoglycemia, and hyponatremia. Flank pain may accompany adrenal infarction or hemorrhage. In some cases, adrenal insufficiency is not evident until the postpartum period (29).

Pregnancy Outcome
Some pregnancies with undiagnosed adrenal insufficiency are associated with fetal growth restriction and neonatal hypoglycemia. Adrenal insufficiency in the neonate has not been reported.

Diagnosis
Maternal baseline cortisol levels may be higher than expected in the nonpregnant state because of the physiologic increase seen during pregnancy. Definitive diagnosis requires an ACTH stimulation test. Basal serum cortisol levels should double within 30 minutes of receipt of 250 μg of Cotrosyn (synthetic ACTH) given intravenously. If this does not occur, adrenal insufficiency is present, and the ACTH level should be measured to distinguish primary from secondary causes. If the clinical picture strongly suggests adrenal insufficiency, diagnostic and therapeutic studies should be done simultaneously (Box 5-6). Dexamethasone is used for glucocorticoid replacement during testing because it is not recognized in the serum cortisol assay and thus will not give falsely elevated readings.

Treatment
During pregnancy, dosage requirements of mineralocorticoids and glucocorticoids do not differ from those in the nonpregnant population. The possible effect on the fetus of synthetic glucocorticoids that differ in maternal-to-fetal transfer rates must be considered (Box 5-7). To limit fetal exposure, hydrocortisone and prednisone are the agents of choice. Glucocorticoid therapy in hu-

man pregnancies is not associated with congenital anomalies, although cleft palate has been reported in animal studies (30). Long-term studies have shown no changes in neurologic development or somatic growth (8).

Parenteral steroids in stress doses are required in pregnancy in times of severe hyperemesis or vomiting from another cause, labor and delivery, other surgical procedures, and other situations of severe stress (see Box 5-7).

Box 5-6 Diagnosis of Adrenal Insufficiency with Concomitant Treatment

1. Draw blood for evaluation of electrolytes, BUN, creatinine, glucose, cortisol, and ACTH (chilled heparinized tube transported on ice).
2. Start IV D5NS rate dependent on volume status.
3. Administer IV dexamethasone 2-4 mg IV.
4. Conduct ACTH stimulation test (250 µg Cortrosyn IV or IM with cortisol measurement at 30 and 60 minutes after injection).
5. Begin hydrocortisone 100 mg IV q8h after last cortisol level is obtained.

Box 5-7 Glucocorticoid Therapy for Labor, Surgery, or Other Severe Stress in Patients with Adrenal Insufficiency

1. Hydrocortisone* 100 mg IM/IV on call to operating room or at onset of labor
2. Hydrocortisone 100 mg IV q8h over course of surgery or labor and delivery
3. Hydrocortisone 50 mg IV q8h postoperative or postpartum Day 1
4. Hydrocortisone 25–50 mg PO or IV q8h postoperative or postpartum Day 2**
5. Hydrocortisone 25 mg PO or IV q8-12h postoperative or postpartum Day 3
   Fludrocortisone (Florinef) 0.1 mg PO daily
6. Hydrocortisone 20 mg PO qA.M. and 10 mg PO qP.M. (or equivalent in other preparation)
   Fludrocortisone 0.1 mg PO daily, thereafter

Adapted from Molitch ME. Endocrine emergencies in pregancy. Baillieres Clin Endocrinol Metab. 1992;6:167-91.
* Hydrocortisone sodium succinate.
** For major procedures, unstable course, or supervening infection, the higher dosages should be used with slower tapering.

Adrenal Medulla

The adrenal medulla is the primary source of circulating catecholamines. Chromaffin cells, which originate from neural crest tissue, form both the adrenal medulla and the sympathetic ganglion. Because of this common embryologic origin, disturbances of chromaffin tissue can be both intra- and extra-adrenal. Pheochromocytomas are tumors of chromaffin cells that overproduce catecholamines.

In pregnancy, plasma and urinary catecholamine levels are unchanged and increase appropriately in stressful situations, such as mental stress, physical illness, labor, and delivery. Pregnancies complicated by hospitalization for preeclampsia or eclampsia have a 1.7-fold to 2.6-fold increase in urinary catecholamines (15). The effect of this increase on fetal well-being is unknown.

Pheochromocytoma

The incidence of pheochromocytoma is approximately 0.002% in the general population. Despite the rarity of the disorder, timely diagnosis is essential for maternal and fetal well being; undiagnosed cases have poor outcome.

Clinical Presentation

The classic presentation of a pheochromocytoma is paroxysms, lasting seconds to hours, of hypertension, headache, diaphoresis, palpitations, anxiety, and chest pain. In about one third of persons, the hypertension is sustained rather than paroxysmal (31). In pregnancy, the incidence of seizures and visual problems seems to be more common (Figure 5-8). Episodes may be precipitated by exercise, urination, bowel movements, abdominal palpation, anaesthesia, fetal movements, uterine contractions, and an enlarging uterus. Antihypertensive treatment with beta-blockers or labetalol (because of the predominance of the beta-blockade effect) may worsen the hypertension because of an unopposed alpha effect.

In pregnancy, the differential diagnosis of severe, labile hypertension includes preeclampsia, thyrotoxicosis, essential hypertension, illicit drug use or drug withdrawal, migraine headaches, and anxiety. A 20% incidence of proteinuria is seen with pheochromocytoma, making it difficult to distinguish pheochromocytoma from preeclampsia.

Most pheochromocytomas are sporadic. However, there are several familial neuroendocrine disorders of which pheochromocytoma is a part. These include multiple endocrine neoplasia (MEN) type IIa, MEN type IIb, von Hippel-Lindau disease, and neurofibromatosis.

It is essential that the patient be examined for the clinical features of the familial disorders and that a detailed family history be obtained.

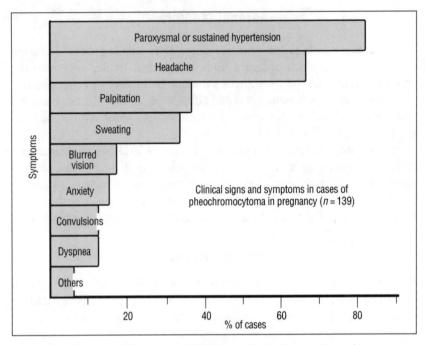

Figure 5-8 Clinical manifestation in 139 cases of pheochromocytoma in pregnancy. (From Shenker JG, Granat M. Pheochromocytoma and pregnancy: an updated appraisal. Aust N Z J Obstet Gynaecol. 1982;22:4; with permission.)

Course in Pregnancy

Pheochromocytoma carries a very high risk for both maternal and fetal death if diagnosis and treatment are delayed. Overall mortality rates have improved significantly in the past decade but continue to be 11% for mothers and 32% for infants (32) (Table 5-10).

Diagnosis

In diagnosing pheochromocytoma, the main caveat is that it should be included in the differential diagnosis. As with most endocrine diagnoses, biochemical confirmation must precede radiographic localization. Use of substances that may interfere with accurate diagnosis must be discontinued before sample collection.

Urinary Catecholamines

The cornerstone of urinary catecholamine diagnosis is a timed urine collection in an acidified medium for catecholamines and their by-products. A baseline 24-hour urine collection should be obtained. If this sample is normal, a

Table 5-10 Maternal and Fetal Mortality in Cases of Pheochromocytoma Diagnosed Prepartum versus Postpartum Since 1980

Time of Diagnosis	Maternal Deaths/Cases (%)	Fetal Deaths/Cases (%)
During pregnancy	1/28 (4)	4/28 (14)
Postpartum	4/16 (25)	10/16 (62)
Total	5/44 (11)	11/44 (32)

Adapted from Keely E. Pheochromocytoma in pregnancy. In. Lee R, ed. Current Obstetric Medicine, v. 3. 1995:73-94.

24-hour collection starting at the onset of a clinical episode should be obtained.   In general, a value greater than two times normal indicates a pheochromocytoma. The most common laboratory method for measurement of these products is high-pressure liquid chromatography. Compared with older methods, this has eliminated the potential for interference from dietary compounds.

Several pharmacologic agents continue to interfere with measurement of catecholamines. These include tricyclic antidepressants, labetalol, levodopa, decongestants, amphetamines, sotalol, methyldopa, ethanol, and benzodiazepines, all of which increase catecholamine values. Clonidine withdrawal also increases them. Use of agents that interfere with catecholamine measurement should be discontinued 7 to 14 days before sample collection (33). Patients with severe renal insufficiency will have elevated urinary catecholamine levels.

Plasma Catecholamines
Baseline measurement of plasma catecholamines has no advantages over measurement of catecholamines in urine. Because of the wide fluctuations from physiologic stimuli (including venipuncture) and the lability of catecholamines in vitro, strict collection protocols must be used.

Pharmacologic Testing
The clonidine suppression test may be used for persons with a moderate increase in urinary catecholamines. A 300-μg dose of clonidine is given, and plasma catecholamines are measured at baseline and 1, 2, and 3 hours after ingestion. Normally, plasma norepinephrine will suppress to less than 2.96 nmol/L or 50% of baseline (34). The risk for significant hypotension makes this test potentially dangerous in pregnancy.

Localization
Anatomic localization is required for definitive treatment once the biochemical diagnosis has been made. In pregnancy, the best choice for anatomic local-

ization is MRI. This imaging method has a sensitivity close to 100% in lesions greater than 1.5 cm, in part because of the high-intensity signal emitted by pheochromocytomas on T_2-weighted images (35). It does not require ionizing radiation and can document extra-adrenal lesions. Ultrasonography lacks sensitivity, and CT requires contrast dye and ionizing radiation. Metaiodbenzulguanidine scanning is contraindicated in pregnancy.

Treatment

Medical Therapy
Medical therapy, in the form of alpha-blockade, should be initiated once a biochemical diagnosis is made, even if localization procedures are not complete. Treatment during pregnancy reduces fetal and maternal mortality rates significantly, regardless of gestational age (Table 5-11). Alpha-blockade is the initial treatment because of its beneficial effects with respect to adrenergic-mediated vasoconstriction. The benefits of alpha-blockade in pregnancy far outweigh any potential unknown teratogenic or long-term effects.

Phenoxybenzamine, a long-acting alpha-blocker, irreversibly binds to alpha-receptors. The initial dose is 10 mg twice daily; this is increased by 10- to 20-mg increments every 2 to 3 days until evidence of an orthostatic decrease in blood pressure is seen. Major maternal adverse effects include nasal stuffiness, sedation, fluid retention, and weakness. There is placental transfer of this drug; the fetal to maternal ratio is 1.6:1. Transient perinatal depression and hypotension may occur, and neonates must be monitored closely (36). Prazosin, a selective alpha-1 antagonist, results in less postural hypotension but is less effective in controlling blood pressure intraoperatively (37).

Beta-blockade should be instituted after alpha-blockade is achieved to avoid intraoperative tachyarrhythmias. The dose should be titrated to achieve a maternal heart rate of 80 to 100 beats/min. The potential fetal risks of beta-

Table 5-11 Effect of Alpha-Blockade on Mortality

	Patients with Alpha-Blockade		Patients without Alpha-Blockade	
	Maternal Deaths/Cases	Fetal Deaths/Cases	Maternal Deaths/Cases	Fetal Deaths/Cases
Time of Diagnosis	(%)	(%)	(%)	(%)
First and second trimester	0/6 (0)	1/6 (17)	2/9 (22)	6/8 (75)
Third trimester	0/10 (0)	0/10 (0)	0/13 (0)	5/12 (42)
Total	0/16 (0)	1/16 (6)	2/21 (9.5)	11/20 (55)

From Burgess GE. Alpha-blockade and surgical intervention of pheochromocytoma in pregnancy. Obstet Gynecol. 1979;53:267; with permission.

blockade include decreased fetal heart rate, neonatal hypoglycemia, neonatal hyperbilirubinemia, and apnea. However, in controlled studies, beta-blockers (especially those that are beta-1–specific and have intrinsic sympathomimetic activity, such as acebutolol) seem to be as safe as other antihypertensive agents. Labetolol has alpha- and beta-blocking properties in a ratio of 1:5. The risk for excessive beta-blockage without adequate alpha-blockade, resulting in worsening hypertension, limits the usefulness of labetolol.

Surgical and Obstetric Management

After adequate medical therapy (usually requiring 10 to 14 days) and localization of the tumor, surgery can be considered. The optimal timing of surgery in pregnancy is controversial. The most important factor in fetal and maternal outcome is adequate alpha-blockade. In the first and second trimesters (before 24 weeks of gestation), it is reasonable to consider surgical excision before fetal maturity. After 24 weeks of gestation, medical therapy should continue until fetal maturity is achieved. At that time, delivery with concurrent or delayed surgical excision should occur. Cesarean section is the delivery method of choice because it is associated with a lower incidence of maternal death (38, 39). Clearly, a skilled team composed of anesthetists, obstetricians, neonatologists, and internists is required. If the pheochromocytoma has not been identified radiographically before delivery, adrenal exploration or metaiodobenzylguanidine scanning may be used postpartum.

REFERENCES

1. **Taylor AL, Fishman LM.** Corticotropin-releasing hormone. N Engl J Med. 1988;319:213-22.

2. **Sasaki A, Shinkawa O, Yoshinaga K.** Placental corticotropin-releasing hormone may be a stimulator of maternal pituitary adrenocorticotropic hormone secretion in humans. J Clin Invest. 1989;84:1997-2001.

3. **Riley SL, Walton JC, Herlick JM, Challis JRG.** The localization and distribution of corticotropin-releasing hormone in the human placenta and fetal membranes throughout gestation. J Clin Endocrinol Metab. 1991;72:1001-7.

4. **Kaplan NM.** Endocrine hypertension. In: Wilson JD, Foster DW, eds. Williams Textbook of Endocrinology, 8th ed. Philadelphia: WB Saunders; 1992:707-31.

5. **Wilson M, Morganti AA, Zervoudakis I, Letcher RL, Romney BM, Oeyon PV, et al.** Blood pressure, the renin-aldosterone system and sex steroids throughout normal pregnancy. Am J Med. 1980;68:97-104.

6. **Gant NF, Daley GL, Chand S, Whalley PJ, MacDonald PC.** A study of angiotensin II pressor response throughout primigravid pregnancy. J Clin Invest. 1973;52:2682-9.

7. **Broughton Pipkin F, Hunter JC, Turner SR, O'Brien PMS, Sant-Cassia LJ, Turner SR.** Effects on the renin-angiotensin system of the administration of prostaglandin E1 and E2 in second trimester in pregnancy. Clin Exp Hypertens. 1983;B2:233-45.

8. **Garner PG.** Disorders of the Adrenal Cortex in Current Obstetric Medicine, v. 2. Lee R, ed. 1993:183-220.

9. **Buescher MA, McClamrock HD, Adashi EY.** Cushing's syndrome in pregnancy. Obstet Gynecol. 1992;79:130-7.

10. **Hadden DR.** Adrenal disorders of pregnancy. Endocrinol Metab Clin North Am. 1995;24:139-51.

11. **Pickard J, Jochen AL, Sadur CN, et al.** Cushing's syndrome in pregnancy. Obstet Gynecol Surv. 1990;45:87-93.

12. **Aron DC, Schanll AM, Sheeler LR.** Cushing's syndrome and pregnancy. Am J Obstet Gynecol. 1990;45:87-93.

13. **Oldfield EH, Doppman JL, Nieman LK, et al.** Petrosal sinus sampling with and without corticotropin-releasing hormone for the differential diagnosis of Cushing's syndrome. N Engl J Med. 1991;325:897-905.

14. **Pinette MG, Pan Y, Oppenhiem D, et al.** Bilateral inferior petrosal sinus corticotropin sampling with corticotropin-releasing hormone stimulation in a pregnant patient with Cushing's syndrome. Am J Obstet Gynecol. 1994;171:563-4.

15. **Keely E.** Endocrine causes of hypertension in pregnancy—when to start looking for zebras. Semin Perinatol. In press.

16. **Pricolo VE, Monchik JM, Prinz RA, et al.** Management of Cushing's syndrome secondary to adrenal adenoma during pregnancy. Surgery. 1990;108:1072-7.

17. **Laurel MT, Kabadi UM.** Primary hyperaldosteronism. Endocrine Practice. 1997;3:47-53.

18. **Solomon CG, Thiet M, Moore F, Seely EW.** Primary hyperaldosteronism in pregnancy—a case report. J Reprod Med. 1996;41:255-8.

19. **Baron F, Sprauve ME, Huddleston JF, Fisher AJ.** Diagnosis and surgical treatment of primary aldosteronism in pregnancy—a case report. Obstet Gynecol. 1995;86:644-5.

20. **Webb JC, Bayliss P.** Pregnancy complicated by primary aldosteronism. South Med J. 1997;90:243-5.

21. **Miller WL.** Genetics, diagnosis and management of 21-hydroxylase deficiency. J Clin Endocrinol Metab. 1994;78:241-6.

22. **Mulaikal RM, Migeon CJ, Rock JA.** Fertility rates in female patients with congenital adrenal hyperplasia due to 21-hydroxylase deficiency. N Engl J Med. 1987;316:178-82.

23. **Feldman S, Billaud L, Thalabard JC, et al.** Fertility in late onset adrenal hyperplasia due to 21-hydroxylase deficiency. J Clin Endocrinol Metab. 1992;74:635-9.

24. **Pang S.** Congenital adrenal hyperplasia. Endocrinol Metab Clin North Am. 1997;26:853-91.

25. **Speiser PW, New MI.** Prenatal diagnosis and management of congenital adrenal hyperplasia. Clin Perinatol. 1994;21:631-45.

26. **Mercado AB, Wilson RC, Cheng KC, Wei J, New M.** Prenatal treatment and diagnosis of congenital adrenal hyperplasia owing to steroid 21-hydroxylase deficiency. J Clin Endocrinol Metab. 1995;80:2014-20.

27. **Seckl JR, Miller WL.** How safe is long-term prenatal glucocorticoid treatment? JAMA. 1994;21:631-45.

28. **Pang S, Clark AT, Freeman LC, et al.** Maternal side effects of prenatal dexamethasone therapy for fetal congenital adrenal hyperplasia. J Clin Endocrinol Metab. 1992;75:249-53.

29. **Molitch ME.** Endocrine emergencies in pregnancy. Baillieres Clin Endocrinol Metab. 1992;6:167-91.

30. **Czeizel AE, Rockenbauer M.** Population-based case control study of teratogenic potential of corticosteroids. Teratology. 1997;56:335-40.

31. **Sheps SG, Jiang NS, Klee GC.** Diagnostic evaluation of pheochromocytoma. Endocrinol Metab Clin North Am. 1988;17:397-415.

32. **Keely E.** Pheochromocytoma in pregnancy. In: Lee R, ed. Current Obstetric Medicine, v. 3. 1995:73-94.

33. **Young WF.** Pheochromocytoma and primary aldosteronism: diagnostic approaches. Endocrinol Metab Clin North Am. 1997;26:801-27.

34. **Sjoberg RJ, Simcic KJ, Kidd GS.** The clonidine suppression test for pheochromocytoma: a review of its utility and pitfalls. Arch Intern Med. 1992;152:1193-7.

35. **Velchik MG, Alavi A, Kressel HY, et al.** Localization of pheochromocytoma: MIBG, CT and MRI correlation. J Nucl Med. 1989;30:328-36.

36. **Santeiro ML, Stromquist C, Wyble L.** Phenoxybenzamine placental transfer during the third trimester. Ann Pharmacother. 1996;30:1249-51.

37. **Nicholson JP, Vaughn ED, Pickering TG, et al.** Pheochromocytoma and prazosin. Ann Intern Med. 1983;99:477-9.

38. **Schenker JG, Granat M.** Pheochromocytoma and pregnancy—an updated appraisal. Aust N Z J Obstet Gynaecol. 1982;22:1-10.

39. **Botachan A, Hauser R, Kupfermine M, Grisaru D, Peyser MR, Lessing JB.** Pheochromocytoma in pregnancy: case report and review of the literature. Obstet Gynecol Surv. 1995;50:321-7.

VII. Calcium and Parathyroid Metabolism
Howard Lippes

Pregnancy creates a formidable challenge for mineral homeostasis in the mother. At term, the newborn possesses an average of 25 to 30 g of calcium and 16 g of phosphorus (1, 2). The accumulation of fetal skeletal mineral places a significant stress on maternal calcium balance. The potential for a negative maternal calcium balance is even greater during lactation. The amount of calcium transferred into milk each day varies from 120 to 500 mg (3). What adaptations and hormonal changes take place during pregnancy to allow an adequate amount of calcium for the fetal skeleton and, at the same time, prevent a negative calcium balance in the mother? What are the risks of some common disease states that interfere with calcium homeostasis if they occur during pregnancy? How can these diseases be identified during pregnancy? How should they be evaluated and treated? These questions are explored in this section. For a more detailed review of this subject, including a discussion of the pathophysiology and comparative and experimental animal studies, the reader is referred to a recent paper by Kovacs and Kronenberg (4).

Maternal serum calcium is tightly controlled by a complex interaction of hormones at regulatory sites: intestine, kidney, bone, placenta, and mammary gland (during lactation). It is clear that significant positive calcium absorption from the gut must occur; otherwise, pregnancy would probably result in the significant transfer of maternal bone mineral to the developing fetus and neonate. Indeed, increased calcium absorption occurs during pregnancy but apparently not during lactation (5).

Our understanding of the hormonal interactions that regulate calcium has been advanced greatly by recent improvements in our ability to accurately measure the hormones involved in calcium homeostasis. The principal hormones involved are parathyroid hormone (PTH), parathyroid hormone–related peptide (PTHrp), and vitamin D. Other important but apparently less dominant roles are played by prolactin, GH, insulin-like growth factor-1, calcitonin, and estrogen.

Parathyroid Hormone

Parathyroid hormone is a principal hormone in the regulation of calcium homeostasis in the nonpregnant state. It is an 84–amino acid polypeptide secreted by the parathyroid glands in response to a decrease in serum calcium ion concentration. Its secretion is suppressed by an elevation in the serum calcium ion concentration (6). The terminal third of the NH_2 terminus of PTH (PTH-[1-84]) is critical for binding to a specific receptor, for activation of adenylate cyclase, and for biological activity (7). Some evidence suggests that the active form of vitamin D, 1,25-$(OH)_2$ vitamin D, suppresses PTH secretion (8), whereas prolactin may stimulate PTH secretion (9). The exact physiologic actions and the relative contribution of each of these hormones is not well established, but the changes that have been demonstrated fit with our current understanding of the alterations that are seen for calcium, 1,25-$(OH)_2$ vitamin D, and PTH during pregnancy and lactation (10).

Physiology of Parathyroid Hormone

The primary function of PTH is to regulate and maintain the extracellular calcium concentration within a narrow range. The hormone accomplishes this through its effect on target tissues (directly on kidney and bone; indirectly on intestinal absorption mediated by 1,25-$(OH)_2$ vitamin D). It is secreted when the serum calcium concentration decreases below a critical set point. A calcium sensor or receptor protein has been identified on the parathyroid cell surface (11). The gross control of calcium is made by the activation of a carrier-mediated transport system for calcium absorption from the gastrointestinal tract. This transport system is activated directly by the active form of vitamin D (1,25-dihydroxyvitamin D). In response to a low-calcium diet, serum levels of 1,25-$(OH)_2$ vitamin D can increase by 50% within 48 hours (12). Parathyroid hormone is the primary regulatory factor in calciferol 1-alpha-hydroxylation (25-hydroxyvitamin D_3-1-alpha-hydroxylase) in the kidney proximal convoluted tubules (13). Other important locations for this enzyme are the placenta, decidua, and granulomatous tissue.

The parathyroid hormone has direct effects on the kidney. First, it activates 25-hydroxyvitamin D_3-1-alpha-hydroxylase and then regulates fine control of calcium by decreasing calcium clearance. In other words, PTH increases the fractional reabsorption of the glomerular filtered load of calcium. This occurs primarily in the thick ascending and distal renal tubule (14). When PTH levels are excessive, as in hyperparathyroidism, urine calcium excretion increases because increased calcium absorbed from the gut will cause the filtered load of calcium to be high.

Parathyroid hormone stimulates both bone formation and bone resorption. However, consistent with its main function—to increase calcium—it has a dominant catabolic effect on bone. It stimulates osteoclasts and increases both resorption of bone mineral and breakdown of bone matrix. Thus, PTH mobilizes both calcium and phosphorus from bone mineral stores. At the same time, an examination of bone after PTH infusion in vivo shows an increase in osteoblast activity and new bone formation (15).

Parathyroid Hormone in Pregnancy

During pregnancy, total serum calcium levels decline slightly; however, proportionally, serum albumin levels decrease to a greater extent. Albumin accounts for 70% of the protein binding of calcium in serum. This suggests that ionized calcium levels should increase during pregnancy (16).

More recent studies, done using the highly sensitive immunoradiometric assay technique, indicate that the intact molecule of PTH (PTH-[1-84]) decreases during normal pregnancy. In a study by Rasmussen and colleagues, PTH declined by approximately 72% in pregnant women relative to a nonpregnant control population (17). The change is seen as early as the first trimester, and the lower level is maintained throughout pregnancy. The lower level of PTH was supported by measurements of lower PTH levels on bioassay (18). This finding is particularly striking because the study population included a higher proportion of black persons and had a higher mean pregravid weight. Black and overweight persons have been shown to have higher levels of serum PTH (19, 20). The finding of lower levels in pregnancy has been confirmed by others (17, 21–23). Seki and co-workers (21) noted that the serum PTH level declined slightly, reaching a nadir between 16 and 20 weeks of gestation and increasing thereafter. In the immediate postpartum period (1 to 2 days after delivery), the PTH level remains low. It is now reasonably certain that older data, indicating an increased PTH level in pregnancy, are flawed by the inaccuracy inherent in traditional RIA for PTH, which not only measured immunologically active fragments of PTH but may have cross-reacted with PTHrp and also measured intact PTH. We are left with a paradox of calcium balance in pregnancy. How do ionized calcium levels remain unchanged in the face of lower PTH levels during pregnancy? What calcitropic hormones maintain maternal serum calcium in pregnancy? What mediates the increase in maternal $1,25\text{-}(OH)_2$ vitamin D levels during pregnancy? Because the PTH level is lower, one would expect a lower maternal $1,25\text{-}(OH)_2$ level. The answers to some of these questions may be found in the recent elucidation of the physiologic actions of PTHrp (24).

Vitamin D

Much evidence suggests that pregnancy is best characterized as a state of absorptive hypercalciuria (21). Levels of $1,25\text{-}(OH)_2$ vitamin D are increased in early pregnancy and continue to increase throughout gestation (23, 25–28). $1,25\text{-}(OH)_2$ vitamin D is the biologically active form of vitamin D and is the principal mediator of increased calcium absorption by the gut. Precursor forms of active vitamin D are synthesized in the skin and ingested in normal diet. Vitamin D is then 25-hydroxylated in the liver, and 25-OH vitamin D is converted to the active form, $1,25\text{-}(OH)_2$ vitamin D, by 1-alpha-hydroxylase. In the nonpregnant person, this enzyme is located almost exclusively in the kidney proximal convoluted tubules and, as indicated above, is principally regulated by PTH. The human and rat placenta have been shown to possess 1-alpha-hydroxylase, converting 25-OH vitamin D to $1,25\text{-}(OH)_2$ vitamin D (29, 30). In the nephrectomized rat model, pregnancy also accompanies the in vivo synthesis of $1,25\text{-}(OH)_2$ vitamin D (31). Therefore, it seems likely that the placenta is responsible for some portion of the increased levels of $1,25\text{-}(OH)_2$ vitamin D during pregnancy, but what regulates the apparent increase in placental 1-alpha-hydroxylase enzyme activity is unclear. Kidney 1-alpha-hydroxylase activity is also increased during pregnancy, despite lower levels of PTH (32, 33). What increases kidney 1-alpha-hydroxylase enzyme activity in pregnancy is also unclear. In animal models, $1,25\text{-}(OH)_2$ vitamin D metabolic clearance is unchanged by pregnancy, and the increased levels in pregnancy are a result of increased production (34, 35).

Parathyroid Hormone–Related Peptide

The identification of PTHrp was made by investigators studying the mechanism of humoral hypercalcemia of cancer. They showed the presence of a factor elaborated by a wide variety of tumors that had actions similar to those of PTH. This factor has now been characterized and its gene cloned (36, 37). More recent investigations have shown that PTHrp may be produced by a wide variety of differentiated cells or tissues and that PTHrp has numerous specialized actions. The concept has been developed that PTHrp is a prohormone and that complex post-translational modifications result in numerous vital peptides with distinct and fundamental developmental and physiologic roles. It may be possible to group these peptides into families on the basis of their position in the prohormone and identification of specific receptors. These peptides have been identified as having important effects during pregnancy (38, 39).

The amino-terminal portion of PTHrp has structural homology with PTH, and this portion of the molecule has been shown to bind to and activate the PTH receptor (7). Hence, the name *PTH-related peptide* or *PTH-like peptide*. The amino-terminal forms of PTHrp, through activation of the PTH receptor, have similar actions on bone and kidney. In addition, amino-terminal PTHrp seems to have smooth muscle relaxant and vasorelaxant activity. It also plays an important role in regulating and promoting the development of many fetal tissues, particularly bone, epithelium, and mammary stroma (40).

Parathyroid hormone–related peptide has emerged as an important candidate for the placental calcium transport hormone. The initial investigations of this action were reported by Australian and British investigators working collaboratively (41–45). From experiments done mostly in sheep, these investigators first hypothesized that fetal parathyroid glands might contain a substance that stimulates the activity of the placental calcium pump. Normally, fetal serum calcium concentrations are an average of 20% to 40% greater than maternal concentrations (46). Early studies showed a rapid loss of the normal calcium gradient between fetal and maternal circulations after fetal thyroparathyroidectomy (replacement T_4 is added) (47). When an extract of fetal lamb or fetal calf parathyroid was added to blood perfusing the placenta of previously thyroparathyroidectomized fetal lamb, the normal calcium gradient was restored (43, 46). In a mouse model, the infusion of PTHrp containing the mid-molecule portion of the peptide also restored the calcium gradient. The amino-terminal portion of PTHrp (1-34) does not restore the calcium gradient. Control of the placental calcium transport against an uphill gradient seems to be primarily dependent on fetal hormone influence (48, 49). Despite the observation that the fetal parathyroid gland is essential for maintaining the fetal–maternal calcium gradient, numerous studies have measured only low or indeterminate levels of immunologic PTH in the fetus (50, 51).

Some experiments have shown that fetal serum has elevated PTH relative to maternal PTH activity if measured by a biologic assay sensitive for PTH (52–55). However, biologic assays for PTH are clearly sensitive to both PTH and PTHrp (56). Moreover, in a rat model of placental calcium transport, both

PTH (1-84) and 1,25-$(OH)_2$ vitamin D have a permissive role in the mainte-nance of maternal–fetal calcium transfer. When these hormones were added to the fetal side of the placenta in a parathyroidectomized rat model deficient in both PTH and 1,25-$(OH)_2$ vitamin D, these hormones could not restore fe-tal calcium to that of a control group of pregnant rats (55). It seemed that an additional factor was needed to restore the normal fetal calcium level and rate of placental calcium transport. Parathyroid hormone–related peptide seems to be the likely candidate for stimulating placental calcium transport and maintaining fetal calcium. More specifically, it is likely that a midregion por-tion of PTHrp that is secreted primarily from the fetal parathyroid gland reg-ulates the placental calcium transport system. Parathyroid hormone related peptide produced at local or placental sites might also contribute to placental calcium pump activity. Because maternal PTHrp has been noted to increase during pregnancy (57, 58) and because it activates the PTH receptor in the kidney, it is speculated that PTHrp may be the stimulus for the increase in 1,25-$(OH)_2$ vitamin D. However, this does not explain the rapid decrease seen in 1,25-$(OH)_2$ vitamin D after parturition.

Calcitonin

Calcitonin is a 32–amino acid single-peptide chain secreted primarily by the parafollicular or "C" cells of the thyroid gland, where the highest concentra-tions of this hormone are found. However, smaller concentrations of calci-tonin are widely distributed in neuroendocrine-type cells, particularly in the lung and scattered along the gut. During pregnancy and lactation, the breast may contribute a substantial quantity of calcitonin to maternal plasma (59). The placenta may also contribute to calcitonin production (60). An increase in serum calcium levels causes release of calcitonin. Inflammatory conditions in the lungs and gut also increase calcitonin levels. Hypermagnesemia in-duces calcitonin release. Despite the identification of calcitonin 30 years ago, the physiologic actions of this peptide remain unknown (61). No evidence suggests that calcitonin plays a role in the fine control of serum calcium in humans. For example, medullary carcinoma of the thyroid (a malignancy of the "C" cells) does not cause hypocalcemia. In vitro studies show that calci-tonin retards bone resorption by inhibiting the action of the bone-resorbing cells, osteoclasts (62). Calcitonin can protect against the bone-resorbing ef-fect of PTH. It has been speculated that calcitonin deficiency may be a signifi-cant cause of osteoporosis (63). Some evidence indicates that calcitonin may increase production of 1,25-$(OH)_2$ vitamin D (64). Pharmacologic doses of calcitonin can be used to treat osteoporosis, hypercalcemia, and osteitis de-formans (Paget disease). As a pharmacologic agent, calcitonin is most effec-tive in states of increased osteoclast activity (high bone turnover).

Calcitonin levels have increased during pregnancy in some studies (62, 65) but have been unchanged in others (26, 66, 67). The physiologic actions of calcitonin remain unknown, so the effect of calcitonin in pregnancy and lactation is purely speculative. It is postulated that calcitonin may serve to defend bone mass during pregnancy (68).

Lactation

During lactation (69), the amount of calcium lost per day is variably estimated to be between 120 to 500 mg. The composition of human milk has been analyzed and remains relatively constant, with a mean calcium concentration of 264 mg/L during the first 6 months of nursing and a slightly smaller concentration in the second 6 months (70, 71). At the end of the first postpartum week, a mother produces 550 mL of milk per day. By 2 to 3 weeks postpartum, this increases to 800 mL/d, and production peaks at 1.5 to 2 L/d. A stress is thus placed on maternal calcium balance, and this stress is even greater than that seen in the third trimester. The hormonal changes that regulate calcium homeostasis during lactation are largely unknown. However, some striking differences between pregnancy and lactation have been shown in the hormonal adaptations that increase calcium absorption, protect maternal bone mass, and make calcium available for the developing fetus or the breastfed newborn. The PTHrp produced by mammary gland tissue is a likely regulator of the calcium content of milk and probably regulates calcium transport from the maternal circulation into breastmilk (72, 73). A survey of rodent tissues found PTHrp mRNA in the lactating breast tissue of mice but not in the breast tissue of a control group of nonlactating mice (74). A cDNA probe for PTHrp has detected significant gene activity in mammary glands, and lesser amounts have been detected in many tissues, including brain, placenta, skeleton, smooth muscle, lymph nodes, spleen, and heart (75). A very high level of immunologically and biologically active PTHrp has been measured in human and animal milk (58, 76, 77). An anecdotal report of systemic hypercalcemia in association with massive mammary hyperplasia suggests that PTHrp does gain access to the maternal circulation (78, 79). In the lactating parturient goat, a significant arterial–venous concentration gradient for plasma PTHrp has been measured across the mammary gland circulation. The level of PTHrp in mammary venous plasma averaged 9% of the level found in milk, supporting the conclusion that PTHrp gains access to the maternal circulation. The level of PTHrp in the mammary venous plasma was reduced by decreasing prolactin production with bromocriptine (80). Prolactin may be one important regulator of mammary PTHrp production (81). The access of PTHrp to the systemic circulation and the effect of prolactin in stimulating its PTHrp production was more recently shown in humans. However, the precise regulation of PTHrp production in mammary tissue remains unknown and seems to be influenced greatly by local (paracrine) factors.

After parturition, 1,25-(OH)$_2$ vitamin D levels decrease from the elevated levels found during pregnancy. This decrease occurs within 2 weeks of delivery and reaches a nadir that is lower than that seen in nonpregnant, nonlactating women (82). Subsequently, 1,25-(OH)$_2$ vitamin D concentrations increase but remain below control levels (26, 83). During lactation, there seems to be a steady decrease in 25-hydroxyvitamin D levels. What mediates these changes in vitamin D during lactation is not known, but the changes may occur independent of PTH (84, 85). The increased maternal requirement for calcium during lactation cannot be balanced solely on the basis of renal conservation, even though urinary calcium excretion declines with lactation (86). With the newer assay for PTH, no difference was found between a group of lactating women and their age-matched controls (87). Because 1,25-(OH)$_2$ vitamin D levels are not elevated during lactation and no difference has been found between lactating and nonlactating women, intestinal absorption may not supply all of the calcium required to balance the loss of the calcium through breast milk. Indeed, study of calcium absorption during lactation shows that the absorption of calcium (levels of which are significantly elevated in the third trimester) rapidly declines after parturition. The calcium absorption of lactating women is no different from that in the control population and cannot offset the calcium lost through breastmilk (5). If this is true, bone mineral must supply the balance of calcium during lactation. Several prospective studies, including one that recruited patients before conception, show a loss of bone density during lactation (67). Lactation-associated bone loss is independent of dietary intake of calcium. Recent U.S.–Canadian nutritional guidelines do not recommend an increase in calcium intake during pregnancy and lactation. These recently published guidelines review the important nutritional balance and hormone changes that were used in formulating the recommendations. Adequate intake of calcium in pregnancy and lactation is 1000 mg/d (25 mmol/d) for women older than 19 years of age. Data for adolescent pregnancy and lactation are sparse, and further study is needed. The requirement during adolescence in women who have not reached peak bone mass is greater, and the recommendation is 1300 mg/d (32.5 mmol/d).

The mediation of maternal bone mineral loss during lactation presumably provides for an adequate amount of calcium and phosphate in milk independent of nutritional factors. The mechanisms responsible for milk mineral homeostasis seem to be teleologically preserved and provide for adequate neonatal nutrition during times of deprivation. It has been speculated that an increase in PTHrp combined with an increase in prolactin and a decrease in estradiol may mediate the maternal skeletal change during lactation (88). Further study of calcium homeostasis during lactation and weaning is required.

Because pregnancy and lactation place a significant stress on maternal calcium balance, it is vital to determine whether pregnancy and lactation contribute to diminished bone mass later in life. Numerous retrospective and longitudinal studies have examined the relation between parity and bone mineral density. These studies have yielded inconsistent results. Few have corrected for breast feeding. Similarly, retrospective studies on the relation between lactation and bone mineral density have yielded inconsistent findings. Probable causes of discrepancies include inaccuracies in bone density measurements (especially those obtained by using older methods), failure to adjust for age, time since menopause, body mass index, cigarette smoking, estrogen use, thiazide use, dietary factors, and duration of breastfeeding. The most critical determinant in these studies may be the age or time at which the bone mineral was studied with respect to weaning.

Several studies have shown a rapid correction in bone mass after weaning (85, 89). These studies and others (90–92) support the idea that the marked turnover of bone seen during lactation is accompanied by a net loss of bone mineral at some anatomic sites (femoral neck, ultradistal radius, and lumbar vertebrae). Kent and co-workers (87) have identified a recovery phase after weaning that is characterized by increased bone formation and a return of bone resorption to normal so that bone mineral content is restored. During this postweaning recovery phase, PTH levels are markedly increased and mediate a continuation of renal conservation of calcium. Curiously, the investigators saw no difference in 1,25-(OH)$_2$ vitamin D levels compared with controls at 2 months after weaning, when PTH levels were highest. Recent studies show a correlation between the magnitude of lactation-related bone loss and higher milk volume. Taller women also had greater bone loss (67). Bone loss did not occur in women who fed their newborns formula. Full restoration of bone mineral lost during weaning would logically depend on nutritional and other factors during the postweaning recovery phase.

Hypercalcemia

An elevated serum calcium level is uncommon in women of childbearing age. Most of the time, such a finding is serendipitous and is the result of a screening comprehensive metabolic profile done using an automated chemical analyzer to screen a panel of serum enzymes, ions, and metabolites. Causes of hypercalcemia are listed in Box 5-8. A complete discussion of each of these causes is beyond the scope of this section, and the reader is referred to other recent work on this subject (93, 94). Most ambulatory outpatient hypercalcemia is caused by hyperparathyroidism. As indicated above, the total serum calcium level declines slightly during pregnancy. This decline is apparent by

---

Box 5-8 Causes of Hypercalcemia

Hyperparathyroidism
  Primary hyperparathyroidism
  Primary hyperparathyroidism associated with multiple endocrine neoplasia
  Hyperparathyroidism associated with chronic renal failure (tertiary)
Malignancy-associated hypercalcemia
  Production of PTH-related peptides
  Local tumor-mediated bone resorption
  Production of 1,25-$(OH)_2$ vitamin D
Granulomatous diseases (excess 1,25-$(OH)_2$ vitamin D)
  Sarcoidosis
  Granulomatous infections (e.g., tuberculosis, histoplasmosis, leprosy)
  Berylliosis
Drugs
  Vitamin D intoxication
  Vitamin A intoxication
  Milk-alkali syndrome
  Thiazide diuretics
  Lithium
Endocrinopathies
  Hyperthyroidism
  Adrenal insufficiency
  Pheochromocytoma
Immobilization
Recovery from acute renal failure

---

18 weeks of gestation and corresponds temporally with the decline in serum albumin and the hydremia of pregnancy (16). Therefore, measurements of total calcium during pregnancy should raise suspicion when they are in the "high normal" range relative to nonpregnant controls.

When hypercalcemia has been discovered serendipitously, close questioning may reveal mild symptoms that can be attributed either to the elevated calcium or to pregnancy itself. The bony pains and body aches that are protean symptoms of hyperparathyroidism are easily confused with the aches and pains of pregnancy (95). The neuromuscular effects of hypercalcemia often lead to anorexia, nausea, and vomiting, which can easily be attributed to hyperemesis gravidarum. Constipation occurs as an effect of hypercalcemia on smooth muscle, but constipation is also common during normal pregnancy (96). Although pregnancy is characterized by elevated urinary calcium and calcium oxalate supersaturation, nephrolithiasis is not increased in normal pregnancy (97).

As hypercalcemia progresses, it interferes with vasopressin action on urinary concentrating ability, and nephrogenic diabetes insipidus occurs. Dehydration becomes severe. In pregnancy, vasopressinase activity is increased so that there is an increased metabolic clearance rate for vasopressin (98). Polyuria and polydypsia may be occasionally be seen in normal pregnancy (99). Clearly, mild symptomatic hypercalcemia may be easily overlooked during pregnancy. Hypercalcemia often develops in a pernicious and insidious manner with the gradual development of nephrocalcinosis and deterioration in renal function. It is possible that with declining renal function, preeclampsia or pregnancy-induced hypertension is more likely. When dehydration and the neuromuscular effects of hypercalcemia develop, this must be recognized and treated as an emergency that threatens both mother and fetus.

Hyperparathyroidism

The incidence of primary hyperparathyroidism in the general population is 1/1000. Hyperparathyroidism is more common in females, but the peak incidence is after childbearing age. The incidence in women of childbearing age is estimated to be 8 cases per 100,000 women per year (100). Despite this reported frequency in the nonpregnant population, fewer than 140 cases of hyperparathyroidism during pregnancy have been reported. Most of these cases have been summarized in reviews (101–104). The discrepancy between the reported incidence of hyperparathyroidism and the few reported cases in pregnancy might be explained in at least two ways: 1) the tendency to report only the most severe and complicated cases and 2) the possibility that mild asymptomatic hyperparathyroidism is overlooked in pregnancy, possibly because total calcium levels and PTH levels are decreased in pregnancy.

Clinical presentations of hyperparathyroidism can be divided into three categories: 1) asymptomatic hyperparathyroidism usually discovered serendipitously in screening blood tests, 2) pernicious and insidious symptomatic hyperparathyroidism presenting with renal stone disease (about 20% of cases), and 3) a severe and more aggressive illness characterized by extreme hypercalcemia and the symptoms listed in Box 5-9. In addition, the effect of elevated PTH on bone includes pain and possibly fracture (osteoporosis and osteites fibrosa cystica). Arthritis caused by gout or pseudogout may occur in hyperparathyroidism. The combined effect of elevated PTH and hypercal-

---

Box 5-9 Complications of Extreme Hypercalcemia

Dehydration
Renal complications
  Nephrolithiasis
  Nephrocalcinosis
  Renal failure
Cardiac complication
  Hypertension
  Arrhythmias
Gastrointestinal complications
  Peptic ulcer
  Pancreatitis
  Constipation
  Anorexia
  Nausea
  Vomiting
Neurologic complications
  Weakness
  Depression
  Impaired memory
  Hyporeflexia
  Psychosis
  Stupor
  Coma

---

cemia can cause neuropathy with marked atrophy of type II muscle fibers and mild or severe proximal muscle weakness (105). Parathyroid hormone causes a decrease in bicarbonate reabsorption in the proximal renal tubule so that hyperchloremic metabolic acidosis may be seen.

A single adenoma is responsible for 80% to 90% of cases of primary hyperparathyroidism. The remaining cases are caused by parathyroid hyperplasia. Parathyroid cancer is a rare cause of hyperparathyroidism and is found in less than 1% of cases. When hypercalcemia is found to be caused by hyperparathyroidism, MEN syndromes (both MEN I and MEN II) should be considered, particularly if parathyroid hyperplasia is ultimately found to cause the hypercalcemia. Because these are both inherited autosomal-dominant diseases, a careful family history may provide the clue to diagnosis of MEN.

Hyperparathyroidism During Pregnancy

Hyperparathyroidism during pregnancy was first described in 1931 (106). It poses a serious risk to fetal and neonatal well-being. Stillbirth, IUGR, premature labor, and, especially, neonatal hypocalcemic tetany are particular risks in persons with symptomatic disease. However, these complications can occur in patients with seemingly asymptomatic hyperparathyroidism. Maternal hyperparathyroidism is often a retrospective diagnosis, made postpartum after the development of neonatal tetany. Postpartum diagnosis after neonatal tetany was made in 3 of 12 patients reported by Kelly (104) and in 10 of 15 patients reported by Gelister and colleagues (107). It is postulated that neonatal tetany develops as a result of fetal and neonatal parathyroid gland suppression caused by fetal hypercalcemia. When maternal hypercalcemia exceeds fetal serum calcium and equilibrates across the placenta, the usual gradient of lower serum calcium in the mother is reversed. Because PTH does not cross the placenta, the situation is analogous to the Petersen hypothesis for fetal complications related to GDM and maternal hyperglycemia during pregnancy.

The risks for fetal and neonatal tetany and death in some of the cases reported are summarized in Table 5-12. This retrospective information indicates that parathyroidectomy is the preferred therapy when hyperparathyroidism is discovered during pregnancy. No satisfactory medical therapy exists for primary hyperparathyroidism (108, 109). However, do all such cases discovered during pregnancy require surgical diagnosis and treatment? Patients with persistent hypercalcemia greater than 11.5 mg% are likely to have significant symptoms and should be considered for surgery during pregnancy. In addition to the symptoms of hypercalcemia listed in Box 5-9, hyperemesis gravidarum that persists after 14 weeks of gestation may be caused by hyperparathyroidism. The serendipitous finding of nephrocalcinosis, kidney stones, or excessive calcification of the placenta during fetal ultrasonography should also raise the suspicion of hyperparathyroidism. Each of these symptoms or findings during pregnancy would define the hyperparathyroid state as "symptomatic." Symptomatic hyperparathyroidism requires definitive surgical diagnosis and treatment. In most cases, this should be done during pregnancy. Surgery during pregnancy is ideally done in the middle of the second trimester, when it is unlikely to stimulate premature labor and the risk of anesthetics to fetal development is minimized.

In at least six cases of hyperparathyroidism during pregnancy, surgical treatment has been done late in the third trimester (34 to 35 weeks of gestation) (110–112). In these cases and in our own experience, the patients went on to deliver at term without the development of neonatal hypocalcemia. These few cases suggest that fetal parathyroid function may recover from its suppressed state within a few weeks after resolution of maternal hyperpara-

Table 5-12 Medical versus Surgical Complications in Hyperparathyroid Pregnancy

Source	Total Cases	Medical Treatment			Surgical Treatment		
		Cases	Cases of Tetany	Deaths	Cases	Causes of Tetany	Deaths
Ludwig (1930–1962)	21	20	4	6	1	0	0
Delmonico (1963–1975)	21	13	7	3	8	2	0
Individual cases (1976–1990)	55	33	15	2	22	2	1
Kelly (1930–1991)	12	4	4	0	8	0	0

thyroidism. If this is true, then surgical intervention late in pregnancy can be done at a time when the stress of surgery or anesthesia might precipitate labor. However, by 35 weeks of gestation, fetal development and lung maturity should be advanced to the extent that the risk for prematurity is minimal, particularly in a modern neonatal unit.

It is likely that the current literature on hyperparathyroidism overestimates fetal and neonatal risk. The risk for neonatal tetany is predictable and transient and can be treated. It is not likely to cause long-term adverse effects. Therefore, asymptomatic patients without extreme hypercalcemia have been and can be managed conservatively with close observation and hydration (113, 114). At the same time, severe neonatal hypocalcemic tetany has occurred several days after delivery in mothers who were probably asymptomatic but who had clear evidence of primary hyperparathyroidism. The choice to proceed with surgical diagnosis and treatment during pregnancy often meets with resistance on the part of the neck surgeon and the patient. A multidisciplinary approach with input from the maternal–fetal specialist, the neck surgeon, and the endocrinologist is advisable.

Hypocalcemia

Hypocalcemia during pregnancy is uncommon. On our service, it is most often seen in association with low serum protein levels (hypoalbuminemia) because 40% to 45% of serum calcium is bound to serum protein. Five percent to 10% of calcium in serum is bound to inorganic ions, and the rest is ionized. It is the latter portion that is important physiologically; therefore a low calcium level in conjunction with hypoproteinemia can be considered pseudohypocalcemia. A commonly used method for estimating corrected total calcium is to add 0.8 mg/dL of calcium for each 1 g/L decrease in the albumin concentration.

Causes of hypocalcemia are listed in Box 5-10. Hypomagnesemia impedes the release of PTH and resistance to PTH action, resulting in hypocalcemia. Low serum magnesium levels occur in cases of acute and chronic alcohol abuse and with severe diarrhea. Hypermagnesemia may cause hypocalcemia in conjunction with magnesium sulfate infusion for the treatment of premature labor or toxemia (115, 116). Fat malabsorption (usually accompanied by steatorrhea) can lead to vitamin D deficiency and hypocalcemia. Inflammatory bowel disease and celiac disease are the usual culprits in women of childbearing age. Massive blood transfusion with citrated blood causes sudden, transient, severe hypocalcemia.

Hypoparathyroidism is very rare in pregnancy. Its most common cause is previous thyroid or parathyroid surgery. Idiopathic hypoparathyroidism occurs sporadically as part of autoimmune polyglandular failure (117).

Box 5-10 Causes of Hypocalcemia

Hypoproteinemia (pseudohypocalcemia)
Hypoparathyroidism
  Postoperative
  Idiopathic (sporadic, autoimmune)
  Reversible (hypomagnesemia, hypermagnesemia)
Resistance to parathyroid hormone
  Pseudohypoparathyroidism
  Hypomagnesemia
Vitamin D deficiency
  Malabsorption (Crohn disease, celiac disease, short-bowel syndrome)
  Dietary deficiency
  Chronic renal failure (1–alpha–hydroxylase deficiency)
  Vitamin D–dependent rickets (1-alpha-hydroxylase deficiency or resistance
    to vitamin D)
Altered binding
  Citrate infusion (transfusion, hemodialysis)
  Hyperphosphatemia
  Phosphate infusion
  Rhabdomyolysis
  Respiratory alkalosis

Symptoms of hypocalcemia include acral and perioral paresthesia, neuro-muscular irritability, and psychiatric disturbance. The hyperventilation of pregnancy may lower the threshold for these symptoms. The Chvostek and Trousseau sign may be elicited. On the electrocardiogram, the QT interval can be prolonged (the upper limit of normal is 440 msec). In acute and severe hypocalcemia tetany, laryngeal spasm and seizure activity develop.

Treatment of severe hypocalcemia requires intravenous calcium infusion. Hypocalcemic crisis is treated with 10 to 20 mL of a 10% solution of calcium gluconate (10 mL contains 1 g of calcium gluconate or 90 mg of elemental calcium), which may be infused over 10 minutes. In severe persistent hypocalcemia, a continuous infusion of 5 ampules of calcium gluconate (1 amp = 10 mL of a 10% solution) in 1 L of fluid given intravenously at an infusion rate of 100 mL/h can be administered. Hypocalcemia cannot be corrected when hypomagnesemia persists.

Maintenance therapy for hypoparathyroidism should be supplemental oral calcium and pharmacologic doses of vitamin D. The usual dosage of calcium required is approximately 2 g of elemental calcium per day in divided doses.

The type of calcium salt chosen is not usually important. All calcium salts dissociate in an acid environment, and calcium absorption is increased when the calcium salt is taken with or just after a meal. Calcium carbonate is significantly cheaper than calcium lactate or gluconate per mg of elemental calcium. Calcitriol (1,25-dihydroxyvitamin D_3), the short-acting and active analogue of vitamin D, should be used. Calcitriol is preferred because it allows for the more rapid adjustment of calcium as nutritional requirements change during gestation. In addition, inadvertent vitamin D intoxication is quickly reversed by withholding the calcitriol. Dosages ranging from 0.025 to 3.0 μg/d may be required. Obviously, frequent monitoring of serum calcium is required and should be targeted to 8.5 mg/dL and no higher. Urinary calcium excretion should also be monitored to ensure adequate maternal calcium absorption and to guard against the development of nephrocalcinosis and nephrolithiasis. Urinary calcium should be maintained between 250 and 450 mg/d. When preeclampsia or overt eclampsia develop, there is an acute decrease in urinary calcium, but this should not confuse the usual monitoring of urinary calcium. Some investigators have suggested that the acute decrease in the fractional excretion of calcium can be used to predict preeclampsia (118, 119).

During pregnancy, the requirements for supplemental calcium and vitamin D used to treat a patient with preexisting hypoparathyroidism usually do not change appreciably. Nevertheless, careful monitoring of serum and urinary calcium, serum albumin, and phosphate should be done. After delivery, more frequent monitoring and a careful reassessment of calcium and vitamin D requirements are essential, particularly in the breastfeeding mother. There are a handful of case reports of postpartum hypercalcemia or "remission" of hypoparathyroidism during lactation (120–123). These reports may be similar to the anecdotal report of systemic hypercalcemia in association with massive mammary hyperplasia referred to earlier (78). These few reports show that it is prudent to reduce or discontinue use of pharmacologic doses of vitamin D after delivery in a hypoparathyroid patient, particularly if she chooses to breastfeed. Calcium balance should be reassessed during lactation.

REFERENCES

1. **Hytten, Leitch.** The Physiology of Human Pregnancy, 2d ed. Oxford: Blackwell Scientific Publications; 1971:368-9, 375.

2. **Pitkin RM.** Calcium metabolism in pregnancy and the perinatal period: a review. Am J Obstet Gynecol. 1985;151:99-109.

3. **Jenness R.** The composition of human milk. Semin Perinatol. 1979;3:225-39.

4. **Kovacs CS, Kronenberg HM.** Maternal-fetal calcium and bone metabolism during pregnancy, puerperium, and lactation. Endocrine Rev. 1997;18:832-72.

5. **Institute of Medicine.** Dietary reference intakes: calcium, phosphorus, magnesium, vitamin D and fluoride. Washington, DC: National Academy Press; 1998:37-48.

6. **Habener JF, Rosenblatt M, Potts JT Jr.** Parathyroid hormone: biochemical aspects of biosynthesis, secretion, action, and metabolism. Physiol Rev. 1984;64:985-1053.

7. **Potts JT Jr, Kronenberg HM, Rosenblatt M.** Parathyroid hormone: chemistry, biosynthesis, and mode of action. Adv Protein Chem. 1982;35:323-96.

8. **Naveh-Many T, Friedlaender MM, Mayer H, et al.** Calcium regulates parathyroid hormone messenger ribonucleic acid (mRNA), but not calcitonin mRNA in vivo in the rat: dominant role of 1,25-dihydroxyvitamin D. Endocrinology. 1989;125:275-80.

9. **Pocotte SL, Ehrenstein G, Fitzpatrick LA.** Regulation of parathyroid hormone secretion. Endocrinol Rev. 1991;12:291-301.

10. **Greenberg C, Kukreja SC, Bower EN, et al.** Parathyroid hormone secretion: effect of estradiol and progesterone. Metabolism. 1987;36:151-4.

11. **Brown EM, Pollack M, Seidman CE, Seidman JG, Chou YH, Riccardi D, Hebert SC.** Calcium-ion-sensing cell-surface receptors. N Engl J Med. 1995;333:234-40.

12. **Adams ND, Gray RW, Lemann J Jr.** The effect of oral $CaCO_3$ loading and dietary calcium deprivation on plasma 1,25-dihydroxyvitamin D concentrations in healthy adults. J Clin Endocrinol Metab. 1979;48:1008-16.

13. **Kawashima H, Kraut JA, Kurokawa K.** Metabolic acidosis suppresses 25-hydroxyvitamin D_3-1-alpha-hydroxylase in the rat kidney. J Clin Invest. 1982;70:135-40.

14. **Dennis VW, Brazy PC.** Divalent anion transport in isolated renal tubules. Kidney Int. 1982;22:498-506.

15. **Tam CS, Heersche JNM, Murray TM, Parsons JA.** Parathyroid hormone stimulates the bone apposition rate independently of its resorptive action: differential effects of intermittent and continual administration. Endocrinology. 1982;110:506-12.

16. **Payne RB, Little AJ, Evans RT.** Albumin-adjusted calcium concentration in serum increases during pregnancy. Clin Chem. 1990;36:142-4.

17. **Rasmussen N, Frølich A, Hornnes PJ, et al.** Serum ionized calcium and intact parathyroid hormone levels during pregnancy and postpartum. Br J Obstet Gynecol. 1990;97:857-9.

18. **Rodda DP, Kubota M, Heath JA, et al.** Evidence for a novel parathyroid hormone-related protein in fetal lamb parathyroid glands and sheep placenta: comparisons with a similar protein implicated in humoral hypercalcemia of malignancy. J Endocrinol. 1988;117:261-71.

19. **Bell NH, Greene A, Epstein S, et al.** Evidence for alteration of the vitamin D-endocrine system in blacks. J Clin Invest. 1985;76:470-3.

20. **Bell NH, Epstein S, Greene A, et al.** Evidence for alteration of the vitamin D-endocrine system in obese subjects. J Clin Invest. 1985;76:370-3.

21. **Seki K, Makimura N, Mitsui C, et al.** Calcium-regulating hormones and osteocalcin levels during pregnancy: a longitudinal study. Am J Obstet Gynecol. 1991;164:1248-52.

22. **Saggese G, Baronecelli GI, Bertelloni S, Cipolloni C.** Intact parathyroid hormone levels during pregnancy, in healthy term neonates and in hypocalcemic preterm infants. Acta Pediatr Scand. 1991;80:36-41.

23. **Okonofua F, Menon RK, Houlder S, et al.** Calcium, vitamin D and parathyroid hormone relationships in pregnant Caucasian and Asian women and their neonates. Ann Clin Biochem. 1987;24:22-8.

24. **Care AD.** The placental transfer of calcium. J Dev Physiol. 1991;15:253-7.

25. **Deluca HF, Schnoes HK.** Metabolism and mechanism of action of vitamin D. Annu Rev Biochem. 1976;45:631-66.

26. **Kumar R, Cohen WR, Silva P, et al.** Elevated 1,25-dihydroxyvitamin D plasma levels in normal human pregnancy and lactation. J Clin Invest. 1979;63:342-4.

27. **Lund B, Selnes A.** Plasma 1,25-dihydroxyvitamin D levels in pregnancy and lactation. Acta Endocrinol. 1979;92:330-5.

28. **Bikle DD, Gee E, Halloran B, Haddad JG.** 1,25-dihydroxyvitamin D levels in serum from normal subjects, pregnant subjects, and subjects with liver disease. J Clin Invest. 1984;74:1966-71.

29. **Tanaka Y, Halloran B, Schnoes HK, et al.** In vitro production of 1,25-dihydroxyvitamin D_3 by rat placental tissue. Proc Natl Acad Sci U S A. 1979;76:5033-5.

30. **Weisman Y, Harrell A, Edelstein S, et al.** 1-alpha, 25-dihydroxyvitamin D_3 and 24,25-dihydroxyvitamin D_3 in vitro synthesis by human decidua and placenta. Nature. 1979;281:317-9.

31. **Gray TK, Lester GE, Lorenc RS.** Evidence for extra-renal 1 alpha-hydroxylation of 25-hydroxyvitamin D_3 in pregnancy. Science. 1979;204:1311-13.

32. **Kubota M, Ohno J, Shiina Y, et al.** Vitamin D metabolism in pregnant rabbits: differences between the maternal and fetal response to administration of large amounts of vitamin D. Endocrinology. 1982;110:1950-6.

33. **Lester GE.** Vitamin D metabolism in small mammals. In: Holick MF et al., eds. Perinatal Calcium and Phosphorus Metabolism. New York: Elsevier Science Publishing; 1983:25-34.

34. **Paulson SK, Ford KK, Langman CB.** Pregnancy does not alter the metabolic clearance rate of 1,25-dihydroxyvitamin D in rats. Am J Physiol. 1990;258:E158-62.

35. **Delvin EE, Gilbert M, Pere MC, et al.** In vivo metabolism of calcitriol in the pregnant rabbit doe. J Dev Physiol. 1988;10:451-9.

36. **Insogna KL.** Humoral hypercalcemia of malignancy: the role of parathyroid hormone-related protein. Endocrinol Metab Clin North Am. 1989;18:779-94.

37. **Mangin M, Webb AC, Dreyer BE, et al.** Identification of a cDNA encoding a parathyroid hormone-like peptide from a human tumor associated with humoral hypercalcemia of malignancy. Proc Natl Acad Sci U S A. 1988;85:597-601.

38. **Wysolmerski JJ, Stewart AF.** The physiology of parathyroid hormone-related protein: an emerging role as a developmental factor. Annu Rev Physiol. 1998;60:431-60.

39. **Orloff JJ, Reddy D, DE Papp AE, Yang KH, Soifer NE, Stewart AF.** Parathyroid hormone-related protein as a prohormone: posttranslational processing and receptor interactions. Endocrine Rev. 1994;15:40-60.

40. **Lee K, Deeds JD, Segre GV.** Expression of parathyroid hormone-related peptide and its receptor messenger ribonucleic acids during fetal development of rats. Endocrinology. 1995;136:453-63.

41. **Abbas SK, Pickard KW, Rodda CP, et al.** Stimulation of ovine placental calcium transport by purified natural and recombinant parathyroid hormone-related peptide (PTHrp). Q J Exp Physiol. 1989;74:549-52.

42. **Caple IW, Health JA, Pham TT, et al.** The role of the parathyroid glands, PTH, PTHrP and elevated placental calcium in bone formation in fetal lambs. J Bone Miner Res. 1989;4:S262.

43. **Rodda DP, Kubota M, Heath JA, et al.** Evidence for a novel parathyroid hormone-related protein in fetal lamb parathyroid glands and sheep placenta: comparisons with a similar protein implicated in humoral hypercalcemia of malignancy. J Endocrinol. 1988;117:261-71.

44. **Care AD, Abbas SK, Caple IW.** Evidence for a novel hormone in the parathyroid glands of fetal sheep. In: Jones DT, ed. Fetal and Neonatal Development. Ithaca, NY: Perinatology Press; 1988:103-6.

45. **Loveridge N, Caple IW, Rodda C, et al.** Further evidence for a parathyroid hormone-related protein in fetal parathyroid glands of sheep. Q J Exp Physiol. 1988;73:781-4.

46. **Mughal MZ, Tsang R.** Calcium, phosphorus, and magnesium transport across the placenta. In: Polin RA, Fox WW, eds. Fetal and Neonatal Physiology. Philadelphia: WB Saunders; 1992:1736.

47. **Care AD, Ross R.** Fetal calcium homeostasis. J Dev Physiol. 1984;6:59-66.

48. **Kovacs CS, Lanske B, Hunzelman JL, Guo J, Karaplis AC, Kronenberg HM.** Parathyroid hormone related peptide (PTHrp) regulates fetal-placental calcium transport through a receptor distinct from the PTH/PTHrp receptor. Proc Natl Acad Sci U S A. 1996;93:15233-8.

49. **Care AD.** Placental transfer of calcium to the ovine fetus and its regulation. Proc Nutr Soc. 1987;46:321-9.

50. **Rubin LP, Posillico JT, Anast CS, et al.** Circulating level of biologically active and immunologically intact parathyroid hormone in human newborns. Pediatr Res. 1991;29:201-7.

51. **Khosla S, Johansen KL, Ory SJ, et al.** Parathyroid hormone-related peptide in lactation and in umbilical cord blood. Mayo Clin Proc. 1990;65:1408-14.

52. **Care AD, Ross R, Pickard DW, et al.** Calcium homeostasis in the fetal pig. J Dev Physiol. 1982;4:85-106.

53. **Care AD, Caple IW, Singh R, et al.** Studies on calcium homeostasis in the Yucatan miniature pig. Lab Anim Sci. 1986;36:389-92.

54. **Allgrove J, Adami S, Manning RM, et al.** Cytochemical bioassay of parathyroid hormone in maternal and cord blood. Arch Dis Child. 1985;60:110-5.

55. **Robinson NR, Sibley CP, Mughal MZ, et al.** Fetal control of calcium transport across the rat placenta. Pediatr Res. 1989;26:109-15.

56. **Goltzman D, Bennett HP, Koutsilieris M, et al.** Studies of the multiple molecular forms of bioactive parathyroid hormone and parathyroid hormone-like substances. Recent Prog Horm Res. 1986;42:665-703.

57. **Salleh M, Ardawi M, Nasrat H AN and BA'Aqueel HS.** Calcium-regulating hormones and parathyroid hormone-related peptide in normal human pregnancy and postpartum: a longitudinal study. Eur J Endocrinol. 1997;137:402-9.

58. **Gallacher SJ, Fraser WD, Owens OJ, Dryburgh FJ, Logue FC, Jenkins A, et al.** Changes in calcitropic hormones and biochemical markers of bone turnover in normal human pregnancy. Eur J Endocrinol. 1994;131:369-74.

59. **Bucht E, Telenius-Berg M, Lundell G, Sjoberg HE.** Immunoextracted calcitonin in milk and plasma from totally thyroidectomized women: evidence of monomeric calcitonin in plasma during pregnancy and lactation. Acta Endocrinol (Copenh). 1986;113:529-35.

60. **Balabanova S, Druse B, Wolf AS.** Calcitonin secretion by human placental tissue. Acta Obstet Gynecol Scand. 1987;66:323-6.

61. **Copp DH, Cameron EC, Cheney BA, et al.** Evidence for calcitonin—a new hormone from the parathyroid that lowers blood calcium. Endocrinology. 1962;70:638-49.

62. **Chambers TJ, Chambers JC, Symonds J, Darby JA.** The effect of human calcitonin on the cytoplasmic spreading of rat osteoclasts. J Clin Endocrinol Metab. 1986;63: 1080-5.

63. **Talmage RV.** Comment on the physiological role of calcitonin. Bone Miner. 1992;16:186.

64. **Jaeger P, Jones W, Clemens TL, Hayslett P.** Evidence that calcitonin stimulates 1,25-dihydroxyvitamin D and intestinal absorption of calcium in vivo. J Clin Invest. 1986; 78:456-61.

65. **Samaan N. et al.** Immunoreactive calcitonin in medullary carcinoma of the thyroid and in maternal and cord serum. J Lab Clin Med. 1973;81:671-81.

66. **Saggese G, Bertelloni S, Baroncelli GI, et al.** Evaluation of a peptide family encoded by the calcitonin gene in selected healthy pregnant women. Horm Res. 1990;34:240-4.

67. **Ritchie LD, Fung EB, Hallorand BP, et al.** A longitudinal study of calcium homeostasis during human pregnancy and lactation and after resumption of menses. Am J Clin Nutr. 1998;67:693-701.

68. **Stevenson JC, et al.** A physiological role for calcitonin: protection of the maternal skeleton. Lancet. 1979;2:769.

69. **National Research Council.** Recommended Dietary Allowances, 10th ed. Washington, DC: National Academy of Science; 1989.

70. **Atkinson SA, Alston-Mills BP, Lonnerdal B, Neville MC, Thompson MP.** Major minerals and ion constituents of human and bovine milk. In: Jensen RJ, ed. Handbook of Milk Composition. San Diego, CA: Academic Press; 1995:593-619.

71. **Jenness R.** The composition of human milk. Semin Perinatol. 1979;3:225-39.

72. **Barlet JP, Champredon C, Coxam VD, et al.** Parathyroid hormone–related peptide might stimulate calcium secretion into the milk of goats. J Endocrinol. 1992;132:353-9.

73. **Law FM, Moate PJ, Leaver DD, et al.** Parathyroid hormone-related protein in milk and its correlation with bovine milk calcium. J Endocrinol. 1991;128:21-6.

74. **Thiede MA, Rodan GA.** Expression of calcium-mobilizing parathyroid hormone-like peptide in lactating mammary tissue. Science. 1988;242:278-80.

75. **Selvanayagam P, Graves K, Cooper C, et al.** Expression of the parathyroid hormone-related peptide gene in rat tissues. Lab Invest. 1991;64:713-7.

76. **Budayr A, Halloran BP, King JC, et al.** High levels of a parathyroid hormone-like protein in milk. Proc Natl Acad Sci U S A. 1989;86:7183-5.

77. **Burtis WJ, Brady TG, Orloff JJ, et al.** Immunochemical characterization of circulating parathyroid hormone-related protein in patients with humoral hypercalcemia of cancer. N Engl J Med. 1990;322:1106-12.

78. **Khosla S, van Heerden JA, Gharib H, et al.** Parathyroid hormone-related protein and hypercalcemia secondary to massive mammary hyperplasia. N Engl J Med. 1990;322: 1157.

79. **Leter L, Grill B, Martin TJ.** Hypercalcemia in pregnancy and lactation associated with parathyroid hormone-related peptide [Letter]. N Engl J Med. 1993;328:666-7.

80. **Ratcliffe WA, Thompson GE, Care AD, et al.** Production of parathyroid hormone-related protein by the mammary gland of the goat. J Endocrinol. 1992;133:87-93.

81. **Theide MA.** The mRNA encoding a parathyroid hormone-like peptide is produced in mammary tissue in response to elevations in serum prolactin. Mol Endocrinol. 1989;3:1443-7.

82. **Wilson SG, Retallack RW, Kent JC, et al.** Serum free 1,25-dihydroxyvitamin D and the free 1,25-dihydroxyvitamin D index during a longitudinal study of human pregnancy and lactation. Clin Endocrinol. 1990;32:613-22.

83. **Greer FR, Tsang RC, Searcy JE, et al.** Mineral homeostasis during lactation: relationship to serum 1,25-dihydroxyvitamin D, 25-hydroxyvitamin D, and parathyroid hormone and calcitonin. Am J Clin Nutr. 1982;38:431-7.

84. **Markstad T, Ulstein M, Bassoe HH, et al.** Vitamin D metabolism in normal and hypoparathyroid pregnancy and lactation: case report. Br J Obstet Gynaecol. 1983;90:971-6.

85. **Sowers MF, Zhang D, Hollis BW, Shapiro B, Janney CA, Crutchfield M, et al.** Role of calciotrophic hormones in calcium mobilization of lactation. Am J Clin Nutr. 1998;67:284-91.

86. **Retallack RW, Jeffries M, Kent GN, et al.** Physiologic hyperparathyroidism in human lactation. Calcif Tissue Res. 1977;22(Suppl):142-6.

87. **Kent GN, Price RI, Gutteridge DH, et al.** Human lactation: forearm trabecular bone loss, increased bone turnover, and renal conservation of calcium and inorganic phosphate with recovery of bone mass following weaning. J Bone Miner Res. 1990;5:361-9.

88. **Brommage R, DeLuca HF.** Regulation of bone mineral loss during lactation. Am J Physiol. 1985:E182-7.

89. **Lamke B, Brundin J, Moberg P.** Changes of bone mineral content during pregnancy and lactation. Acta Obstet Gynecol Scand. 1977;56:217-9.

90. **Drinkwater BL, Chestnut CH.** Bone density changes during pregnancy and lactation in active women: a longitudinal study. Bone and Mineral. 1991;14:153-60.

91. **Hayslip CC, Klein TS, Wray HL, et al.** The effect of lactation on bone mineral content in healthy postpartum women. Obstet Gynecol. 1989;73:588-92.

92. **Chan GM, Slater P, Ronald N, et al.** Bone mineral status of lactating mothers of different ages. Am J Obstet Gynecol. 1982;144:438-41.

93. **Burtis WJ, Yang KH, Stuart AF.** Nonparathyroid hypercalcemia. In: Becker KL et al., eds. Principles and Practice of Endocrinology and Metabolism. Philadelphia: JB Lippincott; 1995:520-32.

94. **Bringhurst RF, Demay MB, Kronenberg HM.** Hormones and disorders of mineral metabolism. In: Wilson et al., eds. Williams Textbook of Endocrinology. Philadelphia: WB Saunders; 1998:1155-1209-1476.

95. **Lee RV, Lippes HA, DiMaggio LA.** Common discomforts ("the aches and pains") complicating normal pregnancy. J Soc Obstet Gynecol Canada. 1992;14:19-37.

96. **Baron TH, Ramirez B, Richter JE.** Gastrointestinal motility disorders during pregnancy. Ann Intern Med. 1993;118:366-75.

97. **Maikranz P, Holley JL, Parks JH, et al.** Gestational hypercalciuria causes pathological urine calcium oxalate supersaturation. Kidney Int. 1989;36:108-13.

98. **Lindheimer MD, Barron WM, Davison JM.** Osmoregulation of thirst and vasopressin release in pregnancy. Am J Physiol. 1989;257:F159-69.

99. **Davison JM, Sheills EA, Barron WM, et al.** Changes in the metabolic clearance of vasopressin and in plasma vasopressinase throughout human pregnancy. J Clin Invest. 1989;83:1313-8.

100. **Heath H 3d, Hodgson SF, Kennedy L.** Primary hyperparathyroidism: incidence, morbidity, and potential economic impact in a community. N Engl J Med. 1980;302:189-93.

101. **Zagola GP, Eil C.** Diseases of the parathyroid glands and nephrolithiasis during pregnancy. In: Brody SA, Ueland K, Kase N, eds. Endocrine Disorders in Pregnancy. Norwalk, CT: Appleton & Lange; 1989:231-46.

102. **Wilson DT, Martin T, Christensen R, et al.** Hyperparathyroidism in pregnancy: case report and review of the literature. Can Med Assoc J. 1983;129:986-9.

103. **Shangold MN, Dor N, Welt S, et al.** Hyperparathyroidism and pregnancy: a review. Obstet Gynecol Surv. 1982;37:217-28.

104. **Kelly TR.** Primary hyperparathyroidism during pregnancy. Surgery. 1991;110:1028-34.

105. **Patten BM, Bilezikian JP, Mallette LE, et al.** Neuromuscular disease in primary hyperparathyroidism. Ann Intern Med. 1974;80:182-93.

106. **Hunter D, Turnbull H.** Hyperparathyroidism: generalized osteitis fibrosa with observations upon bones, parathyroid tumours and the normal parathyroid glands. Br J Surg. 1931;19:203-6.

107. **Gelister JSK, Sanderson JD, Chapple CR, et al.** Management of hyperparathyroidism in pregnancy. Br J Surg. 1989;76:1207-8.

108. **Potts JT Jr.** Management of asymptomatic hyperparathyroidism. J Clin Endocrinol Metab. 1990;70:1489-93.

109. **Shane E.** Medical management of asymptomatic primary hyperparathyroidism. J Bone Miner Res. 1991;6(Suppl 2):S131-4.

110. **Schneider B, Peschgens T, Hornchen H, Schild R, Kutta T, Maurin N.** Primary hyperparathyroidism in the third trimester. Deutsche Medizinische Wochenschrift. 1995;120:1123-6.

111. **Peschgens T, Stollbrink-Peschgens C, Merz U, Schneider B, Maurin N, Kutta T, Hornchen H.** Primary hyperparathyroidism and pregnancy. Aspects of neonatal morbidity. Z Geburtshilfe Perinatol. 1994;198:96-9.

112. **Sanghvi KP, Pinto J, Merchant RH.** Neonatal outcome in maternal hyperparathyroidism. Indian J Pediatr. 1996;33:960-4.

113. **Lowe DK, Orwoll ES, McClung MR, et al.** Hyperparathyroid and pregnancy. Am J Surg. 1983;145:611-4.

114. **Croom RD, Thomas CG.** Primary hyperparathyroidism during pregnancy. Surgery. 1984;96:1100-16.

115. **Cholst IN, Steinberg SF, Tropper PJ, et al.** The influence of hypermagnesemia on serum calcium and parathyroid hormone levels in human subjects. N Engl J Med. 1984;310:1221-5.

116. **Smith LG Jr, Burns PA, Schanler RJ.** Calcium homeostasis in pregnant women receiving long-term magnesium sulfate therapy for preterm labor. Am J Obstet Gynecol. 1992;167:45-51.

117. **Neufeld M, Blizzard RM.** Polyglandular autoimmune disease. In: Autoimmune Aspects of Endocrine Disorders. New York: Academic Press; 1980:357-8.

118. **Huikeshoven FJM, Zuijderhoudt FMJ.** Hypocalciuria in hypertensive disorder in pregnancy and how to measure it. Eur J Obstet Gynecol Reprod Biol. 1990;36:81-5.

119. **Rodriguez MH, Masaki DI, Mestman J, et al.** Calcium/creatinine ratio and microalbuminuria in the prediction of preeclampsia. Am J Obstet Gynecol. 1988;159:1452-5.

120. **Wright AD, Joplin GF, Dixon HG.** Post-partum hypercalcaemia in treated hypoparathyroidism. BMJ. 1969;1:23-5.
121. **Cundy T, Haining SA, Guilland-Cumming DF, Butler J, Danis JA.** Remission of hypoparathyroidism during lactation: evidence for a physiological role for prolactin vitamin D metabolism. Clin Endocrinol (Oxf). 1987;26:667-74.
122. **Caplan RH, Beguin EA.** Hypercalcemia in a calcitriol-treated hypoparathyroid woman during lactation. Obstet Gynecol. 1990;76:485-9.
123. **Rude RK, Haussler MR, Singer FR.** Postpartum resolution of hypocalcemia in a lactating hypoparathyroid patient. Endocriol Japon. 1984;31:227-33.

Chapter 6

Cardiovascular Disease

I. Cardiovascular Hemodynamics of Normal Pregnancy
Athena Poppas, MD

II. Congenital and Acquired Heart Disease
Athena Poppas, MD

III. Arrhythmias
Athena Poppas, MD, and Michael P. Carson, MD

IV. Peripartum Cardiomyopathy
Karen Rosene-Montella, MD, and Athena Poppas, MD

V. Syncope
Karen Rosene-Montella, MD, and Raymond O. Powrie, MD

I. Cardiovascular Hemodynamics of Normal Pregnancy
Athena Poppas

Pregnancy is characterized by dramatic and reversible changes in cardiovascular hemodynamics. The normal heart can adapt to these acute alterations, but pregnancy may impose an excessive strain on the diseased heart. The spectrum of heart disease seen in women of childbearing age is changing as persons with repaired congenital heart disease survive longer; as the incidence of rheumatic heart disease declines; and as women delay childbearing

Key Values and Normal Physiologic Changes for Cardiovascular Disease

	Direction of Change	Percentage Change or Normal Range for Pregnancy
Blood volume	↑	30% to 50% increase
Blood pressure	↓	≤120/80 mm Hg
Cardiac output	↑↑	5 to 7 L/m²/min (40% increase)
Chest radiograph		Straightened left upper cardiac border
		Horizontal position of heart
		Increased lung markings
		Small pleural effusion postpartum
Colloid oncotic pressure	↓	10% to 15% decrease
CPK-MB	↑	>7 (after cesarean section)
Central venous pressure	↔	<13 mm Hg
Ejection fraction	↔	70%
Electrocardiogram		Small Q, inverted P lead III
		Sinus tachycardia, PVC, PAC
		ST-T changes
		Change in QRS axis
		↑ R/S ratio V1/V2
Heart rate	↑	70 to 105 beats/min (increase of 10 to 20 beats/min)
Cholesterol and triglycerides	↑↑	50% to 100% increase
Pulmonary capillary wedge pressure	↔	<13 mm Hg
Pulmonary artery pressure	↔	≤25/12 mm Hg
Stroke volume	↑	70 to 100 mL/beat
Systemic vascular resistance	↓↓	600 to 800 dynes/sec/cm² (25% to 30% decrease)

↑ Increase
↓ Decrease
↔ No change

until their later years, when degenerative cardiovascular disease is more likely. It is imperative that primary care physicians be able to recognize and help treat cardiovascular disease, which can adversely affect the pregnant patient and her offspring.

Cardiovascular Hemodynamics of Normal Pregnancy

One must understand normal pregnancy to appreciate the range and mechanisms of adaptation possible in the cardiovascular system and to have a rational basis for comparison when pregnancy is complicated by pathologic conditions. Using both invasive and noninvasive techniques, numerous investigators have characterized some of the basic physiologic and hemodynamic variables of normal pregnancy (Figures 6-1 and 6-2).

Blood volume increases by 30% to 40%, so that it is 1200 to 1600 mL greater than it is in the nonpregnant state. This increase begins as early as 6 weeks of gestation and plateaus by the third trimester (1, 2). It varies greatly from patient to patient but has been correlated with the size of the products of conception in a given person. It results from an expansion of erythrocytes and an even greater increase in plasma volume. This produces a physiologic anemia of pregnancy. Heart rate increases by 10% to 20%, and stroke volume is significantly increased by as early as the eighth week of pregnancy. A 30% to 60% increase in cardiac output begins to appear early in the first trimester. This dramatic change seems to be driven by increases in preload and stroke volume early in pregnancy and is maintained by an increase in heart rate late in pregnancy (3–7). The inherent myocardial contractility does not seem to be altered by pregnancy when load-independent measures of systolic function are evaluated (4, 8). Particularly in the last trimester, body position can significantly affect these variables. When the patient is in the supine position, the gravid uterus compresses the inferior vena cava, decreasing systemic venous return and preload and causing an acute reduction in cardiac output of

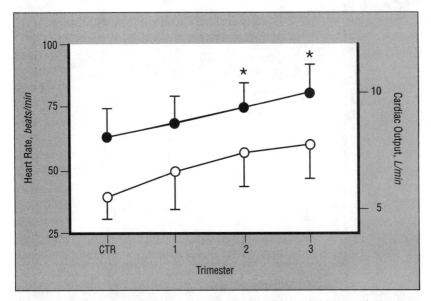

Figure 6-1 Heart rate (*black circles*) and cardiac output (*white circles*) in normal pregnancy.

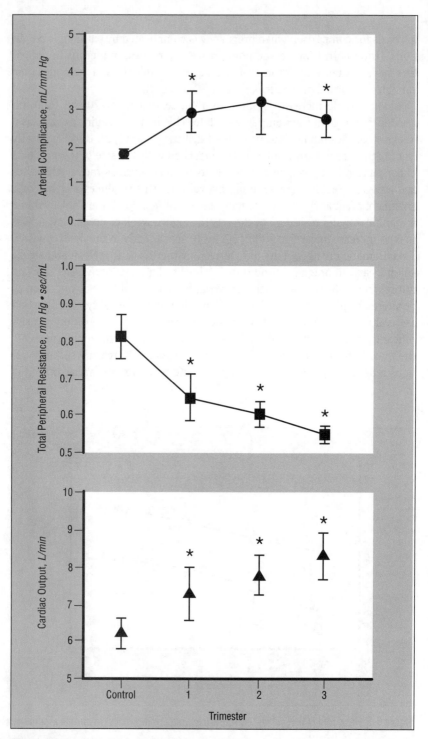

Figure 6-2 Cardiac output, total peripheral resistance, and arterial compliance in normal pregnancy.

up to 25% (9). Use of the left lateral decubitus position can prevent this and allows reliable and reproducible hemodynamic measurements.

The venous and arterial circulations display substantial adaptive changes. The systemic blood pressure decreases, and the diastolic pressure decreases more than the systolic pressure, resulting in a widened pulse pressure (4, 9). Total peripheral resistance has been shown to decrease during gestation, although some older studies reported an increase in the third trimester (5, 8). The compliance of the arterial and venous systems increases in parallel with the expanding blood volume, suggesting that, acting as capacitor, this compliance is one of the body's adaptive mechanisms to accommodate the increase in volume (2, 8). The energy of the cardiovascular system, ventricular—vascular coupling, and power remain unchanged. Despite the alterations in cardiovascular hemodynamics, the cardiac and vascular mechanical properties interact and adapt to maintain the overall efficiency of the system (8). As a result, the cardiovascular system during pregnancy is very dynamic, with a high cardiac output and bounding pulses.

Hemodynamic Effects of Exercise

Compared with nonpregnant women, pregnant women respond differently and with greater variability to the physiologic challenge of exercise. A woman's baseline aerobic fitness affects her ability to respond to exercise during pregnancy. Aerobically fit women normally have an enhanced cardiorespiratory response to acute exercise and, with regular exercise, this is maintained during pregnancy (10). The stage of pregnancy affects the response to exercise. As pregnancy progresses, an attenuated increase in cardiac output with exercise is seen (11). Supine exercise after midgestation decreases venous return and, thus, the ability to augment stroke volume. Numerous studies suggest that well-conditioned recreational athletes who continue regular exercise programs during pregnancy have no significant increases in infertility, abortion, placental abruption, hypertension, fetal anomalies, or poor APGAR scores (12–15). On the other hand, acutely, maximal exertion has been associated with fetal distress as manifested by fetal bradycardia immediately after exercise and possibly during it (16). This may be due to the theoretical ill effects of hyperthermia, blood flow redistribution, and substrate deprivation with acidosis (17). Therefore, in healthy patients with normal pregnancies, continuation of a moderate exercise program to 70% of the maximum predicted heart rate can be recommended. It seems to be well tolerated acutely and chronically by both mother and fetus (16, 17).

Hemodynamic Effects of Labor, Delivery, and the Puerperium Period

Labor, with its cyclic increases in heart rate and volume, dramatically alters cardiovascular loading conditions and demands. With each uterine contraction, approximately 500 cc of blood is briefly diverted from the uterine to the maternal circulation. A resultant increase in cardiac output and mean arterial blood pressure is seen (18, 19). Pain, particularly in the second stage of labor, stimulates the sympathetic nervous system with consequent dramatic increases in heart rate, blood pressure, and myocardial oxygen consumption. The vigorous Valsalva maneuver with pushing exaggerates the increases in blood pressure and myocardial oxygen consumption. Local anesthesia can reduce pain, and epidural anesthesia can further attenuate the increase in cardiac output by causing vasodilatation. Although adequate anesthesia and analgesia can reduce the effects of pain and anxiety, the autotransfusion of blood with each uterine contraction can be averted only by avoiding labor through the use of surgical delivery. On the other hand, blood loss is approximately 300 to 400 cc with a vaginal delivery and increases to twice that with a cesarean section (20). The normal heart can adapt to these acute changes but, depending on the type of lesion, the diseased heart may decompensate. The increase in preload will stress patients with cardiomyopathy or mitral regurgitation, the sudden blood loss will be less tolerated in patients with aortic stenosis, and the increased heart rate may cause decompensation in patients with mitral stenosis.

A few studies have sought to evaluate the cardiovascular changes seen in the puerperium and postpartum periods. Robson and colleagues (5) did serial echocardiographic studies in 15 women from 38 weeks of gestation to 24 weeks postpartum and noted a 33% decrease in cardiac output. Twenty-eight percent of the decrease occurred by 2 weeks after delivery. By 2 weeks after delivery, heart rate and stroke volume had decreased by 20% and left atrial and ventricular end-diastolic dimensions had decreased. By 24 weeks after delivery, all hemodynamic variables had returned to preconception values. Although the numbers were small, Robson and colleagues found no significant difference between lactating and nonlactating women. Similarly, Capeless and Clapp (21) evaluated 13 women before conception and up to 1 year postpartum. At 12 weeks and 6 months, they noted a 19% and a 10% residual increase in stroke volume, respectively, but no increase in heart rate or cardiac output. Values at 1 year were similar to those seen before conception. Thus, women with structural heart disease require continued, close follow-up in the early postpartum period.

Cardiac Evaluation

History and Physical Examination

The normal hemodynamic changes of pregnancy alter the normal physical examination, making it difficult to distinguish pathologic from common physiologic findings. The physical signs and symptoms that can be seen during normal pregnancy are summarized in Table 6-1. The circulatory system in pregnancy is hypervolemic and hyperdynamic, mimicking the circulatory system in disease states that widen pulse pressure, such as aortic insufficiency and hyperthyroidism.

The patient usually seems comfortable. Vital signs show slight increases in heart rate and low-normal blood pressure. Probably as a result of increased blood volume and cardiac output and the more horizontal position of heart, the left ventricular apex is laterally displaced, brisk, and diffuse to palpation, particularly later in pregnancy. The right ventricular impulse is normally palpable along the left sternal border. Yet a sustained heave, like that found in right or left ventricular failure, is not seen (22, 23). The first heart sound is increased in intensity throughout pregnancy with exaggerated splitting that can be mistaken for a fourth heart sound. In the third trimester, the second heart sound is increased in intensity with exaggerated splitting, particularly when the patient is in the left lateral decubitus position. There is debate about the presence of a third heart sound: An older study noted an 84% incidence of this sound after the 20th week of gestation, but newer observations suggest a clear lack of this finding in healthy gravidas (22, 24). A fourth heart sound is rare in normal pregnancy.

Functional flow murmurs may be discovered during pregnancy, and pathologic murmurs may change in intensity because of the hemodynamic burden. A midsystolic, ejection flow murmur without radiation is heard in 96% of patients and is due to increased volume and flow in the right and left ventricular outflow tracts (23). True diastolic murmurs are rare in pregnancy and should prompt a more thorough investigation, usually with echocardiography. Two physiologic, continuous flow murmurs are specific for pregnancy. The first is the cervical or suprasternal hum, which disappears with hyperex-

Table 6-1   Findings on Cardiac Physical Examination in Normal Pregnancy

Signs	Symptoms
Tachycardia	Mild dyspnea
Jugular venous distention	Fatigue
Brisk or bounding peripheral arterial pulses	Orthopnea
Brisk, diffuse, laterally displaced PMI	Palpitations
Palpable RV impulse	
Loud, split S1	
Loud S2 (third trimester)	
Systolic pulmonary flow murmur; tricuspid/regurgitant murmur	
Mammary soufflé	
Suprasternal venous hum	
Lower-extremity edema	

tension of the shoulders or compression of the internal jugular vein. The second, the mammary soufflé, appears in the last trimester or postpartum period. It is heard best over the upper breast area, is loudest in systole, and diminishes with pressure of the stethoscope (25). Pathologic valvular regurgitant murmurs decrease because of the decrease in afterload, whereas stenotic valvular murmurs increase in intensity because of the high cardiovascular flow state. The click associated with mitral valve prolapse usually disappears.

The arterial pulses are usually full, brisk, and even collapsing because of increased vascular volume and compliance with reduced systemic vascular resistance. Jugular venous distention with normal waveforms is common later in pregnancy and is due to increased intravascular volume. This also contributes to lower-extremity edema, which is common later in pregnancy and with advanced maternal age. Other factors that contribute to edema include inferior venal caval compression; decreased oncotic pressure; and, possibly, changes in vascular permeability that occur in normal pregnancy. Pulmonary bibasilar crackles that "open up" with deep inspiration are occasionally heard in late pregnancy and are probably due to raised diaphragms with lower lung compression and atelectasis (24).

Symptoms that are common in normal pregnancy can mimic the symptoms of heart and lung disease. In particular, dyspnea occurs in 50% of women before the 19th week of gestation and in 76% by the 31st week (26, 27). Notably, functional dyspnea is not acute in onset, does not occur at rest, does not interfere with activities of daily living, is not progressive, and usually plateaus in the third trimester. The probable mechanism is the effect of progesterone on the central respiratory center. Fatigue or reduced exercise tolerance is common and is probably due to increased body weight, the demands of the fetus, and anemia. Orthopnea is occasionally noted in late pregnancy and is due to the mechanical disadvantage imposed by the gravid uterus. It is usually alleviated if the patient rests in the lateral decubitus position. If other signs or symptoms suggestive of congestive heart failure are noted, evaluation with echocardiography must be done to exclude peripartum cardiomyopathy (PPCM) or occult valvular disease. Palpitations are reported throughout gestation and, in a structurally normal heart, are rarely associated with arrhythmias.

Although the signs and symptoms common in pregnancy can mimic those of disease states, a careful physical examination that correlates findings with the period of gestation can help. If questions remain, safe, noninvasive testing methods can be used to definitively exclude the presence of high-risk cardiovascular diseases.

Cardiac Testing Methods

Chest radiography can be done with appropriate pelvic shielding. If right heart catheterization is required for hemodynamic monitoring in seriously ill patients, this can be done safely without fluoroscopy, although chest radiography will be necessary after the procedure to exclude complications. Cardiac catheterization and angiography require higher doses of radiation that should be avoided in the first trimester, if possible, but with shielding and limited fluoroscopy, time can be done with a radiation dose of 1 rad or less. In cases where the benefits clearly outweigh the risks (such as acute myocardial infarction), cardiac catheterization has been done successfully (28). Nuclear studies that use radiolabeled tracers can assess ventricular function, infarction, and inducible ischemia, but they are rarely indicated in pregnant patients because echocardiography is a safe, alternative method of evaluation.

Echocardiography can be used for repeated assessment of hemodynamic variables throughout pregnancy with no significant risk to the patient or fetus. The atrial and ventricular chambers and the aortic annulus increase in size by 5% to 15% throughout gestation and return to normal after delivery (4, 6). Small pericardial effusions have been reported in up to 44% of women by the third trimester; these effusions resolve by 6 weeks postpartum and are more common in primigravidas and women with greater weight gain (29). Doppler echocardiography can reliably evaluate cardiac output, shunt flows, and degree of valve regurgitation and stenosis (30). Echocardiography can be used to exclude structural heart disease in symptomatic patients and to evaluate the severity and hemodynamic effects of complex heart defects. Stress echocardiography is the diagnostic procedure of choice for the evaluation of coronary artery disease.

The electrocardiogram may show minor changes during normal pregnancy. The mean QRS axis has been reported to be deviated to the left later in pregnancy because of the elevation of the hemidiaphragm, but others have reported no deviation or a more rightward axis early in pregnancy (31). In addition, minor ST-segment depression and T-wave inversions have been noted in the inferior and lateral leads. Isolated atrial and ventricular premature beats are common (31). Arrhythmias are usually associated with structurally abnormal hearts, and 24-hour Holter monitors or event monitors can be used to better define supraventricular or ventricular arrhythmias in this setting.

REFERENCES

1. **Lund CJ, Donovan JC.** Blood volume during pregnancy. Am J Obstet Gynecol. 1967;98:393.

2. **Pritchard JA.** Changes in the blood volume during pregnancy and delivery. Anesthesiology. 1965;26:393.

3. **Walters WAW, MacGregor WG, Hills M.** Cardiac output at rest during pregnancy and the puerperium. Clin Sci. 1966;30:1.

4. **Katz RM, Karliner JS, Resnik RM.** Effects of a natural volume overload state (pregnancy) on left ventricular performance in normal human subjects. Circulation. 1978;58:434-41.

5. **Robson SC, Hunter S, Moore M, Dunlop W.** Haemodynamic changes during the puerperium: a Doppler and M-mode echocardiographic study. Br J Obstet Gynaecol. 1987;94:1028-39.

6. **Robson SC, Hunter S, Boys RJ, Dunlop W.** Serial study of factors influencing changes in cardiac output during human pregnancy. Am J Physiol. 1989;H1060-5.

7. **Duvekot J, Cheriex E, Pieters F, Menheere P, Peeters L.** Early pregnancy changes in hemodynamics and volume homeostasis are consecutive adjustments triggered by a primary fall in systemic vascular tone. Am J Obstet Gynecol. 1993;169:1382-92.

8. **Poppas A, Shroff S, Korcaz C, et al.** Serial assessment of the cardiovascular system in normal pregnancy: role of arterial compliance and pulsatile arterial load. Circulation. 1997;95:2407-15.

9. **Rubler S, Damani P, Pinto E.** Cardiac size and performance during pregnancy estimated with echocardiography. Am J Cardiol. 1977;40:534.

10. **Privarnik JM, Ayres NA, Mauer MB, Cotton DB, Kirshon B, Dildy GA.** Effects of maternal aerobic fitness on cardiorespiratory responses to exercise. Med Sci Sports Exerc. 1993;25:993-8.

11. **Veille JC, Hellerstein HK, Cherry B, Bacevice AE.** Effects of advancing pregnancy on left ventricular function during bicycle exercise. Am J Cardiol. 1994;73:609-10.

12. **Jarrett JC, Spellacy WN.** Jogging during pregnancy: an improved outcome? Obstet Gynecol. 1984;61:705-9.

13. **Clapp JF.** The effects of maternal exercise on early pregnancy outcome. Am J Obstet Gynecol. 1989;161:1453-7.

14. **Hatch MC, Shu XO, McLean DE, et al.** Maternal exercise during pregnancy, physical fitness, and fetal growth. Am J Epidemiol. 1993;137:1105-14.

15. **Lokey EA, Tran ZV, Wells CL, Myers BC, Tran AC.** Effects of physical exercise on pregnancy outcomes: a meta-analytic review. Med Sci Sports Exerc. 1991;23:1234-9.

16. **Carpenter MW, Sady SP, Hoegsberg B, et al.** Fetal heart rate response to maternal exertion. JAMA. 1988;259:3006-9.

17. **Clapp JF.** Exercise in pregnancy: good, bad or indifferent? Current Obstetric Medicine. 1993;2:25-49.

18. **Uelan K, Hansen JM.** Maternal cardiovascular dynamics. III. Labor and delivery under local and caudal analgesia. Am J Obstet Gynecol. 1969;103:8-18.

19. **Robson SC, Dunlop W, Boys RJ.** Cardiac output during labor. BMJ. 1987;295:1169-72.

20. **Mendelson MA, Lang RM.** Pregnancy and heart disease. In: Barron WM, Lindheimer MD, eds. Medical Disorders during Pregnancy. St. Louis, MO: Mosby; 1995:129-67.

21. **Capeless EL, Clapp JF.** When do cardiovascular parameters return to their preconception values? Am J Obstet Gynecol. 1991;165:883-6.

22. **Cutforth RM, MacDonald CB.** Heart sounds and murmurs in pregnancy. Am Heart J. 1966;71:741-7.

23. **Proctor HW.** Alteration of the cardiac physical examination in normal pregnancy. Clin Obstet Gynecol. 1975;18:51-63.

24. **Warnes CA, Elkayam E.** Congenital heart disease and pregnancy. In: Elkayam U, Gleicher N, eds. Cardiac Problems in Pregnancy. New York: Wiley-Liss; 1998:39-54.

25. **Tabatzink B, Randall TW, Hersch C.** The mammary soufflé of pregnancy and lactation. Circulation. 1960;22:1069-73.

26. **Zeldis SM.** Dyspnea during pregnancy: distinguishing cardiac from pulmonary causes. Clin Chest Med. 1992;13:567-85.

27. **Milne J, Howie A, Pack A.** Dyspnea during normal pregnancy. Br J Obstet Gynaecol. 1978;85:260-3.

28. **Rubler S, Hammer N, Schneebaum R.** Systolic time intervals in pregnancy and the postpartum period. Am Heart J. 1972;86:182.

29. **Abduljabbar HS, Marzouki KM, Zawawi TH, Khan AS.** Pericardial effusion in normal pregnant women. Acta Obstet Gynecol Scand. 1991;70:291-4.

30. **Lee WM, Rokey RM, Cotton DB.** Noninvasive maternal stroke volume and cardiac output determinations by pulsed Doppler echocardiography. Am J Obstet Gynecol. 1988;158:505-10.

31. **Carruth JE, Mirris SB, Brogan DR.** The electrocardiogram in normal pregnancy. Am Heart J. 1981;102:1075-8.

II. Congenital and Acquired Heart Disease
Athena Poppas

Congenital Heart Disease

As a result of significant advances in the accurate identification and treatment of congenital heart disease, women with such disease now live longer into their childbearing years. Although the effect and outcome of pregnancy in these women and their children has improved, pregnancy still carries significant risks. The care and management of patients with congenital heart disease requires an understanding of the how each type of defect responds to the known hemodynamic stresses of pregnancy. Appropriate coordination of diagnostic and therapeutic interventions from preconception counseling through labor and delivery to the postpartum period are necessary.

Preconception counseling about maternal morbidity and mortality and fetal morbidity, mortality, and inheritable risks requires precise, comprehensive characterization of the cardiac abnormalities present and the degree to which the patient has tolerated the condition. Known predictors of poor maternal–fetal outcome include elevated pulmonary artery pressure, depressed right and left ventricular function, cyanosis, and impaired New York Heart Association (NYHA) functional class (1). Overall, the maternal mortality rate is approximately 0.4% for women in NYHA class I-II and may increase to 7% for women in NYHA class III-IV (2). Most experts advise against pregnancy for patients with NYHA class III-IV symptoms or patients with significant pulmonary hypertension (3). Maternal cyanosis most significantly affects fetal outcome: Only 55% of pregnancies result in liveborn infants, and less than 10% of these infants are full term and have normal birthweight (1). Furthermore, counseling should include discussion of the increased risk for congenital heart disease in the fetus. The incidence of congenital heart disease in the general population is 0.7% to 0.8%, but it can be as high as 3.4% to 14.2% (1, 4, 5) for particular lesions. In one report, it was as high as 17.9% to 23% for women with uncorrected lesions, although this finding was confounded by probable genetic syndromes (1). Fetal echocardiography can be done at 18 to 20 weeks of gestation to identify and characterize possible fetal cardiac anomalies in utero.

It is helpful to group the various congenital heart diseases by simple pathophysiologic categories because diseases within these categories have similar outcomes, treatments, and labor and delivery options. In general, delivery should be vaginal with adequate pain control and assistance to shorten the second stage of labor. Cesarean section is usually reserved for obstetric indications (6). The three categories are 1) lesions that produce volume overload, 2) lesions that produce pressure overload, and 3) lesions that produce cyanosis. The volume overload lesions are due to left-to-right shunts and include atrial septal defects (ASDs), ventricular septal defects (VSDs), and patent ductus arteriosus. They are well tolerated in pregnancy unless pulmonary hypertension or right-to-left shunting is present (7). Stenotic lesions produce pressure load on the preceding chamber. They include aortic stenosis, mitral stenosis, coarctation of the aorta, and pulmonary valve stenosis. They are fairly well tolerated in pregnancy unless the obstruction is severe. Cyanotic heart disease results from right-to-left shunts because shunt flow is increased. These patients are usually corrected or palliated at a young age, and uncorrected patients rarely survive to their childbearing years. These diseases include tetralogy of Fallot, Ebstein anomaly, tricuspid atresia, transposition of the great arteries, truncus arteriosus, and univentricles. Patients with severe pulmonary hypertension or the Eisenmenger syndrome have a maternal mortality rate approaching 50% (6). Maternal and fetal outcomes correlate with maternal hematocrit and arterial Po_2. In general, spontaneous or induced vaginal delivery is safer; cesarean section is reserved for obstetric indications. Labor and delivery should be managed with oxygen (particularly in cyanotic patients), cardiac monitoring, the left lateral decubitus position, and adequate pain control. The use of anesthetics, such as epidurals, carries an increased risk for systemic hypotension and may be problematic in patients with pulmonary hypertension and right-to-left shunts. The recommendations given here are based on pathophysiology; no rigorous studies have proven efficacy (8).

Atrial Septal Defects

Atrial septal defects are the most common congenital lesions in adults and are often first diagnosed during pregnancy, when volume is increased and patients come to medical attention. The three types of ASDs are classified by their location and embryology; in descending order of frequency, they are secundum, primum, and sinus venosus defects. The secundum ASD is associated with myxomatous mitral valve disease and prolapse in 20% to 30% of cases. The uncorrected shunt produces a volume load on the right ventricle with enlargement of the right atrium and ventricle. The normal increase in blood volume during pregnancy causes further volume load, although this is usually without a concomitant increase in pressures. Most patients with an isolated ASD tolerate pregnancy well. With larger shunts, there is risk for congestive heart failure, atrial arrhythmias, peripheral venous thrombosis or embolism, cerebral vascular accidents, and shunt reversal with cyanosis from sudden systemic hypotension (9, 10). Congestive heart failure can be treated medically with digoxin, diuretics, and, lastly, surgical or percutaneous closure. Atrial arrhythmias can worsen or precipitate heart failure and should be treated with medications as outlined in Section III. Although no clear data on the practice are available, use of a baby aspirin per day after the first trimester is advocated to prevent venous thrombosis and paradoxical emboli in the relative hypercoagulable state of pregnancy. Systemic hypotension, which can occur during parturition, should be avoided or rapidly corrected with pressors and volume to prevent possible shunt reversal and oxygen desaturation. Notably, bacterial endocarditis prophylaxis is not required for corrected or uncorrected secundum ASDs. Women with significant shunts (a Qp-to-Qs ratio >1.5:1) should have preconception closure if possible.

Ventricular Septal Defects

Ventricular septal defects are common at birth (0.3 to 3 per 1000 live births) but often close by adulthood (11). The size and location of the defect determine the clinical course. Membranous VSDs are the most common and can be associated with aortic insufficiency due to prolapse of the contiguous cusp. Isolated VSDs are usually well tolerated in pregnancy unless the shunt is large. Left ventricular size and function, pulmonary pressures, and functional class help determine risk (10). In hemodynamically significant shunts, complications include congestive heart failure, atrial arrhythmias, pulmonary hypertension, and shunt reversal with cyanosis due to systemic hypotension. In 98 pregnancies resulting in 78 liveborn infants in 50 women with VSDs, no deaths were reported (1). In women with corrected lesions, no increased risks are associated with gestation. Bacterial endocarditis prophylaxis is recommended for patients with uncorrected lesions, residual shunts, or prosthetic patches (Boxes 6-1 and 6-2).

Patent Ductus Arteriosus

Patent ductus arteriosus is common in newborns but rare in adults. The residual embryonic shunt is from the descending aorta at the isthmus to the

---

Box 6-1 American Heart Association Recommendations for Bacterial Endocarditis Prophylaxis

---

High-risk category

Prosthetic cardiac valves (bioprosthetic and homograft)

Previous bacterial endocarditis

Complex cyanotic CHD (single ventricle, transposition of the great vessels, tetralogy of Fallot)

Surgically constructed systemic pulmonary shunts or conduits

Moderate-risk category*

Most other congenital cardiac malformations

Acquired valvular dysfunction (e.g., rheumatic heart disease)

Hypertrophic cardiomyopathy

Mitral valve prolapse with valvular regurgitation or thickened leaflets

Low-risk category[†]

Isolated secundum ASD

Surgical repair of ASD, VSD, or PDA (without residua beyond 6 months)

Previous CABG surgery

MVP without valvular regurgitation

Physiologic, functional, or innocent heart murmurs

Previous Kawasaki disease without valvular dysfunction

Previous rheumatic fever with valvular dysfunction

Cardiac pacemakers and implanted defibrillators

---

* The author of this section and the editors of this book recommend that prophylaxis be used n the moderate-risk category in pregnancy given the woman's altered hemodynamics.
[†] Prophylaxis not recommended.

Box 6-2 Prophylactic Regimens for Bacterial Endocarditis in Mothers with High-Risk Cardiac Lesions*

Standard regimen for high-risk patients

Ampicillin 2 g IM or IV + gentamicin 1.5 mg/kg (up to 120 mg) within 30 min of starting the procedure; 6 hours later, ampicillin 1 mg IM or IV, or amoxicillin 1 g PO[†]

Regimen for high-risk patients with allergy to ampicillin or amoxicillin

Vancomycin 1 g IV or 1 to 2 hours + gentamicin 1.5 mg/kg (up to 120 mg); complete injection or infusion within 30 min of starting the procedure

---

* The author of this section and the editors of this book recommend that these regimens be used for patients who need bacterial endocarditis prophylaxis and who undergo vaginal delivery or cesarean section
[†] Patients requiring surgical prophylaxis will also be adequately covered by this regimen.
Adapted from 1997 AHA Guidelines.

proximal left pulmonary artery. Again, the risks of pregnancy are related to shunt size and degree of pulmonary hypertension. In asymptomatic women with normal pulmonary artery pressures and small shunts, maternal and fetal outcomes are not altered (1). As with other left-to-right shunts, there is still a theoretical risk of shunt reversal and cyanosis from sudden, systemic hypotension. Patients with large shunts have enlargement of the pulmonary artery and left-sided chambers and can develop high-output heart failure. In corrected or uncorrected patent ductus arteriosus, pulmonary hypertension significantly increases maternal and fetal morbidity and mortality rates (10). Bacterial endocarditis prophylaxis is recommended for patients with unrepaired or residual shunts.

Congenital Aortic Stenosis

The most common congenital heart disease found in adulthood is bicuspid aortic valve. Rarer causes of obstruction of left ventricular outflow include unicuspid aortic valves and supra- and subvalvular membranes. Mild-to-moderate valvular aortic stenosis is well tolerated in pregnancy, but severe aortic stenosis (aortic valve area <1.0 cm^2) is associated with increased maternal and fetal morbidity and mortality rates. Studies from the 1970s reported mortality rates of 17% for mothers and 32% for fetuses (12). A 1982 study of 59 pregnancies with 46 liveborn infants in 27 women found no maternal deaths but noted an increased rate of cardiovascular complications in women with worse functional class (1). The most recent study, from 1993, evaluated 25 pregnancies in 13 patients (13). It found no maternal deaths, but 31% of patients had functional deterioration; one patient required percutaneous balloon valvuloplasty, and another required pregnancy termination. Five therapeutic abortions were done. Among the 20 liveborn infants, no perinatal deaths or illnesses were seen. Thus, women with severe valvular aortic stenosis should undergo percutaneous or surgical repair or replacement before conception, if possible, or midgestation (if patient is American Heart Association class III-IV and termination is not an option). Physical exertion, particularly exercise, should be limited. Labor and delivery should be managed with invasive hemodynamic monitoring. Vasodilatory anesthetic agents should be avoided, and hemorrhage should be minimized because hypotension can be rapidly deleterious. Prophylaxis for endocarditis is advised.

Coarctation of the Aorta

An abnormality of the aortic media produces a discreet narrowing of the descending aorta, usually just distal to the left subclavian artery. There is hypertension above the narrowing and hypoperfusion below. Important associated anomalies include bicuspid aortic valve and cerebral aneurysms (11). The risks of pregnancy in women with aortic coarctation include risk for worsening hypertension, new heart failure, and aortic dissection and rupture (1, 3). In patients with aortic or cerebral aneurysms or associated cardiac anomalies, the maternal mortality rate is increased. In the largest study to date of women with corrected and uncorrected coarctation, no maternal deaths occurred, although 9 of 74 pregnant women developed hypertension. Despite the theoretical risks for decreased placental perfusion, fetal morbidity and mortality do not seem to be increased. However, serial fetal monitoring that includes Dopplers may be prudent (2). Treatment includes limitation of physical activity and maintenance of blood pressure close to 140 mm Hg; beta-blockers are the agent of choice. Successful surgical repair has been reported during gestation but should be reserved for patients with uncontrolled hypertension or heart failure. Vaginal delivery is still preferred, although hypertension should be averted during labor by the use of beta-blockers, epidural anesthetics, and assisted delivery (2). Prophylaxis for bacterial endocarditis is advised.

Pulmonary Valve Stenosis

Pulmonary valve stenosis is the most common type of isolated right ventricular outflow tract obstruction. Patients with mild-to-moderate stenosis (gradients less than 80 mm Hg) are usually asymptomatic and tolerate the hemodynamic burden of pregnancy without difficulty. In a study of 46 pregnancies resulting in 36 live births in 24 women with pulmonary stenosis, no maternal deaths occurred, although there was one report of congestive heart failure (1). In patients with more severe obstruction and worsening clinical function, percutaneous balloon valvuloplasty can be done with appropriate abdominal shielding. Ideally, patients with isolated, congenital pulmonary valve stenosis should have percutaneous balloon valvuloplasty before conception. These patients are often left with some degree of insufficiency, which is well tolerated (6). Prophylaxis for bacterial endocarditis is advised by some.

Ebstein Anomaly

Ebstein anomaly is an uncommon congenital heart lesion. The malformed tricuspid valve is apically displaced to a variable extent with resultant tricuspid regurgitation, atrial dilation, and limited ventricular function. Most patients survive to adulthood and often first present as adults. Important lesions often associated with Ebstein anomaly include ASDs and the Wolfe-Parkinson-White syndrome (11). The maternal risks of pregnancy are low and correlate with degree of tricuspid regurgitation, right ventricular function, and presence of cyanosis (14, 15). During gestation, tricuspid regurgitation and right ventricular function may worsen, and atrial arrhythmias may occur.

Fifty percent of women with the Ebstein anomaly have an interatrial shunt, and these women are at risk for paradoxical emboli and cyanosis. In a recent review of 111 pregnancies that resulted in 85 live births in 44 women, no maternal deaths or cardiovascular complications were seen. Increased rates of fetal loss, prematurity, and, in cyanotic patients, lower birthweight were seen (14). Preconception repair is preferable, particularly for patients with an interatrial communication. Prophylaxis for bacterial endocarditis is advised.

Tetralogy of Fallot

Classic tetralogy of Fallot is the most common cyanotic congenital heart defect found in children, adults, and pregnant women. The four findings are a malalignment VSD, overriding aorta, infundibular pulmonic stenosis, and secondary right ventricular hypertrophy (11). Patients with corrected lesions and good residual functional status usually tolerate the increased hemodynamic stress of pregnancy, but the residual risks are for arrhythmias (7). On the other hand, uncorrected or palliated lesions may show clinical deterioration during pregnancy and may lead to increased maternal and fetal complications (3, 16). Maternal risks include increased right-to-left shunting and, thus, cyanosis during gestation and delivery; biventricular heart failure; arrhythmias; and cerebral vascular accidents from paradoxical emboli. Fetal risk is correlated with maternal cyanosis and includes increased risk for prematurity, low birthweight, and spontaneous abortion (9, 16, 17). In a review of 46 pregnancies in 21 uncorrected cyanotic patients, 38% of patients had cardiovascular complications and there were only 15 live births, 60% of which were premature (16). Pregnancy is contraindicated in severe cyanosis, which is defined by a maternal hematocrit greater than 60% and an arterial saturation less than 80%. Preconception repair is preferred to reduce morbidity and mortality, but corrected patients should have a functional assessment to determine risk. Prophylaxis for bacterial endocarditis is advised, and prophylaxis for thrombosis may be indicated.

Complex Cyanotic Congenital Heart Disease

Survival and pregnancy after repair of complex, cyanotic congenital heart disease is now possible albeit rare. In a recent evaluation by mailed questionnaires of patients who had univentricles corrected by the Fontan procedure, 33 pregnancies resulted in 15 live births in 14 women. The only complication was one episode of supraventricular tachycardia (SVT) (18). Similarly, in a review of 26 pregnancies resulting in 8 live births in 10 women with univentricles or tricuspid atresia, no maternal deaths occurred (16). In a report of 15 pregnancies in 9 asymptomatic women with transposition of the great arteries corrected by the Mustard procedure, no cardiovascular complications were seen (19). However, in smaller series of patients with transposition of the great arteries, the morphologic right ventricle deteriorated or preterm delivery ensued, or both (20, 21). In general, complications that should be anticipated include functional deterioration and congestive heart failure due to limited cardiac reserve, bradyarrhythmias, tachyarrhythmias, intracardiac thrombus, and paradoxical emboli (2, 13). Careful obstetric, cardiac, and anesthetic evaluation and management of patients with complex cyanotic congenital heart disease can result in good maternal and fetal outcomes. Prophylaxis for bacterial endocarditis is advised.

Eisenmenger Syndrome and Pulmonary Hypertension

The Eisenmenger syndrome comprises severe pulmonary vascular obstructive disease and hypertension resulting from communication between the systemic and pulmonary circulations. The degree of pulmonary hypertension determines the amount of right-to-left shunting and, thus, cyanosis. The hemodynamic and hemostatic changes of pregnancy and parturition are poorly tolerated in the Eisenmenger syndrome and contribute to the high risk for death. The maternal mortality rate is 39% to 52%; thus, pregnancy is thought to be contraindicated (2, 22). Pregnancy termination carries a relatively lower risk and is recommended. In patients who decline termination, empirical management should include strict limitation of physical activity, oxygen for dyspnea, and heparin prophylaxis throughout pregnancy and for 4 to 6 weeks after delivery. Increased complications have been reported with Swan-Ganz catheterization, and this procedure is not recommended (8). Labor and delivery carry the highest risk. Vaginal delivery has been recommended, but most patients require cesarean section because of maternal or fetal deterioration (7, 23). In mothers who survive, risks to the fetus are substantial. The fetal mortality rate is 40%, and prematurity and intrauterine growth retardation predominate in survivors (9, 22). Sterilization is recommended and can be done laparoscopically.

Acquired Cardiovascular Disease

Rheumatic Mitral Stenosis

Rheumatic fever most often involves the mitral valve and results in leaflet thickening, commissural fusion, and retraction of the chordae tendineae. Mitral stenosis restricts left ventricular inflow, with resultant elevation of the left atrial and pulmonary venous pressures. The hemodynamic changes of pregnancy (increased volume and heart rate) adversely stress patients with rheumatic mitral stenosis; many have clinical deterioration during gestation. Patients with mild-to-moderate or occult mitral stenosis may first become symptomatic during pregnancy and, thus, may first be diagnosed during pregnancy. The risks of mitral stenosis to the mother include risk for atrial arrhythmias, thromboembolic events, and pulmonary edema and are greatest in the third trimester and the puerperal period (7). Treatment should include continued antibiotic prophylaxis for streptococcal pharyngitis and endocarditis prophylaxis at delivery. To reduce heart rate and symptoms in moderate-to-severe mitral stenosis, restriction of physical activity and beta-blockade are useful. Atrial fibrillation will cause clinical deterioration and increased risk for thromboembolism and should be treated aggressively with digoxin, beta-blockade, and anticoagulation (see Section III). In patients with class III-IV symptoms who do not respond to medical therapy, percutaneous balloon valvuloplasty with pelvic shielding is safe (24). In hospitals without expertise in this procedure, surgical commissurotomy carries a maternal mortality rate of approximately 1% to 2% and a fetal mortality rate of 10% (25, 26). Finally, if significant mitral insufficiency precludes commissurotomy, mitral valve replacement can be used, although it leads to increased maternal and fetal morbidity and mortality because of the need for cardiopulmonary bypass (26). In patients with moderate-to-severe mitral stenosis, labor and delivery should be managed with Swan-Ganz catheterization and monitoring, epidural anesthesia, and shortening of the second stage of labor (27).

Mitral and Aortic Insufficiency

Valvular regurgitation may be due to rheumatic disease, endocarditis, prolapse, or connective tissue disease. Even when severe, these lesions are well tolerated in pregnancy because of the favorable effects of decreased systemic vascular resistance and consequent afterload reduction. Regurgitant lesions are not associated with adverse fetal outcome. For the rare patient who is symptomatic, treatment includes digoxin; diuretics; and afterload reduction, preferably with hydralazine (7). Mitral or aortic valve repair or replacement is rarely indicated during pregnancy. Cardiopulmonary bypass surgery done with high flow rates, normothermia, and fetal heart rate monitoring carries a low maternal mortality rate but a 20% fetal mortality rate (26).

Mitral valve prolapse with resultant mitral insufficiency is due to congenital, developmental, or degenerative processes. It is common; the reported incidence is 3% to 6% (28, 29). The characteristic midsystolic click, late systolic murmur, and symptoms are actually lessened during gestation, probably because of the favorable effects of normal hemodynamic changes. Regardless of severity, isolated mitral valve prolapse is well tolerated in pregnancy and has no adverse maternal or fetal effects (29, 30). An increase in supraventricular arrhythmias has been reported by some centers. Antibiotic prophylaxis is indicated for patients with thickened leaflets or significant mitral regurgitation.

Prosthetic Heart Valves

In the patient with mechanical or tissue prosthetic heart valves, pregnancy is associated with significant maternal and fetal morbidity and mortality rates. Maternal risks are for thromboembolism and hemorrhage. Mechanical mitral valves confer a higher risk in both pregnant and nonpregnant patients. In a review of 155 pregnancies in 103 women with prosthetic heart valves, 16 thromboembolic events occurred in 108 mechanical prostheses and 7 premature failures occurred in 74 bioprosthetic valves (31). A study of mechanical valve prosthesis noted no maternal deaths among 140 patients treated with heparin or warfarin, but there were 4 deaths among 68 patients treated with aspirin and dipyridamole alone (32). A review of 60 pregnancies in 49 patients noted four maternal deaths (7%): two were from mechanical valve thrombosis, two were from bioprosthetic valve dysfunction (33). Fetal morbidity and mortality rates are even greater and are, in part, related to type of anticoagulation. Fetal loss and prematurity are increased, and warfarin confers risk for embryopathy, particularly with higher doses and use during the first trimester (32–34).

The choice of anticoagulant and valve type is problematic and fiercely debated (2, 6). There seems to be an increased risk for fatal and nonfatal thrombosis in patients with mechanical valves who are treated with therapeutic heparin, but an increased risk for embryopathy and fetal bleeding is seen in patients treated with warfarin. Low-molecular-weight heparin seems to be relatively safe in pregnancy, but its efficacy in patients with mechanical prosthetic valves has not been determined (6). Furthermore, although mechanical valves carry an increased risk for thromboembolism, bioprosthetic valves confer a higher rate of reoperation because of structural deterioration that may be accelerated in pregnancy (2, 26, 31). In a compliant patient, a mechanical prosthesis and therapeutic heparin in the first trimester and after 34 weeks of gestation combined with warfarin therapy between 12 and 34 weeks of gestation may give the best long-term prognosis for the mother. There is no consensus on valve type or method of anticoagulation, and risks and benefits should be discussed with the patient. Low-molecular-weight heparin at therapeutic doses may result in more consistent therapeutic anticoagulation because of improved bioavailability, but it has been used in only two cases (34a). Prophylaxis against endocarditis is required.

Coronary Artery Disease

Ischemic heart disease rarely complicates pregnancy, although it may become more common with delayed childbearing. Acute myocardial infarction is reported to occur in 1/10,000 deliveries and conveys a high maternal mortality rate (19% to 35%) (35, 36). Approximately half of reported cases are due to atherosclerotic disease in older patients with cardiovascular risk factors, but other cases have been ascribed to oral contraceptives, ergotamine derivatives, cocaine, amphetamines, collagen vascular disease, Kawasaki disease, spontaneous arterial dissection, spasm, thromboembolism, and a hypercoagulable state (35–37). When available, coronary angiograms are normal in 29% to 47% of patients. Most cases, especially cases of coronary artery dissection, occur in the last trimester or the puerperium period.

Medical therapy is the same as that in the nonpregnant patient and includes oxygen, aspirin, beta-blockers, heparin, and nitrates. Thrombolytic agents, particularly streptokinase and tissue plasminogen activator, have been used in pregnancy for massive pulmonary embolism and prosthetic valve thrombosis with no maternal mortality, but significant morbidity from hemorrhage was seen when these agents were used in the peripartum period (38). There are few reports of successful outcome with angioplasty or stent placement during gestation and the postpartum period (39–41). In a patient with a large anterior myocardial infarction, urgent angiography should be considered to define the cause of the infarction and the best treatment options.

There are 20 to 30 reports of successful pregnancies in women after myocardial infarction. Careful preconception evaluation of ventricular function and ischemic burden can help guide recommendations and management. In general, physical activity should be limited and use of cardiovascular medications should be continued (see Drugs for Cardiac Disorders table at the end of this chapter). When left ventricular function is preserved and the patient is vigilantly monitored for cardiovascular complications, maternal and fetal prognosis seem to be good (42, 43).

Cardiomyopathy

Dilated, congestive cardiomyopathy is rare in women of childbearing age. It may be due to ischemic heart disease, hypertension, thyroid disease, valvular disease, toxins (such as alcohol), or viral myocarditis, or it may be idiopathic. Congenital heart disease sequelae are addressed above, and PPCM is addressed in Section IV. Maternal and fetal risks are related to severity of dysfunction. One should expect worsening left ventricular dilation and dysfunction and symptoms due to the metabolic and volume stress of pregnancy and the puerperium period. Other risks include those for thromboembolism, ventricular arrhythmias, sudden death, and shortened life expectancy. Patients who are NYHA functional class III-IV (those who have dyspnea or fatigue at rest or with minimal exertion) should be counseled about the extreme risks of pregnancy (7). Treatment is similar to that in the nonpregnant patient with one important exception: Angiotensin-converting enzyme (ACE) inhibitors cause fetal oligohydramnios and anuria and should be replaced with hydralazine before conception or when pregnancy is diagnosed, if possible. Dietary salt intake should be restricted to less than 2 g/d, and physical exertion should be limited. If clinical deterioration or congestive heart failure ensues, use of digoxin, diuretics, hydralazine, and, in extreme cases, intravenous inotropes should be instituted (see Drugs for Cardiac Disorders table). Heparin anticoagulation should be instituted if prolonged bedrest is required and ejection fraction is significantly decreased (<35%). Management during labor and delivery should include invasive hemodynamic monitoring, which should be continued for 24 to 48 hours postpartum.

Hypertrophic cardiomyopathy is a primary myocardial disorder caused by various mutations of genes for contractile proteins. It can occur sporadically or in an autosomal-dominant pattern of inheritance. It is characterized by ventricular hypertrophy, noncompliance, and outflow tract obstruction with resultant dyspnea, angina, syncope, arrhythmias, and sudden cardiac death (44). Women with hypertrophic cardiomyopathy usually tolerate pregnancy well; the favorable effects of increased preload offset the negative effects of tachycardia and vasodilatation (7). The only fetal risk seems to be the risk for inheriting the disorder. More than 80 case reports describe the maternal gestational problems that may be encountered. These include new or worsening congestive heart failure in 20% of patients and a few reports of chest pain, syncope, ventricular tachycardia (VT), SVT, and sudden cardiac death (45). Treatment should include continuation of cardioselective beta-blockers and verapamil, cautious use of diuretics in symptomatic patients, and avoidance of drugs that increase heart rate, such as tocolytics, sympathomimetic agents, and digoxin (44). Labor and delivery should be managed with electrocardiographic and invasive hemodynamic monitoring, use of the left lateral decubitus position, avoidance of the Valsalva maneuver, and assisted vaginal delivery. Epidural anesthetics should be used only with extreme caution (45). Endocarditis prophylaxis is advised for patients with outflow obstruction or associated mitral regurgitation.

Cardiac Transplantation

Cardiac transplant recipients are now surviving longer and with an improved quality of life. In patients with good ventricular function, pregnancy seems to be well tolerated. Most of the data on outcomes, rejection, and medications come from the larger population of solid-organ transplant recipients, although a review of pregnancy in heart transplant recipients was recently published (46). Cardiac transplantation confers increased risk for hypertension and preeclampsia in the mother and for prematurity in the fetus. Cardiac function and the possibility of rejection should be assessed before conception (47).

Pregnancy does not seem to have an adverse effect with respect to cardiac function or episodes of rejection (46). Immunosuppression must be closely monitored, and medications must be adjusted to achieve the lowest possible therapeutic dose, although they do not seem to confer an increased incidence of congenital anomalies. Labor and delivery should be planned, and vaginal delivery should be attempted. Invasive hemodynamic monitoring is indicated for cesarean section or for patients with significant left ventricular dysfunction.

Marfan Syndrome

Marfan syndrome is a disorder of the connective tissue caused by mutations in the fibrillin gene on chromosome 15. It can occur sporadically but, in most cases, follows an autosomal-dominant pattern of inheritance with a high degree of penetrance (48). The cardiovascular manifestations of the disease include dilation of the aorta, aortic regurgitation, mitral valve prolapse, and regurgitation. Pregnancy in women with the Marfan syndrome carries risk for worsening aortic dilation; regurgitation, heart failure, and, more ominously, acute aortic dissection and death. According to case reports, the mortality rate approaches 50% when patients have an aortic root diameter greater than 4.5 cm or other significant cardiovascular abnormalities, such as aortic regurgitation, left ventricular dilation and dysfunction, hypertension, or coarctation. Pregnancy termination is recommended in these high-risk patients (49). On the other hand, women without cardiovascular complications or aortic dilation seem to tolerate pregnancy with minimal morbidity or mortality (50, 51). The fetus has a 50% chance of inheriting the syndrome. Gestational management includes limitation of physical activity and use of beta-blockers. In low-risk women, vaginal delivery with adequate pain control and a shortened second stage of labor is possible. In high-risk patients with aortic dilation or cardiovascular complications, cesarean section is preferred to avoid deleterious hemodynamic stresses (51).

REFERENCES

1. **Whittemore R, Hobbins JC, Engle MA.** Pregnancy and its outcome in women with and without surgical treatment of congenital heart disease. Am J Cardiol. 1982;50: 641-51.

2. **Warnes CA, Elkayam E.** Congenital heart disease and pregnancy. In: Elkayam U, Gleicher N, eds. Cardiac Problems in Pregnancy. New York: Wiley-Liss; 1998:39-54.

3. **Shime J, Mocarski EJM, Hastings D, Webb GD, McLaughlin PR.** Congenital heart disease in pregnancy: short- and long-term implications. Am J Obstet Gynecol. 1987;156:313.

4. **Dennis NR, Warren J.** Risks to the offspring of patients with some common congenital heart defects. J Med Genet. 1981;18:8-16.

5. **Driscoll DJ, Michels VV, Gersony WM, et al.** Occurrence risk for congenital heart defects in relatives of patients with aortic stenosis, pulmonary stenosis, or ventricular septal defect. Circulation. 1993;87:I114-20.

6. **Perloff JK, Koos B.** Pregnancy and congenital heart disease: the mother and the fetus. In: Perloff JK, Child JS, eds. Congenital Heart Disease in Adults. Philadelphia: WB Saunders; 1998:144-64.

7. **Mendelson MA, Lang RM.** Pregnancy and heart disease. In: Barron WM, Lindheimer MD, eds. Medical Disorders during Pregnancy. St. Louis, MO: Mosby; 1995:129-67.

8. **Perloff JK.** Congenital heart disease in adults. In: Braunwald E, ed. Heart Disease: A Textbook of Medicine, 5th ed. Philadelphia: WB Saunders; 1997:963-87.

9. **Whittemore R.** Congenital heart disease: its impact on pregnancy. Hosp Pract (Off Ed). 1983;18:65-74.

10. **Pitkin RM, Perloff JK, Koos BJ.** Pregnancy and congenital heart disease. Ann Intern Med. 1990;112:445-54.

11. **Perloff JK.** Ventricular septal defects. In: Perloff JK, ed. The Clinical Recognition of Congenital Heart Disease. Philadelphia: WB Saunders; 1994:

12. **Arias F, Pineda J.** Aortic stenosis and pregnancy. J Reprod Med. 1978;4:229-32.

13. **Lao TT, Sermer M, MaGee L, Farine D, Colman JM.** Congenital aortic stenosis. Am J Obstet Gynecol. 1993;169:540-5.

14. **Connolly HM, Warnes CA.** Ebstein's anomaly: outcome of pregnancy. J Am Coll Cardiol. 1994;23:1194-8.

15. **Donnelly JE, Brown JM, Radford DJ.** Pregnancy outcome and Ebstein's anomaly. Br Heart J. 1991;66:368.

16. **Presbitero P, Somerville J, Stone S, Aruta E, Spiegelhalter D, Rabajoli F.** Pregnancy in cyanotic congenital heart disease: outcome of mother and fetus. Circulation. 1994;89:2673-6.

17. **Patton DE, Lee W, Cotton DB, et al.** Cyanotic maternal heart disease in pregnancy. Obstet Gynecol Surv. 1990;45:594-600.

18. **Canobbio MM, Mair DD, van der Velde M, Koos BJ.** Pregnancy outcomes after the Fontan repair. J Am Coll Cardiol. 1996;28:763-7.

19. **Clarkson PM, Wilson NJ, Neutze JM, North RA, Calder AL, Barratt-Boyes BG.** Outcome of pregnancy after the Mustard operation for transposition of the great arteries with intact ventricular septum. J Am Coll Cardiol. 1994;24:190-3.

20. **Lynch-Salamon DI, Maze SS, Combs CA.** Pregnancy after Mustard repair for transposition of the great arteries. Obstet Gynecol. 1993;82:676-9.

21. **Lao TT, Sermer M, Colman JM.** Pregnancy following surgical correction for transposition of the great arteries. Obstet Gynecol. 1994;83:665-8.

22. **Gleicher N, Midwall J, Hochberger D, Jaffin H.** Eisenmenger's syndrome and pregnancy. Obstet Gynecol Surv. 1979;34:721-41.

23. **Avila WS, Grinberg M, Snitcowsky R, et al.** Maternal and fetal outcome in pregnant women with Eisenmenger's syndrome. Eur Heart J. 1995;16:460-4.

24. **Esteves CA, Ramos AL, Braga SL.** Effectiveness of percutaneous balloon mitral valvotomy during pregnancy. Am J Cardiol. 1991;68:930-4.

25. **Vosloo S, Reichard B.** The feasibility of closed mitral valvotomy in pregnancy. J Thorac Cardiovasc Surg. 1987;93:675-9.

26. **Sullivan HJ.** Valvular heart surgery during pregnancy. Surg Clin North Am. 1995;75:59-75.

27.   **Colan SD, Borow KM, Neumann A.** Use of the calibrated carotid pulse tracing for calculation of left ventricular pressure and wall stress throughout ejection. Am Heart J. 1985;109:1306-10.

28.   **Devereux RB, Kramer R, Kligfield P.** Mitral valve prolapse: causes, clinical manifestations and management. Ann Intern Med. 1989;111:305-17.

29.   **Cowles T, Gunik B.** Mitral valve prolapse in pregnancy. Semin Perinatol. 1990;14:34-41.

30.   **Chia YT, Yeoh SC, Viegas OA, Lim M, Ratnam SS.** Maternal congenital heart disease and pregnancy outcome. J Obstetric Gynaecol Res. 1996;22:185-91.

31.   **Hanania G, Thomas D, Michel PL, et al.** Pregnancy and prosthetic heart valves: a French cooperative retrospective study of 155 cases. Eur Heart J. 1994;15:1651-8.

32.   **Salazar E, Zajarias A, Guiterrez N.** The problem of cardiac valve prosthesis, anticoagulants and pregnancy. Circulation. 1984;70:I169-77.

33.   **Born D, Martinez EE, Almeida PA.** Pregnancy in patients with prosthetic heart valves: the effects of anticoagulation on mother, fetus and neonate. Am Heart J. 1992;124:413-7.

34.   **Ginsberg JS, Hirsh J.** Use of anticoagulants during pregnancy. Chest. 1989;95:156S-60S.

34a. **Lee LH.** Low molecular weight heparain for thromboprophylaxis during pregnancy for patients with mechanical mitral valve replacement [Letter]. Thromb Haemost. 1996;76:628-30.

35.   **Badin E, Enciso R.** Acute myocardial infarction during pregnancy and puerperium: a review. Angiology. 1996;47:739-56.

36.   **Hankins GD, Wendel GDJ, Leveno KF.** Myocardial infarction during pregnancy. A review. Obstet Gynecol. 1985;65:139-46.

37.   **Donnelly S, McKenna P, McGing P, Sugrue D.** Myocardial infarction during pregnancy. Br J Obstet Gynecol. 1993;100:781-2.

38.   **Turrentine MA, Braems G, Ramirez MM.** Use of thrombolytics for the treatment of thromboembolic disease during pregnancy. Obstet Gynecol Surv. 1995;50:534-41.

39.   **Cowan NC, deBelder MA, Rothman MT.** Coronary angioplasty in pregnancy. Br Heart J. 1988;59:588-92.

40.   **Giudici MC, Artis AK, Webel RR, Alpert MA.** Postpartum myocardial infarction treated with balloon coronary angioplasty. Am Heart J. 1989;118:614-6.

41.   **Saxena R, Nolan TE, von Dohlen T, Houghton JL.** Postpartum myocardial infarction treated by balloon coronary angioplasty. Obstet Gynecol. 1992;79:810-2.

42.   **Frenkel Y, Barkai G, Reisin L, Rath S, Mashiach S, Battler A.** Pregnancy after myocardial infarction: are we playing it safe? Obstet Gynecol. 1991;77:822-5.

43.   **Vinatier D, Virelizier S, Depret-Mosser S, et al.** Pregnancy after myocardial infarction. Eur J Obstet Gynecol Reprod Biol. 1994;56:89-93.

44.   **Wigle ED, Rakowski H, Kimball BP, William WG.** Hypertrophic cardiomyopathy: clinical spectrum and treatment. Circulation. 1995;92:1680-92.

45.   **Elkayam E, Dave R.** Hypertrophic cardiomyopathy. In: Elkayam U, Gleicher N, eds. Cardiac Problems in Pregnancy. New York: Wiley-Liss; 1998:101-25.

46.   **Wagoner L, Taylor D, Olson S, et al.** Immunosuppressive therapy, management and outcomes of heart transplant recipients during pregnancy. J Heart Lung Transplant. 1993;12:993-1001.

47. **Dildy GA, Clark SL.** Cardiac arrest during pregnancy. Obstet Gynecol Clin North Am. 1995;22:303-14.

48. **Dietz HC, Cutting GR, Pyerutzm RE, et al.** Marfan syndrome caused by a recurrent de dovo missense mutation in the fibrillin gene. Nature. 1991;352:337-9.

49. **Pyertiz RE.** Maternal and fetal complications of pregnancy in the Marfan syndrome. Am J Med. 1981;71:784-90.

50. **Rossiter JP, Repke JT, Morales AJ, Murphy EA, Pyertiz RA.** A prospective longitudinal evaluation of pregnancy in the Marfan syndrome. Am J Obstet Gynecol. 1995;173:1599-606.

51. **Elkayam U, Ostzega A, Shotan A, Mehra A.** Cardiovascular problems in pregnant women with the Marfan syndrome. Ann Intern Med. 1995;123:117-22.

III. Arrhythmias
Athena Poppas and Michael P. Carson

Pregnant women with structural heart disease may experience new or worsening arrhythmias due to the normal hemodynamic alterations of pregnancy. On the other hand, no evidence supports the occurrence of a similar phenomenon in pregnant women with normal hearts. Conventional wisdom held pregnancy to be arrhythmogenic, but this belief was based on older case reports and series in women with organic heart disease (1). Arrhythmia may be the first manifestation of cardiovascular disease; thus, it must be excluded by physical examination or echocardiography. In addition, secondary causes of the symptoms or the arrhythmia must be sought and treated (Figure 6-3). In women with structurally normal cardiovascular systems, arrhythmias are rare. If they do occur, they are often benign and well tolerated.

It should be stressed that fetal well being depends on maternal well being, and pregnancy should not significantly alter the approach to an arrhythmia. Advanced Cardiac Life Support protocols for hemodynamically unstable rhythms should be followed. In fact, pregnancy should lower the threshold for intervention for an unstable rhythm that could result in diversion of blood flow away from the fetus. Cardioversion has been done safely in pregnant women, but one should remove all fetal monitoring devices to prevent arcing and should use appropriate maternal analgesia (2).

Palpitations

During pregnancy, women seem to be more aware of their heart beat, and this may be because heart is shifted closer to the anterior chest wall (3). A history

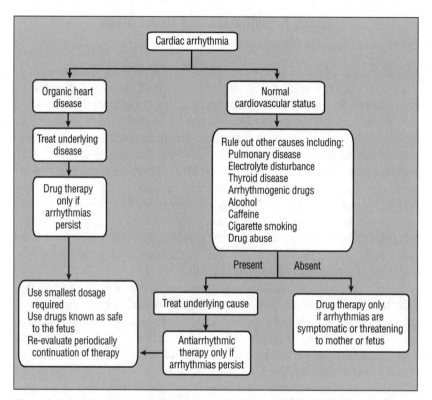

Figure 6-3 Cardiac arrhythmia. (From Rotmensh HH, Rotmensch S, Elkayam U. Management of cardiac arrhythmias during pregnancy: current concepts. Drugs. 1987;33:623–33; with permission.)

of a rapid heart rate with exertion that improves with rest is most consistent with sinus tachycardia. A careful history may distinguish benign atrial or ventricular ectopic beats, which need no further evaluation, from more serious tachyarrhythmias (4). A description of a spontaneously fast or slow heart rate needs further evaluation with a 24-hour Holter monitor or a 30-day transtelephonic event monitor. If cardiac examination suggests regurgitant or stenotic valvular disease, hypertrophic cardiomyopathy, or left ventricular dysfunction, echocardiography should be done to characterize the structural abnormality. Psychiatric disorders have been reported in 20% to 43% of nonpregnant patients with palpitations. However, in a series of 107 patients with documented supraventricular tachycardia (SVT), 67% also met the criteria for panic, stress, or an anxiety disorder (4, 5). Therefore, psychiatric diagnoses should be considered only after organic cardiac disease has been reasonably excluded.

Sinus Arrhythmias and Heart Block

Sinus bradycardia is unusual during pregnancy because of the physiologic changes noted above. Common benign causes of sinus bradycardia include vagal stimulation during the second stage of labor, pain, and cardioactive medications. In the absence of these factors, structural heart disease should be excluded. Symptomatic bradycardia can be treated with brief use of atropine or with a temporary or permanent pacemaker, and safe implantation and use during pregnancy have been reported (6). Pacemakers are most often required in women with congenital heart block. There are more than 100 reports of women with congenital or acquired complete heart block who have had successful pregnancy (6, 7). Pregnant women with complete heart block with or without pacemakers may occasionally become symptomatic, particularly during labor and delivery. Treatment is directed at increasing the pacing heart rate, usually by 10% to 20%. Any pacemaker malfunction should be treated as it would in a nonpregnant patient.

Sinus tachycardia per se does not require therapy. In a study of 93 asymptomatic pregnant women, 58% of those with a body mass index greater than 30 mg/m^2 and no underlying cardiopulmonary disease had mild sinus tachycardia at rest (100 to 120 beats/min) during routine antenatal visits (8). However, sinus tachycardia can be a marker for underlying cardiac or systemic disease, and these conditions must be excluded in women with persistent tachycardia and normal body mass index (see Figure 6-3).

Supraventricular Arrhythmias

Supraventricular Tachycardia

Supraventricular tachycardia is generally well tolerated in pregnant and nonpregnant patients. In the absence of cardiac disease, new onset of SVT during pregnancy is rare. In one study of 207 consecutive women who had electrophysiologic testing for the evaluation of SVT, only 3.9% had their first onset of symptoms during pregnancy. However, 22% of those patients had an increase in the frequency of symptoms during gestation; this finding has been confirmed by others (9, 10). In addition, SVT has been reported in association with the use of sympathomimetic tocolytics to inhibit preterm labor and is increased during pregnancy in patients with mitral valve prolapse and preexcitation syndromes.

Treatment of SVT is the same in pregnant and nonpregnant women and includes vagal maneuvers, such as carotid sinus pressure, cough, or the Valsalva maneuver. Intravenous adenosine has been used to diagnose and terminate

SVT during pregnancy, including SVT associated with the Wolfe-Parkinson-White syndrome. Patients often have brief flushing, lightheadedness, sweating, and nausea, but no adverse maternal or fetal outcomes have been reported (11). Other medications that have been used safely for SVT in pregnancy include metoprolol, verapamil, diltiazem, and digoxin (see Drugs for Cardiac Disorders table at the end of this chapter). A digoxin-like immunoreactive substance is produced during pregnancy and may falsely elevate the serum digoxin level on radioimmunoassay (12). In the absence of hemodynamic instability or structural heart disease, long-term medical treatment is rarely needed. However, recurrent SVTs at rates that exceed 180 beats/min jeopardize uretoplacental blood flow and should be treated.

Atrial Fibrillation and Flutter

Atrial fibrillation and flutter usually occur in the presence of structural heart disease, which must be excluded by physical examination and echocardiography. Hyperthyroidism must also be excluded. In particular, 25% of patients with rheumatic mitral stenosis first present with atrial fibrillation during pregnancy (3). In these patients, atrial fibrillation can lead to acute pulmonary edema, necessitating urgent heart rate control and possibly cardioversion. The ventricular response should be controlled with beta-adrenergic blockers, digoxin, or calcium-channel blockers. Procainamide and quinidine have been used safely in pregnancy to convert to sinus rhythm and, if necessary, to prevent recurrence (see Drugs for Cardiac Disorders table). Pregnancy is a relatively hypercoagulable state, and anticoagulation is therefore necessary for persistent atrial fibrillation with cardiac disease. There is considerable debate about the relative risks and benefits of warfarin and heparin therapy (see sections on thromboembolism and prosthetic valves), but heparin is preferred in patients without prosthetic heart valves.

Ventricular Arrhythmias

Ninety percent of ventricular tachycardias (VTs) are associated with organic heart disease, such as cardiomyopathy or valvular disease, although they have been reported in pregnant patients with acute, severe hypertension and with use of prescription or illicit drugs. The normal increase in catecholamine levels in pregnancy may contribute to VTs, and the arrhythmia may be responsive to beta-adrenergic blockers (13). Synchronized cardioversion should not be withheld if hemodynamic instability dictates its use. However, electrophysiologic studies may be delayed if medical therapy successfully controls the arrhythmia. If necessary, these studies can be done under echocardiographic guidance to avoid the radiation exposure encountered with prolonged fluoroscopy (14). Lidocaine, procainamide, quinidine, or beta-adrenergic blockers are the drugs of choice (see Drugs for Cardiac Disorders table). In women with hereditary long-QT syndrome, the incidence of cardiac events is significantly increased in the postpartum period, and beta-adrenergic blockers may decrease that risk (15). Ventricular fibrillation is a rapidly fatal arrhythmia that requires immediate cardioversion and cardiopulmonary resuscitation (CPR). During CPR, a wedge or pillow should be placed under the patient's right hip so that the uterus will not further compromise preload through compression of the inferior vena cava (2).

Internal cardioverter-defibrillators (ICDs) are used for symptomatic VT or ventricular fibrillation. A series of 44 women who had ICDs implanted before pregnancy showed no increase in the incidence of obstetric complications (cesarean section, growth restriction, or spontaneous loss), device-related complications (generator migration or lead fracture), or ICD discharges (16). (Of note, the ICD must be turned off during surgery if electrocautery is to be used.) The authors of the report on this study concluded that it is unreasonable to prohibit pregnancy simply because of the presence of an ICD.

Cardiovascular Medications

The Drugs for Cardiac Disorders table can be used as a reference when a clinical setting dictates treatment with one of the medications listed. Decisions about medication use in pregnancy should be made on the basis of the benefit-to-risk ratio and with consideration of the fact that fetal well being depends on maternal well being. Of note, because of the increased volume of distribution and the increased hepatic and renal clearance of drugs during pregnancy, patients beyond the first trimester may require a higher dosing frequency or a higher dose than nonpregnant patients do. In addition, only 1% to 2% of the maternal dose of most medications is secreted in breastmilk, so the amount ingested by the fetus tends to be diminutive. The American Academy of Pediatrics considers most medications to be compatible with breastfeeding, and we encourage physicians to confirm a possible risk before precluding this activity.

REFERENCES

1. **Szekely P, Snaith L.** Paroxysmal tachycardia in pregnancy. Br Heart J. 1953;15:195-8.
2. **Dildy GA, Clark SL.** Cardiac arrest during pregnancy. Obstet Gynecol Clin North Am. 1995;22:303-14.
3. **Mendelson MA, Lang RM.** Pregnancy and heart disease. In: Barron WM, Lindheimer MD, eds. Medical Disorders during Pregnancy. St. Louis, MO: Mosby; 1995:129-67.

4. **Zimetbaum P, Josephson ME.** Evaluation of patients with palpitations. N Engl J Med. 1998;338:1369-73.

5. **Lessmeier TJ, Gamperling D, Johnson-Liddon V.** Unrecognized paroxysmal supraventricular tachycardia: potential for misdiagnosis as panic disorder. Arch Intern Med. 1997;157:537-43.

6. **Jaffe R, Gruber A, Fejgin M, Altaras M, Ben-Aderet N.** Pregnancy with an artificial pacemaker. Obstet Gynecol Surv. 1987;42:137-9.

7. **Perloff JK, Koos B.** Pregnancy and congenital heart disease: the mother and the fetus. In: Perloff JK, Child JS, eds. Congenital Heart Disease in Adults. Philadelphia: WB Saunders; 1998:144-64.

8. **Carson MP, Powrie RO, Rosene-Montella K.** Sinus tachycardia in pregnancy: a normal finding [Abstract]. Am J Obstet Gynecol. 1998;178:S61.

9. **Lee S, Chen S, Wu T, Chiang C, Cheng C, Tai C.** Effects of pregnancy on first onset and symptoms of paroxysmal supraventricular tachycardia. Am J Cardiol. 1995;76:675-8.

10. **Tawam M, Levine J, Mendelson M, Goldberger J, Dyer A, Kadish A.** Effect of pregnancy on paroxysmal supraventricular tachycardia. Am J Cardiol. 1993;72:838-40.

11. **Hagley MT, Cole PL.** Adenosine use in pregnant women with supraventricular tachycardia. Ann Pharmacother. 1994;28:1241-2.

12. **Phelps SJ, Cochran EC, Gonzalez-Ruiz A, Tolley EA, Hammond KD, Sibai BM.** The influence of gestational age and preeclampsia on the presence and magnitude of serum endogenous digoxin-like immunoreactive substance(s). Am J Obstet Gynecol. 1988;158:34-9.

13. **Brodsky M, Doria R, Allen B, Sato D, Thomas G, Sada M.** New-onset ventricular tachycardia during pregnancy. Am Heart J. 1992;123:933-41.

14. **Lee MS, Evans SJ, Blumberg S, Bodenheimer MM, Roth SL.** Echocardiographically guided electrophysiologic testing in pregnancy. JASE. 1994;7:182-6.

15. **Rashba EJ, Andrews M, Schwartz PJ, Locati EH, Robinson J, Hall WJ.** Influence of pregnancy on the risk of cardiac events in patients with hereditary long QT syndrome. Circulation. 1998;97:451-6.

16. **Natale A, Davidson T, Geiger MJ, Newby K.** Implantable cardioverter-defibrillators and pregnancy: a safe combination? Circulation. 1997;96:2808-12.

IV. Peripartum Cardiomyopathy
Karen Rosene-Montella and Athena Poppas

Epidemiology

Peripartum cardiomyopathy is a dilated cardiomyopathy of uncertain cause that is most often seen in the third trimester and in the first 6 months after delivery. It is rare, and its incidence varies greatly by region. It occurs in 1/15,000 pregnancies in the United States, 1/6000 pregnancies in Japan, and

1/1000 pregnancies in South Africa (1–3). The unusually high incidence reported in Nigeria is thought to be due to the Hausa tradition of ingesting kanwa (dried lake salt) while lying on heated mud beds twice daily for 40 days postpartum and thus is probably related to pure volume overload. Because earlier reports of postpartum cardiomyopathy (PPCM) included a heterogeneous group of patients with clinical and radiographic signs of heart failure, the true incidence of PPCM may be hard to determine.

Risk factors thought to be associated with PPCM include advanced maternal age, multiple gestation, and African descent. Long-term tocolytic therapy, hypertension, and preeclampsia were also previously thought to be risk factors. Although pulmonary edema is a reported complication of tocolytic therapy, it is not thought to be due to a true cardiomyopathy (see Chapter 7). Similarly, although acute systolic left ventricular dysfunction can occur in the setting of severe hypertension or preeclampsia, it seems to resolve more quickly than PPCM and is probably not related to this condition.

Cause

The cause of PPCM is unknown but may be multifactorial. The clustering of a rare illness that 1) appears peripartum in patients with no evidence of underlying heart disease and 2) recurs in subsequent pregnancies implies that PPCM is a distinct entity. It is tempting to invoke the hemodynamic stress of pregnancy as a contributing factor, but PPCM may present long after blood volume and heart rate have returned to prepregnancy levels, as much as 6 months after delivery.

Numerous studies have looked at possible immunologic and infectious causes of PPCM, but none have found an individual inciting agent. Endomyocardial biopsy may show a high incidence of myocarditis, with resolution of myocarditis on repeated biopsy correlating with clinical improvement in ventricular function (4–7). One recent study, however, did not corroborate these findings (8). Thus, biopsy is usually not recommended when PPCM is suspected.

Diagnosis

The diagnostic criteria for PPCM, established in 1971 by Demakis and coworkers (9), include 1) development of cardiac failure in the last month of pregnancy or within 5 months after delivery, 2) the absence of a determinable cause of cardiac failure, and 3) the absence of demonstrable heart disease before the last month of pregnancy. More recent epidemiologic data have shown onset both earlier in gestation and after 5 months postpartum. Therefore, PPCM should be considered in the differential diagnosis of left ventricular systolic dysfunction at any time in association with pregnancy. To exclude other causes of heart failure, we recommend that echocardiography confirming global left ventricular systolic dysfunction be added to the diagnostic criteria for PPCM (Box 6-3).

The signs and symptoms of PPCM are indistinguishable from those of other forms of congestive heart failure (Table 6-2). A cardiac arrhythmia may be the initial manifestation in PPCM, as it is in other forms of cardiomyopathy. Chest radiography and electrocardiography should be done to seek other causes of dyspnea, and the diagnosis should be confirmed by echocardiography. Because most patients with PPCM are young and have no comorbid cardiopulmonary conditions, they may be clinically well, even in the presence of

---

Box 6-3 Diagnostic Criteria for Peripartum Cardiomyopathy

Development of cardiac failure during pregnancy or within 6 months of delivery

Absence of a determinable cause for cardiac failure (i.e., valvular heart disease, ischemia, pericardial disease)

Impairment in left ventricular systolic function on echocardiography

Absence of heart disease before pregnancy

Adapted from Elkayam U, Gleicher N, eds. Cardiac Problems in Pregnancy. New York: Wiley-Liss; 1998.

Table 6-2 Signs and Symptoms of Peripartum Cardiomyopathy

Symptoms	Signs
Dyspnea	Normal or increased blood pressure
Cough	Increased jugular venous pressure
Orthopnea	Cardiomegaly
Paroxysmal nocturnal dyspnea	Third heart sound
Fatigue	Loud pulmonic valve component of second heart sound
Palpitations	Mitral or tricuspid regurgitation
Hemoptysis	Pulmonary rales
Chest pain	Peripheral edema
Abdominal pain	Ascites
	Arrhythmias
	Embolic phenomena
	Hepatomegaly

Adapted from Elkayam U, Gleicher N, eds. Cardiac Problems in Pregnancy. New York: Wiley-Liss; 1998.

significant left ventricular dysfunction; thus, a high index of suspicion is required for prompt diagnosis. The coexistence of intracardiac and venous thromboembolism is common, occurring in up to 50% of patients with PPCM, and should be thoroughly investigated as described in Chapter 8. Thyroid disease should be ruled out because hypothyroidism can result in diffuse ventricular dysfunction.

Treatment

Treatment of PPCM should be the same as for that of other forms of congestive heart failure and cardiomyopathy. Medical therapy should include restriction of sodium intake, use of digoxin (for its inotropic effect and for rate control in the presence of atrial fibrillation), diuresis, and afterload reduction. Hydralazine should be used in place of ACE inhibitors for afterload reduction while the patient is still pregnant; ACE inhibitor therapy can be substituted for vasodilator therapy postpartum. Antepartum thromboprophylaxis with heparin should be instituted as soon as the diagnosis is made; warfarin may be substituted after delivery. Therapeutic anticoagulation should be instituted if the ejection fraction is less than 35% or if evidence of mural thrombosis is seen.

Immunosuppressive agents have been tried when myocarditis is suspected, but these agents cannot be routinely recommended because small controlled trials have failed to confirm that they have any benefit. Patients with severe, progressive heart failure may require an intra-aortic balloon pump for stabilization. All patients with progressive deterioration or persistence of significant left ventricular dysfunction over months should have early evaluation for cardiac transplantation.

Prognosis

The prognosis for patients with PPCM may be better than previously thought; 30% of patients recover to baseline ventricular function within 6 months of delivery. However, it is now known that even patients who have recovered resting left ventricular size and performance have decreased contractile reserve on dobutamine stress echocardiography (10). This means that although standard echocardiograms return to normal, a patient may have a suboptimal response to hemodynamic stress, including stress from subsequent pregnancies.

Approximately 50% of patients have marked improvement in clinical symptoms and left ventricular function within 6 months of presentation. The

Table 6-3 Maternal and Fetal Oucome in 67 Subsequent Pregnancies in 63 Patients with a History of Peripartum Cardiomyopathy

Group*	Maternal Outcome, %			Fetal Outcome, %		
	Normal	LV Dysfunction	Death	Live Birth	Abortion	Stillbirth
A	74	23	2	93	5	2
B	37	54	8	83	17	0

*Group A: 43 pregnancies in 40 patients with history of PPCM who had recovery of left ventricular function. Group B: 24 pregnancies in 23 patients with history of PPCM and persistent left ventricular dysfunction.

Adapted from Elkayam U, Gleicher N, eds. Cardiac Problems in Pregnancy. New York: Wiley-Liss; 1998.

other 50% continue to have varying degrees of persistent dysfunction ranging from mild compensated congestive heart failure to rapid hemodynamic deterioration and death. Recovery of cardiac function is least likely in patients whose initial left ventricular dysfunction was severe, patients with a significant increase in left ventricular dimension, or patients with marked increases in pulmonary artery and wedge pressures. Age and multiparity may also be adverse prognostic factors. However, the only consistently predictive indicator seems to be the severity of disease at the time of initial presentation.

Recommendations for Subsequent Pregnancies

Recommendations for subsequent pregnancies in patients with a history of PPCM are controversial. Most authors agree that 1) patients with the highest risk for illness and death in future pregnancy are those who have had persistent left ventricular dysfunction and 2) pregnancy is relatively contraindicated in this group.

It was initially thought that even patients with previous PPCM who had recovered completely were at significant risk for recurrence in subsequent pregnancies. Recent data do not support this assumption (11). The results of a recent survey by Ostrzega and Elkayam (12) are summarized in Table 6-3. Seventy-eight percent of fully recovered patients and only 37% of patients with persistent left ventricular dysfunction had a normal maternal outcome. On the basis of this information and the study of contractile reserve mentioned previously, we recommend that four things be done before a pregnancy is started in a patient with previous PPCM:

1. The patient should undergo echocardiography and, if the results of echocardiography are normal, dobutamine stress echocardiography.
2. Patients with persistent left ventricular dysfunction on echocardiography should be advised against pregnancy.
3. Patients with normal results on echocardiography but decreased reserve on stress testing should be warned that they may not tolerate the hemodynamic stresses associated with pregnancy.
4. Patients with full recovery should be told that, although they have a small chance for recurrence, the mortality rate is low and they have a good chance of an uneventful pregnancy.

REFERENCES

1. **Cunningham FG, Pritchard JA, Hankins GD, Anderson PL, Lucas MJ, Armstrong KF.** Peripartum heart failure: idiopathic cardiomyopathy or compounding cardiovascular events? Obstet Gynecol. 1986;67:157-68.

2. **Desai D, Moodley J, Naidoo D.** Peripartum cardiomyopathy: experience at King Edward VIII Hospital, Durban, South Africa and review of the literature. Trop Doct. 1995;25:118-23.

3. **Sanderson JE, Adesanya CO, Anjorin FL, Parry EO.** Postpartum cardiac failure: heart failure due to volume overload. Am Heart J. 1979;97:613-21.

4. **Melvin KR, Richardson PJ, Olsen EG, Daly K, Jackson G.** Peripartum cardiomyopathy due to myocarditis. N Engl J Med. 1982;307:731-4.

5. **Sanderson JE, Olsen EG, Gatei D.** Peripartum heart disease: an endomyocardial biopsy study. Br Heart J. 1986;56:289-91.

6. **Midei MG, DeMent SH, Feldman AM, Hutchins GM, Baughman KL.** Peripartum myocarditis and cardiomyopathy. Circulation. 1990;81:922-8.

7. **Rizeq MN, Rickenbacher PR, Fowler MB, Billingham ME.** Incidence of myocarditis in peripartum cardiomyopathy. Am J Cardiol. 1994;74:474-7.

8. **Poppas A, Shroff S, Korcaz C, et al.** Serial assessment of the cardiovascular system in normal pregnancy: role of arterial compliance and pulsatile arterial load. Circulation. 1997;95:2407-15.

9. **Demakis JG, Rhimtoola SH, Sutton GC, Meadows R, Szanto PB, Tobin JR, Gunnar RM.** Natural course of peripartum cardiomyopathy. Circulation. 1971;44:1053-61.

10. **Lampert MB, Weinert L, Hibbard J, Korcarz C, Lindheimer M, Lang RM.** Contractile reserve in patients with peripartum cardiomyopathy and recovered left ventricular function. Am J Obstet Gynecol. 1997;176:189-95.

11. **Sutton MS, Cole P, Piappert M, Saltzman D, Goldhaber S.** Effects of subsequent pregnancy on left ventricular cardiomyopathy. Am Heart J. 1991:121:1776-8.

12. **Ostrzega E, Elkayam U.** Risk of subsequent pregnancy in women with a history of peripartum cardiomyopathy: results of a survey [Abstract]. Circulation. 1995;92(suppl I):I-333.

V. Syncope
Karen Rosene-Montella and Raymond O. Powrie

Syncope or near-syncope during pregnancy is a common reason for referral by obstetricians for consultation. In a retrospective review, dizziness accounted for 10% of consultation requests in an obstetric medicine service. Although true syncope is relatively rare, near-syncope and postural dizziness are both common. Numerous normal physiologic changes in pregnancy converge to make syncope a multifactorial event.

Marked venodilatation and venous pooling are seen, beginning early in pregnancy and persisting until term. When combined with other factors, this can cause a significant decrease in preload. This decrease is exacerbated by standing for long periods, hyperemesis with dehydration, and anemia. Systemic vascular resistance decreases by as much as 30% simultaneous with resistance to the vasoconstrictive effect of angiotensin II, making compensatory mechanisms to postural hypotension limited in normal pregnancy.

The most common cause of syncope in otherwise healthy young adults is neurocardiogenic syncope (also known as *vasovagal* or *vasodepressor syncope*). Classic neurocardiogenic syncope is precipitated by emotional stress, fatigue, prolonged standing, fear, or pain. However, many episodes occur with no obvious precipitant. Classic neurocardiogenic syncope is usually associated with lightheadedness, nausea, pallor, and diaphoresis. It typically occurs in the setting of decreased venous return (such as that in pregnancy),

Table 6-4 Evaluation of Pregnant Patient with Syncope: History

Finding	Most Likely Diagnosis	Further Evaluation/Comments
Precipitating features: Emotional stress Prolonged standing Fear Pain	Neurocardiogenic syncope	
Family history of: Recurrent syncope Cardiac disease Sudden death	Consider inherited hypertrophic cardiomyopathy	Requires echocardiogram for diagnosis Congenital prolonged QT syndrome apparent on electrocardiogram
History or symptoms of concomitant heart disease Risk factors for ischemic heart disease present Arrhythmia Palpitations: rapid, regular, prolonged	Consider cardiovascular cause of syncope, such as arrhythmia	Holter monitor Cardiac event monitor Electrocardiography
History of: Seizure disorder Postictal phase after syncope	Seizure Consider eclampsia if seizure occurs during last half of pregnancy or first week postpartum	EEG and/or CT/MRI of head
History of migraines	Vertebral basilar migraines	This diagnosis is rare and should be made only in conjunction with a neurologist
Any history of syncope	–	All patients presenting with syncope should undergo screening for psychiatric disorders (especially depression and anxiety disorders), domestic violence, and substance abuse (including alcohol) and provide a complete medication history

which leads to a sudden compensatory increase in sympathetic stimulation to the heart. In predisposed persons, this sympathetic stimulation can lead to a centrally mediated increase in parasympathetic tone that causes inappropriate peripheral vasodilatation and relative bradycardia manifesting as sudden syncope.

Another common type of syncope in pregnancy is postural or orthostatic syncope. This type of syncope occurs when a person moves from the supine to an upright posture. The mechanism of this postural syncope is similar to that of neurocardiogenic syncope but always involves a change in posture. A pregnancy-related decrease in sensitivity to the vasoconstrictive effects of angiotensin II further impedes any compensatory response to postural hypotension.

The supine hypotensive syndrome is a common cause of syncope in pregnancy. It occurs in 0.5% to 11.2% of women in the third trimester. As the name of the syndrome suggests, these women develop lightheadedness, nausea, pallor, and hypotension when lying flat on their backs. The syndrome is caused by mechanical compression of the inferior vena cava and aorta by the gravid uterus. Care should be taken to keep pregnant women out of the supine position so that true syncope does not occur (1).

Although most cases of syncope in pregnancy are probably cases of neurocardiogenic or postural syncope, the complete differential diagnosis of sudden loss of consciousness is extensive and important. Because of the possibility of life-threatening causes, all pregnant patients with syncope require a careful history (Table 6-4), physical examination (Table 6-5), and laboratory testing (Table 6-6) to screen for features that would suggest the need for additional

Table 6-5 Evaluation of Pregnant Patient with Syncope: Physical Examination

Finding	Most Likely Diagnosis	Further Evaluation/Comments
Focal neurologic signs	Cerebrovascular disease Seizure disorder	Focal findings suggest need for consideration of head CT/MRI, lumbar puncture, and/or EEG
Carotid massage if strong carotid pulse with no bruit	Check for carotid sinus hypersensitivity	Carotid sinus massage; carotid sinus hypersensitivity is a very rare cause of syncope, especially in young persons
Careful cardiac examination	Need to rule out: Aortic stenosis Hypertrophic cardiomyopathy Congenital heart disease Suspicious murmur	Presence of suspicious murmur suggests need for echocardiography
Orthostatic hypotension	Benign postural syncope	Tilt testing contraindicated in pregnancy

Table 6-6 Evaluation of Pregnant Patient with Syncope: Laboratory Investigations

Laboratory Variable	Recommendation
Hemoglobin testing	Look for possible contribution of anemia
Stool testing	Look for occult blood
Electrocardiography	Look for evidence of myocardial ischemia, short QT syndrome, short PR interval, evidence of congenital heart disease, or evidence of cardiomyopathy
PIH labs: CBC, platelet count, AST, ALT, BUN, creatine, uric acid, urinalysis	If patient is beyond 20 weeks of gestation and history suggests seizure

studies. A casual assumption that sudden loss of consciousness is a normal manifestation of pregnancy is not justifiable and may be very hazardous to a patient (2–4).

REFERENCES

1. **Shotan A, Ostrzega E, Mehra A, et al.** Incidence of arrhythmia in normal pregnancy and relation to palpitations, dizziness and syncope. Am J Cardiol. 1997;79:1061-4.
2. **Linzer M, Yang EH, Estes NAM, Wang P, Vorperian VR, Kapoor WN.** Diagnosing syncope. Part 1: Value of history, physical examination and electrocardiography. Ann Intern Med. 1997;126:989-96.
3. **Linzer M, Yang EH, Estes NAM, Wang P, Vorperian VR, Kapoor WN.** Diagnosing syncope. Part 2: Unexplained syncope. Ann Intern Med.
4. **Kinsella SM, Lohmann G.** Supine hypotensive syndrome. Obstet Gynecol. 1994;83:774.

APPENDIX: DRUGS FOR CARDIAC DISORDERS

The drug table on page 386 is for reference when there is a clinical indication for treatment with one of the medications listed. Decisions about medication use in pregnancy should be made on the basis of a benefit-to-risk ratio, avoiding unnecessary treatment of symptoms but with consideration of the fact that fetal well-being depends on maternal well-being. Because the U.S. Food and Drug Administration is working on a new classification system of medications used in pregnancy, we have classified medications as follows:

Data Suggest Drug Use May Be Justified When Indicated
When data and/or experience supports the safety of the drug.

Data Suggest Drug Use May Be Justified in Some Circumstances
When less extensive or desirable data are reported, but the drug is reasonable as a second-line therapy or may be used on the basis of the severity of maternal illness.

Data Suggest Drug Use Is Rarely Justified
Use drug only when alternatives supported by more experience and/or a better safety profile are not available.

Pregnancy pharmacokinetics may necessitate a significant increase in dose or dosing frequency, and dosing recommendations may require modification according to individual circumstances.

Drugs for Cardiac Disorders

Drug	Use May Be Justified When Indicated	Use May Be Justified in Some Circumstances	Use Is Rarely Justified	Comments/Dose Adjustment
ACE inhibitors			√	Use only in scleroderma renal crisis
Adenosine	√			No change in fetal heart rate when used for maternal SVT
Amiodarone			√	Fetal hypothyroidism, prematurity
Amlodipine		√		
Aspirin (≤ 81 mg/d)	√			With low dose, no increased risk for bleeding or closure of patent ductus arteriosus
Atenolol		√		Low birthweight, IUGR
Digoxin	√			Shortened maternal half-life, need increased dose and frequency
Diltiazem		√		
Disopyramide		√		Case reports of PTL
Diuretics		√		Use for volume overload only
Esmolol		√		More pronounced bradycardia has been seen in pregnancy
Flecainide*		√		Inadequate data but used for fetal arrhythmia
Hydralazine†	√			Vasodilator of choice
Labetalol†	√			No effect on uterine blood
Lidocaine	√			
Metoprolol†	√			Shortened maternal half-life
Nitroprusside			√	Potential for fetal thiocyanate toxicity
Organic nitrates	√			No apparent increased risk
Phenytoin		√		See Chapter 12, Section III
Procainamide*	√			
Propafenone*		√		Inadequate data but used for fetal arrhythmias
Propranolol		√		Some IUGR but use when indicated
Quinidine†	√			Increases digoxin levels
Sotalol*		√		Inadequate data for maternal use
Verapamil*		√		Fetal distress, maternal hypotension with rapid IV infusion

* Used for fetal arrhythmias
† Preferred drug in class.

CHAPTER 7

Pulmonary Disease

I. Asthma
Linda Anne Barbour, MD, MSPH

II. Acute Lung Injury
Raymond O. Powrie, MD

III. Chronic Lung Disease
Jeffrey Pickard, MD

I. Asthma
Linda Anne Barbour

Asthma, which affects at least 4% of pregnancies, is one of the most common serious medical complications seen during pregnancy (1). It is estimated that 10% of the population have airway hyperresponsiveness, and the prevalence of asthma increased by 60% from 1980 to 1989. The rate of death from asthma has also increased, and asthma has emerged as the most common chronic disease of childhood, affecting one in seven children in Great Britain. Given these worrisome trends and the observation that prenatal and postnatal exposure to indoor allergens may be major determinants of the development of airway responsiveness, pregnant women and their children are more likely to face asthma than any other chronic disease. Furthermore, poorly con-

387

Key Values and Normal Physiologic Changes for Pulmonary Disease

	Direction of Change	Percentage Change or Normal Range for Pregnancy
ABGs		
pH	↑	7.44 to 7.45
Pco$_2$	↓	28 to 32 mm Hg
Po$_2$	↑	95 to 105 mm Hg
Hco$_3$	↓	18 to 22 meq/L
Chest radiograph	See Cardiac Table (p 346)	
Functional residual volume	↓	
Peak expiratory flow rate	↔	
Forced expiratory volume in 1 second	↔	
Forced vital capacity	↔	
Minute ventilation	↑	0% to 50% increase
Oxygen consumption	↑	20% increase
Respiratory rate	↔	12 to 16 breaths/min
Tidal volume	↑	40% increase

↑ Increase
↓ Decrease
↔ No change

trolled asthma in pregnancy is associated with preterm labor, preterm birth, intrauterine growth restriction (IUGR), and increased perinatal mortality rates.

Physiologic Changes in Pregnancy

Numerous anatomic changes occur in the chest when a woman is pregnant. The lower ribs flare out, and the subcostal angles increase as the transverse diameter of the chest increases by about 2 cm (2). The diaphragm rises by about 4 cm, but this affects functional residual capacity (FRC) rather than inspiratory capacity, so the ability to move air in and out of the lungs is not significantly impeded (3). The increase in progesterone stimulates the respiratory center in the brain to produce hyperventilation and a mild sensation of dyspnea. Hyperventilation decreases alveolar CO_2 tension and arterial Pco$_2$, producing respiratory alkalosis. This is compensated for by a decreased plasma bicarbonate level, so little change is seen in the pH. As a result, a Pco$_2$ of 35 mm Hg or more is of great concern in an asthmatic pregnant woman with an acute exacerbation and may represent respiratory decompensation and impending failure.

Pulmonary function tests during pregnancy can be very useful, and the Key Values table on page 388 shows the effects of pregnancy on lung functions and blood gases. Tidal volume increases in pregnancy, as do minute ventilation and oxygen consumption, but the respiratory rate is not significantly altered. Forced expiratory volume in one second (FEV_1), forced vital capacity, and peak expiratory flow rate are not appreciably affected by pregnancy and should be used to determine a patient's baseline respiratory function and the severity of an asthma attack (4). There is concern that hypocarbia may result in decreased uterine blood flow and cause dissociation of oxygen from fetal hemoglobin. Hypoxemia (PaO_2 <60 mm Hg) results in decreased fetal oxygen saturation and fetal hypoxia and distress.

Effect of Pregnancy on Asthma

The pathophysiology of asthma and its manifestations is no different in pregnancy than outside of pregnancy. It is now well known that chronic inflammation is the primary cause of airway hyperresponsiveness, which manifests as recurrent episodes of wheezing, breathlessness, chest tightness, or coughing, particularly at night or early in the morning. However, pregnancy may have a variable effect on asthma, and in a prospective study of 198 pregnant women (5) 40% needed the same amount of medication that they had needed before pregnancy, 42% needed more medication, and only 18% needed less medication. Hospital admission rates may be high, and it has been estimated that 40% to 50% of pregnant women with asthma are hospitalized (6,7). There is a trend for the effect of pregnancy on asthma to be similar in subsequent pregnancies in the same woman (8). Pregnancy-induced hyperemia and edema of the tracheobronchial tree may exacerbate asthma as well as the increased gastroesophageal reflux and sinusitis associated with pregnancy. Table 7-1 lists some factors that may improve or worsen asthma during pregnancy.

Effect of Asthma on Pregnancy Outcome

Data are now sufficient to support the hypothesis that women with well-controlled mild or moderate asthma do not have a significantly higher rate of adverse pregnancy outcomes than women without asthma do. This was shown in two case–control studies in which asthma was actively managed in approximately 400 pregnant women (6, 9). However, pregnancy outcomes in women with more severe asthma, especially if the disease is not optimally controlled, may be less favorable. Such women have increased risk for preterm labor, preterm birth, IUGR, neonatal hypoxia, and perinatal death. In a retrospective case–control study of 81 asthmatic patients who were receiving long-term medications (7), the 31 women receiving long-term steroids had higher incidence rates of preterm labor, premature rupture of membranes, preterm delivery, and gestational diabetes. Fetal hypoxia can result in IUGR and fetal distress. Therefore, the severity of asthma probably contributes more to adverse fetal outcome than long-term steroid use does. Eighty-seven percent of prednisone is metabolized by the placenta before it reaches the fetus, but systemic steroids may contribute to premature rupture of membranes and gestational diabetes (10). Preeclampsia has also been associated with severe asthma, but underlying chronic hypertension and use of steroids (resulting in increased blood pressure and edema) have not been adequately controlled. Themes common to both the pathogenesis of severe asthma and the pathogenesis of preeclampsia include vascular endothelial dysfunction and altered reactivity in the constriction of smooth muscle, but it is not clear whether severe asthma is an independent risk factor for preeclampsia.

Management

In 1993, The National Heart, Lung, and Blood Institute (NHLBI) of the National Institutes of Health published a report of the Working Group on Asthma and Pregnancy (11) as part of the National Asthma Education Program (NAEP). The report strongly recommended that asthma be treated as aggressively in pregnant women as in nonpregnant patients.

The 1997 NAEP guidelines (12) recommend that determinations of the severity of asthma should be based on objective measures and symptoms in

Table 7-1 Factors That May Affect Asthma in Pregnancy

Factor	Effect on Asthma
Progesterone-mediated bronchodilatation	Improves
Prostaglandin E–mediated bronchodilatation	Improves
Hormonally mediated increased beta-receptor responsiveness	Improves
Increase in serum-free cortisol levels	Improves
Increase in gastroesophageal reflux	Worsens
Increase in rhinitis, sinusitis, and estrogen-mediated nasal mucosal edema	Worsens
Increase in prostaglandin $F_{2\alpha}$-mediated bronchoconstriction	Worsens
Decrease in functional residual volume	Worsens
Decrease in cell-mediated immunity predisposing to viral infection	Worsens
Tissue refractoriness to cortisol due to increases in progesterone and aldosterone	Worsens

pregnant as well as nonpregnant persons (Table 7-2). A shift away from reactive management has led to the use of proactive maintenance therapy as the current standard of care, and the NAEP recommends that management be based on 1) objective measures for monitoring maternal lung function and fetal well being, 2) avoiding or controlling asthma triggers, 3) pharmacologic therapy, and 4) patient education.

Objective measures to monitor both mother and infant include peak flows, checked twice daily, in patients with mild persistent, moderate, or severe asthma. It is recommended that the FEV_1 be measured at the initial office assessment. Patients must determine their personal best peak expiratory flow rates during a 1- to 2-week period when their asthma is well controlled. In this way, diurnal fluctuation can be determined and an asthma action plan can be devised on the basis of percentage decrements in predicted peak flow.

Table 7-2 Classification of Asthma Severity and Appropriate Treatment*

Severity of Asthma	Symptoms	Lung Function	Treatment
Mild intermittent asthma	≤ 2 time/wk (daytime) ≤ 2 times/mo (night-time)	FEV_1 or PEFR >80% PEFR variation <20%	No daily treatment Inhaled beta$_2$-agonists up to twice per week
Mild persistent asthma	> 2 times/wk but < 1 time/d > 2 times/mo (night-time) < 1 time/wk	FEV_1 or PEFR >80% PEFR variation 20% to 30%	Low-dose inhaled steroids or cromolyn or nedocromil daily preferred over theophylline
Moderate persistent asthma	Daily symptoms Daily use of beta-2 agonists Exacerbations ≥2 times/wk Night-time symptoms > 1 time/wk	FEV_1 >60% to <80% PEFR >60% to <80% PEFR variation >30%	Med-high dose inhaled steroids or low-med dose inhaled steroids and long-acting beta$_2$-agonists or sustained-release theophylline
Severe persistent asthma	Continual symptoms Limited physical activity Frequent exacerbations Frequent night-time symptoms	FEV_1 or PEFR <60% PEFR variation >30%	High-dose inhaled steroids and long-acting beta$_2$-agonists or sustained-release theophylline and oral steroids if necessary

* Presence of one of the features of severity is sufficient to place a patient in the most severe category. A patient at any level of severity can have mild, moderate, or severe exacerbations. Leukotriene modifiers are not discussed because they are not alternatives in pregnancy. Daily use of short-acting beta$_2$-agonists indicates the need for additional long-term control therapy.

Adapted from the National Asthma Education and Prevention Program. Guidelines for the diagnosis and management of asthma expert panel, report II. 1997:NIH publication no. 97-4051.

In addition, it is recommended that fetal monitoring, including sequential ultrasonographic testing for fetal growth, nonstress testing, and daily kick counts, be done in pregnant women with moderate to severe asthma. Electronic fetal heart monitoring during acute asthma exacerbations is advised. The fetus is an important "barometer" of the severity of the exacerbation because fetal heart rate tracings may indicate fetal distress even if the mother is not overtly hypoxic.

Given that environmental triggers affect at least 85% of asthmatic patients, it is imperative to identify and control triggers, including house dust mites, cockroach antigens, animal danders, pollen, mold spores, and tobacco smoke (13). In addition, pregnant asthmatic patients should be asked about sulfite and aspirin sensitivity, rhinitis and sinusitis, gastroesophageal reflux disease (GERD), exercise- or cold-induced asthma, and nocturnal asthma. Most pregnant women have GERD because of progesterone-induced smooth muscle relaxation and increased mechanical upward pressure on stomach contents, and GERD is likely to worsen and exacerbate asthma as pregnancy progresses. Elevating the head of the bed and eating smaller meals earlier in the evening can be helpful. Bacterial sinusitis is 5 to 6 times more common in pregnancy and needs to be aggressively treated, as does chronic sinusitis (14). Most asthmatic patients, including pregnant women, have a nocturnal worsening in peak flow that needs to be appropriately identified and treated.

Almost all pharmacologic agents used to treat asthma can be used during pregnancy (15). The exceptions are leukotriene modifiers and iodide (Table 7-3). Of the inhaled steroids, beclamethasone is preferred because it has been used most often in pregnancy, but limited data are available on the use of tri-

Table 7-3 Preferred Drugs for Treating Asthma in Pregnancy*

Drug Class	Preferred Agent
Anti-inflammatory	Cromolyn sodium
	Beclamethasone
	Prednisone
Bronchodilator	Albuterol or metaproterenol
	Theophylline (8 to 12 µg/mL)
Antihistamine	Chlorpheniramine
	Tripelennamine
Decongestant	Pseudoephedrine
	Oxymetazoline
Antitussive	Guaifenesin
	Dextromethorphan

Adapted from the National Asthma Education Program, National Heart, Lung and Blood Institute, National Institutes of Health. Report of the Working Group on Asthma and Pregnancy. 1993: NIH publication no. 93-3279A.

amcinolone, budesonide, and fluticasone (11). Like nonpregnant persons, pregnant patients should use inhaled steroids if they consistently use inhaled bronchodilators more than twice a week; this is because beta$_2$-agonists have no effect on airway hyperresponsiveness. Beclamethasone decreased the hospital readmission rate by 55% in a randomized, controlled trial of 84 pregnant women with asthma exacerbations who required hospitalization (16). In another trial of 504 pregnant asthmatic patients (17), those who had not been initially treated with inhaled steroids had a fourfold increase in acute exacerbations during pregnancy. Exacerbations occurred most often between 17 and 24 weeks of gestation. Among the 257 patients who used inhaled steroids (beclamethasone or budesonide) throughout pregnancy, there was no difference in prematurity or low birthweight in asthmatic patients compared with healthy controls, but asthmatic patients had a slightly higher risk for preeclampsia. Triamcinolone was found to be superior to beclamethasone in a very small trial (18).

Other agents, including prednisone, theophylline, beta$_2$-agonists, and cromolyn, also seem to be safe for the treatment of asthma in pregnancy. No short-term effect on maternal circulation was seen when maximum doses of inhaled albuterol were used (19). In a prospectively monitored cohort of 824 pregnant women with asthma and 678 pregnant women without asthma (20), no significant relation was seen between major congenital malformations and first-trimester use of beta$_2$-agonists, theophylline, cromolyn, corticosteroids, antihistamines, and decongestants. However, it should be noted that beclamethasone and prednisone were the primary steroids used; metaproterenol, terbutaline, and albuterol were the primary beta$_2$-agonists; pseudoephedrine and intranasal oxymetazoline were the primary decongestants; and chlorpheniramine and tripelennamine were the primary antihistamines. The study had adequate power to detect an odds ratio of approximately 2.0. When theophylline is used during pregnancy, a serum level of 8 to 12 mg/mL should be the target to avoid both maternal and fetal toxicity. The half-life of theophylline is increased in pregnancy, and clearance is decreased, especially in the third trimester (14). Because theophylline seems to have some immunomodulatory properties, the NHLBI is conducting a randomized, double-blind trial comparing beclamethasone with theophylline for mild asthma in pregnancy. Sustained-release theophylline given at 8:00 P.M. or salmeterol may be especially useful in nocturnal asthma. Cimetidine, ranitidine, and metoclopramide can all be used safely in pregnant women with GERD who need pharmacologic treatment. Inhaled ipratropium is probably safe but usually adds little to inhaled beta$_2$-agonists in the treatment of acute asthma.

Patient education includes development of an asthma action plan; this is recommended for all asthmatic patients with the possible exception of those with mild, intermittent asthma (defined primarily on the basis of peak flows).

If the peak flow decreases to less than 70% of predicted, a clear plan must be in place so that the patient knows what additional medications to take and when to call a physician or be evaluated. In addition, the NAEP (12) recommends use of a spacer to improve delivery of both inhaled steroids and beta$_2$-agonists. This is because most asthmatic patients do not use their inhalers correctly, and spacers have been shown to decrease dysphonia and thrush. Patient education should emphasize the relative safety and benefit of medication use over the risks of poorly controlled asthma.

Hospitalization

Hospitalization should be recommended to all asthmatic patients whose peak flows are less than 40% of predicted or remain between 40% to 70% of predicted despite aggressive treatment for 4 hours. Treatment of an acute exacerbation in pregnancy is nearly identical to that outside of pregnancy. Intravenous methylprednisone and nebulized beta$_2$-agonists every 20 minutes may be warranted. Blood gases should be checked because a Po$_2$ less than 60 mm Hg signifies severe maternal hypoxemia that can result in fetal hypoxia and distress. As mentioned, a Pco$_2$ of 35 mm Hg or more is an ominous sign of respiratory fatigue and impending failure and warrants immediate consideration of intubation (14). Fetal monitoring should be initiated in all cases of asthma exacerbation. Almost 50% of asthma-related deaths occur in the hospital and, in 85% of cases, the final episode lasts at least 12 hours. Risk factors for potentially fatal asthma are shown in Box 7-1, and it should be noted that a patient who has a marked circadian variation in lung function, has a large bronchodilator response, and is overreliant on bronchodilator

---

Box 7-1 Characteristics of Patients with Potentially Fatal Asthma

Marked circadian variation in lung function
Large bronchodilation response
Psychosocial instabilities or noncompliance
Use of three or more medications or need for long-term oral steroids
Frequent visits to emergency department or recurrent hospitalization
Previous life-threatening attacks
Previous mechanical ventilation
Inability to perceive airflow obstruction until quite severe
Over-reliance on bronchodilator therapy
Use of illicit drugs

therapy is strongly at risk. Prognosis is poor after a near-fatal event, and 10% of patients die within 1 year of such an event. Some patients cannot sense the presence of marked airway obstruction, and others have a blunted hypoxic ventilatory drive. Thus, peak flow monitoring is imperative.

Labor and Delivery and Postpartum Management

Approximately 10% of pregnant women have an asthma exacerbation during labor or delivery. Peak flows should be checked in women with moderate or severe asthma on admission and every 4 hours. Hydrocortisone 100 mg every 8 hours should be used in women who used oral steroids for more than 2 to 3 weeks within 1 year before delivery and in women who have had repeated oral steroid tapers (Box 7-2). It should also be considered in women receiving high-dose inhaled steroid therapy because adrenal suppression can occur at doses of 1500 µg/d. Prostaglandin E_2 is safe for cervical ripening, as is oxytocin (14). The agent 15-methyl prostaglandin $F_{2\alpha}$, used to treat postpartum hemorrhage, should be avoided because it is a bronchoconstrictor. Fentanyl is preferred to morphine and meperidine, which can release histamine. Epidural anesthesia is optimal because it decreases oxygen consumption and minute ventilation. Cesarean section may be associated with a greater postpartum exacerbation of asthma (6), so peak flows should continue to be monitored in the postpartum period. All asthma medications that are safe in pregnancy are compatible with nursing. Breastfeeding should be encouraged. It seems to protect against the development of asthma in the neonate, and it changes the T-helper response to environmental agents.

Box 7-2 Asthma Exacerbation in Labor and Delivery

Hydrocortisone 100 mg every 8 hours if superphysiologic doses have been used for ≥3 weeks within past year

Peak expiratory flow rate measured on admission and every 4 hours if asthma is moderate or severe

Fetal heart monitoring if asthma is severe

Avoid 15-methyl prostaglandin $F_{2\alpha}$ for postpartum hemorrhage

Avoid morphine and meperidine; fentanyl is preferred

Prostaglandin E_2 and oxytocin are safe

Epidural is optimal because it decreases oxygen consumption and minute ventilation

Pregnancy requires that practitioner be aware of several considerations that can affect the course of asthma in the antepartum and peripartum periods. However, for the most part, the treatment of asthma in pregnancy is the optimal treatment of asthma. Poor control of maternal asthma poses unacceptable risks to the mother and leads to chronic and episodic fetal hypoxia, which is thought to be an important cause of perinatal illness and death.

REFERENCES

1. **Dombrowski MP.** Pharmacologic therapy of asthma during pregnancy. Obstet Gynecol Clin North Am. 1997;24:559-74.
2. **Elkuj R, Popovich J.** Respiratory physiology in pregnancy. Clin Chest Med. 1992;13: 555-65.
3. **American College of Obstetricians and Gynecologists.** ACOG Technical Bulletin. Pulmonary disease in pregnancy. Int J Gynecol Obstet. 1996;187-96.
4. **Venkataraman MT, Shanies HM.** Pregnancy and asthma. J Asthma. 1997;34:265-71.
5. **Stenius-Aarniala B, Riikonen S, Teramo K.** Asthma and pregnancy: a prospective study of 198 pregnancies. Thorax. 1988;43:12-8.
6. **Mabie WC, Barton JR, Wasserstrum N, Sibai BM.** Clinical observations on asthma in pregnancy. J Mat Fet Med. 1992;1:45-50.
7. **Perlow JH, Montgomery D, Morgan MA.** Severity of asthma and perinatal outcome. Am J Obstet Gynecol. 1992;167:963-7.
8. **Witlin AG.** Asthma in pregnancy. Semin Perinatol. 1997;21:284-97.
9. **Schatz M, Zeiger R, Clement P, et al.** Perinatal outcomes in the pregnancies of asthmatic women: a prospective controlled analysis. Am J Respir Crit Care Med. 1995;151: 1170-4.
10. **Mabie WC.** Asthma in pregnancy. Clin Obstet Gynecol. 1996;5:21-38.
11. **National Asthma Education Program, National Heart, Lung and Blood Institute, National Institutes of Health.** Report of the Working Group on Asthma and Pregnancy. 1993: NIH publication no. 93-3279A.
12. **National Asthma Education and Prevention Program.** Guidelines for the diagnosis and the management of asthma expert panel, report II. 1997: NIH publication no. 97-4051.
13. **Becklake MR, Ernst P.** Environmental factors and asthma. Lancet. 1997;350(suppl 2):10-3.
14. **Schatz M, Zeigler RS.** Asthma and allergy in pregnancy. Clin Perinatol. 1997;24:407-32.
15. **Rosene Montella K.** Pulmonary pharmacology in pregnancy. Clin Chest Med. 1992;13:587-95.
16. **Wendel PJ, Ranin SM, Barnett-Hamm C, et al.** Asthma treatment in pregnancy: a randomized controlled study. Am J Obstet Gynecol. 1996;175:150-4.
17. **Stenius-Aarniala BSM, Hedman J, Teramo KA.** Acute asthma during pregnancy. Thorax. 1996;51:411-4.
18. **Dombrowski MP, Brown CL, Berry SM.** Preliminary experience with triamcinolone acetonide during pregnancy. J Mat Fet Med. 1996;5:310-3.

19. **Rayburn WF, Atkinson BD, Gilbert K, Turnbull GL.** Short-term effects of inhaled albuterol in maternal and fetal circulations. Am J Obstet Gynecol. 1994;171:770-3.

20. **Schatz M, Zeiger RS, Harden K, Hoffman CC, Chilingar L, Petitti D.** The safety of asthma and allergy medications during pregnancy. J Allergy Clin Immunol. 1997; 100:301-6.

II. Acute Lung Injury
Raymond O. Powrie

Medical providers should be familiar with the causes and management of acute lung injury (ALI) in the gravid woman because ALI is surprisingly common in obstetric patients. Fortunately, most cases of ALI in pregnancy respond readily and rapidly to appropriate therapy and, when properly managed, do not usually proceed to full acute respiratory distress syndrome (ARDS) requiring prolonged mechanical ventilation. Familiarity with the management and causes of ALI in pregnancy can help avert unnecessary investigations and treatments in pregnant women with acute respiratory failure and can help ensure a good outcome for the patient and her child (1) (Box 7-3).

Physiologic Changes in Pregnancy That Predispose to Acute Lung Injury

As a result of numerous normal physiologic changes that occur in pregnancy, pregnant women have a unique predisposition to ALI. These changes are "contributing" factors that increase the likelihood that a pregnant woman with a particular insult or condition will develop ALI, but they do not, in themselves, cause ALI. These changes are summarized in Box 7-4.

Box 7-3 Diagnostic Criteria for Acute Lung Injury and Acute Respiratory Distress Syndrome

Acute onset
Bilateral infiltrates on chest radiography
PCWP <18 mm Hg or no evidence of left atrial hypertension
Impaired oxygenation manifested by a Pao_2/Fio_2 <300 torr (<40 kPa) for ALI and <200 torr (<27 kPa) for ARDS

Decrease in Plasma Colloid Osmotic Pressure

Pregnancy is associated with a significant expansion of blood volume that occurs predominantly through an increase in plasma free water. The increase in plasma free water leads to a progressive decrease in the concentration of plasma proteins (e.g., albumin), and plasma colloid osmotic pressure (PCOP) thus decreases as gestation advances. The decrease in PCOP creates an increased propensity for fluid to move out of the intravascular spaces and into the interstitium (2).

The pregnancy-associated decrease in PCOP seen throughout gestation has been shown to continue in the puerperium period. The mechanism of this further decrease is multifactorial but involves normal peripartum blood loss, the "autotransfusion" of blood into the circulation that occurs with each uterine contraction, and the sudden increase in preload that occurs when compression of the inferior vena cava by the gravid uterus is alleviated. Preeclampsia is also associated with an additional decrease in PCOP; this partly explains the increased risk for ALI seen with preeclampsia (3).

Increase in Blood Volume and Cardiac Output

Normal pregnancy is characterized by a progressive increase in blood volume and cardiac output, which peaks at 26 to 32 weeks of gestation. Fever, pain, preeclampsia, and multiple gestations can further increase cardiac work and lead to an increase in pulmonary artery occlusion pressure (PAOP) that, although within the "normal" range (<18 mm Hg), can lead to pulmonary edema in a patient with low PCOP or endothelial damage.

Decrease in Functional Residual Capacity

Increased minute ventilation and an elevation of the diaphragm by the gravid uterus make the FRC about 18% lower in pregnant women than in nonpregnant persons. Therefore, at end expiration, the pregnant woman is closer to her critical closing volume (the volume at which alveoli collapse on them-

---

Box 7-4 Normal Physiologic Changes of Pregnancy That Predispose To, and May Exacerbate, Acute Lung Injury

20% decrease in colloid osmotic pressure
50% increase in blood volume and cardiac output
Decreased functional residual capacity

selves) than the nonpregnant woman is. Some investigators believe that the decreased FRC increases the ease with which small airways and alveoli collapse when small amounts of pulmonary edema are present and may thereby contribute to a progressive worsening of oxygenation when intra-alveolar fluid is present.

Precipitating Causes of Acute Lung Injury and Acute Respiratory Distress Syndrome

Despite the predisposition (due to low colloid osmotic pressure and increased cardiac work) of pregnant women to ALI, the occurrence of ALI still requires an inciting agent or event to "tip the balance" and allow fluid to move into the interstitial spaces of the lung (Box 7-5). Some of these inciting agents or events have clear, causative relationships; for others, the links are not readily apparent. Some are unique to pregnancy, whereas others are common to both pregnant and nonpregnant persons. In all cases, the presence of anemia or multiple gestation seems to further increase the risk that a particular inciting event will lead to ALI. In addition, the routine administration of generous amounts of crystalloid fluids to provide hydration during labor may have ill effects because patients with another predisposition to ALI may not be able to compensate for this excess volume.

Box 7-5 Some Causes of Acute Lung Injury in Pregnancy

More likely in setting of multiple gestation, anemia, and fluid overload

Tocolytic therapy

Preeclampsia or eclampsia

Sepsis (especially pyelonephritis, chorioamnionitis, endometritis, septic abortion, and appendicitis)

Aspiration

Mendelson syndrome

Severe hemorrhage (especially related to systemic inflammatory response, low plasma colloid osmotic pressure, and, rarely, leukoagglutination in the lung)

Amniotic fluid embolism

Venous air embolism

High-dose opiates (in susceptible patients)

Neurogenic pulmonary edema after eclamptic seizure

Tocolysis

Internists may not know that beta-adrenergic agonists (such as terbutaline) used for tocolysis (medical inhibition of uterine contractions in preterm labor) are a relatively common cause of ALI (4). Although beta-mimetics have been used extensively to treat asthma in nonpregnant patients without precipitating ALI, there is a clear association in the obstetric literature between beta-adrenergic agonists and ALI. The cause of the association remains unclear. Possible contributing factors include a primary cardiogenic component related to barometric-induced myocardial fatigue or altered capillary permeability (5). Fluids routinely given in association with tocolysis may be responsible for some cases, and beta-mimetics themselves can decrease PCOP beyond the decrease normally seen in pregnancy. The altered physiology of normal pregnancy must contribute to the effects of beta-mimetics because this complication is not seen in nonpregnant persons who use beta-mimetics for other indications. The risk for ALI is further increased with steroid use or in the presence of infection (6).

Preeclampsia

Preeclampsia, or pregnancy-induced hypertension (PIH), occurs in approximately 5% of pregnant patients and is an important cause of ALI. Three percent of patients with preeclampsia develop ALI during the course of their illness (7). Thirty percent of cases of ALI associated with preeclampsia occur antepartum, and 70% occur postpartum, usually within the first 72 hours after delivery. The maternal mortality rate may be as high as 10% and the perinatal mortality rate may be as high as 50% in the presence of ALI associated with preeclampsia. The alarmingly high fetal mortality rate may be related to placental abruption, an associated complication of preeclampsia, and may reflect the severity of the PIH more than the presence of ALI itself.

It is believed that PIH causes ALI by a variety of mechanisms. In some cases, the ALI is due to the decrease in PCOP that occurs in preeclampsia and is in excess of the normal decrease seen in pregnancy (8). This additional decrease may be enough, in some cases, to allow fluid to move into the interstitial spaces of the lungs. In other cases, evidence suggests that the endothelial damage characteristic of severe preeclampsia may disrupt the normal endothelial barrier in the lungs (as in early sepsis or "leaky capillary syndromes"), allowing fluid to escape into the alveoli and interstitium. In some cases, a stiff left ventricle resulting from chronic hypertension with significant diastolic dysfunction may be an important factor contributing to ALI in preeclamptic patients who have a sudden and dramatic increase in afterload due to intense vasospasm and increased systemic vascular resistance. Finally, many cases of ALI in the setting of preeclampsia can be attributed to left ventricular systolic dysfunction. The occurrence of this dysfunction in pre-eclampsia is well described but poorly understood (9, 9a). Presumably, the intense vasospasm and endothelial damage that characterize preeclampsia significantly affect myocardial oxygen supply and, thereby, myocardial contractility (10).

Sepsis

Sepsis is a very important cause of ALI in pregnancy. Pneumonia can progress to ALI and ARDS and is an important reason for prolonged mechanical ventilation in pregnant women. However, it seems that any systemic bacterial infection can lead to ALI in pregnant women. This increased incidence of sepsis-related ALI in pregnancy seems to be related to a combination of decreased PCOP, altered capillary permeability, and increased sensitivity to endotoxins. The best-described example of this is the occurrence of ALI in as many as 10% of women who have pyelonephritis in pregnancy. The greatly increased incidence of pyelonephritis in pregnancy makes this infection a particularly important cause of ALI and argues against the outpatient management of pyelonephritis in pregnant women (11).

Aspiration Syndromes

Aspiration syndromes are common in pregnancy because of the delayed gastric emptying and decreased lower esophageal sphincter pressure seen in all pregnant women. In the setting of altered mental status resulting from drugs, anesthesia, or seizures, stomach contents can be aspirated and can lead to Mendelson syndrome or bacterial aspiration pneumonia.

Mendelson syndrome usually occurs in association with a difficult intubation or in the postanesthetic period, when the gag reflex may be depressed. It can also occur de novo in pregnant women. Gastric juice is aspirated into the lungs and leads to intense pulmonary inflammation that proceeds rapidly to full ALI over 8 to 24 hours. The patient becomes tachypneic, hypoxic, and febrile. Chest radiograph classically shows a complete "white out." Despite rapid and marked deterioration, the syndrome generally resolves without antibiotics within 48 to 72 hours, unless bacterial superinfection intervenes (12).

Bacterial aspiration pneumonia usually has a more insidious onset, with clinical manifestations—persistent fever, sputum, and leukocytosis—presenting 48 to 72 hours after aspiration. Classically, chest radiograph findings are localized to the basilar segments if the patient aspirated while upright and to the posterior segment of the upper lobe or the superior segment of the lower lobe if the patient aspirated while supine. The bacterial infection is generally polymicrobial, with mouth anaerobes predominating. Treatment with penicillin or clindamycin is advisable.

Massive Hemorrhage

Massive red blood cell transfusion for antepartum or postpartum hemorrhage can result in ALI. The mechanism of this is often multifactorial and can include volume overload, decrease in PCOP resulting from the replacement of lost whole blood with packed red blood cells and crystalloids, endothelial damage from a systemic inflammatory response to massive hemorrhage, and, rarely, leukoagglutination in the lung.

Amniotic Fluid Embolism

Amniotic fluid embolism (AFE) is a rare but catastrophic complication of pregnancy that may present as ALI but often proceeds to full ARDS. Its incidence is variably cited as being between 1/8000 and 1/80,000 pregnancies (13). Prolonged labor, multiparity, increased maternal age, meconium staining of the amniotic fluid, and use of forceps are risk factors for AFE. It is usually seen at the time of delivery but has been reported to occur antepartum. It is associated with a mortality rate greater than 50% and is responsible for 10% of maternal deaths in the United States (14).

Patients with AFE usually present with sudden onset of agitation and dyspnea followed by symptomatic hypotension, hypoxia, and disseminated intravascular coagulation resulting in massive obstetric hemorrhage. Seizures can be seen with acute AFE. The diagnosis is difficult to establish with certainty but should be considered in any woman who is near term (especially if she is in labor) who has sudden cardiorespiratory failure. Although the entry of amniotic fluid into the maternal circulation through endocervical veins or uterine tears is an important prerequisite of AFE, animal studies indicate that it is not enough, in itself, to cause the catastrophic reaction seen in patients with AFE. For this reason, many researchers would prefer the term *anaphylactoid lung of pregnancy* to describe AFE to emphasize the importance of the maternal immunologic response in this syndrome (15).

Clinical Findings in Acute Lung Injury in Pregnancy

Symptoms and Signs

The symptoms and signs of ALI in pregnancy are similar to those of ALI in the general medical population. Early signs and symptoms of ALI may be few and mild, and it can therefore be difficult to distinguish ALI from other causes of cardiopulmonary problems seen in pregnancy. One of the most common mistakes that we have noted at our institution is delayed diagnosis of ALI. Diagnosis is often delayed when the mild symptoms of ALI in pregnancy are attributed to less serious and more common causes of dyspnea, such as respiratory tract infection, asthma, or dyspnea of pregnancy. This may occur because the absence of comorbid conditions in most pregnant women makes patients "look" better and maintain respiratory and cardiovascular stability longer than the typical medical patient with ALI.

Tachypnea is an important clinical sign that a woman has more than just the increased shortness of breath normally seen with exertion in pregnancy. The chest may initially be clear to auscultation early in the course of evolving ALI, especially in the otherwise well pregnant woman. The patient often has some degree of anxiety related to mild dyspnea or hypoxia. Eventually, as the condition progresses and the alveoli fill with fluid, diffuse crackles, wheezing, and cough appear. Tachycardia is common, but the heart rate should be interpreted with the knowledge that a resting pulse of 100 beats/min is not unusual in normal pregnancy (16).

Arterial Blood Gas, Chest Radiography, and Electrocardiography Findings

Initially, patients with ALI typically show a decrease in both Pao_2 and $Paco_2$. As the condition worsens, the Pao_2 decreases further but the $Paco_2$ increases because the patient can no longer maintain adequate ventilation and respiratory failure ensues. It is worth emphasizing that a Pao_2 of 70 mm Hg or a $Paco_2$ of 40 mm Hg in a pregnant woman is very abnormal and strongly suggests ventilatory failure.

The initial chest radiograph in ALI is often normal. Subsequently, pulmonic infiltrates and (in some cases) pleural effusions appear. Although classic ALI and ARDS are associated with diffuse chest radiograph changes, the damage may be patchy in some cases of ALI and ARDS. The radiation necessary to obtain a proper chest film is well below the maximal levels of radiation exposure recommended for pregnancy; therefore, an indicated chest radiograph should never be withheld because of concern about the effects of radiation on the fetus.

Additional tests that should be routinely done in patients with suspected ALI are complete blood count (CBC) and measurement of creatinine and blood urea nitrogen levels. This is because anemia and renal failure may be contributing factors. Urinalysis and tests for aspartate aminotransferase and uric acid (see Chapter 4) should also be done.

Treatment of Acute Lung Injury in Pregnancy

The treatment of ALI in pregnancy is a medical emergency (Box 7-6). Regardless of the cause of ALI, the immediate goal is to maintain adequate maternal oxygenation (Pao_2 ≥70 mm Hg) to avoid fetal hypoxia. It is recommended that maternal oxygen saturation be kept above 95%. The second goal is to treat the underlying causes of the edema, and the third goal is to relieve symptoms to improve patient comfort.

Careful monitoring of fluid balance should be initiated. The use of intravenous morphine sulfate to reduce maternal anxiety and decrease pulmonary congestion is safe if used cautiously. Clear, reassuring communication with both the patient and her support person is also important in decreasing ma-

---

Box 7-6 Management of Acute Lung Injury in Pregnancy

Provide supplemental oxygen to maintain Pao_2 >70 mm Hg

Have patient sit at 45° if possible

Minimize intravenous fluids

If patient is maintaining blood pressure and placental perfusion is not in question, consider administration of intravenous furosemide (at a dose of 10 mg if patient has not received furosemide in the past)

Control pain and allay patient's anxiety with small doses of morphine as needed and good communication

Carefully review history, cardiac examination, and electrocardiogram for cardiogenic causes such as ISHD, PPCM, and valvular heart disease; obtain echocardiogram semi-emergently if cardiogenic cause is suspected; consider screening for cocaine use

Consider possibility of primary pneumonia by questioning patient about presence of a prodromal illness, fever, chills, rigors, and sputum and by reviewing chest radiograph for localized findings suggestive of pneumonia; treat empirically if suspicion of pneumonia is strong

Remove or treat underlying causes: discontinue tocolytic therapy; evaluate for presence of preeclampsia, begin active efforts toward delivery if patient has preeclampsia; evaluate for presence of infection (especially pyelonephritis) and treat if present; protect airway if aspiration is suspected; check INR, aPTT, and CBC if AFE suspected

If oxygenation cannot be maintained, consider use of intermittent positive-pressure nasal ventilation or semi-elective intubation

Consider central hemodynamic monitoring if 1) cardiac cause is suspected and patient unresponsive to diuretics, 2) urine output is poor despite diuretic administration, or 3) hypotension is present

Consider use of inotropic and vasoactive agents to maximize cardiac output in a minority of cases (therapy should be guided in this setting by central hemodynamic monitoring)

ternal distress. Finally, although most patients with ALI in pregnancy do not have volume overload, diuresis—to try to achieve the lowest possible PAOP that still supports normal blood pressure—is advisable. Pregnant patients with ALI who do not have cardiac or renal disease will respond dramatically to doses of intravenous furosemide as low as 10 mg. Use of the lowest possible dose of diuretics has additional importance in patients with preeclampsia, who are relatively volume contracted despite having massive peripheral edema and ALI. Overdiuresis in these patients can lead to intravascular hypovolemia that can impair placental perfusion and lead to fetal distress.

Differential Diagnosis of Acute Lung Injury in Pregnancy

Other causes of respiratory failure in pregnancy should be routinely considered part of the differential diagnosis of ALI (Table 7-4) (17). The diagnosis of cardiogenic pulmonary edema from peripartum cardiomyopathy (18), ischemic heart disease, or occult valvular heart disease should be ruled out by a careful history, cardiac examination, and electrocardiography. When any doubt exists, echocardiography is indicated to discern whether the ALI is actually congestive heart failure.

Drug screening should be done, although the vast majority of patients with cocaine-associated pulmonary edema are notable for severe hypertension.

The possibility of acute infectious pneumonia should also be considered. Features suggestive of pneumonia include prodrome, fever, purulent sputum, chills, rigors, and localized findings on chest radiography. Blood and sputum cultures should be obtained in any patient with ALI and fever, and empirical antibiotic use pending culture results is often advisable in the initial 48 hours.

Table 7-4 Causes of Respiratory Failure in Pregnancy To Be Considered in the Differential Diagnosis of Acute Lung Injury

Causes of Respiratory Failure	Comment
Cardiac disease	Peripartum cardiomyopathy Ischemic heart disease Valvular heart disease
Cocaine-associated pulmonary edema	
Pneumonia	*Streptococcus* infection, *Hemophilus* infection, *Klebsiella* infection, *Staphylococcus* infection, bacterial aspiration pneumonia, *Mycoplasma* infection, *Legionella* infection, influenza A, varicella, measles
Drug-related pneumonitis	Nitrofurantoin, commonly used as urinary tract infection prophylaxis in pregnancy, can cause an acute pulmonary reaction

A careful drug history should be taken. Drug-induced pneumonitis is a rare but reversible cause of respiratory failure and has been reported to occur with the antibiotic nitrofurantoin, which is commonly used as prophylaxis for urinary tract infections during pregnancy.

Removing or Treating the Underlying Cause

Tocolytic-Related Acute Lung Injury
Most important in the management of ALI in pregnancy is treatment of the underlying cause of ALI. If the cause is tocolytic therapy, this therapy should be stopped. Deciding whether this should be done can be difficult for the obstetrician if the patient is in labor at a very early point in gestation. The decision becomes easier when one recognizes that 1) fetal well-being is dependent on maternal well-being and 2) the tocolytic agents that cause ALI have limited proven efficacy for significant prolongation of gestation.

Preeclampsia-Related Pulmonary Edema
Delivery is the treatment of choice for edema related to preeclampsia. Clues to the presence of preeclampsia are reviewed in Chapter 4. Even in the absence of typical feature of preeclampsia, consideration of PIH as a possible cause of ALI is required. Blood pressure should be decreased to less than 160/100 mm Hg in the setting of preeclampsia-associated ALI because a decrease in afterload may help decrease pulmonary edema. The intravenous infusion of magnesium sulfate (used for seizure prophylaxis in patients with preeclampsia) requires high doses of fluids. For this reason, we recommend considering the use of phenytoin to prevent seizures in the setting of PIH in selected patients with pulmonary edema. We make this recommendation despite recent research indicating that phenytoin may not be as effective as magnesium in preventing seizures. In addition, there are case reports of magnesium-associated pulmonary edema occurring when magnesium has been used for tocolysis.

Infection-Related Pulmonary Edema
Sepsis-related ALI is indicated by the presence of fever and should be treated with broad-spectrum antibiotics. As in suspected pneumonia, it is generally advisable to initiate empirical antibiotic use pending culture results. Any abdominal pain and tenderness should prompt consideration of the possibility of appendicitis and chorioamnionitis or endometritis, and signs of pyelonephritis should be evaluated.

Amniotic Fluid Embolism
Other than supportive management, no specific treatment is available for AFE. No pathognomonic findings or diagnostic tests "prove" this diagnosis,

but few conditions (other than acute pulmonary embolism) present so suddenly with such severe manifestations. Tests for disseminated intravascular coagulation must be done when a diagnosis of AFE is being considered. Treatment is supportive. It should begin with aggressive volume administration to maintain blood pressure but will almost always include intubation, mechanical ventilation, and vasopressor support of blood pressure. Hemorrhage should be treated with fresh frozen plasma and cryoprecipitate as needed (14).

Endotracheal Intubation

If oxygenation cannot be maintained above a PaO_2 of 70 mm Hg or if the patient shows evidence of respiratory muscle fatigue (by subjective evidence based on findings of accessory muscle use, intercostal indrawing, and abdominal breathing or on the basis of an increasing $PaCO_2$), a trial of spontaneous breathing with supplemental oxygen and positive end-expiratory pressure (PEEP) administered through a tight-fitting mask should be done (17). Noninvasive nasal intermittent positive-pressure ventilation may also be used, but concern about its use in the setting of pregnancy-associated upper airway edema and the propensity of pregnant women to aspiration pneumonia may limit its use in critical care obstetrics.

Intubation (Box 7-7) is generally required if a patient does not respond to therapy and has signs of respiratory failure (PaO_2 <70 mm Hg or $PaCO_2$ >45 mm Hg on 100% oxygen administered through a tight-fitting mask and a nonrebreathing mask). In "borderline" cases, it is worth remembering that it is always better to intubate a patient in an elective manner than to delay intubation until it is required emergently. This is particularly true in pregnant women for several reasons. First, the upper airway in pregnant women is often difficult to visualize because of soft tissue swelling related to a physiologic hyperemia of mucosal tissues. Second, pregnant women are at high risk for aspiration because of the lower gastroesophageal sphincter tone and delayed gastric emptying that are normal in pregnancy. Third, because pregnant women have decreased FRC, their lungs have less available oxygen with which to maintain PaO_2 between periods of "bagging." Preoxygenation with 100% oxygen should always be done before and between any attempts to intubate a pregnant woman. Finally, there is reason to believe that the fetus tolerates maternal hypoxia poorly and that a prolonged period of time "off" of the manual inflation bag and supplemental oxygen necessary for intubation may harm the fetus. It is therefore paramount that intubation of the pregnant woman be done by the most experienced person available and that every effort be made to ensure that all equipment is available and functioning properly before an attempt at intubation is started. The rate of failed elective intubation attempts in pregnant patients is eight times greater than that in general surgical patients (19).

Box 7-7 Equipment and Medications Necessary for Intubation of Pregnant Woman

---

Continuous EKG monitoring

Blood pressure monitor on patient's arm

Pulse oximeter

High-flow oxygen source

Secure large-bore intravenous access in place

Most experienced intubationist available, with assistant

Mask (that fits securely) and manual inflation bag

Oropharyngeal suction equipment

Endotracheal tubes with tested inflatable cuff; oral intubation (rather than nasal) with a smaller endotracheal tube than would be used in a similar nonpregnant patient is preferable because of upper airway narrowing in pregnancy

Laryngoscope with light

Stylet

Medications for sedation and (if necessary) paralysis of patient (e.g., thiopental 3–5 mg/kg IV, for sedation; etomidate 0.3 mg/kg IV over 60 seconds, for muscle relaxation; and succinylcholine 1–1.5 mg/kg up to 150 mg IV, for paralysis)

Method ready to assess that endotracheal placement is not esophageal (listener with stethoscope or CO_2 detector*)

Chest radiography done shortly after intubation to ensure that endotracheal tube is properly placed 4 to 7 cm above the carina

Gloves, mask, goggles, and gown for intubationist

Plan in place for next step if intubation attempt fails

---

*Self-inflating bulbs or syringes have been found unreliable in pregnant women.

Mechanical Ventilation

Mechanical ventilation in the pregnant woman with ALI or ARDS should be the same as that in nonpregnant patients. A reasonable way to start is to improve arterial oxygenation with volume-cycled ventilation in the assist-control mode with PEEP added in increments of 3 to 5 cm H_2O. Tidal volumes should be set at 12 to 15 mL/kg. The Fio_2 should be kept at less than 60% if possible. There is little reason to use PEEP greater than 15 to 20 cm H_2O. The $Paco_2$ should ideally be kept at 28 to 32 mm Hg to mimic the respiratory function seen in normal pregnancy. Respiratory alkalosis from overventilation should be avoided, however, because alkalemia can adversely affect uterine blood flow. Some advocates in critical care suggest use of smaller tidal volumes (<6 mL/kg), pressure-limited ventilation (rather than volume-cycled ventilation), PEEP at 17 cm H_2O, and a "permissive hypercapnia," but the experience with such an approach in pregnant women is limited, and there are theoretical reasons to believe that the fetus may not tolerate the acidosis necessary to this approach. Inverse-ratio ventilation has also been used in pregnant women. Clinicians should know that the degree of sedation or paralysis necessary for this type of ventilation makes fetal test results uninterpretable.

Positive-pressure ventilation in pregnancy-associated ALI often results in marked and rapid patient improvement because the positive pressure helps move fluid out of the interstitium. If a patient requires intubation, it is important to correct the underlying problem before extubation because patients who are prematurely extubated may simply slip back into ALI once they are no longer under the therapeutic effects of positive-pressure ventilation (20).

Pulmonary Artery Occlusion Pressure Monitoring

In most cases of ALI in pregnancy, central hemodynamic monitoring is not necessary for diagnostic purposes. In the absence of preeclampsia and in the absence of history, physical examination, or electrocardiogram findings suggestive of cardiac disease, it can generally be assumed that the PAOP is unlikely to be greater than 18 mm Hg in a young pregnant woman (21). The patient with preeclampsia is an exception because severe preeclampsia may be associated with diastolic or systolic dysfunction. If cardiac dysfunction is suspected, bedside echocardiography can be very useful in deciding whether PAOP monitoring may be helpful.

In the absence of a prompt clinical response to oxygen, diuresis, and morphine, invasive hemodynamic monitoring may be indicated to aid management. The goal of invasive monitoring in ALI in pregnancy is to 1) guide therapy aimed at reducing the pulmonary capillary wedge pressure (PCWP) and 2) improve and optimize left ventricular performance. In general, however, it must be remembered that a PCWP that is normal in a nonpregnant patient may be too high in the setting of preeclampsia or in the postpartum period. Because the most important factor is not the absolute PCWP but the relation of the PCWP to the COP, therapeutic decisions may be difficult in some circumstances. If the COP is very low, as it is in preeclampsia and in the postpartum period, a "normal" PCWP can still be associated with significant pulmonary edema. In general, trends in the PCWP may be more useful than absolute numbers. However, most authors have found that in the absence of cardiac disease or sepsis, hemodynamic monitoring in the setting of ALI in pregnancy is not generally necessary (22).

Vasoactive and Inotropic Medications

Use of vasoactive substances to help maintain cardiac output at a lower PCWP may be helpful in some cases of ALI in pregnancy in which cardiac dysfunction is present. The Drugs for Pulmonary Disorders table at the end of this chapter lists some commonly used vasoactive agents and data on their use in pregnancy. In the setting of critical illness, it is important not to withhold any potentially beneficial treatment from a pregnant woman because of concern about possible fetal effects. However, the paucity of human data on the effects of most of these medications on placental blood flow should caution against the use of these agents to "fine tune" maternal hemodynamic variables.

Conclusions

Internists should know that acute lung injury occurs with increased frequency in pregnant women despite the rarity of cardiopulmonary disease in this population. It is associated with the tocolytic treatment used for preterm labor and with pyelonephritis. It can be precipitated by entities unique to pregnancy, such as peripartum cardiomyopathy, amniotic fluid embolism, or, most commonly, preeclampsia. Management of ALI in pregnancy is similar to that outside of pregnancy but requires 1) added consideration of the specific entities that cause ALI in pregnancy and 2) prompt attention to fetal oxygen requirements. Both intubation and invasive hemodynamic monitoring may have roles in patients who do not respond to diuresis and oxygenation. Good maternal and fetal outcomes can be expected with prompt recognition and treatment.

REFERENCES

1. **Hook JW.** Acute respiratory distress syndrome in pregnancy. Semin Perinatol. 1997;21:320-7.
2. **Nguyen HN, Clark SL, Greenspoon J, et al.** Peripartum colloid osmotic pressure: correlation with serum proteins. Obstet Gynecol. 1986;68:807-10.
3. **Cotton DB, Gonik B, Spillmann T, Dorman KF.** Intrapartum to postpartum changes in colloid osmotic pressure. Am J Obstet Gynecol. 1984;149:174-7.
4. **Benedetti TJ, Hargrove JC, Rosene KA.** Maternal pulmonary edema during premature labor inhibition. Obstet Gynecol. 1982;59(6 Suppl):335-75.
5. **Pisani RJ, Rosenow EC 3d.** Acute lung injury associated with tocolytic therapy. Ann Intern Med. 1989;110:714-8.
6. **Ingemarsson I, Arulkomoran S, Kottegoda SR.** Complications of beta mimetic therapy in preterm labour. Aust N Z J Obstet Gynecol. 1985;25:182-9.
7. **Benedetti TJ, Kates R, Williams V.** Hemodynamic observations in severe pre-eclampsia complicated by acute lung injury. Am J Obstet Gynecol. 1985;152:330-4.

8. **Zinaman M, Rubin J, Lindheimer MD.** Serial plasma oncotic pressure levels and echoencephalography during and after delivery in severe pre-eclampsia. Lancet. 1985.

9. **Mabie WC, Hackman BB, Sibai BM.** Acute pulmonary edema associated with pregnancy: echocardiographic insights and implications for treatment. Obstet Gynecol. 1993;81:227-34.

9a. **Mabie WC, Ratts TE, Ramanathan KB, Sibai BM.** Circulatory congestion in obese hypertensive women: a subset of acute lung injury in pregnancy. Obstet Gynecol. 1988;72:553-8.

10. **Gottlieb JE, Darby MJ, Gee MH, Fish JE.** Recurrent non-cardiac acute lung injury accompanying pregnancy-induced hypertension. Chest. 1991;100:1730-2.

11. **Cunningham FG, Lucas MJ, Hankins GDV.** Pulmonary injury complicating antepartum pyelonephritis. Am J Obstet Gynecol. 1987;156:797-807.

12. **Soreide E, Bjornstad E, Steen PA.** An audit of perioperative aspiration pneumonia in gynecological and obstetric patients. Acta Anaesthesiol Scand. 1996;40:14-9.

13. **Clark SL, Hankins GDV, Dudley DA, Dildy GA, Porter TF.** Amniotic fluid embolism: analysis of the national registry. Am J Obstet Gynecol. 1995;172:1158-69.

14. **Martin RW.** Amniotic fluid embolism. Clin Obstet Gynecol. 1996;39:101-6.

15. **Burrows A, Khoo SK.** The amniotic fluid embolism syndrome: 10 years' experience at a major teaching hospital. Aust N Z J Obstet Gynaecol. 1995;35:245-50.

16. **Catanzarite VA, Willms D.** Adult respiratory distress syndrome in pregnancy: report of three cases and review of the literature. Obstet Gynecol Surv. 1997;52:381-92.

17. **Deblieux PM, Summer WR.** Acute respiratory failure in pregnancy. Clin Obstet Gynecol. 1996;39:143-52.

18. **Cunningham FG, Pritchard JA, Hankins GDV, Anderson PL, Lucas MJ, Armstrong KF.** Peripartum heart failure: idiopathic cardiomyopathy or compounding cardiovascular events? Obstet Gynecol. 1986;67:157-68.

19. **Lapinsky SE, Kruczynski K, Slutsky AS.** Critical care in the pregnant patient. Am J Respir Crit Care Med. 1995;152:427-55.

20. **Rizk NW, Kalassian KG, Gilligan T, Druzin MI, Daniel DL.** Obstetric complications in pulmonary and critical care medicine. Chest. 1996;110:791-809.

21. **Nolan TE, Wakefield ML, Devoe LD.** Invasive hemodynamic monitoring in obstetrics, a critical review of its indications, benefits, complications, and alternatives. Chest. 1992;101:1429-33.

22. **Matthay MA, Chatterjee K.** Bedside catheterization of the pulmonary artery: risks compared with benefits. Ann Intern Med. 1988;109:826-34.

III. Chronic Lung Disease
Jeffrey Pickard

Various chronic lung diseases can complicate pregnancy. Unfortunately, data on care for the pregnant woman with chronic lung disease are limited. Most of the available information is based on case reports and a few observational studies. Nevertheless, some recommendations can be made.

Cystic Fibrosis

Increasing numbers of women with cystic fibrosis (CF) are reaching their childbearing years. Although fertility is compromised in women with CF, the health care of these patients is improving and their life expectancy is increasing, and more and more of them are becoming pregnant. Many men and women are heterozygous carriers of the CF gene and can pass CF to their children without knowing it. However, carrier testing is available and, depending on the population in which it is used, can be very accurate. Practitioners who care for women of childbearing age must be able to counsel patients about the likelihood of having a child affected with CF and may be called on to participate in the care of patients with CF who become pregnant.

Fertility

More than 95% of men with CF are infertile because of morphologic abnormalities of the reproductive tract that cause obstructive azoospermia. Although testicular histologic findings are normal and sperm formation occurs, sperm are not expressed in the semen (1). Because a small percentage of men with CF are fertile, all men with CF must undergo sperm analysis. Men who are infertile and wish to have children generally adopt or use artificial insemination of donor sperm. It may be possible for sperm to be aspirated from the epididymis of a man with CF and used for in vitro fertilization.

Women with CF have anatomically normal reproductive tracts, but many are infertile. This is most often because of the thick, tenacious cervical mucus that they produce; it impedes the passage of sperm through the cervical os. Women with CF who do not wish to become pregnant must use contraception. Although there may be concern about the use of oral contraceptives in CF, the overall experience with these agents has been favorable and without significant adverse events. Intrauterine insemination may be used in women with CF who are infertile because of abnormal cervical mucus (1).

Genetics

Cystic fibrosis is the most common serious recessive genetic disorder among white persons in the United States. It occurs in 1 in 3000 persons. Approximately 4% of Caucasians are heterozygous for the mutant gene and thus are asymptomatic carriers (1, 2). With a negative family history, the risk for being a CF carrier depends on ethnic background. It is approximately 2% for Hispanic-Americans, 1.5% for African-Americans, and less than 1% for Asian-Americans (3). Current screening tests in the United States detect 85% to 90% of carriers in the white non–Ashkenazi Jewish population and about

97% of Ashkenazi heterozygotes (3–5). The CF gene itself was originally identified in 1989 on the long arm of chromosome 7 and has been cloned. The gene product is an ion transport protein that is known as CFTR (cystic fibrosis transmembrane conductance regulator) and is located in the cell membrane (3, 6, 7). The most common mutation (ΔF508) makes up about two thirds of the mutations present in patients with CF, and the next five most common mutations each account for 1% to 2.5% (3, 7, 8). To date, more than 750 mutations have been identified (7). Assuming that the prevalence is 4% and that a DNA diagnostic laboratory identifies 90% of all mutations, a white person who is not an Ashkenazi Jew, has no family history, and screens negative has about a 1 in 250 chance of being a carrier. If one partner screens negative and the other positive, the risk for a child with CF is about 1 in 1000. If both partners screen negative, the risk for an affected child is about 1 in 250,000. If the mother has CF and the father screens negative, the risk for an affected child is about 1 in 500 and all unaffected children will be carriers. It is important to emphasize to the parents that although the risk for CF is low, it is not zero, and that the genetic screening test is not 100% sensitive. Not all mutations result in the same phenotypic expression of the disease; thus, some affected children of unsuspecting carriers may have mild disease and may not be diagnosed until they are adults themselves. The median survival is 29 years in patients with CF who have pancreatic (exocrine) insufficiency and 56 years in patients with CF who have sufficient pancreatic function (7).

Effect of Pregnancy on Cystic Fibrosis

Pulmonary disease accounts for most of the morbidity and mortality seen in CF (1). Pancreatic disease is also important and eventually leads to diabetes in many patients. Pregnant women with CF should be screened early for preexisting and gestational diabetes. Malabsorption, gut motility disorders, and hepatic and biliary diseases also occur in CF. The physiologic stresses of pregnancy can lead to significant maternal and fetal morbidity. In pregnancy, the increased workload on the respiratory system and the altered gas exchange can contribute to hypoxemia and pulmonary decompensation in women with CF (1). Women with CF who have pulmonary hypertension may not be able to handle the increased blood volume that occurs with normal pregnancy and delivery. Women with CF who have underlying cor pulmonale may not be able to adequately augment their cardiac output as needed for normal gestation (1, 6, 9).

Information on the effect of pregnancy on CF is derived mostly from limited observation, case reports, chart reviews, and the North American Cystic Fibrosis Foundation registry (4, 6, 10–12). Overall, women with CF who become pregnant and do not have severe disease tolerate pregnancy without significant untoward events (1, 6, 9–14). The maternal mortality rate does not exceed that in age-matched controls if airflow obstruction is mild and pancreatic function is sufficient (1, 6, 9–14). An FEV_1 greater than 70% is generally considered to define mild airflow obstruction. An FEV_1 less than 50% has generally been considered a contraindication to pregnancy, but there are reports of women with CF and an FEV_1 less than 50% who have had successful pregnancies without significant adverse affects on their disease (1, 10, 13). Pulmonary function may decline during pregnancy, but for most patients who have stable disease before conception, this decline does not seem to be greater than that of age-matched controls (10, 11). Pregnant women with CF often require hospitalization for acute exacerbation of their pulmonary disease and often need parenteral antibiotics (11, 13). Pulmonary hypertension, especially if cor pulmonale exists, poses substantial risk to the patient with CF who becomes pregnant (1, 6, 9). Because of underlying progressive disease of the pancreas, pregnant women with CF have an increased incidence of glucose intolerance and gestational diabetes, especially if they need corticosteroids for exacerbations of obstructive pulmonary disease. Pancreatic insufficiency may also present problems for the woman with CF who becomes pregnant; this is because of the increased nutritional demands of pregnancy and because malabsorption may lead to diminished absorption of fat-soluble vitamins (6, 9).

Effect of Cystic Fibrosis on Pregnancy

Because no prospective studies have been done and because the rate of infertility is increased in women with CF, it is difficult to know whether the incidence of early fetal loss is increased in these women. The overall perinatal mortality rate (7.9% to 11%) seems to be increased and is directly related to the severity of CF (6, 12). Most of the increase in fetal mortality is related to the increased likelihood of prematurity (24% to 35%). Women with CF also have an increased risk for IUGR. In general, pregnancy outcome depends on disease severity and stability at the time of conception. Some use the Schwachman scoring system to assess disease status. This system assigns quantitative values in four categories—physical findings, general activity, nutritional status, and chest radiography—and produces a total score that many consider to be unhelpful and outdated (6). Clinical severity is generally assessed on the basis of pulmonary status (pulmonary function test results, arterial blood gases, colonization or infection with multidrug-resistant organisms such as *B. cepacia*, and evidence of pulmonary hypertension or right heart failure), degree of pancreatic insufficiency, and overall nutritional status (6, 9–14). Inadequate weight gain during pregnancy is a poor prognostic sign in women with CF (10, 12).

Care of the Pregnant Patient with Cystic Fibrosis

Maintenance therapy and routine respiratory management should be continued throughout gestation as needed (1, 13). Certain medications may be substituted for others during the first trimester (for example, H_2-antagonists may be substituted for proton-pump inhibitors). Daily exercise may be helpful in mobilizing pulmonary secretions. Inhaled steroids may be used as indicated during pregnancy. Office spirometry should be done at each prenatal visit. Antibiotics, such as aminoglycosides and antipseudomonal penicillins and cephalosporins, are often necessary to treat recurrent pulmonary infections and have been used safely during pregnancy (1, 11, 13). Maternal weight gain and general nutritional status should be continuously managed. Patients with severe pancreatic insufficiency and malnutrition may need supplemental parenteral nutrition. Some recommend periodically checking the international normalized ratio as an indicator of vitamin K absorption (1). Fetal growth and well-being may be monitored by serial ultrasonography and nonstress tests beginning at 28 weeks of gestation. Labor may need to be induced if evidence of IUGR is seen, and the pregnancy may need to be terminated if the mother's life is at risk because of severe worsening of disease (1, 9). In the past, breastfeeding by mothers with CF was discouraged because of fear that the normally low sodium concentration in breastmilk might be elevated, just as the sweat of most patients with CF is hypernatremic. However, milk from patients with CF has been analyzed and found to contain normal concentrations of electrolytes and macronutrients (15).

Sarcoidosis

Sarcoidosis is a disease of unknown cause that commonly affects young adults and, therefore, women of childbearing age. The characteristic noncaseating granulomas may be found in almost any organ but are most common in the lung, lymph nodes, eyes, and skin. Typically, the diagnosis of sarcoidosis is made in an asymptomatic person as a result of a routine chest radiograph, although patients may have dyspnea, nonproductive cough, and atypical chest pain. Abnormal laboratory test results include a decreased lymphocyte count, hyperglobulinemia, an elevated sedimentation rate, and an elevated angiotensin-converting enzyme level. Other laboratory abnormalities depend on the organs involved. The lung is almost always involved, and a chest radiograph usually shows bilateral hilar adenopathy with or without interstitial or alveolar infiltrates. Occasionally, only the infiltrates are seen (16). Pulmonary function tests typically show decreased lung volume with normal flow rates and an abnormal diffusing capacity.

Fertility is unaffected by sarcoidosis (16). Sarcoidosis does not increase fetal or obstetric complications and usually does not alter management of pregnancy, labor, or delivery (16). Pregnancy usually has no effect on the course of the disease, but it may result in a temporary improvement. Relapse may occur 3 to 6 months postpartum (16). There are case reports of women with sarcoidosis whose disease worsens during pregnancy, but this is uncommon (17). Symptomatic disease usually responds to corticosteroids. Women who are using steroids at the time of conception usually require the same or smaller doses during gestation (16) and will require stress doses during labor and delivery.

Connective Tissue Disorders

The most common type of lung disease seen in patients with connective tissue disease (CTD) is a chronic interstitial lung disease (ILD) that is indistinguishable from idiopathic pulmonary fibrosis (16). This ILD occurs in up to 20% of patients with rheumatoid arthritis. Other CTDs that may show ILD are scleroderma, systemic lupus erythematosus, Sjögren syndrome, polymyositis, and dermatomyositis. It is unclear whether the pregnancy affects the pulmonary disease or vice versa, but pregnancy usually has little effect on CTDs in general.

Idiopathic Pulmonary Fibrosis

Idiopathic pulmonary fibrosis usually has onset in the sixth or seventh decade of life and is therefore distinctly uncommon in women of childbearing age (16). It usually presents with cough and dry rales. Chest radiographs show diffuse interstitial infiltrates. Pulmonary function tests show a restrictive pattern with decreased diffusing capacity and hypoxemia. Mean survival is 4 to 6 years after diagnosis (16). Because of poor prognosis and because cytotoxic agents are often needed for treatment, pregnancy is usually discouraged. However, if a woman can improve her oxygen consumption threefold over resting levels, she will probably be able to tolerate pregnancy and delivery (16).

Lymphangioleiomyomatosis

Lymphangioleiomyomatosis (LAM) affects only women and may occur during the childbearing years. It is characterized by dyspnea, cough, chest pain, and hemoptysis. Chylous pleural effusions, when present, strongly suggest the diagnosis, but open-lung biopsy is usually required for confirmation (16). The onset or exacerbation of the disease may coincide with pregnancy. Sex hor-

mones, especially estrogen, may play a role in pathogenesis. Estrogen receptors are not seen in normal lungs but are present in lungs of patients with
LAM (16). Most women with LAM are advised to avoid pregnancy and oral
contraceptive use for fear of exacerbating the disease (16).

Pulmonary Histiocytosis X

Also known as eosinophilic granuloma of the lung, pulmonary histiocytosis X
occurs almost exclusively in current or former smokers between 20 and 40
years of age. It probably has little effect on pregnancy unless diabetes insipidus supervenes (18).

Kyphoscoliosis

The bony deformity of the spine known as *kyphoscoliosis* is of unknown cause
and is more common in women than in men. Its incidence in pregnancy is
less than 1 in 1000. It may cause prematurity but does not seem to increase
other complications of pregnancy. Pregnancy probably has little or no effect
on the disease (16).

Other Lung Diseases

Obstructive sleep apnea may be present in women who become pregnant, but
it seems to be well tolerated by the fetus, even when the mother requires continuous positive airway pressure and supplemental oxygen (19, 20). Pregnant
women reported a higher incidence of snoring during pregnancy in one uncontrolled study, but the snoring was not associated with daytime sleepiness
or compromised fetal outcome (21).

Chronic obstructive lung disease is rare in women of childbearing age.
One case report (22) described a woman with bullous emphysema secondary
to alpha$_1$-antitrypsin deficiency who delivered a healthy baby despite a spontaneous pneumothorax that required a chest tube at 21 weeks of gestation.

Pregnancy has been reported in women with Wegener granulomatosis. Cyclophosphamide and corticosteroids have been used successfully to treat this
disease during pregnancy, but it is preferable to withhold cyclophosphamide
until the second trimester because of potential teratogenicity. To minimize
the duration of exposure to cyclophosphamide, delivery should probably occur as soon as the fetal lungs are mature (23, 24).

Lung cancer in women of childbearing age is rare but may increase as
more young women smoke. Non–small-cell cancer stage I, II, and IIIA can be

surgically resected in the second trimester. Postoperative radiation may be given, if necessary, with abdominal shielding. To date, no cases of metastatic disease to the fetus have been reported. Inoperable tumors can be treated with radiation and chemotherapy, usually during the second trimester, to reduce risk to the fetus. Because of the very aggressive nature of small-cell lung cancer, chemotherapy should be instituted at the time of diagnosis, regardless of gestational age. Fetal growth restriction is a concern and should be monitored with serial ultrasonography. Corticosteroids may be used to hasten fetal lung maturity starting at 24 weeks of gestation. Fetal well-being should be monitored with biweekly nonstress tests beginning at 26 to 28 weeks of gestation. Amniocentesis should be done at 35 weeks of gestation, and the baby should be delivered as soon as the lungs are mature (25).

REFERENCES

1. **Kotloff RM, FitzSimmons SC, Fiel SB.** Fertility and pregnancy in patients with cystic fibrosis. Clin Chest Med. 1992;13:623-35.

2. **Brock DJ.** Prenatal screening for cystic fibrosis: 5 years' experience reviewed. Lancet. 1996;347:148-50.

3. **Doksum T, Bernhardt BA.** Population-based screening for cystic fibrosis. Clin Obstet Gynecol. 1996;39:763-71.

4. **Holmes LB, Pyeritz RE.** Screening for cystic fibrosis (Letter). JAMA. 1998;279:1068-9.

5. **Eng CM, Schecter C, Robinowitz J, Fulop G, Burgert T, Levy B, et al.** Prenatal genetic carrier testing using triple disease screening. JAMA. 1997;278:1268-72.

6. **Hilman BC, Aitken ML, Constantinescu M.** Pregnancy in patients with cystic fibrosis. Clin Obstet Gynecol. 1996;39:70-86.

7. **Durie PR.** Pancreatitis and mutations of the cystic fibrosis gene. N Engl J Med. 1998;339:687-8.

8. **Doherty RA, Bradley LA, Haddow JE.** Prenatal screening for cystic fibrosis: an updated perspective. Am J Obstet Gynecol. 1997;176:268-70.

9. **Canny GJ.** Pregnancy in patients with cystic fibrosis. Can Med Assoc J. 1993;149:805-6.

10. **Frangolias DD, Nakielna EM, Wilcox PG.** Pregnancy and cystic fibrosis: a case-controlled study. Chest. 1997;111:963-9.

11. **Canny GJ, Corey M, Livingstone RA, Carpenter S, Green L, Levison H.** Pregnancy and cystic fibrosis. Obstet Gynecol. 1991;77:850-3.

12. **Kent NE, Farquharson DF.** Cystic fibrosis in pregnancy. Can Med Assoc J. 1993;149:809-13.

13. **Edenborough FP, Stableforth DE, Webb AK, Mackenzie WE, Smith DL.** Outcome of pregnancy in women with cystic fibrosis. Thorax. 1995;50:170-4.

14. **Stableforth DE, Mackenzie WE.** Pregnancy in women with cystic fibrosis. BMJ. 1995;311:822-3.

15. **Shiffman ML, Seale TW, Flux M, Rennert OR, Swender PT.** Breast-milk composition in women with cystic fibrosis: report of two cases and a review of the literature. Am J Clin Nutr. 1989;49:612-7.

16. **King TE.** Restrictive lung disease in pregnancy. Clin Chest Med. 1992;13:607-22.

17. **Haynes de Regt R.** Sarcoidosis and pregnancy. Obstet Gynecol. 1987;70:369-72.

18. **DiMaggio LA, Lippes HA, Lee RV.** Histiocytosis X and pregnancy. Obstet Gynecol. 1995;85:806-9.

19. **Lewis DF, Chesson AL, Edwards, MS, Weeks JW, Adair CD.** Obstructive sleep apnea during pregnancy resulting in pulmonary hypertension. South Med J. 1998;91:761-2.

20. **Charbonneau M, Falcone T, Cosio MG, Levy RD.** Obstructive sleep apnea during pregnancy: therapy and implications for fetal health. Am Rev Respir Dis. 1991;144: 461-3.

21. **Loube MDI, Poceta JS, Morales MC, Peacock MMD, Mitler MM.** Self-reported snoring in pregnancy: association with fetal outcomes. Chest. 1996;109:885-9.

22. **Atkinson AR.** Pregnancy and alpha-1 antitrypsin deficiency. Postgrad Med J. 1987; 63:817-20.

23. **Luisiri P, Lance NJ, Curran JJ.** Wegener's granulomatosis in pregnancy. Arthritis Rheum. 1997;40:1354-60.

24. **Dayoan ES, Dimen LL, Boylen CT.** Successful treatment of Wegener's granulomatosis during pregnancy: a case report and review of the medical literature. Chest. 1998;113:836-8.

25. **Van Winter JT, Wilkowske MA, Shaw EG, Ogburn PL, Pritchard DJ.** Lung cancer complicating pregnancy: case report and review of literature. Mayo Clin Proc. 1995; 70:384-7.

APPENDIX: DRUGS FOR PULMONARY DISORDERS

The drug table on page 421 is for reference when there is a clinical indication for treatment with one of the medications listed. Decisions about medication use in pregnancy should be made on the basis of a benefit-to-risk ratio, avoiding unnecessary treatment of symptoms but with consideration of the fact that fetal well-being depends on maternal well-being. Because the U.S. Food and Drug Administration is working on a new classification system of medications used in pregnancy, we have classified medications as follows:

Data Suggest Drug Use May Be Justified When Indicated
When data and/or experience supports the safety of the drug.

Data Suggest Drug Use May Be Justified in Some Circumstances
When less extensive or desirable data are reported, but the drug is reasonable as a second-line therapy or may be used on the basis of the severity of maternal illness.

Data Suggest Drug Use Is Rarely Justified
Use drug only when alternatives supported by more experience and/or a better safety profile are not available.

Pregnancy pharmacokinetics may necessitate a significant increase in dose or dosing frequency, and dosing recommendations may require modification according to individual circumstances.

Drugs for Pulmonary Disorders

Drug	Use May Be Justified When Indicated	Use May Be Justified in Some Circumstances	Use Is Rarely Justified	Comment/Dose Adjustment
Anti-inflammatory agents				No known adverse effects
Cromolyn sodium	√			
Beclomethasone (inhaled)	√			
Prednisone	√			
Anti-inflammatory agents				
Triamcinolone		√		
Fluticasone		√		
Antihistamines (first trimester)		√		
Chlorpheniramine		√		
Tripelennamine		√		
Diphenhydramine		√		
Antihistamines (second and third trimester)	√			
Diphenhydramine preferred	√			
Antitussives	√			
Guaifenesin	√			
Dextromethorphan	√			
Bronchodilators	√			No known adverse effects
Albuterol	√			
Metaproterenol	√			
Theophylline	√			
Bronchodilators (inhaled)		√		
Salmeterol		√		
Ipratropium		√		
Decongestants				
Pseudoephedrine				
Nasal steroids	√			
Ephedrine			√	Adverse effect on placental flow
Leukotriene modifiers			√	
Prostaglandin $F_{2\alpha}$			√	Used for uterine constriction Can cause severe bronchoconstriction Contraindicated in asthmatic patients
Nonsedating antihistamines (all trimesters)		√		
Cetrizine				
loratidine				
Fexofandine				

CHAPTER 8

Hematology

I. Thromboembolic Disease and Hypercoagulable States
Karen Rosene-Montella, MD, and Linda Anne Barbour, MD, MSPH

II. Bleeding Disorders
Janis Bormanis, MD

III. Platelets and Platelet Disorders
Robert F. Burrows, MD, and Elizabeth A. Burrows, BA, MBA

IV. Anemia
Janis Bormanis, MD

V. Hemoglobinopathies
Kathryn Hassell, MsD

VI. Maternal Isoimmunization
Erin Keely, MD

I. Thromboembolic Disease and Hypercoagulable States
Karen Rosene-Montella and Linda Anne Barbour

Thrombosis during pregnancy presents diagnostic and therapeutic challenges. Venous thromboembolism (VTE) complicates 0.5 to 3.0 of every 1000 pregnancies and is the leading nonobstetric cause of maternal death (1–4). In the United States, 50% of all cases of VTE in women younger than 40 years of age are associated with pregnancy. Pulmonary embolism (PE) was responsible for 11% of pregnancy-related deaths in the United States in the years 1987 to 1990 (5).

Key Values and Normal Physiologic Changes for Hematologic Disorders

	Direction of Change	Percentage Change or Normal Range for Pregnancy
Anti-Xa assay (heparin)	↔	
B$_{12}$	↔	
Clotting factors	Most ↑	See Table 8-1
FE	↓	
Ferritin	↔	If ↓, need ↑ iron replacement
Fibrinogen	↑↑	500 to 600 mg/dL
Folate	↓	
Hb (hemoglobin)	↓	10 to 13 g/dL
Plasma volume	↑↑	30% to 50%
Platelet count	↓ gradual to term	150,000 to 200,000
Protein S	↓ free	Progressive ↓ to term
PT, PTT, INR	↔	
RBC mass	↑	20%
Sedimentation rate (ESR)	↑	1 to 80 mm/h
TIBC	↑	
WBC	↑	10,000 to 16,000/mm^3

↑ Increase
↓ Decrease
↔ No change

The mortality rate for patients with untreated PE is 15% to 40%. The risk for embolization from untreated proximal deep venous thrombosis (DVT) is 20% to 40%, and the incidence of postphlebitic syndrome after DVT during pregnancy is 32% to 49% (6). It is imperative to prevent thromboembolism when feasible. If thromboembolism is suspected, diagnosis and treatment should be immediate and effective. Most practitioners hesitate to use standard diagnostic and therapeutic tools in pregnant women; the correct approach to VTE during pregnancy may seem counterintuitive. The goal of this section is to translate current information about VTE and thrombophilia into practical guidelines for management of these conditions during pregnancy.

Predisposing Factors

Pregnancy alone confers a five- to six-fold increase in the risk for thromboembolism relative to the nonpregnant state. This is due to a combination of two factors: 1) stasis due to hormonal and mechanical effects on the venous system and 2) hypercoagulability associated with the normal increase in clotting factors and decreased fibrinolysis (Table 8-1). A history of VTE further in-

Table 8-1 Some Effects of Pregnancy on Coagulation

Factor*	Effect of Pregnancy
Platelets	Slow decrease during pregnancy; further decrease after delivery; marked increase postpartum day 3 to 5; increase in aggregation
Fibrinogen	Marked increase during antepartum period; no change during labor but prompt decrease after placental delivery; increase to predelivery level by postpartum day 3 to 5 with slow decrease thereafter
Prothrombin	No change
Factor V	Immediate increase after placental delivery; slow decrease to normal by postpartum day 7
Factor VII, IX, X	Progressive increase during pregnancy; gradual decrease in puerperium
Factor VIII	Progressive increase during pregnancy; decrease after delivery with secondary increase and then gradual decrease
Factor XI, XIII	Decrease during pregnancy; gradual increase to normal in puerperium
Fibrin split products	Increase in labor and immediately postpartum
Fibrinolysis	Decrease after first trimester with prompt increase to normal after delivery
Protein S	Gradual decrease in free levels during pregnancy
Protein C	No change
Antithrombin III	No change or decrease; decrease in presence of preeclampsia or nephrotic syndrome
Activated protein C resistance: functional assay	Increased by PTT-based assay
Activated protein C resistance: genetic assay (PCR for factor V Leiden)	No change

*Clotting factors return to normal by 8 weeks postpartum.
Adapted from Rosene-Montella K, Ginsberg JS. Thromboembolic disease in pregnancy. In: Elkayam U, Gleicher N, eds. Cardiac Problems in Pregnancy. New York: Wiley-Liss; 1998:223-35.

creases this risk; the rate of recurrence is estimated at 7.5% to 12% (7, 8). No clear data stratify risk for recurrence on the basis of the circumstances in which the previous event occurred, and this makes it difficult to assign absolute risk in a given person. The data emerging from nonpregnant persons support the idea that a clot that arises de novo with no obvious associated risk factors may have particular significance for recurrence risk. It is not yet known, however, whether this is the case in pregnant women. The presence of an underlying hypercoagulable state can further increase the risk for recurrence to 25% to 70%, depending on the specific thrombophilia (9). Other predisposing factors include cesarean section or other surgical procedure, obesity, prolonged hospitalization and bedrest, and advanced age and parity.

Hypercoagulability as a Predisposing Factor

Our knowledge about thrombophilia has grown enormously in the past 5 years and has had a tremendous effect on current recommendations for the investigation of VTE during pregnancy. Each of the known thrombophilias has been detected in association with thrombosis during pregnancy, and each is known to increase the risk for VTE (Table 8-2). It is important to keep in mind that thrombosis can occur not only in the deep venous and systemic arterial circulation but also in the placental bed. Thus, anything that can cause thrombosis during pregnancy can cause placental thrombosis, which may lead to intrauterine growth restriction (IUGR), fetal demise, and early-onset, severe preeclampsia. It was previously believed that antiphospholipid antibodies (including lupus anticoagulant) were the primary cause of placental thrombosis, but it now appears that the factor V Leiden mutation (conferring activated protein C [APC] resistance) may be an even more common contributor to placental infarction (10). Deficiencies in protein C, protein S, antithrombin III, and hyperhomocystinemia have also been reported in association with placental thrombosis (Table 8-3). A history of pregnancy

Table 8-2 Risk for Recurrence of Thrombosis (Percent) in Pregnancy with Previous Venous Thromboembolism

Previous VTE only	7.5–12
AT III deficiency	50–70
Protein C deficiency	16–25
Protein S deficiency	10–20
APC resistance	30–40
Hyperhomocystinemia	No data

Table 8-3 Placental Vascular Complications Associated with Thrombophilia

	Miscarriages	IUFD	Preeclampsia	HELLP Syndrome
Antithrombin III deficiency	DA	DA	PA	
Protein C deficiency	PA	DA	PA	
Protein S deficiency	PA	DA	PA	PA
Dysfibrinogenemia	PA	DA	PA	
Activated protein C resistance	PA	DA	DA	
Factor V Leiden mutation	PA	DA	DA	PA
Hyperhomocystinemia	PA	PA	PA	PA
Antiphospholipid syndrome	DA	DA	DA	PA
Combined defects	DA	DA	PA	PA

IUFD = intrauterine fetal death; DA = definite association; PA = possible association.
Adapted from Brenner B, Blumenfeld A. Thrombophilia and fetal loss. Blood Rev. 1997;11:72-9.

complications that suggest placental thrombosis may be as important as family history when the likelihood of an inherited or acquired thrombophilia is being considered.

It is important to understand the timing of thrombosis associated with a hypercoagulable state. Fifty percent of VTE episodes occur in patients younger than 35 years of age. Moreover, in at least 50% of patients with an underlying hypercoagulable state, a first episode of thrombosis will occur in association with an additional risk factor. In young women, this additional risk factor is most often pregnancy or use of oral contraceptives. In recent studies of a subgroup of patients whose venous thrombosis occurred during pregnancy or in the puerperium, the incidence of APC resistance was 40% to 78% (11). This new information makes it clear that thrombosis should not be dismissed as resulting from pregnancy, oral contraceptive use, surgery, or other provoking events until the presence of an underlying hypercoagulable state has been excluded. This information is essential to informed recommendations for long-term care, has implications for future pregnancies and need for prophylaxis, and is essential for adequate genetic counseling. Obstetric and nonobstetric indications for evaluation for thrombophilia are outlined in Box 8-1.

Location and Timing of Venous Thromboembolism

In pregnancy, DVT has an overwhelming propensity to occur in the left leg (12). The reason for this is not known but is assumed to be exaggerated compression of the left iliac vein by the right iliac artery, which exacerbates the normal venous stasis associated with pregnancy.

Box 8-1 Indications for Diagnostic Evaluation for Thrombophilia

Nonobstetric
  Family history of thrombophilia
  Early-onset venous thromboembolism
  Recurrent thrombosis
  Thrombosis at unusual site
Obstetric
  Early-onset severe preeclampsia
  Fetal demise
  Intrauterine growth restriction
  Placental thrombosis
  Previous child with cerebral palsy
  Neural tube defect (marker for hyperhomocystinemia)

Excellent data support the conclusion that VTE is not primarily a third-trimester and postpartum phenomenon. On the contrary, most cases of DVT occur before delivery, and the events are evenly distributed among the trimesters (Table 8-4) (13). In a study of 17,000 pregnancies (3), 75% of DVTs were antepartum, and half of these had occurred by 15 weeks of gestation. In the same study, 66% of pulmonary emboli occurred postpartum, and 80% of these occurred after cesarean section. Any recommendations about prophylaxis must take into account the timing and nature of this risk for thrombosis, which is present throughout gestation and the postpartum period.

Diagnosis of Deep Venous Thromboembolism and Pulmonary Embolism

Diagnostic Problems

The clinical diagnosis of DVT and PE is unreliable in nonpregnant patients and is further complicated during pregnancy. Nonthrombotic causes of leg pain and swelling are common in pregnancy, and the compressive effects of the gravid uterus can make interpretation of diagnostic tests difficult. Furthermore, isolated iliac vein thrombosis, which may not be detected by routine diagnostic methods, occurs with increased frequency during pregnancy. Finally, the mean age of pregnant patients with PE is much lower than that of nonpregnant patients with PE. This means that pregnant patients with PE are less likely than nonpregnant patients with PE to have comorbid conditions. They are likely to look clinically "well" and to have normal arterial blood gases, even in the presence of significant PE. In a recent retrospective review (14), 58% of 17 pregnant patients with documented PE had normal A-a gradients.

Diagnostic Testing for Deep Venous Thromboembolism

Compression ultrasonography (CUS) is the noninvasive test of choice for the diagnosis of DVT during pregnancy. It is very sensitive for proximal DVT in symptomatic outpatients; the most reliable finding is a noncompressable venous segment (15). The safety of withholding anticoagulation if CUS results remain normal within 7 days of presentation has been shown in nonpregnant patients. Because pregnant patients often present earlier in the course of illness, it may be reasonable to repeat CUS 3 to 7 days after a negative result and again at 14 days in patients with persistent symptoms. Although CUS is very sensitive for thrombi in the common femoral, superficial femoral, and

Table 8-4 Timing of Deep Venous Thrombosis and Pulmonary Emboli in Pregnancy

Author	Events (n)	DVT Antepartum (%)	Antepartum Events (%) Occurring During Trimester:			DVT Postpartum (%)	PE Antepartum (%)	PE Postpartum (%)
			One	Two	Three			
Aaro	77	36	12	35	53	64	23	77
Hellgren	23	78	33	33	33	22		
Bergqvist	17	Only antepartum events reported	24	41	35			
Tengborn	12	67	37	*	*	33		
Rutherford	93	75	51	*	*	25	34	66†
Ginsberg	60	Only antepartum events reported	22	47	31			

DVT = deep venous thrombosis; PE = pulmonary emboli.

*Only the percent of antepartum events occurring during the first trimester are reported.

†82% of postpartum emboli occurred after cesarean delivery.

From Barbour LA. Current concepts of anticoagulant therapy in pregnancy. Obstet Gynecol Clin North Am. 1997;24:499-521; with permission.

popliteal veins, it may be insensitive to isolated iliac DVT. It is also insensitive to calf DVT, which may propagate in pregnancy. If calf DVT is suspected, serial CUS, impedance plethysmography, or limited venography may be necessary. Patients in whom iliac DVT is suspected (patients who have severe back or flank pain with or without cramping abdominal pain in association with unilateral leg swelling or swelling of an entire extremity) should have further diagnostic testing (Figure 8-1). Magnetic resonance imaging (MRI) or indirect

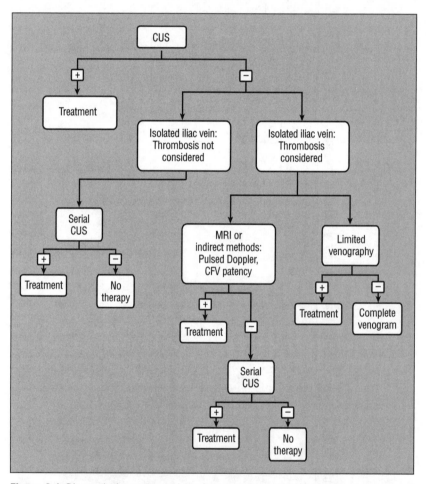

Figure 8-1 Diagnosis by compression ultrasonography (CUS) of clinically suspected deep venous thrombosis during pregnancy. Plus signs indicate positive results; minus signs indicate negative results. CFV = compressed femoral vein; MRI = magnetic resonance imaging. (Adapted from Rosene-Montella K, Ginsberg JS. Thromboembolic disease in pregnancy. In: Elkayam U, Gleicher N, eds. Cardiac Problems in Pregnancy. New York: Wiley-Liss; 1998:223-35.)

approaches, such as measurement of the diameter of the iliac vein or application of pulsed Doppler sampling of the common femoral vein, should be used to detect iliac vein thrombosis. If neither MRI nor an indirect approach is available, limited venography with pelvic shielding that does not obscure visualization of the iliac vein is an acceptable alternative.

Diagnostic Testing for Pulmonary Embolism

The tests that are useful in patients with clinically suspected PE are ventilation–perfusion lung scanning, pulmonary angiography, and the tests described above for the diagnosis of DVT. The tests for DVT are used because the detection of DVT in a patient with clinically suspected PE is enough to allow the diagnosis of PE and treatment with anticoagulation without further testing (16). Chest radiography and electrocardiography should be used to exclude other diagnoses. The most common electrocardiographic abnormality other than sinus tachycardia is T-wave inversion in the anterior leads, especially V1–V4. Recent echocardiographic data showed right ventricular hypokinesis in 40% of patients with PE who were evaluated, so the electrocardiogram changes are thought to represent reciprocal changes from the inferoposterior ischemia that occur when the right coronary artery is compressed by the volume- or pressure-overloaded right ventricle (17).

Ventilation–perfusion lung scanning is the diagnostic test of choice for pregnant patients in whom PE is suspected. The amount of radiation absorbed by the fetus is about 0.2 rads, an amount well below the 5 rads recommended by the National Commission on Radiation Protection (NCRP) as the maximum allowable exposure for the entire pregnancy. Given the maternal mortality rate associated with untreated PE, the benefit of making the diagnosis clearly outweighs the risks of the scanning procedure. In nonpregnant patients, the positive predictive value of a normal or high-probability perfusion scan (segmental or large subsegmental defect with normal ventilation) is 90%, so diagnostic evaluation can end at this point. If the lung scan is normal, PE is excluded; if the scan is high probability, PE is diagnosed (Figure 8-2). Unfortunately, at least half of all patients have neither a normal nor a high-probability scan but a nondiagnostic, intermediate, or indeterminate scan. The prevalence of PE in both nonpregnant and pregnant patients with such scans is still approximately 25%, so further investigation is clearly indicated. Pulmonary angiography can and should be done in pregnant patients in this category if evaluation of the lower extremities has not detected DVT. Fetal radiation exposure can be minimized by using the brachial or internal jugular approach when possible; if the femoral approach is used, fluoroscopy over the pelvis should be minimized. Table 8-5 summarizes the radiation exposure to the fetus associated with various diagnostic procedures.

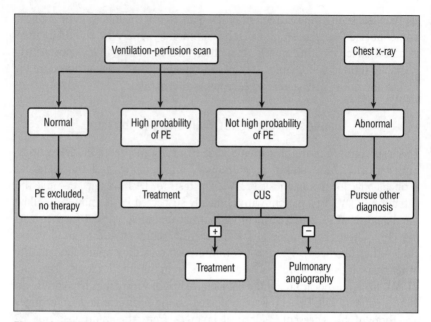

Figure 8-2 Diagnosis of clinically suspected pulmonary embolism (PE) during pregnancy by means of ventilation-perfusion scan/plain chest radiography. CUS = compression ultrasonography. (Adapted from Rosene-Montella K, Ginsberg JS. Thromboembolic disease in pregnancy. In: Elkayam U, Gleicher N, eds. Cardiac Problems in Pregnancy. New York: Wiley-Liss; 1998:223-35.)

Other Thromboses

The final consideration in diagnostic investigation for thrombosis during pregnancy should be an awareness of unusual thromboses that can occur during pregnancy (1). *Ovarian vein thrombosis*, which has a right-side preponderance, presents with flank, back, or groin pain and is often seen in the setting of postpartum endometritis with persistent fever (3). Because propagation into the inferior vena cava and embolization have been seen with this thrombosis, it should be viewed as a true DVT and treated accordingly (2). A clinical diagnosis of septic pelvic thrombophlebitis is no longer acceptable. When septic pelvic thrombophlebitis is suspected, MRI, magnetic resonance with venography (MRV), or computed tomography should be done.

Cerebral sinus venous thrombosis occurs with increased frequency during pregnancy and the postpartum period and may present as severe headache with or without neurologic findings. When this diagnosis is suspected, MRI/MRV should be used. Mutations in the prothrombin gene and the factor V gene are associated with a further increase in risk for cerebral venous thrombosis.

Table 8-5 Estimated Fetal Exposure to Radiation from Various Diagnostic Procedures

Procedure	Estimated Fetal Radiation Exposure (rads)
Bilateral venography without abdominal shield	0.628
Unilateral venography without abdominal shield	0.314
Limited venography	<0.050
Pulmonary angiography via femoral route	0.221–0.374
Pulmonary angiography via brachial route	<0.050
Perfusion lung scan using ^{99m}Tc-MAA:	
3 mCi	0.018
1–2 mCi	0.006–0.012
Ventilation lung scan using:	
^{133}Xe	0.004–0.019
^{99m}Tc-DTPA	0.007–0.035
^{99m}Tc-SC	0.001–0.005
Radioisotope venography using ^{99m}Tc	0.001–0.005
^{125}I-fibrinogen leg scan	2.000
Chest X-ray	<0.001

^{99m}Tc-MAA = technetium-labelled macroaggregated albumin. ^{99m}Tc-DPTA = technetium-labelled diethylene-triamine pentaacetic acid. ^{99m}Tc-SC = technetium-labelled sulfur colloid. ^{133}Xe = xenon-133 (the isotope itself) (gas).
From Rosene-Montella K, Ginsberg JS. Thromboembolic disease in pregnancy. In: Elkayam U, Gleicher N, eds. Cardiac Problems in Pregnancy. New York: Wiley-Liss; 1988:223-35; with permission.

An unusually high incidence of *subclavian vein thrombosis* in the absence of intravenous catheter use has been reported in association with ovarian hyperstimulation. The ovarian hyperstimulation syndrome, which occurs with hormonal therapy used in conjunction with assisted reproductive technology, is characterized by ascites, pleural effusions, and azotemia and often includes DVT.

Treatment of Venous Thromboembolism

Choice of Anticoagulant

Fetal Considerations
Heparin is the anticoagulant of choice during pregnancy because it does not cross the placenta and its safety for the fetus is clearly established (18). By enhancing the action of antithrombin III, heparin prevents further thrombus formation and allows time for fibrinolysis to dissolve established clot. Risks of heparin therapy are to the mother only and include risks for bleeding, under-

or over-anticoagulation, thrombocytopenia, and osteoporosis. Warfarin, however, crosses the placenta and therefore poses significant risk for both bleeding of the fetus and teratogenicity. An embryopathy similar to chondromalacia punctata (stippled epiphyses and nasal and limb hypoplasia) has been reported in at least 5% to 10% of infants exposed to warfarin between 6 and 12 weeks of gestation (19). Although prevention of first-trimester exposure may avert skeletal embryopathy, the risk for fetal bleeding persists throughout gestation, resulting in a high rate of fetal loss. Fetal central nervous system (CNS) abnormalities that are probably secondary to bleeding (including dorsal and ventral midline dysplasias and midline cerebellar atrophy) may result from warfarin exposure at any point in gestation. These conditions present as microcephaly, optic atrophy, or mental retardation. Warfarin is further contraindicated toward term, when the combination of delivery-induced trauma and anticoagulation can cause serious bleeding in the neonate. Warfarin use during pregnancy is usually restricted to patients with mechanical heart valves between 12 and 34 weeks of gestation because of the high failure rates seen with therapeutic doses of standard heparin in these patients (see Chapter 6).

Maternal Considerations

The major maternal considerations in heparin therapy are bleeding and risk for inadequate anticoagulation. The rate of major bleeding in a cohort study of pregnant patients receiving therapeutic heparin was 2%; this is consistent with the reported rates of bleeding associated with heparin therapy in nonpregnant patients and with warfarin therapy for DVT (20). The risk for inadequate anticoagulation is enhanced by increased heparin requirements and the difficulty of maintaining anticoagulation with subcutaneous heparin (see Chapter 9). Some patients need up to 40,000 U/d to prolong the activated partial thromboplastin time (aPTT); dosages as high as 20,000 U every 8 hours may be required to maintain adequate levels during subcutaneous administration (21). When pregnant patients have unusually high heparin requirements, the aPTT may not be the best way to monitor dose requirements. When monitoring was done by using anti-factor Xa levels instead of aPTTs in a similar nonpregnant group (21), lesser doses were required and unnecessary dose escalation was avoided.

Other possible maternal complications of heparin therapy include heparin hypersensitivity manifesting as skin reactions, heparin-induced thrombocytopenia, and heparin-induced osteoporosis.Thrombocytopenia is a well-recognized complication of heparin therapy. It occurs in 1% to 3% of patients, and two forms of it have been described (22). An early nonimmune thrombocytopenia can occur 2 to 5 days after the start of heparin therapy as a result of direct activation by unfractionated heparin but is not associated with adverse clinical effects and does not necessitate discontinuation of therapy. The immune form of heparin-induced thrombocytopenia is caused by heparin-induced IgG platelet antibodies, which lead to serotonin-induced platelet aggregation and significant risk for thrombotic complications. This form of thrombocytopenia is seen at 5 to 15 days but can occur earlier in patients previously exposed to heparin. Careful monitoring of platelet counts during the first 3 weeks of heparin therapy is necessary. Thrombocytopenia is much less likely to occur with low-molecular-weight heparin (LMWH), so use of LMWH is a possible alternative (23).

Heparin-induced osteoporosis is a more common complication of long-term therapy with standard heparin (24, 25). Although the risk for fracture is low (<2%), most studies confirm a subclinical reduction in bone density of 5% to 10% in up to 20% to 30% of pregnant patients. The effects are thought to be at least partly reversible, and no dose-response relation is evident. In pregnant patients exposed to heparin, postpartum bone density measurements, with recommendations for calcium, vitamin D, and weightbearing exercise if osteopenia is detected, should be considered. This complication may be less common with LMWH, but this is not certain.

Low-Molecular-Weight Heparin

In nonpregnant patients, LMWH has been shown to be at least as effective and safe as unfractionated heparin for the treatment of acute VTE and for the prevention of VTE in patients undergoing general or orthopedic surgery (26). Numerous studies confirm that LMWH does not cross the placenta; this implies that LMWH should be as safe for the fetus as standard heparin. In addition, LMWH has the advantages to the mother of a longer half-life and less binding to proteins, macrophages, and endothelium; these advantages lead to better bioavailability and a more predictable dose response, allowing the drug to be given in fixed doses without laboratory monitoring in nonpregnant patients. In pregnant patients, pharmacokinetic studies show increasing LMWH requirements with increasing gestation; thus, LMWH therapy must be monitored in all pregnant patients (27). Various LMWH preparations may differ in anti-factor Xa activity, so monitoring may need to be tailored to the individual preparation. Furthermore, good evidence suggests that LMWH has a minimal effect on platelets and vascular permeability and, therefore, a decreased incidence of thrombocytopenia and major bleeding (23). Studies of osteoporosis are inconclusive but suggest a decrease in the incidence of osteoporosis with LMWH.

Experience with LMWH in pregnancy is confined to case reports and retrospective chart reviews (23). Results of the use of LMWH for thromboprophylaxis and for chronic-phase treatment (after initial use of intravenous standard heparin) are available for about 500 patients, mostly in the United

Kingdom and Canada, where LMWH use has replaced unfractionated heparin use in most nonpregnant populations. Trials now underway are using LMWH for acute thrombosis without first using intravenous standard heparin; this allows acute DVT to be treated on an outpatient basis. Rates of bleeding and treatment failure do not seem to be increased with LMWH relative to the rates seen with standard heparin in uncontrolled reports. Twice-daily dosing and monitoring of anti-factor Xa activity are required because the pharmacokinetics are altered by pregnancy. A multicenter trial comparing Enoxaparin with unfractionated heparin for prophylaxis is underway in the United States. In this trial, LMWH is given at 30 mg twice daily until 28 weeks of gestation and then at 40 mg twice daily. To date, no trials have compared enoxaparin and heparin for use in pregnant women. We use LMWH in pregnancy only for patients who cannot use standard heparin; patients with hypersensitivity reactions; patients in whom a steady therapeutic level of standard heparin cannot be established; and patients who need but cannot tolerate three-times-daily injections. In the United Kingdom and in Canada, LMWH has become the standard of care in the pregnant population.

Treatment of Established Venous Thromboembolism

The acute treatment of VTE is similar in pregnant and nonpregnant patients. The major questions in pregnancy involve the dose and duration of heparin therapy for established DVT because the dose of heparin required to achieve a given anticoagulant effect increases as gestation advances. This decrease in bioavailability, seen especially with subcutaneous heparin, is due to pregnancy-related changes in pharmacokinetics. Increases are seen in heparin-binding proteins (such as von Willebrand factor [vWF]), plasma volume, renal clearance, and heparin degradation by the placenta. In addition, the pregnancy-related increase in factor VIII levels may prevent prolongation of the PTT, even at adequate heparin levels.

Patients who develop venous thrombosis during gestation should receive full-dose intravenous heparin for 5 to 10 days and then adjusted-dose subcutaneous heparin every 8 to 12 hours for at least 3 months to prolong the PTT into the therapeutic range or to achieve a therapeutic heparin level (0.2 to 0.4) (Box 8-2). In some circumstances, LMWH is an acceptable alternative. No studies have compared therapeutic with prophylactic doses after 3 months, but heparin therapy should be continued for the remainder of the pregnancy. One way to avoid an anticoagulant effect of adjusted-dose subcutaneous heparin at delivery is to replace subcutaneous heparin therapy with intravenous heparin therapy near term and induce labor 12 to 24 hours later. Recent data showed prolongation of the PTT at delivery in patients who received adjusted-dose subcutaneous heparin within the previous 24 hours, but these patients

---

Box 8-2 Treatment of Acute Venous Thromboembolism in Pregnancy

- Give full-dose intravenous heparin for 5 to 10 days.
- Follow with subcutaneous injections every 8 to 12 h to:
  Prolong mid-interval PTT to 1.5 to 2 times control or maintain 2 to 3 h peak at 2 to 2.5 times control; trough 10 to 15 s prolonged or midinterval anti-Xa level 0.2 to 0.6.
- If LMWH used, maintain peak (3 h) anti-Xa activity at 0.5 to 1.0 or midinterval 0.2 to 0.6.
- After 3 months, maintain therapeutic PTT or drop to prophylactic dose.

Management peripartum
- Stop subcutaneous heparin 24 h before delivery.
- Stop IV heparin 4 to 6 h before delivery.
- When hemostasis established, start IV heparin or subcutaneous heparin followed by warfarin. Discontinue warfarin 4 to 6 weeks postpartum if the patient has been treated for 3 months with therapeutic anticoagulation.

---

had no evidence of bleeding (28). Reports of epidural hematoma in elderly patients who received preoperative LMWH for surgical prophylaxis have increased concerns about anesthesia. However, there have been no similar reports for epidural anesthesia in pregnant women receiving LMWH for thromboprophylaxis. Nonetheless, the American Society of Regional Anesthesia recently recommended that LMWH be withheld for at least 24 hours before a patient receives epidural anesthesia.

As soon as hemostasis is achieved after delivery, heparin therapy (full-dose intravenous or adjusted-dose subcutaneous) and warfarin therapy, at doses that do not exceed 5 mg initially, should be started. Heparin therapy can be discontinued once a therapeutic international normalized ratio (INR) of 2.0 to 3.0 is achieved; warfarin therapy should be continued for 4 to 6 weeks postpartum or until the patient has received therapeutic anticoagulation for 3 months. Some data in nonpregnant patients show that prolonged anticoagulant therapy (for up to 2 years) may help prevent recurrences. Warfarin is not excreted in breast milk and does not pose a risk for bleeding in the neonate.

Thrombolytic Therapy

Worldwide, 172 pregnant patients who have received thrombolytic therapy have been reported. When these cases are combined, the maternal mortality rate is 1.2%, the bleeding rate is 8.1%, and the incidence of fetal loss is 5.8%

(29). Streptokinase at therapeutic doses was not associated with a fibrinolytic effect in cord blood, and neither streptokinase nor urokinase seems to be teratogenic. Hemorrhagic complications, when they occur, are most often seen intrapartum or postpartum when fibrinolytic therapy has been given near delivery. Tissue plasminogen activator is being used with increasing frequency, is not teratogenic, and seems to be the safest fibrinolytic drug in pregnancy. It should be considered for use in the presence of a hemodynamically threatening PE or thrombosis of a prosthetic heart valve. It is not indicated for DVT because of increased hemorrhagic complications, potential fetal risk, and an absence of proven efficacy in decreasing the incidence of the postphlebitic syndrome.

Hypercoagulable States

It is now estimated (as a result of the recent discovery of the factor V mutation, which results in APC resistance) that almost half of patients with thrombosis have an identifiable thrombotic disorder. Hypercoagulable states may be inherited or acquired (Box 8-3) and are important causes of venous, arterial,

---

Box 8-3 Classification of Hypercoagulable States

Acquired
  Antiphospholipid antibody syndrome
  Antithrombin III deficiency (ATIII)
    Nephrotic syndrome
    Preeclampsia
  Medical illness
    Cancer
    Systemic lupus erythematosus
  Drugs
    Estrogen-containing compounds
Congenital
  Protein C deficiency
  Protein S deficiency
  ATIII deficiency
  Activated protein C resistance
  Factor V Leiden mutation
  Fibrinolytic defects
  Prothrombin gene mutation

and placental thrombosis. Diagnostic tests for hypercoaguable states and the effects of pregnancy are given in Table 8-6.

Mutations in the Factor V and Prothrombin Genes

The factor V mutation, the most common form of which is the factor V Leiden mutation, results from a single point mutation in the factor V gene that renders the gene resistant to cleavage and inactivation by APC. Currently, APC resistance is the most common inherited cause of an underlying predisposition to thrombosis in both pregnant and nonpregnant patients (30). It is ten times more common than deficiencies of protein C, protein S, and antithrombin III; accounts for 40% to 70% of venous thrombosis in pregnant women; and accounts for 20% to 30% of venous thrombosis in oral contraceptive users (31). A recent study of 120 women attending a pregnancy loss clinic (32) showed that 20% of patients with second-trimester loss but only 4% to 5% of those with first-trimester loss or no loss had APC resistance. When 39 patients with recurrent fetal loss (stillbirth or second-trimester loss) of unknown cause were reviewed by a group in Israel, 48% were found to have APC resistance; this implies that the factor V Leiden mutation may be the most common cause of placental thrombosis.

Oral contraceptive use and pregnancy may increase the frequency of APC resistance, even in the absence of the factor V Leiden mutation. In addition,

Table 8-6 Diagnostic Evaluation for Hypercoagulable States

	Effect of Pregnancy or Oral Contraceptives	Other Effects
Antithrombin III	↔	↓ by preeclampsia ↓ by nephrotic syndrome ↓ by heparin
Protein C	↔	↓ by warfarin ↓ by acute thrombosis
Protein S (free)	↓	↓ by warfarin ↓ by acute thrombosis
Activated protein C resistance:		
On PTT-based assay	↓	↔
On genetic assay (factor V Leiden mutation)	↔	
Antiphospholipid antibodies:	↔	↔
Anticardiolipin antibody	↔	
Lupus anticoagulant	↔	
Homocysteine levels	↔	If high, check folate, B_6, B_{12}
Prothrombin gene mutation	↔	

↓ = Decrease; ↔ = No effect.

the APC resistance screening test (the functional aPTT-based assay) is affected by pregnancy, so mutational analysis (polymerase chain reaction genetic assay) is required to detect APC resistance during pregnancy (33). Inheritance is autosomal dominant, and assessment of risk in a given person depends partly on identification of the person as heterozygous or homozygous. Patients who are homozygous for the factor V Leiden mutation have a 30-fold increase in the relative risk for thrombosis with the use of oral contraceptives.

Of great interest is the newly described association of some cases of cerebral palsy with the presence of the factor V Leiden mutation in the fetus. The palsy is thought to result from fetal stroke related to thrombosis of the fetal placental vessels.

A single-point mutation in the gene for prothrombin (transition from guanine to adenine at position 20210) was recently identified. Prothrombin gene mutation is emerging as a common cause of DVT in the lower extremities in nonpregnant patients and of cerebral venous thrombosis, particularly in oral contraceptive users (34).

Protein C, Protein S, and Antithrombin III

Protein C, protein S, and antithrombin III deficiency account for approximately 10% to 15% of cases of heritable thromboses, and these patients have a lifetime risk for recurrence of 50% to 60%. Like APC resistance, these deficiencies have autosomal-dominant inheritance with variable penetrance. Patients with a personal and family history of thrombosis often have more than one thrombophilic state and therefore should be tested for these deficiencies as well as for factor V mutations.

Patients with antithrombin III deficiency seem to have the highest risk for thrombosis during pregnancy, and 40% to 70% of these patients have VTE during pregnancy. An increased risk for fetal loss, with an estimated fivefold increase in the rate of stillbirth, has also been reported (10). Acquired antithrombin III deficiencies may be present in preeclampsia and the nephrotic syndrome. Protein C deficiency and protein S deficiency have, less often, been associated with thrombosis during pregnancy. Both have been shown to be associated with an increased risk for intrauterine fetal demise, which results from placental thrombosis and infarction.

Hyperhomocystinemia

Hyperhomocystinemia is emerging as an important cause of hypercoagulability and a risk factor for VTE. It has been known for some time that in the severe form of hyperhomocystinemia, which is related to an inborn error of metabolism, both arterial and venous thrombosis can occur. However, it was discovered only recently that mild acquired hyperhomocystinemia resulting from folic acid, vitamin B_6, or vitamin B_{12} deficiency; renal failure; or certain drugs was also associated with an increased risk for thrombosis (35). Hyperhomocystinemia is associated with a threefold increase in risk for VTE and was found in 18% of young patients with recurrent or early VTE and 10% of patients with an initial DVT. It has also been associated with spontaneous abortion, placental infarction, and placental abruption. Of note is the association between neural tube defects and hyperhomocystinemia; this association may partly explain the decrease in the risk for neural tube defects seen with folic acid supplementation.

Antiphospholipid Antibodies

The presence of antiphospholipid antibodies, anticardiolipin antibody and lupus anticoagulant, is a risk factor for both VTE and placental thrombosis. The antiphospholipid antibody syndrome is present when recurrent fetal loss or thrombosis manifests in a patient who has 1) antiphospholipid antibodies of adequate titer and 2) no evidence of an overt systemic autoimmune process, such as systemic lupus erythematosus. A full discussion of antiphospholipid antibodies is presented in Chapter 9.

Compound Heterozygotes

The coexistence of multiple inherited risk factors has recently been appreciated. In one study (30), approximately 15% of patients with protein C deficiency and 39% of patients with protein S deficiency were positive for the factor V Leiden mutation, and this positivity greatly increased the likelihood of expression of thrombosis. Similarly, coinheritance of hyperhomocystinemia and the factor V Leiden mutation may manifest as severe thrombotic events. The coexistence of antiphospholipid antibodies and any of the other defects increases the likelihood of both thrombosis and fetal loss. A study of 85 women with a history of severe, early-onset preeclampsia (36) showed protein S deficiency in 25% of the women, anticardiolipin antibody in 29%, hyperhomocystinemia in 18%, and APC resistance in 8%.

Prophylaxis for Thromboembolic Disease

The optimal management of pregnant patients with previous thromboembolism has not been defined in randomized, controlled trials. In the absence of adequate data, consensus panels have offered numerous, often conflicting recommendations (Table 8-7) that result in varying patterns of prophylaxis. A summary of what we know should provide a more rational basis for recommendations:

1. The risk for VTE is 5 to 6 times higher in pregnant than in nonpregnant patients and is further increased by cesarean section.
2. A history of a thromboembolic event increases the risk for VTE in any subsequent pregnancy well beyond the increased risk seen with pregnancy alone.
3. No data support a highest-risk period for VTE, given that antepartum events may be more common than postpartum events and that antepartum events are evenly distributed throughout gestation. The postpartum period may carry a higher risk for PE, largely because of the increased risk related to cesarean section.

Table 8-7 Prophylactic Options for Anticoagulation Based on Consensus Panels

American College of Chest Physicians (1995 Grade C Recommendations)

Previous thromboembolic event	Heparin 5000 U q12h *or*
	Heparin adjusted to level of 0.1–0.2 IU/mL *or*
	Clinical surveillance and periodic CUS
	and
	Warfarin prophylaxis postpartum for 4–6 weeks
Mechanical prosthetic valves	Subcutaneous heparin q12h to prolong 6-h post-injection APTT into therapeutic range *or*
	Adjusted-dose heparin until 13th week
	Warfarin (target INR, 2.5–3.0) until middle of 3rd trimester, then adjusted-dose heparin until delivery
	and
	Low-dose aspirin (80–100 mg/d) should be considered with either regimen

British Society for Haematology Guidelines (1992)

Previous thromboembolic event	Heparin 5000 U q12h 1st and 2nd trimesters
	Increase in 3rd trimester to prolong midinterval APTT 1.5 times *or*
	Heparin 10,000 U q12h throughout pregnancy unless heparin level >0.3 IU/mL

Maternal and Neonatal Haemostasis Working Party of the Haemostasis Thrombosis Task Force (1992)

Previous single event without thrombophilia or risk factors	Careful antenatal surveillance with prophylaxis intrapartum and 6 weeks postpartum *or*
	Heparin 7500–10,000 q12h throughout pregnancy (and prophylaxis postpartum)

CUS = compression ultrasonography; INR = international normalized ratio.

4. No data indicate which previous events, in the absence of thrombophilia, confer the highest risk for recurrence. This is because no available data in pregnant women stratify risk for recurrence according to the predisposing event.
5. The dose of heparin needed to achieve a given anticoagulant effect increases with increasing gestation. Heparin levels may be undetectable in the second and third trimesters at some of the recommended doses.

We recommend that pregnant patients with a history of VTE, even without a known hypercoagulable state, receive prophylaxis. We recognize that there are consensus panel recommendations to the contrary. The assumption the risk for recurrence is lower in women whose initial event occurred in the presence of a transient risk factor (such as surgery or trauma) than in women who had an "idiopathic" VTE is based on data from nonpregnant patients whose follow-up did not include subsequent pregnancy. As more and more genetic thrombophilias (such as the factor V and prothrombin gene mutations) are identified, more and more patients will move into a clearly defined high-risk group. Furthermore, at least 50% of the time, patients with an underlying hypercoagulable defect will present with their initial VTE in association with a transient risk factor. For this reason, we recommend that pregnant patients with a history of a single thromboembolic event—even without evidence of a detectable hypercoagulable state, recurrent thrombosis, or other indications for lifelong anticoagulation—should receive heparin prophylaxis as outlined in Table 8-8. An acceptable alternative is to use LMWH in a dosage equivalent to enoxaparin, 30 to 40 mg every 12 to 24 hours, or in a dose designed to achieve prophylactic anti-factor Xa levels (Table 8-9) (37).

Thromboprophylaxis in Patients with Previous Venous Thromboembolism and Thrombophilia

Better agreement exists among authorities on the best prophylactic regimen for patients with identified hypercoagulable states and previous VTE. All agree that heparin prophylaxis is necessary, but dosing recommendations vary on the basis of a perceived variation in risk with specific disorders (see Table 8-7).

The highest risk for recurrence seems to be in patients with antithrombin III or protein C deficiency, patients homozygous for the factor V Leiden mutation, and patients with VTE and the antiphospholipid antibody syndrome. These patients may require antepartum heparin therapy with the aPTT maintained at 1.5 times normal throughout the dosing interval. This is accomplished by 1) dosing every 8 to 12 hours and monitoring the PTT as described in Box 8-2 and 2) switching to intravenous heparin peripartum and then to

Table 8-8 Protocols for Thromboprophylaxis in Pregnancy

Category	Risk Factors	Prophylactic Regimen
Group 1 (lower risk)	Previous VTE (no thrombophilia) Protein S deficiency Heterozygote factor V Leiden mutation Recurrent pregnancy loss with thrombophilia (APA syndrome add ASA)	a) Heparin 5000 U q12h 1st trimester, 7500 U q12h 2nd trimester, and 10,000 U q12h 3rd trimester unless PTT prolonged *or* b) 10,000 U q12h throughout pregnancy unless aPTT elevated *or* c) Heparin to keep 3 h peak anti-Xa level 0.1–0.2 U/mL *or* d) LMWH to keep 3-h peak anti-Xa level 0.1–0.25 Continue heparin postpartum until INR is 2.0, then give warfarin for 6 weeks
Group 2 (higher risk)	Recent thrombosis Recurrent thrombosis Previous VTE with: Protein C deficiency AT III deficiency Homozygote factor V Leiden mutation Antiphospholipid antibodies	a) Therapeutic heparin q8–12h to keep aPTT at least 1.5× control throughout dosing interval (Box 8-2) *or* b) LMWH to achieve peak anti-Xa activity of 0.2–0.5 Continue heparin postpartum until INR is 2.0–3.0, then give warfarin for 6 weeks

warfarin postpartum. Patients with a history of recurrent thrombosis or other indications for lifelong anticoagulation should also be treated in this way.

Patients with protein S deficiency or heterozygotes for the factor V Leiden mutation may be given prophylaxis as described in Table 8-8, given their somewhat lower risk for recurrence. Other patients who are candidates for thromboprophylaxis during pregnancy are patients undergoing prolonged bedrest, patients undergoing surgery, and patients with the nephrotic syndrome and acquired antithrombin III deficiency. Patients who have known thrombophilias detected because of an affected family member with early or

Table 8-9 Optimum Anti-Xa Activity for Use of Low-Molecular-Weight Heparin

	Peak Anti-Xa Activity (IU/ml)
Prophylaxis for moderate risk patient	0.10–0.25
Prophylaxis for high risk patient	0.20–0.50
Treatment of established deep venous thrombosis or pulmonary embolism	0.50–1.0

Adapted from Samama MM, Monasterio J. Symposium on LMWH [Editorial]. Haemostasis. 1996;26S: 315–30..

recurrent thrombosis but who do not yet have a personal history of thrombosis may also fall into this category. Patients with recurrent pregnancy loss and antiphospholipid antibodies should receive low-dose aspirin in addition to prophylactic heparin (see Chapter 9).

Oral Contraceptives and Hormone Replacement Therapy in Patients with Venous Thromboembolism

A final question that often arises in any discussion of pregnancy-related thrombosis is whether patients with a previous history of VTE are candidates for estrogen-containing oral contraceptives or for hormone replacement therapy. Patients with a history of thrombosis should not use oral contraceptives, given the three- to four-fold increase in thrombosis seen in patients who use these agents (38). In addition, patients with thrombophilias, especially APC resistance, have an unacceptably high risk for thrombosis during oral contraceptive use (39). Estrogen replacement therapy (ERT) doubles the risk for VTE. Of note, the risk for VTE is greater at the onset of therapy and decreases over time with regular use (39). As is true of therapy with oral contraceptives, current but not previous use is associated with this increased risk. It is possible that transdermally administered estrogen (because it bypasses hepatic metabolism) may avoid the estrogen-related increase in clotting factors that is seen with oral preparations. Use of ERT should be individualized and should be weighed against the risks of withholding therapy, especially in women who have multiple risk factors for coronary disease or women with known osteopenia. Data are not yet available on whether estrogen receptor modulators, such as raloxifene, are a safer alternative in patients with a history of thrombosis.

Summary

Clearly, further trials that include pregnant women are needed to elucidate risk and optimize therapeutic and prophylactic regimens. When VTE is suspected during pregnancy, diagnosis and treatment must not be withheld unnecessarily. It is important to recognize that isolated iliac vein thrombosis may occur and that the presentation of PE may be more subtle in the pregnant population. In both pregnant and nonpregnant patients, LMWH may replace standard heparin as the agent of choice.

Heritable thrombophilia and the antiphospholipid syndrome are major causes of VTE and fetal loss. Laboratory evaluation is indicated in pregnant women with previous VTE and in women with recurrent fetal loss so that obstetric thromboprophylaxis can be offered.

REFERENCES

1. **Kaunitz AM, Hughes JM, Grimes DA, Smith JC, Rochat RW, Kafrissen ME.** Causes of maternal mortality in the U.S. Obstet Gynecol. 1985;65:605-12.

2. **DHSS.** Report on confidential inquiries: maternal deaths in England and Wales 1986-1988. London: Her Majesty's Station Office; 1991.

3. **Rutherford S, Montoro M, McGehee W, Strong T.** Thromboembolic disease associated with pregnancy: an 11 year review [Abstract]. Am J Obstet Gynecol. 1991;164:286.

4. **Dixon JE.** Pregnancies complicated by previous thromboembolic disease. Br J Hosp Med. 1987;37:449-52.

5. **Berg CJ, Atrash HK, Kounin CM, Tucker M.** Pregnancy-related mortality in the United States 1987-1990. Obstet Gynecol. 1996;88:161-7.

6. **Lindhagen A, Bergqvist A, Bergqvist D, Halbook T.** Late versus function in the leg after deep venous thrombosis occurring in relation to pregnancy. Br J Obstet Gynaecol. 1986;93:348-52.

7. **Badaracco MA, Vessey M.** Recurrent venous thromboembolic disease and use of oral contraceptives. BMJ. 1994;1:215-7.

8. **Tengborn L, Bergqvist D, Matzsch T, Bergqvist A, Hedner U.** Recurrent thromboembolism in pregnancy and puerperium: is there a need for thrombo prophylaxis? Am J Obstet Gynecol. 1989;160:90-4.

9. **Bauer KA.** Management of patients with hereditary defects predisposing to thrombosis including pregnant women. Thromb Haemost. 1995;74:94-100.

10. **Brenner B, Blumenfeld Z.** Thrombophilia and fetal loss. Blood Rev. 1997;11:72-9.

11. **Hallak M, Senderowicz J, Cassel A, Shapira C, Aghai E, Auslender R, Abramovici H.** Activated protein C resistance (factor V Leiden) associated with thrombosis in pregnancy. Am J Obstet Gynecol. 1997;176:889-93.

12. **Ginsberg JS, Brill-Edwards P, Burrows RF, Bona R, Prandoni P, Butler HR, Lensing A.** Venous thromboembolism during pregnancy: leg and trimester of presentation. Thromb Haemost. 1992;67:519-20.

13. **Barbour LA.** Current concepts of anticoagulant therapy in pregnancy. Obstet Gynecol Clin North Am. 1997;24:499-521.

14. **Powrie RO, Larson L, Abraca M, Barbour LO, Trujilli N, Rosene-Montella K.** Alveolar-arteriolar oxygen gradient in acute pulmonary embolism in pregnancy. Am J Obstet Gynecol. 1998;178:394-6.

15. Lensing AWA, Prandoni P, Brandjes D, Huisman PM, Vigo M, Tomasella G, et al. Detection of deep-vein thrombosis by real-time B-mode ultrasonography. N Engl J Med. 1989;320:342-5.

16. Hull RD, Hirsh J, Carter CJ, Jay RM, Dodd PE, Ockelfield PA, et al. Pulmonary angiography, ventilation lung scanning and venography for clinically suspected pulmonary embolism with abnormal perfusion lung scan. Ann Intern Med. 1983;98: 891-9.

17. Goldhaber SZ. Pulmonary embolism. N Engl J Med. 1998;339:93-104.

18. Ginsberg JAS, Hirsh J, Turner DC, Levine MN, Burrows R. Risks to the fetus of anticoagulant therapy during pregnancy. Thromb Haemost. 1989;61:197-203.

19. Hall JG, Pauli RM, Wilson KM. Maternal and fetal sequelae of anticoagulation during pregnancy. Am J Med. 1980;68:122-40.

20. Ginsberg JS, Kowalchuk G, Hirsh J, Brill-Edwards P, Burrows R. Heparin therapy during pregnancy: risks to the fetus and mother. Arch Intern Med. 1989;149:2233-6.

21. Levine MN, Hirsh J, Gent M, Turpie AG, Cruickshank M, Weitz J, et al. Trial comparing activated thromboplastin time with heparin assay in patients with acute venous thromboembolism requiring large daily doses of heparin. Arch Intern Med. 1994;154:49-56.

22. Hirsh J, Raschke R, Warkentin TE, Dalen JE, Deykin D, Poller L. Heparin: mechanism of action, pharmacokinetics, dosing considerations, monitoring, efficacy and safety. Chest. 1995;108:258S-75S.

23. Warkentin TE, Levine MN, Hirsh J, Horsewood P, Roberts RS, Gent M, Kelton JG. Heparin-induced thrombocytopenia in patients treated with low-molecular weight heparin or unfractionated heparin. N Engl J Med. 1995;332:1330-5.

24. Barbour L, Kick SD, Steiner JF, LoVerde ME, Heddleston LN, Lear JL, et al. A prospective study of heparin-induced osteoporosis in pregnancy using bone densitometry. Am J Obstet Gynecol. 1994;170:862-9.

25. Dahlman TC, Sjoberg HE, Ringertz H. Bone mineral density during long-term prophylaxis with heparin in pregnancy. Am J Obstet Gynecol. 1994;170:1315-20.

26. The Columbus Investigators. Low molecular weight heparin in the treatment of the patient with venous thromboembolism. N Engl J Med. 1997;337:657-62.

27. Casele H, Laifer S. Prospective evaluation of bone density changes in pregnant women on low molecular weight heparin [Abstract]. Am J Obstet Gynecol. 1998;178: S65.

28. Anderson DR, Ginsberg JS, Burrows R, Brill Edwards P. Subcutaneous heparin therapy during pregnancy: a need for concern at the time of delivery. Thromb Haemost. 1991;65:248-50.

29. Turrentine MA, Braems G, Ramirez MM. Use of thrombolytics for the treatment of thromboembolic disease during pregnancy. Obstet Gynecol Surv. 1995;50:534-41.

30. Florell SR, Rodgers GM. Inherited thrombotic disorders: an update. Am J Hematol. 1997;54:53-60.

31. Hellgren M, Svensson PJ, Dahlback B. Resistance to activated protein C as a basis for venous thromboembolism associated with pregnancy and oral contraceptives. Am J Obstet Gynecol. 1995;173:210-3.

32. Rai R, Regan L, Hadley E, Dave M, Cohen H. Second trimester pregnancy loss is associated with activated protein C resistance. Br J Haematol. 1996;92:489-90.

33. **Walker MC, Garner PR, Kelly EJ, Rock GA, Reis MD.** Changes in activated protein C resistance during normal pregnancy. Am J Obstet Gynecol. 1997;177:162-9.

34. **Martinelli I, Sacchi E, Landi G, Taioli E, Duca F, Mannucci PM.** High risk of cerebral-vein thrombosis in carriers of a prothrombin-gene mutation and in users of oral contraceptives. N Engl J Med. 1998;338:1793-7.

35. **Bakker RC, Brandjes DPM.** Hyperhomocystinemia and associated disease. Pharm World Sci. 1997;19:126-32.

36. **Dekker GA, deVries JI, Doelitzsch PM, Huijgens PC, Von Blomberg BM, Jakobs C, Van Gfeijn HP.** Underlying disorders associated with early-onset severe preeclampsia. Am J Obstet Gynecol. 1995;173:1042-8.

37. **Nelson-Piercy C, Letsky EA, deSwiet M.** Low-molecular weight heparin for obstetric thrombo prophylaxis: experience in sixty-nine pregnancies in sixty-one women at high risk. Am J Obstet Gynecol. 1997;176:1062-8.

38. **Farmer RDT, Lawrenson RA, Thompson CR, Kennedy JG, Hambleton IR.** Population-based study of the risk of venous thromboembolism associated with various oral contraceptives. Lancet. 1997;349:83-8.

39. **Vandenbroucke JP, Helmerhorst FM.** Risk of venous thrombosis with hormone replacement therapy. Lancet. 1996;348:972.

II. Bleeding Disorders
Janis Bormanis

Uncontrolled bleeding problems in pregnancy are often dramatic and can be stressful for patient, physician, and family. They may occur abruptly, and quick recognition and assessment are necessary to prevent tragedy. Disseminated intravascular coagulation (DIC) is a common component of these conditions.

Hemostasis results from a sequence of events that is dependent on platelet aggregation, fibrin clot formation, and clot dissolution (fibrinolysis). Normal changes in hemostasis in pregnancy include an increase in coagulation factors, a decrease in fibrinolytic activity, and, sometimes, a decrease in platelet count. When assessing possible abnormal hemostasis in pregnancy, it is important to realize that changes may reflect a decrease from the physiologic high levels normal for pregnancy to lower levels that would be normal in nonpregnant patients.

The effects of pregnancy on coagulation factors can be detected by the third month of pregnancy. The most important of these effects are increases in factor VII, VIII, and X levels and a marked increase in fibrinogen levels, which double by late pregnancy and delivery (see Key Values table). Both factor VIII and vWF levels increase, and a greater increase in factor VIII coagulant activity is seen. Fibrinolytic activity is reduced during a healthy pregnancy and returns to normal quickly after delivery; this is thought to be due to the abundance of placenta-derived plasminogen activator inhibition. D-dimer levels indicate the presence of ongoing coagulation and fibrinolysis. These levels are often used to aid in the diagnosis of thromboembolic disease and DIC in nonpregnant patients. However, in pregnancy, they are elevated by the third trimester and increase 50% to 100% in the peripartum state and therefore are less reliable indicators (1).

The increases in coagulation factors ensure adequate hemostasis at delivery. At placental separation during birth, a blood flow of 500 to 800 mL/min must be stopped within seconds. This is best accomplished through myometrial contraction, which stems the flow rapidly at the terminal end of spiral arteries. The placental implantation site is then rapidly covered with a fibrin mesh after delivery so that, in normal circumstances, blood loss is minimal.

Coagulation quickly begins to return to normal after delivery. The fibrinolytic changes disappear within hours because of the loss of placental plasminogen inhibitors. After delivery, there is evidence of activation of coagulation: increases in platelet counts, fibrinogen levels, and factor VIII levels, which revert to normal by the fourth postpartum week.

Bleeding disorders in pregnancy may be known before pregnancy (e.g., von Willebrand disease [vWD]) or may occur as a result of pregnancy or a disease associated with pregnancy such as amniotic fluid embolism (AFE). This section discusses the approach to both pre-existing disease and new-onset hemostasis disorders.

Disseminated Intravascular Coagulation

Most bleeding disorders in pregnancy involve DIC, which is triggered by the release of large quantities of placental or fetal tissue thromboplastin substances into the circulation or by shock of any kind. In a system primed for response, these conditions require quick recognition, diagnosis, and therapy.

Diagnosis

In DIC, consumption of coagulation factors and platelets is caused by activation of the clotting cascade. Fibrin is laid down in small vessels, resulting in erythrocyte shear forces and creating the hallmark fragmented erythrocyte, a sign of microangiopathic hemolysis. Activation of the fibrinolytic system is also seen. In pregnancy, DIC most often occurs in the setting of an obstetric complication, such as abruptio placenta or AFE. The manifestations of DIC comprise excess bleeding from venipuncture sites, nose, gums, surgical wounds, vagina, bladder, and rectum. Blood loss may be sufficient to result in hemorrhagic shock.

The diagnosis of DIC is confirmed with laboratory testing (Table 8-10). Fibrinogen and D-dimer levels are increased in normal pregnancy, and this must be taken into account when results are interpreted. A fibrinogen level less than 100 mg/dL is generally required for a woman to have clinically significant bleeding (2).

Therapy

The main goal of therapy is to correct the underlying cause of bleeding. In pregnancy, this usually means evacuating the uterus of the fetus and retained products of conception. Supportive resuscitative care for shock and specific blood product replacement, when needed, are quickly initiated. The blood products often required include packed red blood cells, fresh frozen plasma, or cryoprecipitate, which is rich in fibrinogen and platelets.

Coagulation factors should be replaced only if bleeding is present and should not be given to correct abnormal test results without evidence of bleeding. It can be difficult to remember formulas for factor replacement. If one thinks of replacing 50% of plasma volume with a known quantity of coagulation factor, it is relatively easy to increase the level of factors by 40% to 50%, an amount sufficient for normal hemostasis. Thus, for fresh frozen plasma that contains about 250 mL of plasma per unit, 6 to 8 U is enough for most patients with a plasma volume of 2.5 to 3.0 L. Cryoprecipitate contains approximately 250 mg of fibrinogen and, thus, 10 to 15 U will increase the serum fibrinogen level by 80 to 120 mg%. The expected increase for platelets is about 5000 to 8000 per unit of platelets. Replacement must be given in sufficient quantity to decrease bleeding and must always be given in conjunction with definitive procedures, such as supportive care and delivery.

In the treatment of bleeding disorders in pregnancy, no controlled trials have compared possible therapies. Even with advances in obstetric care and

Table 8-10 Laboratory Testing for Disseminated Intravascular Coagulation

Laboratory Test	Description
International normalized ratio	Test of extrinsic system; replacing PT; increased in DIC
Partial thromboplastin time	Measures intrinsic system; sensitive to heparin, single-factor deficiency, VIII, IX; increased in DIC
Thrombin time	Sensitive to low fibrinogen, FDP heparin; increased in DIC
Serum fibrinogen level	Circulating fibrinogen measured as mg%; decreased in DIC
Fibrin degradation products, D-dimer	Markers of fibrinolysis, fibrin degradation products; increased in DIC
	Decreased in DIC
Platelet count	Microscopic evaluation for RBC fragmentation (shistocytes);
Blood film	evidence of microangiopathic hemolysis may appear in DIC

transfusion services, hemorrhage in pregnancy with or without DIC is still a major factor in maternal death and illness.

Associated Conditions

The clinical scenarios that most often lead to DIC are abruptio placentae, AFE, retained products of conception, induced abortion, sepsis, and acute fatty liver of pregnancy. In addition, DIC can be an important feature of preeclampsia. A discussion of the clinical features, diagnosis, and treatment of these specific entities follows. More detailed discussions of acute fatty liver of pregnancy and preeclampsia can be found in Chapters 4 and 10.

Abruptio Placentae

Premature separation of the placentae, or *abruptio placentae*, is probably the most common cause of coagulation failure in obstetric medicine. It can occur in apparently healthy women with no clinical warning, can occur in the context of severe hypertension or preeclampsia, and is seen with increased frequency in association with smoking and chronic hypertension. The degree of hemostatic abnormality seems to be related to the degree of placental separation. If the separation is small and there is evidence of only mild hemostatic failure, the fetus will probably survive. If no fetal heart can be heard and the uterus is tense and tender, separation and retroplacental hemorrhage are probably extensive. The amount of vaginal bleeding is not a predictor of the amount of hemorrhage because most of the bleeding is concealed and vast amounts of blood can be lost quickly without obvious overt bleeding.

In this situation, shock develops rapidly and blood is almost incoagulable. Tests typically show a DIC pattern with elevation of INR, PTT, and TT; low fibrinogen levels and platelet counts; and the presence of fibrin degradation products (FDPs). Quick resuscitation of volume with crystalloid is paramount. This resuscitation may be followed by the use of erythrocytes, fresh frozen plasma, and cryoprecipitate if the fibrinogen level is less than 100 mg%. The presence of FDPs is also thought to inhibit myometrial contraction and, thus, further inhibit normal hemostatic processes.

Once stabilization is accomplished, the viability of the fetus is determined. If the fetus is dead, prompt vaginal delivery is facilitated. After the emptying of the uterus, myometrial contraction will greatly reduce bleeding from the placental site; this, along with fluid resuscitation and factor replacement, may save the mother's life. Postpartum hemorrhage may be a further complication and is the most common cause of death associated with abruptio placentae. If the fetus is alive and the abruption is small, prompt cesarean section may save the child if vaginal delivery is not possible or imminent. Appropriate replacement of blood products is an important adjunct in all cases.

Even though extensive bleeding occurs in the uterine myometrium, uterine contraction after removal of the fetus, placenta, and retroperitoneal clot is often sufficient to establish hemostasis. Hysterectomy as a means to control bleeding should be delayed as long as possible because it may lead to delayed internal bleeding. Gelfoam embolization of the uterine arteries, if available, may be lifesaving and may obviate hysterectomy. Adjuncts to treatment may include antifibrinolytic agents such as epsilon aminocaproic acid and nexamic acid. These agents should be used only if prolonged fibrinolysis is contributing to bleeding. Aprotinin has also been used and may have some advantages, but experience with it is anecdotal and it should be used specifically and in conjunction with expert consultation. The mainstays of therapy are still rapid recognition, volume and blood product support, and uterine evacuation.

Amniotic Fluid Embolism

Fortunately, AFE is rare, but when it occurs it is the most dangerous and untreatable condition in obstetrics. Its estimated incidence is between 1/8000 and 1/80,000 pregnancies; it is associated with a maternal mortality rate as high as 80%; and it accounts for 10% of all maternal deaths (3, 4). Amniotic fluid enters the maternal circulation through endocervical veins as a result of uterine trauma at delivery. Lethal AFE is most often associated with small tears in the uterus, cervix, or vagina without complete rupture of the wall. It occurs more often in older, multiparous patients with large babies during or after a short but strenuous labor that often necessitates uterine stimulants. It seems to be associated with stronger contractions and particularly with a single bolus of an oxytocic drug, but the trend remains unclear.

The consequences of AFE are acute and dramatic. The presenting feature is often agitation or sudden shock with cyanosis due to pulmonary vessel occlusion. The main differential diagnosis in acute AFE is PE. The mortality rate is very high in the initial resuscitation period; patients who survive may have massive DIC and bleeding. There may be profound uterine bleeding that is intractable because of a massive release of tissue thromboplastin substances (richly present in amniotic fluid) directly into the maternal circulation. This results in profound intravascular consumption. Treatment is supportive, as described above.

Retention of Dead Fetus

If the fetus is retained after intrauterine fetal death, gradual changes in coagulation are evident by 3 to 4 weeks. Most women (80%) proceed to spontaneous abortion within 3 weeks of fetal death. This abortion occurs as thromboplastin-like substances from dead fetal tissues in the uterus are released into the maternal circulation. This triggers a chronic DIC process with a much greater depletion of fibrinogen and a lesser effect on coagulation factors and platelets. This condition is becoming less common as fetal death is diagnosed earlier and delivery occurs before hemostatic abnormalities develop. However, when there are multiple gestations and a single dead fetus, expectant management may be complicated by this disorder. All patients with fetal demise should be tested for coagulation abnormalities because the duration of demise may be uncertain at the time of presentation. Any significant hemostatic abnormalities should be corrected before delivery.

If time allows or in the setting of multiple gestations, this is one of the few situations in which heparin can stop the chronic activation and reverse the DIC process (5). The necessary dose of heparin is low; 1000 U/h without a loading dose is sufficient. Increases in fibrinogen levels and platelet counts should be seen within 48 hours. If time is paramount, the infusion of cryoprecipitate will correct the fibrinogen enough to allow delivery. If delivery must occur in a patient receiving heparin, heparin therapy should be discontinued. Reversal of effect with protamine is not necessary unless abnormal bleeding is present. It is important to stipulate that this is a special form of chronic DIC and one of the few indications for the use of heparin in DIC.

Abortion

Patients who undergo abortion, especially if hypertonic saline is used, have a risk (658 in 100,000) for DIC resulting from the release of tissue factor into the maternal circulation from damage induced by the hypertonic saline (6). This release can lead to DIC with subsequent massive hemorrhage. Diagnosis and therapy are the same as those for DIC of other causes in pregnancy. Treatment is resuscitation and support, and the DIC process reverses fairly quickly with uterine evacuation.

Intrauterine Infection

Septic abortion and antepartum or postpartum intrauterine infection can occur. They are usually caused by gram-negative and anaerobic organisms. These organisms may subsequently release endotoxin, resulting in sepsis that may initiate DIC and cause cardiovascular collapse. Features of DIC should resolve as sepsis and hypotension are controlled with antibiotics and fluid resuscitation. Laboratory features of DIC may be present but, unless bleeding occurs, the use of blood products is not necessary. A search for, and evacuation of, any retained products of conception are also required.

Acute fatty liver of pregnancy can be associated with DIC and is covered in Chapter 10.

Pre-Existing Bleeding Disorders

Von Willebrand Disease

Von Willebrand disease is a heterogeneous group of disorders characterized by a quantitative or qualitative defect of vWF, which is produced in the endothelium and exists as many different multimers within the circulation. Its role is to 1) facilitate hemostasis by adhering platelets to damaged endothelium and 2) prevent removal of activated factor VIII from the circulation. These two functions are mediated by different parts of the vWF molecule.

Von Willebrand disease is the most common inherited bleeding disorder (frequency, 0.8% to 1.6%) (7). As such, it is probably one of the more common bleeding disorders seen in pregnancy. Diagnosis is based on a history of bleeding, which is usually mucosal rather than deep (due primarily to a platelet effect), and a family history suggesting autosomal-dominant inheritance. Patients with moderate or severe disease are diagnosed in childhood or adolescence by a history of epistaxis, gingival bleeding, or menorrhagia. Those with mild disease may escape diagnosis until an event, such as surgery or delivery, suggests a bleeding problem.

There are three types and many subtypes of vWD, defined by the type of defect present (Table 8-11). It is important to define the type of vWD before pregnancy because treatment and outcome vary according to type. Type 1, the most common type, accounts for 70% to 80% of cases. The estimated frequency of the most severe type of vWD (type III) is only one in a million.

The type and severity of vWD are defined by laboratory tests, which can be confusing because of the terminology of the various investigations (Table 8-

Table 8-11 Von Willebrand Disease in Pregnancy*

	Laboratory Findings					
Type	Factor VIII	vWF Antigen	Ristocetin Cofactor Activity	Bleeding Time	Effect of Pregnancy	Treatment
I	↓	↓	↓	Low or normal	Improves	Responds to DDAVP
IIA	↓ or normal	Low normal	↓	Prolonged	No improvement, bleeding likely	Responds to DDAVP
IIB	↓ or normal	Low normal	↓ or normal	Prolonged	May cause thrombocytopenia	DDAVP contraindicated
III	1–10%	<3%	Absent	Prolonged	Rare	

*In mild cases, all test results can be normal. Bleeding time correlates with platelet vWF level.

12). The disturbance common to all forms of vWD is prolonged bleeding time due to decreased platelet adhesion. Another test for platelet function is measurement of ristocetin cofactor activity. Under normal circumstances, ristocetin (an antibiotic) causes agglutination of platelets in the presence of vWF. Ristocetin cofactor activity is normal in less than 10% of persons with vWD and is thus one of the sensitive tests for diagnosis of vWD (8). Other tests include measurement of factor VIII levels (factor VIII:C activity), measurement of vWF antigen, measurement of vWF activity, and analysis of the multimeric pattern, which defines which forms are absent. The expert advice of a hematologist is often required for interpretation.

Pregnancy Outcome

Factor VIII levels increase during pregnancy and, by the third trimester, factor VIII levels, vWF antigen levels, and vWF activity are two- to three-fold higher than nonpregnant values (9). This increase does not occur until after the first trimester and quickly disappears postpartum. Thus, women with vWD who have a quantitative defect (type 1 vWD) may have fewer bleeding problems during pregnancy, but they remain at risk in the first trimester (especially after spontaneous abortion) and in the postpartum period. The amount of increase or normalization of vWF activity during pregnancy is not predictable in an individual woman. In women with type 2 or type 3 vWD, pregnancy does not result in improved hemostasis. In women with type 2B vWD, thrombocytopenia may worsen during pregnancy because of increased spontaneous platelet aggregation.

The incidence of spontaneous loss is not increased in vWD, but the reported incidence of first-trimester vaginal bleeding is increased twofold; this may represent either increased reporting or increased incidence (9). Postpartum hemorrhage occurs in up to 20% of women with vWD; most cases occur

Table 8-12 Terminology for von Willebrand Disease

Term	Description
Factor VIII	Coagulation test; level expressed as % of activity; the anti-hemophilic factor depressed in classic hemophilia and von Willebrand disease
vWD	Von Willebrand disease
vWF	Von Willebrand factor activity – necessary for normal platelet adhesion and bleeding time
vWF:ag	Von Willebrand antigen – immunoassay of the whole molecule
vWF multimers	Electrophoresis separates vWF into multimers useful in diagnosis
Ristocetin cofactor activity	Property of vWF that supports ristocetin-induced agglutination of washed or fixed normal platelets

in women with levels less than 50 IU/dL who did not receive prophylaxis during labor. Bleeding may occur several days after delivery, when the physiologic changes of pregnancy are reversing (9). Women with excessive postpartum bleeding of no apparent cause should be screened for vWD because they may be experiencing an initial presentation of vWD. The risks of epidural anesthesia and spinal hematoma are a concern. In a series of eight women who received regional anesthetic, no complications were seen. Each woman must be assessed individually, and anesthetists may have different comfort levels, but if the clotting factor concentrations exceed 50 IU/dL and the bleeding time is normal, these procedures are not prohibited.

Because most types of vWD have autosomal-dominant transmission, it must be assumed that the fetus is affected until proven otherwise. Cord blood should be obtained for diagnosis, but mild forms of vWD may not be apparent until as late as 6 months of age, when adult levels are achieved (10). Excessive trauma at delivery, use of scalp electrodes, and instrumental delivery should be avoided if possible. Neonatal procedures such as intramuscular injections and circumcision should be postponed until a definitive diagnosis is made.

Treatment

The need for treatment during pregnancy is assessed on an individual basis according to factor VIII levels, vWF antigen levels, ristocetin cofactor activity, vWF activity, bleeding time, and platelet count (for women with type 2B vWD). The risk for antenatal bleeding, outside of a first-trimester loss, is low; thus, prophylaxis is reserved for preparation for delivery and the postpartum period. A vaginal delivery in a woman with mild vWD (factor VIII level >25%) may proceed without prophylaxis, but care should be taken to avoid episiotomy and intramuscular injections. All patients requiring cesarean section should be treated to a factor VIII level greater than 50%.

Treatment options to normalize bleeding time include 1-desamino-8-D-arginine vasopressin (DDAVP), factor VIII concentrates, and cryoprecipitate. Treatment with DDAVP causes release of factor VIII antigen from endothelial cells. Patients with mild type I or type IIA vWD respond best to DDAVP, which is given as an intravenous infusion of 0.3 μg/kg over 20 to 30 minutes; the maximum effect is seen at 90 to 120 minutes. It should be given during labor and not earlier because its effect wanes. Administration of it may be repeated every 24 hours; tachyphylaxis occurs if it is used more frequently. The intranasal preparation is approximately one tenth as potent and may be used. Hyponatremia and water intoxication are theoretical risks that have not been reported with the use of DDAVP in vWD.

Each bag of cryoprecipitate contains approximately 100 U of factor VIII. Thus, ten bags will increase the factor VIII level by about 30%. Although the level continues to increase over 24 hours, the bleeding time is corrected for only 12 to 18 hours, so replacement must be done close to the time of delivery. Recombinant factor VIII should not be used because it does not contain vWF, and concentrates that contain sufficient vWF should be used. These concentrates are packaged with the units of factor VIII clearly marked, so it should be a straightforward matter to calculate the expected increase in VIII:C. For example, 1000 U would increase the factor VIII level by about 30% (1000 U in 3000 cc of plasma)

The mother should be observed postpartum and treated if bleeding persists. Because this is a hereditary condition, cord blood should be examined upon delivery and risk for the fetus should be determined.

Hemophilia A

This is an X-linked condition with a carrier state. Obligate carriers are female offspring of hemophilic fathers or females with more than one hemophilic son. The main concern is that the infant will be affected. As factor VIII levels increase during pregnancy, diagnosis may be difficult. Ordinarily, the female carrier has about 50% of normal activity. In a situation of massive bleeding, the level may decrease and contribute to more bleeding. They generally do not require replacement therapy, particularly if the factor VIII level is greater than 50%. The problem is likely to be in a male fetus who has the potential for a low factor VIII level and severe bleeding.

REFERENCES

1. **Betlart J, Calabert R, Pontcuberta J, Carreras E, Miralles RM, Cabero L.** Coagulation and fibrinolysis parameters in normal pregnancy and in gestational diabetes. Am J Perinatol. 1998;15:479-86.

2. **Richey ME, Gilstrap LC, Ramin JM.** Management of disseminated intravascular coagulopathy. Clin Obstet Gynecol. 1995;38:514-20.

3. **Richey ME, Gilstrap LC, Ramin SM.** Management of disseminated intravascular coagulopathy. Clin Obstet Gynecol. 1995;38:514-20.

4. **Weeks JW.** Disorders of blood coagulation factors. In: Gleicher, ed. Principles and Practice of Medical Therapy in Pregnancy. Stamford, CT: Appleton & Lange; 1998: 1192-8.

5. **Romero R, Duffy TP, Berkowitz RL, Chang E, Hobbins JC.** Prolongation of a preterm pregnancy complicated by death of a single twin in utero and disseminated intravascular coagulation: effects of treatment with heparin. N Engl J Med. 1984;310:772-4.

6. **Kafrissen ME, Barke MW, Workman P, Schulz K, Grimes DA.** Coagulopathy and induced abortion methods: rates and relative risks. Am J Obstet Gynecol. 1983;147:344.

7. **Rodeghiero F, Castaman G, Dini E.** Epidemiological investigation of the prevalence of von Willebrand's disease. Blood. 1987;69:454-9.

8. **Duerbeck NB, Chaffin DG, Coney P.** Platelet and hemorrhagic disorders associated with pregnancy: a review. Part II. Obstet Gynecol Surv. 1997;52:585-95.

9. **Kadir RA, Lee CA, Sabin CA, Pollard D, Economides DL.** Pregnancy in women with von Willebrand's disease or factor XI deficiency. Br J Obstet Gynaecol. 1998;105:314-21.

10. **Andrew M, Paes B, Milner R, et al.** Development of the human coagulation system in the full-term infant. Blood. 1987;70:165-72.

III. Platelets and Platelet Disorders
Robert F. Burrows and Elizabeth A. Burrows

Thrombocytopenia, defined as a platelet count less than $150 \times 10^9/L$, is the most common hemostatic abnormality identified in pregnancy. Clinicians often focus on the direct risks of thrombocytopenia—maternal bleeding and potential thrombocytopenia in the neonate—but these events are distinctly uncommon. The emphasis should be on identifying and reacting appropriately to the cause of the maternal thrombocytopenia, which is often more significant than the hemostatic abnormality.

Platelets, derived from megakaryocytes, have a lifespan of 7 to 10 days before they are cleared by the reticuloendothelial system. Thrombocytopenia in pregnancy, as in the nonpregnant state, can result from reduced production, increased sequestration, or increased destruction of platelets. Most pathologic conditions in pregnancy are due to increased destruction. In response to platelet destruction, immature platelets are released that have an increased mean platelet volume and may be better functioning (i.e., "stickier"). This section discusses 1) common disorders related to thrombocytopenia in pregnancy and 2) the management of these disorders. It is not a complete compendium of all possible thrombocytopenic disorders and their relation to pregnancy.

Maternal Thrombocytopenia

Most laboratories perform complete blood counts (CBCs) with automated particle counters. Thus, almost all pregnant women have platelet counts done. A low platelet count in a pregnant woman may have been identified before the pregnancy began, may be found incidentally through an automated CBC, or may be identified as a result of specific investigation spurred by the presence of other maternal conditions or drug ingestions.

Before embarking on extensive investigations or treatment, it is important to consider the benign condition *pseudothrombocytopenia*. Pseudothrombocytopenia is a laboratory artifact in which the platelet count is spuriously low because the platelets "clump" after collection (1). Unexpected thrombocytopenia should always be confirmed by visual inspection of the peripheral smear.

The differential diagnosis of thrombocytopenia is extensive (Box 8-4). Reduced platelet production is normally associated with decreased production of all bone marrow elements, resulting in anemia and leukopenia as well as thrombocytopenia. Defective bone marrow production of platelets occurs with vitamin B_{12} or folate deficiency, myeloproliferative disorders, and bone marrow suppression after chemotherapy or radiation therapy. Thrombocytopenia caused by platelet sequestration is usually associated with massive splenomegaly. All of the above, except for folate deficiency, are

---

Box 8-4 Differential Diagnosis of Maternal Thrombocytopenia in Pregnancy

Reduced production
  Vitamin deficiency
    Folate*
    Vitamin B_{12}
  Myeloproliferative disorders
  Drugs
  Chemotherapy
  Alcohol
  Radiation
Increased sequestration
  Hypersplenism
Increased destruction
  Immune
    Idiopathic thrombocytopenia*
    Systemic lupus erythematosus
    Drugs (e.g., heparin, H_2-antagonist, sulfonamites, penicillin)
    Infections (e.g., HIV infection, mononucleosis)
    Lymphoproliferative disease
  Consumptive
    Disseminated intravascular coagulation
    Thrombotic thrombocytopenic purpura
  Preeclampsia/HELLP syndrome*
  Incidental thrombocytopenia*

*Most common.

rare causes of thrombocytopenia, and most require consultation with hematology specialists.

Increased platelet destruction is the most common cause of thrombocytopenia in pregnancy. The most serious types of consumptive thrombocytopenia in pregnancy—thrombocytopenia caused by sepsis, thrombocytopenia caused by obstetric-related DIC (discussed in the previous section, Bleeding Disorders), and thrombocytopenia associated with preeclampsia—are usually part of an identifiable disease process. Less obvious causes of reduced platelet count, thrombotic thrombocytopenic purpura (TTP) and acute fatty liver of pregnancy, should be considered when typical obstetric scenarios do not explain the condition.

Isolated consumptive thrombocytopenia in an otherwise healthy pregnant woman is usually idiopathic thrombocytopenia (ITP) or drug-induced or incidental thrombocytopenia. Drug-induced thrombocytopenia is relatively uncommon in pregnancy, probably because many physicians are reluctant to prescribe drugs that might cause it. Any drug is suspect (2) and in pregnancy antibiotics (penicillin, ampicillin, and sulfonamides) and heparin are the most common offenders.

Maternal Risks from Thrombocytopenia

Risks to the woman with thrombocytopenia include risk for spontaneous bleeding (specifically intracerebral bleeding), limited analgesic options, and increased risk for bleeding postpartum. The condition causing the thrombocytopenia (e.g., preeclampsia) may also confer risk. In general, a platelet count greater than $10,000 \times 10^9/L$ rarely results in spontaneous bleeding. A count greater than $40,000 \times 10^9/L$ is safe for vaginal or surgical delivery, but most anesthetists require a platelet count greater than $80,000 \times 10^9/L$ for epidural insertion.

Fetal Risks from Thrombocytopenia

Maternal thrombocytopenia can adversely affect the fetus in two ways. First, in immune-mediated destruction of platelets (such as that seen in ITP), IgG antibodies may cross the placenta, resulting in fetal thrombocytopenia. This puts the fetus at risk for intracranial hemorrhage in utero and neonatal bleeding. However, diagnosis in utero has little benefit. Second, the underlying condition associated with the thrombocytopenia (e.g., infection, systemic lupus erythematosus, APS) may have an important effect on the pregnancy.

We have reviewed our experience at McMaster University (Hamilton, Ontario, Canada) over a 10-year period (January 1986 to December 1995) with regard to the frequency, cause, and prognosis of thrombocytopenia in the fetus or neonate in relation to the maternal platelet count at delivery. The methods of our cross-sectional survey are reported elsewhere (3, 4). Maternal thrombocytopenia was considered to be present if the mother's platelet count was 150×10^9/L or less. A neonatal cord-blood platelet count of 50×10^9/L or less was considered to be the threshold below which risk began. In infants with platelet counts below this threshold, ultrasonography was done to identify any intracranial hemorrhages. During the 10-year period, there were 21,723 deliveries of 22,167 liveborn infants in our obstetric unit.

Neonatal thrombocytopenia was recorded in 41 infants (15%); but severe thrombocytopenia ($<50 \times 10^9$/L) was seen in only 4 infants. The rate of severe thrombocytopenia did not correlate with severe maternal thrombocytopenia; all mothers of the severely affected infants had platelet counts greater than 60×10^9/L It was noted that in normal mothers and mothers with ITP neonatal thrombocytopenia was not significantly affected by the maternal platelet count. Hypertensive mothers with a normal maternal platelet count had a significantly reduced rate of severe newborn thrombocytopenia compared with hypertensive mothers with thrombocytopenia ($P < 0.001$). In women who were thrombocytopenic and hypertensive, the maternal platelet count did not predict severe newborn thrombocytopenia. We have found the frequency of severe neonatal thrombocytopenia to be 0.06% in mothers with normal platelet counts, 0.7% in mothers with platelet counts of 101 to 150×10^9/L, and 1.4% in mothers with platelet counts less than 100×10^9/L. In the group with normal platelet count, only a history of ITP increases the probability of severe neonatal thrombocytopenia; in the mothers with platelet counts of 101 to 150×10^9/L, a history of ITP or a diagnosis of hypertension increases the probability. Once the mother's platelet count is below 100×10^9/L, no history or physical finding increases the probability.

Although cord-blood platelet counts at delivery are helpful in predicting risk to the neonate in the setting of maternal thrombocytopenia, the neonatal platelet count does not reach its nadir until 2 to 3 days postpartum. Platelet counts must therefore be rechecked at that time.

Thrombocytopenia and Platelet
Disorders Unrelated to Pregnancy

Idiopathic Thrombocytopenia Purpura

Idiopathic thrombocytopenic purpura is a common autoimmune disorder in women of childbearing age, but it is uncommon in any obstetric population. It was identified in only 71 of 21,732 deliveries (0.3%) in our 10-year survey and can present in three ways. In some cases, there is an abrupt onset of hemostatic impairment with petechiae, purpura, and nose bleeds; this onset is often precipitated by ingestion of an antiplatelet agent, aspirin, or alcohol or by an upper respiratory tract infection. In the second presentation, the patient has a long history of insidious and relatively mild hemostatic impairment with easy bruising and prolonged bleeding after mild abrasions. A third presentation is identification of asymptomatic thrombocytopenia during routine laboratory testing. This is not an uncommon means of identifying patients with ITP, especially pregnant patients with ITP.

The primary differential diagnosis of ITP in pregnancy is incidental thrombocytopenia. Currently, no diagnostic test for ITP exists (5, 6). The measurement of bound or circulating platelet-associated IgG is, unfortunately, neither specific nor sensitive. Elevated levels may be seen in both immune and nonimmune thrombocytopenia and are not useful in predicting affected infants. Tests for HIV antibodies, lupus anticoagulant, and anticardiolipin antibodies; thyroid function tests; and coagulation tests may be appropriate in selected patients. Liver function tests have been recommended by the American Society of Hematology (5), but some clinicians believe that in patients with no epigastric pain, normal blood pressure, and normal results on urinalysis, the yield may not be worth the effort or cost. New thrombocytopenia in the third trimester should trigger investigation for preeclampsia.

The first and probably most important issue in the treatment of ITP is whether the patient needs treatment at all. Any patient with generalized petechiae and purpura and any patient with potentially life-threatening bleeding needs urgent treatment. The urgency of the intervention is based on the type of bleeding. Bruising or mild petechiae indicates the need for immediate, but not urgent, treatment; potentially life-threatening bleeding (such as intracranial or major gastrointestinal bleeding) requires emergency intervention. These premises are unchanged by pregnancy. In the asymptomatic patient, we concur with the American Society of Hematology and would not offer therapy for a platelet count greater than 50×10^9/L (5). With a platelet count less than 10×10^9/L, therapy should be offered. There is no consensus about therapy for patients with platelet counts of 10 to 50×10^9/L. The American Society of Hematology states that no therapy is appropriate for counts of 30 to 50 $\times 10^9$/L in the first or second trimester but that therapy is indicated for counts less than 30×10^9/L in the second or third trimester. They make no statement about counts of 10 to 20 $\times 10^9$/L in the first trimester or about counts of 30 to 50×10^9/L in the third trimester. Although our inclination is to not treat asymptomatic patients with platelet counts greater than 10 $\times$ 10^9/L, regardless of trimester, many authors recommend treatment and, as term approaches, treatment is needed to ensure adequate hemostasis and the availability of all analgesic options (including epidural analgesia) at delivery. A platelet count of 50×10^9/L is usually considered hemostatic for most obstetric interventions, but a count closer to 80 to 100×10^9/L is most often the threshold for epidural analgesia and cesarean section.

The prevalence of antepartum hemorrhage is not increased in ITP, but the frequency of postpartum hemorrhagic complications is. These hemorrhagic complications are not usually due to uterine bleeding (because uterine hemostasis is achieved by contraction of the uterus) but rather are secondary to lacerations, episiotomies, and bleeding from surgical sites.

Fetal thrombocytopenia is the other reason for treatment during pregnancy. One review (7) found that the prevalence of neonatal platelet counts less than 50×10^9/L at delivery was 10% and that the prevalence of severe thrombocytopenia (platelet count $<20 \times 10^9$/L) was less than 5%. In our 10-year survey, 7.0% of infants born to mothers with ITP had cord-blood platelet counts less than 50×10^9/L and none had counts less than 20×10^9/L. Intrauterine intracranial hemorrhage has not been reported in association with maternal ITP, and extrauterine misadventures have been reported only when platelet examination was delayed in the neonatal period (7). The method of delivery for the infant who is potentially thrombocytopenic and at risk is controversial. Cesarean section has been traditional for pregnant patients with ITP. There is no evidence that this procedure improves outcomes for the fetus or neonate, but there is evidence that it increases maternal morbidity rates. Little evidence supports the idea that vaginal delivery is harmful to the fetus, provided that a cord-blood platelet count is done at the time of delivery and appropriate interventions are initiated (1, 8–10). Over the years, many tests, interventions, and predictors have been proposed to dictate the mode of delivery. It has been suggested that maternal splenectomy increases the probability of neonatal thrombocytopenia. Our review of the literature (11) suggests that this may be true, but only in mothers who have had splenectomy and still have a platelet count less than 100×10^9/L. Although this group may be a unique at-risk group, this observation had not been substantiated in clinical practice. It has been suggested that maternal platelet count could be used to determine the safety of vaginal delivery, but it is now recognized that the maternal platelet count does not correlate with the fetal platelet count and thus does not have predictive properties (11–13). Cordocentesis before delivery offers absolute proof of fetal thrombocytopenia and, when done within 5 days of delivery, correlates with platelet counts at birth (14–16). In experienced hands, mortality and morbidity rates can be very low, but fetal distress, bradycardia, bleeding, and death do occur (14, 17, 18). Cordocentesis should be offered only by centers of excellence. We argue, however, that given the small likelihood of a negative outcome from ITP, cordocentesis can bring harm and offers no benefit. The American Society of Hematology (5) does not support the use of cordocentesis regardless of maternal platelet count or history. It does acknowledge that information from this test, if done, would influence their decision about the preferred route of delivery: If the fetal platelet count were known to be less than 20×10^9/L, it would recommend cesarean section over vaginal birth. However, a review of the literature (8) found no neonatal deaths or increased morbidity when vaginally delivered infants were compared with those delivered by cesarean section (no prospective studies have been done). Difficult forceps deliveries are not done, and low midcavity delivery forceps are preferred to vacuum extraction, although these actions are not based on any evidence of harm or benefit.

Several studies have found that fetal scalp sampling in clinical practice has not performed well. Inadequate samples and platelet clumping have led to no information or—worse—unnecessary interventions (19). The American Society of Hematology (5) does not recommend fetal scalp sampling and considers that a history of a previous infant with a platelet count less than 50×10^9/L after birth was important in estimating risk for fetal thrombocytopenia. This is substantiated by Christiaens and colleagues (20), who showed correlations between the platelet counts of siblings. These correlations have little clinical usefulness to the clinician, and all infants of mothers with ITP should have a cord-blood platelet count done immediately at birth, regardless of history. Treatment of the neonate is based on absolute and subsequent platelet counts with the knowledge that the nadir of the neonate's platelet count will appear 2 to 3 days after delivery.

Therapy in pregnancy is limited, and the best treatment—glucocorticoids or intravenous IgG—is controversial (Table 8-13). The American Society of Hematology has not decided whether glucocorticoids are more or less appropriate than intravenous IgG in pregnant patients. Options other than these two treatments include anti-D, platelet transfusion, and other immunosup-

Table 8-13 Comparison of Intravenous Immunoglobulin (IV IgG) and Glucocorticoids for Idiopathic Thrombocytopenia

Variable	IV IgG	Glucocorticoids
Dosage	1 g/kg	Prednisone 1 mg/kg daily
Cost	Very expensive	Inexpensive
Time to determine response	24–48 hours	2–4 weeks
Response rate	60–80%	~ 66%
Adverse effects	Risk of transmission of infectious organisms Chest pain Fever, chills, flushing Headache	Hypertension Adrenal insufficiency Hyperglycemia Osteoporosis Increased striae Postpartum psychosis

pressants. Splenectomy is generally reserved for patients in the first or second trimester who have not responded to glucocorticoids and intravenous IgG, have a platelet count less than 10×10^9/L, and are bleeding.

Glucocorticoids are usually initiated at a dosage of 1 mg of prednisone per kg per day. The platelet count may begin to increase within a few days, but 2 to 4 weeks is required to see whether the patient responds (21–23). Thus, glucocorticoid therapy must be started 4 weeks before the expected due date. Approximately two thirds of patients will respond to this therapy, but the response will be sustained in only one third of patients. The prednisone dose can then be tapered, and the minimum dose can be used to maintain a reasonable platelet count (approximately 50×10^9/L). Minimal dosing is essential in pregnancy because corticosteroid use in pregnancy is associated with increased prevalences of preeclampsia, gestational diabetes, postpartum psychosis, and osteoporosis. Because about 90% of the administered dose of prednisone is metabolized by placental enzymes and does not reach the fetus (22), the fetus is generally unaffected by this intervention.

Intravenous IgG is the other standard therapy. It is produced from pooled serum specimens from more than 100 donors who are screened for HIV, hepatitis B virus, and hepatitis C virus, so that risk for infection (a major concern to pregnant women) is reduced. The manufacturing process reduces HIV infectivity 10^{15}-fold, but HIV antibody is not affected and, thus, some patients may receive passive immunization that lasts less than 1 month (24). Other adverse effects of intravenous IgG include chest pain, fever, chills, flushing, headache, and malaise in less than 5% of patients. Patients with migraine headaches may be at increased risk for aseptic meningitis. Intravenous administration and cost are other major disadvantages. The platelet count will increase in most patients (60% to 80%) after intravenous IgG administration. A typical dose is 1 g/kg administered over 8 hours on a single day. If response has been minimal, an additional 1g/kg can be given two days later. The response to therapy is usually rapid (appearing in 24 to 48 hours); such a response provides an early indication of efficacy and the need for use only in the late stages of pregnancy. The duration of platelet response is 1 to 3 weeks, and administration may need to be repeated if delivery has not occurred.

The relative benefits of corticosteroids and intravenous IgG in increasing neonatal platelet counts are controversial (24–28), and no randomized controlled trials have been done to show which treatment is most effective. Given the overall low prevalence of neonatal thrombocytopenia, treatment should be given for maternal reasons only.

The American Society of Hematology (5) states that platelet transfusions to prevent maternal bleeding are unnecessary for 1) asymptomatic women with platelet counts greater than 30×10^9/L who are having vaginal delivery and 2) asymptomatic women with platelet counts greater than 50×10^9/L who are having cesarean section. Some believe that a count greater than 30 × 10^9/L is adequate for cesarean section. The policy in most centers has been to transfuse patients with platelet counts less than 30 × 10^9/L for cesarean section and to transfuse for clinical indications for either vaginal or cesarean delivery.

Our proposed management of ITP in pregnancy is to investigate minimally on the basis of history and physical examination, monitor the maternal platelet count, and offer treatment as we would for nonpregnant patients. If treatment is necessary, we prefer intravenous IgG because of its safety and patients' rapid response to it, but we recognize the usefulness of glucocorticoids. Delivery is conducted solely according to obstetric indications. Maternal platelet counts less than 100 × 10^9/L at term are modified by intravenous IgG to give the patient all analgesic options. If the platelet count is modified, we generally also offer induction because of cost and the desire to expedite delivery during the window of opportunity. The neonatal cord-blood platelet count is done immediately at birth. All persons involved in the care of ITP pregnancies should read the excellent consensus statement of the American Society of Hematology (5).

Thrombotic Thrombocytopenic Purpura

Thrombotic thrombocytopenic purpura is a rare condition that is classically described as a pentad of microangiopathic hemolytic anemia, thrombocytopenia, fever, and CNS and renal impairment. Because of the thrombocytopenia and the CNS and renal impairments, TTP in pregnancy may mimic preeclampsia. Unlike preeclampsia, TTP is usually not associated with hypertension and, with delivery, the platelet count and clinical condition worsen rather than improve. Although the cause of TTP has not been determined, aggressive treatment with plasmapheresis has improved prognosis for the mother. The fetus is not affected by TTP, and fetal prognosis is based on gestational age at delivery. An excellent review of the experience with and prognosis of TTP in pregnancy has been recently published and is highly recommended (29). Platelet transfusions are contraindicated in TTP because they can precipitate thrombosis and worsen clinical status.

Human Immunodeficiency Virus Infection

Infection with HIV will be associated more often with pregnancy as it spreads into the female population. In a recent report (30), a platelet count less than 100 × 10^9/L was seen in 9 (8%) of 112 prospectively followed pregnant patients with HIV infection. Thrombocytopenia in the HIV-infected mother may be due to various causes, including immune-mediated bone marrow suppression from opportunistic infections (especially fungal and mycobacterial infections), lymphoma, and drugs.

In another report, of 890 HIV-infected pregnant patients (31), 29 mothers had platelet counts less than $100 \times 10^9/L$ (3.2%). Most were responsive to either zidovudine therapy or intravenous IgG. Of the resulting 30 infants, only one had a cord-blood platelet count less than $100 \times 10^9/L$ (it was $71 \times 10^9/L$), and none had a negative result that could have been related to thrombocytopenia.

Both of these reports were published before it was recommended that zidovudine therapy be used to reduce perinatal transmission in pregnant HIV carriers. It is likely that the prevalence of maternal thrombocytopenia will be reduced by this intervention. The available evidence indicates that no specific intervention needs to be planned for the potential neonatal thrombocytopenia and may be moot because cesarean section is the preferred route of delivery for HIV-infected mothers. Mothers with unresponsive severe thrombocytopenia can be offered intravenous IgG to ensure obstetric options at birth and reduced hemorrhagic complications.

Systemic Lupus Erythematosus

Mild thrombocytopenia is seen in patients with systemic lupus erythematosus (32, 33), but it is not usually a clinical problem for the mother. The cause of the maternal thrombocytopenia is an IgG autoantibody that readily crosses the placenta, but the maternal thrombocytopenia is rarely associated with severe neonatal thrombocytopenia. Again, this has been our experience.

Thrombocythemia

Thrombocythemia is considered to be present when the platelet count exceeds $600 \times 10^9/L$. The condition is classified as primary or secondary. Primary thrombocythemia is a chronic myeloproliferative disorder in which qualitative abnormalities of platelets may be seen and, thus, the patient may be at risk for excessive bleeding with trauma or at delivery. In addition, primary thrombocythemia has been associated with recurrent late abortion (34), but the platelet count at which any of these events occurs is undefined. Anecdotally, the use of antiaggregating agents in such patients may lead to normal pregnancy outcome (34). Secondary thrombocytosis is associated with chronic iron deficiency, postsplenectomy, acute hemorrhage, hemolysis, infection, and chronic inflammatory bowel disease. If possible, secondary thrombocytosis should be treated by correction of the underlying disorder.

The patient with isolated thrombocythemia, thrombocythemia associated with another chronic myeloproliferative disease, or secondary thrombocythemia should be followed by both an obstetrician and a hematologist. No platelet count is uniformly associated with a negative outcome, although a count greater than 1 million increases risk for both thrombosis and bleeding. Therapeutic options include doing nothing and using low-dose aspirin, full-dose aspirin, or platelet pheresis. No trials have been done, so the patient and physician must decide on the degree of intervention on the basis of history and the patient's and provider's perceptions of risk. At a minimum, low-dose aspirin seems reasonable; its safety in pregnancy has been clearly shown.

Thrombocytopenia Related to Pregnancy

Incidental Thrombocytopenia

Most hospitals have automated particle counters for the performance of CBC. Platelet counts are now being done in large numbers in otherwise well, pregnant patients, many of whom are found to have thrombocytopenia (incidental thrombocytopenia). This initially caused confusion because these patients, who were otherwise well, were thought to have subclinical ITP. In our 10-year survey (3), we identified 1055 patients classified as normal (no hypertension, medical disorders, or obvious cause of thrombocytopenia). These 1055 patients represented 5.4% of this normal population. Ninety-four percent of all patients ($n = 990$) had platelet counts of 101 to 150 $\times$ 10^9/L, and 6% ($n = 65$) had counts less than 100 $\times$ 10^9/L. Less than 1% had counts less than 70 $\times$ 10^9/L. More importantly, we noted no "illness" to account for this level of platelet count, these patients had no bleeding complications, most patients who were serially followed returned to normal postpartum, and risk for thrombocytopenia in the infants born to these women was minimal (0.2%) and appeared unrelated to the maternal cause of thrombocytopenia (e.g., Down syndrome or parvovirus infection).

Increased platelet size and resolution after delivery suggest that these women have increased platelet destruction despite lack of correlation with platelet-associated antibodies. Whether they represent the tail of a normal distribution or have a separate pathophysiology remains to be determined. Thus, incidental thrombocytopenia can be defined as asymptomatic thrombocytopenia that 1) occurs in the last half of pregnancy in a woman with no history of thrombocytopenia (except in previous pregnancy), 2) is not associated with fetal thrombocytopenia, and 3) resolves spontaneously postpartum. Minimal management is required. Because a platelet count less than 100 $\times$ 10^9/L is rare, most patients are followed with serial platelet counts. Those with counts much less than 50 $\times$ 10^9/L are offered corticosteroids or intravenous IgG as term and delivery approach (see section on Idiopathic Thrombocytopenia Purpura). Delivery is done according to obstetric indication. The cord-blood platelet count is done in all neonates to establish a normal count or to produce an appropriate referral if the platelet count is decreased.

Preeclampsia

Preeclampsia is the most common pathologic cause of thrombocytopenia encountered in obstetric practice. Almost every study has reported thrombocytopenia associated with preeclampsia (35, 36). In one longitudinal study (37), the platelet count decreased before the serum urate increased; this suggests that increased platelet destruction is an early event in preeclampsia. For the individual patient, however, a decrease in the platelet count is not inevitable, even with the onset of eclampsia. A rapid decrease in the platelet count suggests progression of the preeclamptic process, but because interventions are usually made when this decrease is seen, we do not know to which clinical correlate this may be related. In addition to decreased platelet counts in preeclampsia, there is in vivo and in vitro evidence of platelet activation (38–40), increased mean platelet volume (41), decreased platelet lifespan (42, 43), and increased megakaryocytic activity in the bone marrow (44), all of which provide evidence of increased platelet use. Whether the increased turnover of platelets is an extension of the normally increased platelet turnover seen during pregnancy or stems from an entirely different cause is uncertain. Whether platelets are involved primarily or secondarily in preeclampsia is also unresolved.

Infants of hypertensive mothers are at risk for platelet counts less than 150 $\times$ 10^9/L (45). The rate of neonatal thrombocytopenia was 9.2% in hypertensive mothers and 2.2% in normotensive mothers. Premature infants, especially those with IUGR, seem to be at greatest risk for thrombocytopenia. Term infants of hypertensive mothers were no more likely to be thrombocytopenic than control infants were. Although obstetric interventions are not indicated, the rate of thrombocytopenia in preterm infants of hypertensive mothers justifies neonatal scrutiny.

In the management of preeclampsia, we believe that a platelet count is an essential component of the initial investigation. Patients with counts greater than 100 $\times 10^9$/L should have repeated counts to establish trends; counts less than 100 $\times$ 10^9/L indicate increased severity. Temporary resolution of severe thrombocytopenia has been seen in response to corticosteroids given for lung maturation of the fetus, and corticosteroids have recently been used therapeutically, both before and after birth, for this purpose (45, 46). This temporary resolution often provides an opportunity for a hemostatically competent delivery. It is prudent to try to avoid prophylactic platelet transfusion, reserving transfusion for the correction of perceived hemostatic impairment, generally at the time of cesarean section. Almost all platelet counts normalize spontaneously in the postpartum period, and patients need no specific treatment (47).

Acute Fatty Liver of Pregnancy

Acute fatty liver of pregnancy is a rare but potentially lethal complication of pregnancy (48). The presentation often includes mild hypertension, proteinuria, hyperuricemia, and thrombocytopenia and thus mimics preeclampsia. Unlike preeclampsia, acute fatty liver of pregnancy is often associated with coagulation abnormalities (an elevated INR), hypoglycemia, diabetes insipidus, and jaundice. Computed tomography has been reported to show fat in the liver (49), but it remains to be seen whether this technique can be used reliably to diagnose acute fatty liver of pregnancy. As in preeclampsia, delivery often resolves the pathologic condition, but patients with advanced hepatic encephalopathy, hepatorenal failure, and DIC may not recover. In these circumstances, liver transplantation may be considered. While awaiting delivery (which does not have to be by cesarean section), patients should be stabilized and supported by glucose and coagulation factor infusions. Many clinicians (50) consider acute fatty liver of pregnancy to be a variant of preeclampsia because of its rapid improvement with delivery and other clinical similarities.

Role of Platelet Transfusion in Obstetrics

Platelet transfusions are given to prevent or control bleeding. The usual dose of random donor platelets (platelets collected from different persons) is 6 to 8 units per transfusion, and this should increase the platelet count by 5 to 10 $\times$ 10^9/L per unit given, provided that the platelets are not destroyed in the patient's circulation. Therapeutic platelet transfusion can be given to any patient with life-threatening bleeding due to any quantitative or qualitative platelet defect, except in TTP, where transfusions can make the clinical situation worse. Prophylactic platelet transfusion is not recommended for a patient with isolated thrombocytopenia who is hemostatically stable. If it is given to patients with ITP, intravenous IgG must also be given to avert rapid destruction of the transfused platelets. Risks include those for transmission of infectious organisms (HIV, cytomegalovirus, and hepatitis C virus) and for possible antibody formation to platelet-specific antigens. Platelet-specific antibodies may complicate future platelet transfusions and may increase the frequency of alloimmune neonatal thrombocytopenia.

Neonatal Alloimmune Thrombocytopenia

Alloimmunization to platelets, which is analogous to Rh disease, occurs when the mother lacks the target antigen on her platelets and the baby inherits the antigen from the father. The most common immunizing event is pregnancy. A previous blood transfusion has been implemented but is rare. The IgG antibodies formed by maternal sensitization then cross back over the placenta, producing fetal thrombocytopenia. But, unlike Rh disease, neonatal alloimmune thrombocytopenia (NAIT) affects the first pregnancy in 33% to 50% of identified cases (51–53). Because the antigens are present on the fetal platelet at 16 weeks of pregnancy (53) and because fetomaternal mixing of blood is not uncommon, it is not surprising that sensitization occurs; what is surprising is that sensitization is not more common.

Prevalence

The prevalence of NAIT ranges from 1/1000 to 1/3000 deliveries (54–56). The most common sensitizing antigen is PlA1; it occurs in 80% of reported cases. Depending on geographic region, other antigens (Ko, Bak, Yuk, Pen, and Br) have variable prevalence. Between 2% and 3% of all pregnant women are PlA1 negative, with an 85% chance that each fetus is PlA1 positive; thus, the prevalence of NAIT is much lower than would be predicted by the phenotypic frequency. This may be because only certain maternal HLA types respond to the antigenic stimulus (57, 58). A DR3-positive mother is 76.5 times more likely than a DR3-negative mother to develop antibody response (59).

Natural History

Typically, the diagnosis of NAIT is suggested when an infant within hours of birth shows petechiae and purpura, has thrombocytopenia, and responds poorly to a random-donor platelet transfusion. The platelet count usually ranges from 5 to 25 $\times$ 10^9/L but may decrease further within the first 24 hours after birth. The platelet count returns to normal slowly over the subsequent weeks as maternal antibody is cleared. Although most infants recover completely, intracranial hemorrhages do occur, and the frequency of these hemorrhages has been estimated to be as high as 10% to 20% in cases of PlA1 incompatibility (60).

An index pregnancy alerts the clinician and family to the possibility of recurrence in a subsequent pregnancy. Intracranial hemorrhages in utero can occur as early as 16 weeks of gestation (61), but most occur at 30 to 35 weeks of gestation. Prenatal ultrasonography can identify the effects of these bleeds (61, 62); after-the-fact but a negative ultrasonographic examination does not rule out an event in utero (61).

Although the presence of antibody is correlated with infant thrombocytopenia (63), the level of antibody is not correlated with degree of severity, and changes in titer are not correlated with the severity of NAIT. Furthermore, the absence of antibody does not predict a normal platelet count. Although identification of the antibody is important, its identification lacks clinical usefulness.

Management

Diagnosis of NAIT in the first affected child has often been problematic. Today, an otherwise well child who has petechiae or purpura at or shortly after birth should be considered to have alloimmune neonatal thrombocytopenia until it is proven otherwise. The thrombocytopenia is usually severe (typical platelet count, 5 to 25×10^9/L), but this may only be seen in the infant with signs of NAIT; lesser degrees of thrombocytopenia remain unrecognized and unreported because platelet counts are not routinely done in neonates. The leukocyte count and hemoglobin concentration are normal unless bleeding has been excessive. Although the differential diagnosis of thrombocytopenia is extensive, the differential diagnosis of thrombocytopenia in a well infant is not. Once identified, NAIT responds rapidly to washed, irradiated maternal platelets and responds more slowly to intravenous IgG. Other therapies have been used, including exchange transfusion and corticosteroids (64, 65). However, we believe that the mainstay of therapy is maternal platelets and intravenous IgG to block the neonatal reticulocyte endothelial system.

The efficacy of prenatal treatments in subsequent pregnancies is uncertain because the condition is rare, the clinical course is variable, and the subsequent rate of severe complications in the untreated patient is unknown. After an index case is identified and the probably antigenic site responsible is isolated, the father can be typed to determine zygosity. This can be done for many common antigens today. For P1A1 specifically, we recognized that 28% of white P1A1-positive persons are heterozygous. In this population, 50% of the next infants will be P1A1 negative and not at risk. From amniocytes collected at 16 to 20 weeks of gestation, the genotype of the fetus for P1A1 status can be determined. If the fetus is P1A1 negative, no further interventions are done and a nonthrombocytopenic infant can be expected. For those who are P1A1 positive, therapeutic options can be discussed.

Most investigators are comfortable offering an antenatal intervention, with its inherent risks, to a woman who becomes pregnant after the birth of a severely thrombocytopenic infant with an in utero intracranial event. There is no clear consensus about offering a potentially lethal intervention to a mother–fetus pair in which the index event is only thrombocytopenia and some petechiae in the neonate. Determining the presence or absence of antibodies and following patients with antibody titers has not been shown to be useful and therefore has academic but not clinical interest. Serial ultrasonography in utero will not identify an infant with thrombocytopenia or predict intercranial events.

Central to most antenatal interventions is cordocentesis or percutaneous umbilical blood sampling. These procedures are used to confirm the diagnosis and determine the degree of thrombocytopenia and are sometimes used as a route for platelet transfusion. Because of the platelet lifespan, the therapeutic benefits of platelet transfusion are short-lived and transfusions must be repeated weekly. In addition, it has been estimated that each transfusion carries a 1% to 2% risk for fetal loss. The cumulative risk for loss during a potential 15 procedures (one procedure per week for 20 to 34 weeks) could be as high as 13% to 23% and must be weighed against the potential risk to the fetus from the disease. Needless to say, serial transfusions require operator skills and blood bank expertise that are not available to all, and they create financial and emotional stress for the mother and her family. Thus, apart from high-risk patients with infants who have had an intracranial hemorrhage in utero, repeated platelet transfusions are rarely indicated as the sole therapeutic intervention.

Isolated cordocentesis is justified in high-risk patients, but its benefit in low-risk patients is still questionable. It is now recommended that after determination of the platelet count and before removal of the needle, infants with NAIT should be given a platelet transfusion because the risk for bleeding from the puncture site without transfusion is substantial (66).

Maternally administered fetus-directed therapies are now under evaluation. Weekly intravenous gamma globulin and dexamethasone or weekly intravenous gamma globulin alone has been reported to increase platelet counts in infants with NAIT compared with historic controls, but the benefit can be modest (67). Some investigators do not believe that intravenous gamma globulin is beneficial (68–70). The risks for the fetus or neonate may be a matter of degree. If the index patient had an intracranial event, death, or residual in utero, extremes of therapy may be justified and intravenous IgG, cordocentesis, repeated platelet transfusions, and steroids in combinations may be offered. If the index patient had a neonatal intracranial event, interventions centered on the neonate may be more appropriate. If the index patient had only thrombocytopenia, interventions centered on the neonate may again be appropriate.

Optimal management is in evolution, and the appropriate and best therapy is uncertain. The clinician must evaluate, from the history of the index pregnancy and the type of antigen involved in the NAIT, the risk for the next child. On the basis of this risk, interventions that do not impose greater risk should be considered. For some mother–fetus pairs, this may mean no interventions until the infant is born.

Screening

It is now feasible to determine the P1A1 status of all pregnant (or prenatal) patients and then assess the risk for production of anti-P1A1—that is, paternal P1A1 phenotype and maternal HLA status. Having the immunogenic potential to produce an antibody response does not ensure the production of antibody and the appearance of an affected infant. Many persons have risk for antibody production, but few fulfill this potential. Screening is not justified until 1) the link between antigen status and manifestation of the potential for antibody production through an affected infant is clarified, 2) antenatal treatment is effective and feasible, and 3) risks of intervention are substantially reduced.

REFERENCES

1. **Pegels JG, Bruynes ECE, Engelfriet CP, von dem Borne AE.** Pseudothrombocytopenia: an immunologic study on platelet antibodies dependent on ethylene diaminetetraacetate. Blood. 1982;59:157-61.

2. **Hackett T, Kelton JG, Powers P.** Drug-induced platelet destruction. Semin Thromb Hemost. 1982;8:116-37.

3. **Burrows RF, Kelton JG.** Fetal thrombocytopenia and its relationship to maternal thrombocytopenia. N Engl J Med. 1993; 329:1463-6.

4. **Burrows RF, Kelton JG.** Incidentally detected thrombocytopenia in healthy mothers and their infants. N Engl J Med. 1988;319:142-5.

5. **George JN, Woolf SH, Raskob GE, et al.** Idiopathic thrombocytopenic purpura: a practice guideline developed by explicit methods for the American Society of Hematology. Blood. 1996;88:3-40.

6. **Browning J, James D.** Immune thrombocytopenia in pregnancy. Fetal Med Rev. 1990;2:143-50.

7. **Burrows RF, Kelton JG.** Pregnancy in patients with idiopathic thrombocytopenic purpura: assessing the risks for the infant at delivery. Obstet Gynecol Surv. 1993;48:781-8.

8. **Cook RL, Miller RC, Katz VL, Cephalo RC.** Immune thrombocytopenic purpura in pregnancy: a reappraisal of management. Obstet Gynecol. 1991;78:578-83.

9. **Burrows RF, Kelton JG.** Thrombocytopenia at delivery: a prospective survey of 6715 deliveries. Am J Obstet Gynecol. 1990;162:731-4.

10. **Territo M, Finklestein J, Oh W, Hobel C, Kattlove H.** Management of autoimmune thrombocytopenia in pregnancy and in the neonate. Obstet Gynecol. 1973;41:579-84.

11. **Burrows RF, Kelton JG.** Low fetal risks in pregnancies associated with idiopathic thrombocytopenic purpura. Am J Obstet Gynecol. 1990;163:1147-50.

12. **Aviles A, Coute G, Ambriz R, Sinco A, Pizzuto J.** Lack of relationship between maternal and fetal platelet counts. N Engl J Med. 1981;305:830.

13. **Wenske G, Gaedicke G, Heyes H.** Idiopathic thrombocytopenic purpura in pregnancy and neonatal period. Blut. 1984;48:377-82.

14. **Moise KJ, Carpenter RJ, Cotton DB, Wasserstrum N, Kirshon B, Cano L.** Percutaneous umbilical cord blood sampling in the evaluation of fetal platelet counts in pregnant patients with autoimmune thrombocytopenia purpura. Obstet Gynecol. 1988;72:346-50.

15. **Kaplan C, Daffos F, Forrestier F, Tertian G, Catherine N, Pons JC, Tchernia G.** Fetal platelet counts in thrombocytopenic pregnancy. Lancet. 1990;336:979-82.

16. **Garmel SH, Craigo SD, Morin LM, Crowley JM, D'Alton ME.** The role of percutaneous umbilical blood sampling in the management of immune thrombocytopenic purpura. Prenat Diagn. 1995;15:439-45.

17. **Pielet BW, Socol ML, MacGregor SN, Ney JA, Dooley SL.** Cordocentesis: an appraisal of risks. Am J Obstet Gynecol. 1988;159:1497-50.

18. **Scioscia AL, Grannum AT, Copel JA, Hobbins JC.** The use of percutaneous umbilical blood sampling in immune thrombocytopenic purpura. Am J Obstet Gynecol. 1988;159:1066-8.

19. **Christiaens GCML, Helmerhorst FM.** Validity of intrapartum diagnosis of fetal thrombocytopenia. Am J Obstet Gynecol. 1987;157:864-5.

20. **Christiaens GCML, Nieuwenhuis HK, Bussel JB.** Comparison of platelet counts in first and second newborns of mothers with immune thrombocytopenic purpura. Obstet Gynecol. 1997;90:546-52.

21. **Karpatkin M, Porges RF, Karpatkin S.** Platelet counts in infants of women with autoimmune thrombocytopenia: effect of steroid administration to the mother. N Engl J Med. 1981;305:936-9.

22. **Blanchette V, Freeedman J, Garvey B.** Management of chronic immune thrombocytopenic purpura in children and adults. Semin Hematol. 1998;35(suppl 1):36-51.

23. **Smith BT, Torday JS.** Steroid administration in pregnant women with autoimmune thrombocytopenia. N Engl J Med. 1982;306:744-5.

24. **Clark AL, Gall SA.** Clinical uses of intravenous immunoglobulin in pregnancy Am J Obstet Gynecol. 1997;176:241-53

25. **Newland AC, Boots MA, Patterson KG.** Intravenous IgG for autoimmune thrombocytopenia in pregnancy. N Engl J Med. 1984;310:261-2.

26. **Tomiyama T, Mizutani H, Tsubakio T, Kurata Y, Yonezawa T, Tarui S.** High-dose intravenous IgG before delivery for idiopathic thrombocytopenic purpura: transplacental treatment of the fetus. Acta Haematol Jpn. 1987;50:890-4.

27. **Adderley RJ, Rogers PC, Shaw D, Wadsworth LD.** High-dose intravenous therapy with immune globulin before delivery for idiopathic thrombocytopenic purpura. Can Med Assoc J. 1984;130:894-6.

28. **Davies SV, Murray JA, Gee H, Giles H McC.** Transplacental effects of high-dose immunoglobulin in idiopathic thrombocytopenia (ITP). Lancet. 1986;1:1098-9.

29. **Dashe JS, Ramin SM, Cunningham FG.** The long term consequences of thrombotic microangiopathy (thrombotic thrombocytopenic purpura and hemolytic uremic syndrome) in pregnancy. Obstet Gynecol. 1998;91:662-8.

30. **Taylor U, Gascon P, Apuzzio J, et al.** HIV-associated immune thrombocytopenia in pregnancy [Abstract]. Am J Obstet Gynecol. 1992;166:390.

31. **Mandelbrot L, Schlienger I, Bongain A, et al.** Thrombocytopenia in pregnant women infected with human immunodeficiency virus: maternal and neonatal outcome. Am J Obstet Gynecol. 1994;171:252-7.

32. **Rothfield N.** Clinical features of systemic lupus erythematosus. In: Kelley WN, Harris ED, Ruddy S, et al., eds. Textbook of Rheumatology. Philadelphia: WB Saunders; 1981:1106-32.

33. **Cowchock S.** The role of antiphospholipid antibodies in obstetric medicine. In: Lee RV, Barron WM, Cotton DB, et al., eds. Current Obstetric Medicine. St. Louis: Mosby–Year Book; 1991:229-47.

34. **Snethlage W, Ten Gate JW.** Thrombocythemia and recurrent late abortions: normal outcome of pregnancies after antiaggregating treatment. Case report. Br J Obstet Gynaecol. 1986;93:386-8.

35. **Pritchard JA, Ratnoff DD, Weisman R.** Hemostatic defects and increased red cell destruction in pre-eclampsia and eclampsia. Obstet Gynecol. 1954;4:159-64.

36. **Burrows RF.** Thrombocytopenia in the hypertensive disorders of pregnancy. Clin Exp Hypertens Preg. 1990;B9:199-209.

37. **Redman CWG, Bonnar J, Berlin L.** Early platelet consumption in preeclampsia. BMJ. 1978;1:467-9.

38. **Whigham KAE, Howie PW, Drummond AH, et al.** Abnormal platelet function in preeclampsia. Br J Obstet Gynecol. 1978;85:28-32.

39. **Hoche C, Kefalides A, Dadak C, et al.** Platelet sensitivity to prostacyclin in pregnancy and puerperium. In: Lewis PJ, ed. Prostacyclin in Pregnancy. New York: Raven Press; 1983:189-93.

40. **Burrows RF, Hunter DJS, Andrew M, et al.** A prospective study investigating the mechanism of thrombocytopenia in preeclampsia. Obstet Gynecol. 1987;70:337-8.

41. **Giles C, Ingles TCM.** Thrombocytopenia and macrothrombocytosis in gestational hypertension. Br J Obstet Gynecol. 1981;88:1115-9.

42. **Inglis TCM, Stuart J, George AJ, et al.** Hemostatic and rheological changes in normal pregnancy and preeclampsia. Br J Haematol. 1982;50:461-5.

43. **Pekonen F, Rasi V, Ammala M, et al.** Platelet function and coagulation in normal and preeclamptic pregnancy. Thromb Res. 1986;43:553-60.

44. **Thiagarajah S, Bourgeois FJ, Harbert GM, et al.** Thrombocytopenia in preeclampsia: associated abnormalities and management principles. Am J Obstet Gynecol. 1984;150: 1-7.

45. **Magann EF, Perry KG, Meydrech EF, Harris RL, Chauhan SP, Martin JN.** Postpartum corticosteroids: accelerated recovery for the syndrome of hemolysis, elevated liver enzymes, and low platelets (HELLP). Am J Obstet Gynecol. 1994;171:1154-8.

46. **Magann EF, Bass D, Chauhan SP, Sullivan DL, Martin RW, Martin JN.** Antepartum corticosteroids: disease stabilization in patient with the syndrome of hemolysis, elevated liver enzymes and low platelets (HELLP). Am J Obstet Gynecol. 1994;171:1148-53.

47. **Martin JN, Files JC, Blake PG, Perry KG, Morrison JC, Norman PH.** Postpartum plasma exchange for atypical preeclampsia as HELLP syndrome. Am J Obstet Gynecol. 1995;172:1107-27.

48. **Burroughs AK, Seong NG, Dojcinov DM, et al.** Idiopathic acute fatty liver of pregnancy in 12 patients. QJM. 1982;51:481-97.

49. **Mabie WC, Dacus JV, Sibai BM, et al.** Computed tomography in acute fatty liver of pregnancy. Am J Obstet Gynecol. 1988;158:142-5.

50. **Riely CA.** Case study in jaundice of pregnancy. Semin Liver Dis. 1988;7:191-9.

51. **Shulman NR, Marder VJ, Hiller MC, et al.** Platelet and leukocyte isoantigens and their antibodies: serologic, physiologic, and clinical studies. Prog Hematol. 1964;8:222-304.

52. **Reznikoff-Etievant MF.** Management of alloimmune neonatal and antenatal thrombocytopenia. Vox Sang. 1988;55:193-201.

53. **Pearson HA, Shulman NR, Marder VJ, et al.** Isoimmune neonatal thrombocytopenic purpura: clinical and therapeutic considerations. Blood. 1964;23:154-77.

54. **Blanchette VS, Peters MA, Pegg-Feige K.** Alloimmune thrombocytopenia. Curr Stud Hematol Blood Transfus. 1986;52:87-96.

55. **Mueller-Ekhardt C, Mueller-Eckhardt G, Willen-Ohff H, et al.** Immunogenicity of and immune response to the human platelet antigen Zwa is strongly associated with HLA-B8 and DR3. Tissue Antigens. 1985;26:71-6.

56. **Taaning E, Skibsted L.** The frequency of platelet alloantibodies in pregnant women and the occurrence and management of neonatal alloimmune thrombocytopenia purpura. Obstet Gynecol Surv. 1990;45:521-5.

57. **Reznikoff-Etievant MF, Dangu C, Lobet R.** HLA-B8 antigen and anti-P1A1 alloimmunization. Tissue Antigens. 1981;18:66-8.

58. **Reznikoff-Etievant MF, Muller JY, Julien F, et al.** An immune response gene linked to MCH in man. Tissue Antigens. 1983;22:312-4.

59. **Muller JY.** Neonatal alloimmune thrombocytopenias: clinical immunology and allergy. In: Engelfreit CP, von dem Borne AEGK, eds. Alloimmune and Autoimmune Cytopenias. Philadelphia: Balliere Tindall; 1987:427-42.

60. **Mueller-Eckhardt C, Grubert A, Weisheit M, et al.** Three hundred and forty-eight cases of suspected neonatal alloimmune thrombocytopenia. Lancet. 1989;1:363-6.

61. **Burrows RF, Caco CC, Kelton JG.** Neonatal alloimmune thrombocytopenia: spontaneous in utero intracranial hemorrhage. Am J Hematol. 1988;28:98-102.

62. **Herman JH, Jumbelic MI, Ancona RJ, Kickler TS.** In utero cerebral hemorrhage in alloimmune thrombocytopenia. Am J Pediatr Hematol Oncol. 1986;8:312-7.

63. **McFarland JG, Frenzke M, Aster RH.** Testing of maternal sera in pregnancies at risk for neonatal alloimmune thrombocytopenia. Transfusion. 1989;29:128-33.

64. **Meuller-Eckhardt C, Kiefel V, Grubert A.** High-dose IgG treatment for neonatal alloimmune thrombocytopenia. Blut. 1989;59:145-6.

65. **Bussel JB, Schreiber AD.** Immune thrombocytopenia purpura, neonatal alloimmune thrombocytopenia, and post-transfusion purpura. In: Hoffman R, Benz EJ, Shattil SJ, et al., eds. Hematology: Basic Principles and Practice. New York: Churchill-Livingstone; 1991:1485-94.

66. **Bussel JB, Kaplan C, McFarland JG, and the Working Party on Neonatal Alloimmune Thrombocytopenia of the Neonatal Hemostasis Subcommittee of the Scientific and Standardization Committee of the ISTH.** Recommendations for the evaluation and treatment of neonatal autoimmune and alloimmune thrombocytopenia. Thromb Haemost. 1991;65:631-4.

67. **Bussel JB, Berkowitz RI, Lunch L, et al.** Antenatal management of alloimmune thrombocytopenia with intravenous Y-globulin: a randomized trial of the addition of low-dose steroid to intravenous Y-globulin. Am J Obstet Gynecol. 1996;174:1414-23.

68. **Kroll H, Kiefel V, Giers C, et al.** Maternal intravenous immunoglobulin treatment does not prevent intracranial hemorrhage in fetal alloimmune thrombocytopenia. Transfus Med. 1994;4:293-6.

69. **Mir N, Samson D, House MJ.** Failure of antenatal high-dose immunoglobulin to improve fetal platelet count in neonatal allo-immune thrombocytopenia. Vox Sang. 1988:55:188-9.

70. **Nicolini U, Tannirandorn Y, Gonzalez P, et al.** Continuing controversy in alloimmune thrombocytopenia: fetal hyperimmunoglobulinemia fails to prevent thrombocytopenia. Am J Obstet Gynecol. 1990;163:1144-6.

IV. Anemia
Janis Bormanis

The diagnosis and effects of anemia in pregnancy are not always entirely clear. Women may be known to have anemia before pregnancy, may be first diagnosed by routine screening at the initial prenatal visit, or may develop anemia during pregnancy. Routine screening at the initial prenatal visit identifies women at risk for anemia so that diagnostic and therapeutic interventions can be initiated. Iron deficiency is by far the most common cause of anemia in both pregnant and nonpregnant women. Folic acid deficiency is less common but may, in the preconception period, be more important because of its relation to neural tube defects. Vitamin B_{12} deficiency may also occur but is uncommon in areas without malnutrition. These and other, less common causes of anemia are reviewed here.

Normal Physiologic Changes

Normal physiologic changes occur in erythrocyte mass and plasma volume during gestation. Plasma volume begins to increase by the sixth week of gestation: An initial rapid increase is followed by a more gradual increase to a peak by week 30, with a total of 1250 mL by term. This reflects an increase as great as 50%. The greatest increase in plasma volume occurs in patients whose pregnancies involved assisted reproductive technology (because the high hormone level from ovarian hyperstimulation causes tremendous fluid retention and plasma volume expansion) and in patients with multiple gestations. The erythrocyte mass increases, but more slowly than the plasma volume, to a total increase of 18% to 30%, or approximately 400 mL, depending on iron replacement. These changes result in a dilutional effect that is referred to as the *physiologic anemia of pregnancy* (1).

Parturition results in blood loss of 500 to 1000 mL. This leads to a temporary further decline in hemoglobin concentrations, but as plasma volume decreases, the hematocrit reaches predelivery levels by postpartum day 5 to 7 (2).

Diagnostic Criteria

If the 2-SD limit for biological variation is applied, the lowest hemoglobin concentration occurs at week 25 to 26 of gestation and ranges from 9.8 to 10.4 g/dL (3). It is commonly accepted that 10 g/dL is the lower limit of normal hemoglobin concentration in pregnancy, and only a few women (3% to 5%) have slightly lower levels. A patient should be considered anemic if the hemoglobin concentration is less than 11 g/dL in the first trimester and less than 10 g/dL in the late second and third trimesters.

Effect of Anemia on the Fetus and Mother

The effect of anemia on the pregnancy is primarily determined by the severity of the anemia. Mild anemia, although it may be a marker for poor nutritional status, rarely has untoward effects. However, when the hemoglobin concentration is 6 to 7 g/dL, the mother is at risk for high-output cardiac failure and extreme fatigue. To compensate for decreased oxygen delivery, the placenta hypertrophies to increase oxygen extraction (4, 5). Some evidence indicates that iron deficiency may cause decreased fertility, IUGR, preterm delivery, and perinatal death (4, 6).

Diagnosis

Anemia is investigated in the same way in pregnant and nonpregnant patients. Complete blood count, which includes investigation of hemoglobin, erythrocyte size (mean corpuscular volume [MCV]), erythrocyte number, variation in erythrocyte size, and calculated erythrocyte indices is obtained, and an initial classification by erythrocyte size is done. Normocytic patients have a normal MCV, microcytic patients have an MCV less than 80, and macrocytic patients have an MCV greater than 100 (Box 8-5). The MCV, as a

---

Box 8-5 Differential Diagnosis of Anemia in Pregnancy

Microcytic patients (MCV < 80)
 Iron deficiency
 Anemia of chronic disease
 Sideroblastic
 Thalassemia
Normocytic patients (MCV normal)
 Hemolytic anemia (see Table 8-16)
 Anemia of chronic disease
 Renal disease
 Hypothyroidism or hypoadrenalism
Macrocytic patients (MCV > 100)
 Folate deficiency
 Vitamin B$_{12}$ deficiency

MCV = mean corpuscular volume.

---

mean value, may be normal if the patient has a dimorphic population of cells (as when iron deficiency and folate deficiency co-exist). In this situation, the variation in erythrocyte size is increased and the smear has evidence of megaloblastic changes (i.e., hypersegmented polymorphs).

Although the CBC is automated, the blood film (peripheral smear) remains a manual procedure that is done when an abnormality is seen in the numbers on an automated CBC. Erythrocyte morphologic study and a reticulocyte count add important clues to the cause of anemia, particularly in hemolytic syndromes. The reticulocyte count should be increased in any case of hemolytic anemia or blood loss but should be unchanged in patients with bone marrow production problems. Tables 8-14 and 8-15 provide glossaries of morphologic terms and their associations; they are meant to be a reference guide for further testing when an abnormal blood film is seen.

The tests for hematinic substances are also fairly standard. For iron, measurement of the serum ferritin level (a measure of iron stores) is preferred; measurements of serum iron and iron-binding capacity are less specific. A ferritin level greater than 35 µg/L is not consistent with iron deficiency (7). For macrocytic anemias, assessment of folate deficiency is best done with the erythrocyte folate, which reflects stores of folic acid better than the serum folate does (serum folate can change significantly with dietary variation alone). Serum B_{12} levels may be difficult to interpret, and repeated testing for clarification may be indicated. Bone marrow examination may be needed and can

Table 8-14 Red Cell Glossary

Term	Definition
Rouleaux	Hypergammaglobulinemia (usually polyclonal; if monoclonal, myeloma is possible), may need serum protein electrophoresis
Agglutination	Red cell clumping, cold antibody, possible hemolysis
Microcytes	Iron deficiency, thalassemias, anemia of chronic disease
Macrocytes	Vitamin B_{12} and folate deficiency, liver disease, myeloma, agglutination if oval, macrocytes more specific for B_{12} or folate
Ovals	May be nonspecific but found in iron deficiency
Targets	Liver disease, thalassemias, hemoglobinopathy, hypersplenism
Acanthocytes	Severe liver disease and hyposplenism
Burr	Renal failure
Spherocytes	Immune hemolysis, hereditary spherocytosis
Blister (bite)	Oxidative hemolysis (G6PD, Dapsone)
Tear drop	Thalassaemia, myelofibrosis, severe anemia
Fragment	DIC, PIH, prosthetic valves, hyposplenism, TTP (the term *microangiopathic hemolysis* may be used)
Sickle	Sickle-cell disorders
Inclusions	Howell-Jolly bodies, Pappenheim stain, malaria

be done safely in pregnancy when the cause of anemia is not indicated by simpler tests.

Iron Deficiency

Iron deficiency is the most common cause of anemia in pregnancy. Women are more prone to iron depletion because of menstrual blood loss. Thus, they may begin pregnancy in a depleted state. A short interval between pregnancies further contributes to poor iron stores in some women. In North America, poor dietary intake alone is rarely a cause of iron deficiency.

In the nonpregnant state, approximately 1 to 2 mg of iron is lost each day and must be replaced through the diet. Throughout the course of pregnancy, an additional 1 g of iron per day is needed. This is used both for the increase in maternal erythrocyte mass and for fetal hematopoieses (Table 8-16). In addition, maternal blood loss occurs at delivery. By the third trimester, there is need for an additional 6 mg/d, and a negative iron balance will result if no iron supplementation is given. Breastfeeding causes a further loss of about 0.5 mg of iron per day.

Table 8-15 White Cell Glossary

Term	Definition
Hypersegmentation	Megaloblastic anemias, Vitamin B_{12}, folate
Lymphocytosis	Atypical, variant, viral illness, infectious mononucleosis with smudge cells, chronic lymphocytic leukemia
Eosinophilia	Allergic conditions, parasitic infections
Monocytosis	Myeloproliferative disorders, infections, cancer
Blasts	Usually signifies acute leukemia and must be taken in context
Nucleated RBC	Seen in rapid marrow turnover (bleeding hemolysis); also metastatic disease, myeloproliferative disorders
Leukoerythroblastic	Primitive WBC and primitive RBC, marrow infiltration or myelofibrosis (NRBC and myelocytes)

Table 8-16 Iron Loss Related to Pregnancy

Factor	Iron Loss (mg)
Increase in red cell mass	400–500
Transfer to fetus	250
Placenta	100
Blood loss	50 (225–250 mg of iron per unit of blood)

A careful history and an assessment of iron stores (serum ferritin level) easily estimate the initial iron status of a mother and identify the risk for anemia due to a lack of iron during pregnancy. Depleted iron exists when stores are gone but anemia has not developed because daily intake is sufficient to maintain base production. At this time, the serum iron level is normal but the serum ferritin level is less than normal. As iron stores are further depleted, serum iron levels decrease, serum iron-binding capacity increases, and anemia develops. At this point, the MCV is still at the lower limit of normal. With further iron loss, more significant anemia develops and cells become microcytic and hypochromic. This is *iron-deficiency anemia.* This progression of early iron depletion to true iron-deficiency anemia can easily occur during pregnancy (8).

Iron is actively transported across the placenta. The fetus takes iron from the mother at a very efficient rate, and the placenta becomes more and more efficient in removing iron at a decreasing gradient, even as the mother becomes more anemic, because the number of transferrin receptors available to bind iron in the placenta increases. Except in cases of extreme maternal iron deficiency, the fetus can extract sufficient iron to allow relatively normal erythropoiesis. However, the neonate may have lower ferritin levels.

Although iron-deficiency anemia leads to more weakness and fatigability and more pronounced dyspnea on exertion, there is no evidence of long-term physical harm to the mother from iron deficiency. The classic symptoms of pica, including cravings for ice, clay, and starch, may be present.

Routine iron replacement is recommended in the second and third trimesters because most women's diets are insufficient to meet the increased demand. Oral iron is best absorbed in the stomach and duodenum in a mildly acidic medium, so enteric-coated or sustained-release iron preparations are inefficient (many are also expensive). Iron absorption is inhibited by antacids. Iron is best taken without food because phytates, phosphates, and tannates in food bind iron and impair its absorption. Iron absorption is enhanced by ascorbic acid, even as little as 250 mg administered at the time of iron administration. The upper gastrointestinal discomfort and constipation experienced by some patients relates best to the amount of elemental iron present in the iron salt. For example, 300 mg ferrous sulfate contains 60 mg elemental iron, ferrous gluconate 35 mg, and ferrous fumarate 100 mg. If an incremental increase of oral iron is indicated, liquid iron can be used to gradually increase dosing. The use of parenteral iron, such as iron dextran, is usually not warranted during pregnancy and carries a risk for anaphylaxis (5).

The length of time needed for treatment is determined by the extent of loss and the time needed to replete iron stores. Initially, hemoglobin concentrations increase in response to treatment, and iron stores then gradually build up over months. A seesaw effect is often seen when hemoglobin concentrations increase because patients feel better and may stop taking their iron. Consequently, no stores are developed and, if losses are the same as before, the cycle starts over. The necessary duration of iron replacement depends on all of these factors, on tolerance, and on prediction of future need, as in lactation or future pregnancies. Iron supplementation should be continued until iron stores, as reflected by ferritin levels, are replete.

Megaloblastic Anemias

Folic Acid

Folic acid has received much attention both in the lay press and the scientific literature in the past few years. A deficiency in folic acid is the second most common cause of anemia in pregnancy. This deficiency is most important in the preconception period because folate deficiency at conception and early in gestation is associated with neural tube defects. The main dietary source of folic acid is green leafy vegetables. Folic acid is absorbed in the jejunum without a specific carrier and is needed for DNA synthesis and homocysteine metabolism. Lack of it results in a macrocytic anemia that may be associated with a decrease in leukocyte and platelet counts. Diagnosis is suggested by anemia with an elevated MCV and a peripheral blood smear showing oval macrocytes and hypersegmented neutrophils. Measurement of erythrocyte folate confirms the diagnosis.

The major cause of folate deficiency in pregnancy is the increased demand caused by fetal growth and increased erythropoiesis. There is a net increase in the folate requirement of 50 to 100 µg/d (9). Increased metabolic demand due to an increase in catabolism (10) and an inhibitory effect on absorption due to increased levels of estrogen and progesterone may also contribute to folate deficiency. Risk factors for folate deficiency include poor diet, multiple pregnancies, hemolytic anemia, urinary tract infections, and use of drugs that impair folate metabolism (such as trimethoprim, ethanol, and dilantin) (9). It is important to remember that dual deficiencies of folate and iron can result from poor nutrition. This is very important in alcoholic women, who have poor nutrition and further metabolic demand. Folate deficiency usually manifests in the third trimester with mild macrocytic changes, but frank megaloblastic anemia is rare.

Effect on the Fetus and the Pregnancy

Women with a low mean daily folate intake at 28 weeks of gestation had an approximately twofold greater risk for preterm delivery and low-birthweight infants after maternal characteristics, energy intake, and other correlated nutrients were controlled for (11).

It has been shown that dietary supplementation with 0.4 mg of folic acid can decrease the risk for a baby with a neural tube defect by as much as 48% (12). Studies of how this happens have pointed to higher levels of homocysteine and methylmalonic acid in women who have children with neural tube defects. Both substances, especially methylmalonic acid, are toxic to neural tissue. This has given rise to a suggestion that to further prevent neural tube defects, vitamin B_{12} supplementation may be necessary (13), but this has not yet been adequately studied.

Folate Supplementation

Supplementing the diets of women of childbearing potential with folic acid 0.4 mg/d would effectively increase erythrocyte folate to levels associated with a low risk for folate-responsive neural tube defects. Protective levels of erythrocyte folate may also be obtained by ample consumption of vegetables, fruits, and folic acid–fortified breakfast cereals. This well-studied effect has led the U.S. government to fortify foods in an effort to prevent neural tube defects. Although this is a well-intentioned measure, it needs to be associated with an education program to reach the women with the highest risk. In the United Kingdom, investigators examined dietary habits in adolescents 16 to 19 years of age. They found that at least one fourth of students had a dietary folate intake less than that needed to prevent neural tube defects. Only 14% of an undergraduate group but 41% of more senior students knew about folate and neural tube defects (14). Although this study was done in a European population, the results are probably transferable to young women in North America. Efforts to increase folic acid supplementation and folate consumption in women of childbearing potential must go beyond fortification of refined cereal and grain products and must reach women in all educational and income groups.

Current recommendations are that the normal diet should be embellished with at least 0.4 mg of folic acid per day (12). Some investigators believe that higher doses are needed, and recommendations vary from 1 to 5 mg/d in women contemplating pregnancy. In the rare patient with vitamin B_{12} deficiency, replacement of folate at a dosage of 1 to 5 mg/d could mask a true deficiency and facilitate neurologic damage.

Vitamin B_{12}

It is interesting that a decrease in vitamin B_{12} levels is seen during pregnancy, even though B_{12} requirements increase. Storage of B_{12} is predominately in the liver and, in contrast to folic acid, B_{12} has a storage time of up to 2 years.

As such, true B_{12} deficiency is unusual. The clinical manifestations of B_{12} deficiency include the general symptoms of fatigue and dyspnea but can also include neurologic symptoms, such as memory loss, paresthesias, and ataxia. The hematologic changes of B_{12} deficiency are indistinguishable from those of folic acid deficiency: macrocytic anemia with varied degrees of leukopenia and thrombocytopenia. Peripheral blood smears show oval macrocytes and hypersegmented neutrophils. The serum vitamin B_{12} level will be low in the presence of normal folate. In a pregnant woman, the cause of a true B_{12} deficiency may be pernicious anemia, and treatment should be started if clinically indicated. Treatment consists of the subcutaneous injection of cyanocobalamin at a dose of 100 µg, as in pernicious anemia in the nonpregnant state. If a woman is truly deficient, an increase in hemoglobin concentration and reticulocytosis will be seen within 3 to 5 days. Treatment should be continued until after delivery and lactation, when definitive diagnosis with a Schilling test can be safely done.

Hemolytic Anemias

Premature destruction of erythrocytes—hemolysis—is the result of either an abnormal intravascular environment or abnormal erythrocytes. The defect may be acquired, as in immune hemolytic anemias, or may be hereditary, as in glucose-6-phosphate dehydrogenase (G6PD) deficiency. Box 8-6 outlines the differential diagnosis of hemolytic anemia.

All causes of hemolysis lead to either erythrocyte lysis in the vasculature or removal of erythrocytes by the spleen. The clinical manifestations common to all forms of hemolytic anemia include hyperbilirubinemia, which may cause icterus, elevated levels of lactate dehydrogenase (especially in intravascular causes), splenomegaly, and reticulocytosis. The demand for folate is higher because of increased erythrocyte turnover. Depending on the underlying cause, peripheral smears may show spherocytes, fragmented erythrocytes (schistocytes), and target cells (in the thalassemias and sickle-cell disease) (15).

Intrinsic Hemolytic Anemia

Intrinsic hemolytic anemia is the result of abnormal structure or metabolism of erythrocytes. Inherited membrane defects, such as spherocytosis, lead to increased sequestration in the spleen. Intrinsic hemolytic anemia is an autosomal-dominant syndrome in 75% of cases and is acquired in the other 25% (16). Increased permeability of the erythrocyte membrane to sodium results in osmotically fragile cells. Pregnancy does not affect clinical course. The treatment of choice in affected persons is splenectomy to prevent destruction of affected cells.

Box 8-6 Differential Diagnosis of Hemolytic Anemia in Pregnancy

---

Intrinsic
Abnormal interior of erythrocytes
  Enzyme defects
    Glucose-6-phosphate dehydrogenase
    Pyruvate kinase deficiency
  Thalassemias
  Hemoglobinopathies
Abnormal erythrocyte membrane
  Hereditary spherocytosis, elliptocytosis, poikiloctyosis, stomatocytosis
  Paroxysmal nocturnal hemoglobinopathy
  Liver disease (spur cell anemia)
Extrinsic
Hypersplenism
Microangiopathic hemolytic anemia
  HELLP syndrome
  Disseminated intravascular coagulation
  Thrombotic thrombocytopenic purpura
  Malignant hypertension
  Acute glomerulonephritis
Immune-mediated
  Idiopathic
  Drugs (e.g., Aldomet, penicillin, quinidine)
  Collagen vascular disease (e.g., systemic lupus erythematosus,
    polyarteritis nodosa, rheumatoid arthritis)
  Lymphoproliferative disorders
  Cold agglutinin disease
    Secondary to mycoplasma, mononucleosis, lymphoproliferative
    disorders, and others

Erythrocyte enzyme defects are the other major category of intrinsic hemolytic anemias. Deficiency of G6PD is an X-linked disorder most prevalent in persons of West African, Mediterranean, Middle Eastern, or Southeast Asian descent. Approximately 25% of African-American women are heterozygous and may have normal, moderately reduced, or clearly deficient G6PD activity (16). Hemolysis generally occurs acutely when there is a superimposed oxidative stress, such as infection or use of oxidative drugs (e.g., antimalarial agents, sulfas, or nitrofurantoin), and is self-limited. The oxidated hemoglobin precipitates the formation of Heinz bodies, which are phagocytosed by the spleen. In pregnancy, G6PD activity decreases during the second and third trimester. This may result in increased hemolysis in affected persons. There is an increased risk for stillbirth, IUGR, and neonatal jaundice (17). An acute hemolytic reaction from an oxidative drug may precipitate an acute in utero fetal hemolysis resulting in hydrops (16). In the setting of fetal nonimmune hydrops, it is possible to perform cordocentesis and measure fetal G6PD activity (16).

Abnormal hemoglobin structure (hemoglobinopathies and thalassemias) may also lead to hemolytic anemias. These are discussed in a separate section.

Extrinsic Hemolytic Anemia

Extrinsic hemolytic anemia results from influences other than erythrocyte structure. There is a wide range of potential sources of erythrocyte destruction. In pregnancy, microangiopathic hemolytic anemia is most common. Fibrin deposition in the small vessels leads to fragmentation of erythrocytes and, often, thrombocytopenia. The peripheral smear shows evidence of schistocytes, nucleated erythrocytes, and thrombocytopenia. The lactate dehydrogenase level is usually markedly elevated. The HELLP (*h*emolysis, *e*levated *l*iver enzyme levels, and *l*ow *p*latelet count) syndrome is the most common cause, but the differential diagnosis includes TTP, DIC, malignant hypertension, and acute glomerulonephritis.

Paroxysmal nocturnal hemoglobinuria is an acquired increased sensitivity to complement-mediated hemolysis. It is probably secondary to a deficiency of decay-accelerating factor (15) that is usually present on erythrocyte membranes. It is also associated with a hypercoagulable state.

In pregnancy, the risk for thrombotic events is increased, but heparin should be avoided because it can increase hemolytic events. Warfarin, however, should be given in the postpartum period (16, 18).

Hypoplastic Anemias

Insufficient bone marrow function leads to pancytopenia, resulting in infection, bleeding, and anemia. The differential diagnosis includes nutritional depletion of folate and vitamin B_{12}; marrow suppression from exogenous factors, such as alcohol, drugs, and radiation; infections; consumptive coagulopathies, such as DIC; and marrow infiltration from lymphoproliferative cancer (19). Pure erythrocyte aplasia is most often due to parvovirus infection. There are reports of aplastic anemia limited to pregnancy that have recurred in subsequent pregnancies associated with the occurrence of thymomas (19).

REFERENCES

1. **Whittaker PG, Mcphail S, Lind T.** Serial hematologic changes and pregnancy outcome. Obstet Gynecol. 1995;88:33-9.
2. **Williams MD, Wheby MS.** Anemia in pregnancy. Med Clin North Am. 1992;76:631-47.
3. **Garn SM, Ridella A, Petzold SA, Falkner F.** Maternal hematologic levels and pregnancy outcomes. Semin Perinatol. 1981;5:155.
4. **Murphy JE, O'Riorda J, Newcombe RG, et al.** Relation of haemoglobin levels in first and second trimester to outcome of pregnancy. Lancet. 1986;1:992.
5. **Mani S, Duffy TP.** Anemia of pregnancy. Clin Perinatol. 1995;22:593-607.
6. **Garn SM, Ridella SA, Petzold AS, et al.** Maternal hematologic levels and pregnancy outcomes. Semin Perinatol. 1981;5:155.
7. **Puolakka J.** Serum ferritin as a measure of iron stores during pregnancy. Acta Obstet Gynecol Scand Suppl. 1980;95:1-63.
8. **Kaufer M, Casaneuva E.** Relation of pregnancy serum ferritin levels to hemoglobin levels throughout pregnancy. Eur J Clin Nutr. 1990;44:709-15.
9. **Williams MD, Wheby MS.** Anemia in pregnancy. Med Clin North Am. 1992;76:631-47.
10. **McPartlin J, Halligan A, Scott JM, Darling M, Weir DG.** Accelerated folate breakdown in pregnancy. Lancet. 1993;341:148-9.
11. **Scholl TO, Hediger ML, Schall JI, Khoo CS, Fischer RL.** Dietary and serum folate: their influence on the outcome of pregnancy. Am J Clin Nutr. 1996;63:520-1.
12. **Daly LE, Kirke PN, Molloy A, Weir DG, Scott JM.** Folate levels and neural tube defects: implications for prevention. JAMA. 1995;6274:1698-702.
13. **Mills JL, McPartlin JM, Kirke PN, Lee YJ, Conley MR, Weir DG, Scott JM.** Homocysteine metabolism in pregnancies complicated by neural-tube defects. Lancet. 1995;345:149-51.
14. **Wild J, Schorah CJ, Maude K, et al.** Folate intake in young women and their knowledge of preconceptual folate supplementation to prevent neural tube defects. Eur J Obstet Gynecol. Reprod Biol. 1996;70:185-9.
15. **Tabbara IA.** Hemolytic anemias—diagnosis and management. Med Clin North Am. 1992;76:649-68.
16. **Roberts WE.** Hemolytic anemias. In: Gleicher, ed. Principles and Practice of Medical Therapy in Pregnancy. Stamford, CT: Appleton & Lange; 1998:1173-6.
17. **Perkins RP.** The significance of glucose-6 phosphate dehydrogenase deficiency in pregnancy. Am J Obstet Gynecol. 1976;125:215.
18. **Hurd WW, Modovnik M, Stys SJ.** Pregnancy associated with paroxysmal nocturnal hemoglobin urea. Obstet Gynecol. 1982;60:742.
19. **Stewart FM.** Hypoplastic/aplastic anemia: role of bone marrow transplantation. Med Clin North Am. 1992;76:683-97.

V. Hemoglobinopathies
Kathryn Hassell

Erythrocytes contain two major forms of hemoglobin, hemoglobin A_1 ($\alpha_2\beta_2$) and hemoglobin A_2 ($\alpha_2\delta_2$). Fetal hemoglobin ($\alpha_2\gamma_2$) is the major hemoglobin produced in utero, but it is replaced in the newborn by hemoglobin A_1 by the age of 2 to 3 months. Inherited abnormalities of the hemoglobin molecule include structural hemoglobinopathies and thalassemias. Almost all hemoglobin mutations have minimal clinical significance, but production of abnormal hemoglobin chains can result in altered hemoglobin chemistry, inducing polymerization (hemoglobin S), crystallization (hemoglobin C), or abnormal hemoglobin function (altered oxygen affinity). Underproduction of normal hemoglobin chains, termed *thalassemia*, alters erythrocyte function and shortens erythrocyte survival. In women with hemoglobinopathies or thalassemia, pregnancy is often possible and successful but increased attention is needed to detect and avoid maternal and fetal complications.

Hemoglobinopathies

Sickle-Cell Diseases

Care of the pregnant woman with a sickle-cell disease should be given by a team of health care professionals who are familiar with the disease itself and with the early recognition and management of obstetric and fetal complications. Co-management by a hematologist–internist and an obstetrician familiar with sickle-cell diseases and high-risk obstetric care can result in a successful pregnancy for most women with sickle-cell diseases.

Pathophysiology
Erythrocytes that contain sickle hemoglobin ($\alpha_2\beta^S_2$) are deformed into sickle shapes when the hemoglobin in the cell polymerizes. This polymerization is initially reversible, but eventually the cell becomes irreversibly sickled and is destroyed, resulting in chronic hemolytic anemia and an elevated reticulocyte count. Even when unsickled, the erythrocytes of patients with sickle-cell disease seem to be "sticky" and can adhere to the walls of small blood vessels. When the blood vessel wall itself is activated (e.g., in the setting of infection or inflammation), increased numbers of erythrocytes may adhere to the vessel wall, resulting in occlusion of the vessel. Acutely, this may cause ischemia, resulting in a vasoocclusive pain event or "crisis." Even in the absence of pain, intermittent microvascular occlusion may cause chronic vascular injury and chronic organ damage.

Types

At least 17 types of hemoglobinopathies are called *sickle-cell disease,* which is defined as a hemoglobinopathy in which at least one β-globin gene has the "sickle" mutation ($\beta^{6(glu \cdot val)}$) and the other β-globin gene has a mutation resulting in an abnormal β chain (as in hemoglobin C disease) or underproduction of the β-chain (as in β-thalassemia). Sickle-cell trait (hemoglobin AS disease), in which there is one sickle β-globin gene and one normal β-globin gene, is a genetic carrier state and does not result in a sickle-cell disorder. The more common sickle-cell diseases are outlined in Table 8-17. Other, less common types of sickle-cell disease include hemoglobin SE, hemoglobin SO, and hemoglobin SD disease. Diagnosis of the type of sickle-cell disease is made by hemoglobin electrophoresis; sickle-cell screening tests (such as "Sickledex") are inadequate because they do not detect other hemoglobin variants (such as hemoglobin C) or thalassemias and do not distinguish between sickle-cell diseases and sickle-cell trait.

Maternal Death

The maternal mortality rate is said to be increased in women with sickle-cell disease compared with women without sickle-cell disease. This conclusion seems to be based on retrospective data from limited numbers of patients in the 1960s and 1970s. Since 1975, at least nine series have reported results in more than 1100 pregnancies in which the maternal mortality rate has been less than 1% (1, 2). In the largest and most recent series (2), two maternal deaths were seen among 445 pregnancies; only one death was related to sickle-cell disease, and this death occurred 3 weeks postpartum. Most reported deaths occur in women with sickle-cell anemia (hemoglobin SS disease) and not the milder forms of sickle-cell disease.

Table 8-17 Characteristics of Common Sickle-Cell Diseases

Disease	Baseline Hemoglobin Concentration (g/dL)	Mean Corpuscular Volume (MCV)	Baseline Reticulocyte (%)	Relative Clinical Severity
Hb SS (sickle-cell anemia)	6.0–9.0	Normal	5–30	++++
Hb S-β-0-thalassemia	6.0–9.0	Low	5–30	++++
Hb SC (sickle-hemoglobin C disease)	10–13	Normal	3–4	+++
Hb S-β-(+)-thalassemia	10–14	Low	3–4	++
Hb AS (sickle-cell trait)	14–16	Normal	0–1	0

Obstetric Complications

The rate of spontaneous abortion in women with sickle-cell disease is unclear. It seems to be higher than that in African-American women without sickle-cell disease, but the older literature suggesting very high rates is based on retrospective data from 1950 to 1980. A randomized transfusion study done from 1978 to 1986 showed that 55% to 65% of women with sickle-cell anemia, hemoglobin SC disease, and sickle-β-thalassemia compared with 41% of healthy African-American women had a history of spontaneous or elective abortion (3). The Cooperative Study of Sickle Cell Disease (2) reported a miscarriage rate of 6.5% in women with sickle-cell anemia, hemoglobin SC disease, sickle-β-0-thalassemia, and sickle-β-(+)-thalassemia in 445 pregnancies.

Preterm labor, abruptio placenta, and preeclampsia may occur more often in women with sickle-cell anemia than in healthy African-American women without sickle-cell anemia. Table 8-18 summarizes the frequency of obstetric complications using the results of a prospective study (3) and the experience of the Cooperative Study of Sickle Cell Disease (2). Although probably more common in sickle-cell anemia, these complications occur in women with milder forms of sickle-cell disease, and awareness, early detection, and appropriate treatment of these complications can reduce maternal morbidity rates.

Fetal Implications

Perinatal mortality rates have been reported to be as high as 53% for babies born to women with sickle-cell anemia. These rates have decreased dramatically over the past three decades as obstetric and neonatal care have improved. Since 1980, the neonatal mortality rate is reported to be 0% to 5%

Table 8-18 Frequency of Obstetric Complications in Women with Sickle-Cell Diseases

	Transfusion Study (1978–86)*				Cooperative Study (1979-86)[†]
	Control	SS	SC	Sâthal	
No. of pregnancies	8981	100	66	23	225
Gestational age at delivery (wks)	40	37.5	38.6	37.1	37.7
Preterm labor (%)	17	26	15	22	9
Placenta previa (%)	0.4	1	2	4	–
Abruptio placenta (%)	0.5	3	2	4	–
Toxemia (%)	4	18	9	13	11
Cesarean section (%)	14	29	30	26	–

*Data from Koshy M, Burd L, Wallace D, et al. Prophylactic red-cell transfusions in pregnant patients with sickle cell disease: a randomized cooperative study. N Engl J Med. 1988;319:1447-52.
[†]Data from Smith JA, Espeland M, Bellevue R, et al. Pregnancy in sickle cell disease: experience of the Cooperative Study of Sickle Cell Disease. Obstet Gynecol. 1996;87:199-204.

(1), and a mean Apgar score of 9 at 5 minutes has been seen in babies born to women with all types of sickle-cell disease (2). In babies affected with sickle-cell disease, no manifestations are seen antenatally, perinatally, or in the immediate postpartum period because fetal hemoglobin ($\alpha_2\gamma_2$) continues to be produced until 2 months of age, when production of normal adult hemoglobin A_1 or sickle hemoglobin ($\alpha_2\beta^s_2$) predominates.

In women with sickle-cell anemia, factors that may affect fetal growth include chronic anemia and placental damage due to vascular occlusion. Birthweights average 2.5 to 2.8 kg for babies born to women with sickle-cell anemia and 2.7 to 3.0 kg for babies born to women with hemoglobin SC disease, women with sickle-β-(+)-thalassemia, and healthy African-American women (2–4). However, at least two reports have found no correlation between birthweight and degree of anemia in women with sickle-cell disease (2, 5). These data include women with hemoglobin values as low as 6.0 g/dL during pregnancy. There is an increased frequency of abnormal placentas in women with sickle-cell disease, and the placentas often show infarcted areas with fibrosis. This suggests the possibility of hypoxic or vasoocclusive stresses. In a study of 15 pregnancies (6), third-trimester Doppler flow velocimetry showed a correlation between decreased uterine and umbilical flow and birthweight. Third-trimester Doppler flow velocimetry, when combined with ultrasonography (the "ultradop index"), had a sensitivity of 89% and a positive predictive value of 89% for small-for-gestational-age infants in one series of 27 women with sickle-cell anemia (7). However, uteroplacental Doppler velocimetry showed no change after transfusion therapy, despite a significant reduction in sickle hemoglobin (8).

Despite 1) theoretical concerns about diminished blood flow to the placenta during sickle-cell pain episodes due to increased erythrocyte adherence and vascular occlusion and 2) apparent increased uterine vascular resistance, studies have shown no change in umbilical artery flow during these episodes (9). Monitoring of fetal well-being during a pain episode is complicated by the use of opioids to treat sickle-cell pain; opioids may affect nonstress testing and biophysical profile scores (Table 8-19). Caution must be used in interpreting the results of these tests during acute pain episodes because they may not be predictive of increased perinatal morbidity and mortality rates in the absence of other findings.

Management of Pregnancy

Pregnant women with sickle-cell disease should be followed closely by medical personnel familiar with high-risk obstetrics and sickle-cell diseases. In the first trimester, prevention of dehydration and control of nausea may reduce the risk for sickle-cell pain episodes. Prenatal diagnosis may be discussed in pregnancies in which the father of the child is unknown or is

Table 8-19   Frequency of Abnormal Findings in Fetal Surveillance at Mean Gestational Age of 36 Weeks During 39 Sickle-Cell Pain Events in 24 Women

	Abnormal Findings During Pain Episode (%)	Abnormal Findings after Pain Episode (%)
Nonreactive nonstress test	58.9	10.3*
Biophysical profile score <8	33.3	7.7*
Decreased fetal movement	33.3	7.7*
Decreased fetal breathing	10.3	7.7
Fetal tone	7.7	5.1

*Statistically significant difference.
Adapted from Anyaegbunam A, et al. Antepartum fetal surveillance tests during sickle cell crisis. Am J Obstet Gynecol. 1991;165:1081-3.

known to carry an abnormal hemoglobin gene. If the father is available and his hemoglobin status is unknown, he can be tested by hemoglobin electrophoresis. The presence of sickle-cell disease in the fetus can be determined by amniocentesis or chorionic villous sampling, even though the fetus does not yet produce sickled erythrocytes (10). In the second and third trimesters, twice-monthly visits to educate the mother about and monitor for preterm labor, placental abruption, placenta previa, and sickle-cell disease activity may permit early detection and treatment of these possible complications. A CBC and a reticulocyte count should be done at each visit. Prenatal vitamins, without iron in regularly transfused patients, and additional folate (1.0 mg/d) are given. Patients using long-term pain treatments, including methadone therapy, should be discouraged from abrupt discontinuation of these regimens because maternal withdrawal symptoms may significantly affect the fetus (11). Starting at 24 to 28 weeks of gestation, monthly ultrasonography is recommended to assess fetal growth, and patients should be instructed in how to do daily fetal movement counts. Nonstress tests and biophysical profile testing should be considered weekly beginning at 32 to 34 weeks of gestation; Doppler ultrasonography to assess umbilical artery flow and ratios of systolic to diastolic pressure as a predictor of IUGR may be a useful adjunct. Unless otherwise obstetrically indicated, pregnancy should be allowed to proceed to term with spontaneous onset of labor (1). During labor, adequate hydration and oxygenation should be maintained. Doses of analgesia may exceed those usually required for obstetric pain because of an increased tolerance to pain medications. Vaginal delivery is preferred; cesarean section should be reserved for obstetric indications. If cesarean section is planned, an exchange transfusion should be done first, if possible, in the untransfused patient to avoid perioperative sickle-cell complications (12).

Treatment of Pain Episodes

Most women have some increase in the frequency of sickle-cell pain episodes during pregnancy, but in the Cooperative Study of Sickle-Cell Disease (2), this averaged only one to two episodes (2). Careful surveillance for the development of complications from sickle-cell pain events, which can rapidly become life-threatening, is necessary. These complications most often include the acute chest syndrome, in which diffuse microvascular vasoocclusion occurs with sequestration of erythrocytes in the lungs, resulting in progressive hypoxia, capillary leak, and often a significant decrease in hemoglobin concentrations. Acute sequestration or infarction of the spleen may occur in women with milder forms of sickle-cell disease whose spleen is still present in adulthood. Acute multiorgan failure may also occur, with rapid declines in pulmonary, hepatic, and renal function. Early recognition of these complications, with supportive care and judicious use of transfusion therapy, can halt the progression of these complications and prevent significant illness and death.

The goal of treatment for an uncomplicated sickle-cell pain episode is to restore and maintain normal physiologic conditions to reduce sickling, limit erythrocyte adherence to vessels, and control pain. As outlined in Box 8-7, intravenous fluids and oxygen therapy are used to maintain normal intravascu-

---

Box 8-7 Management of Acute Sickle-Cell Pain Episodes in the Pregnant Woman

1. Intravenous fluids: correct dehydration, then maintain euvolia
2. Oxygen therapy: maintain normal oxygen saturation
3. Investigation and treatment of infection
4. Pain control: intravenous therapy on a regular schedule (not "prn")
   Narcotics (IV)
     Morphine sulfate
     Hydromorphone
     Fentanyl
   Non-narcotic adjuncts (1st–2nd trimester)
     Ibuprofen
     Naproxen
   Antihistamines
     Diphenhydramine
5. Monitor for complications of sickle-cell disease
   Daily complete blood count, reticulocyte count, pulse oximetry
   Baseline chemistry profile, repeat as needed to evaluate clinical deterioration
6. Fetal monitoring if > 26 weeks of gestation

lar volume status and oxygenation. The administration of large volumes of intravenous fluids has no proven benefit once dehydration has been corrected. Some experience suggests that excessive fluid administration may worsen or precipitate the acute chest syndrome, with progressive pulmonary failure as noncardiogenic pulmonary edema develops as a result of sequestration of erythrocytes in the microvasculature of the lung. Excessive oxygen therapy has not been shown to lessen the severity of crisis and may diminish reticulocyte production with subsequent worsening of anemia. Infection may trigger pain episodes by enhancing a local or systemic inflammatory response that increases erythrocyte adherence to the vasculature. Recognition and treatment of infection may shorten sickle-cell pain episodes. Pain medication in doses adequate to control pain should be giving on a routine schedule (not "as needed" or "prn"), intravenously, through a patient-controlled analgesia pump when available and appropriate. Opioids are not associated with teratogenicity, congenital malformations, or toxic effects other than transient suppression of movement and variability in fetal heart tones (13). Chronic exposure to opioids, as in women who require methadone maintenance or routine medications to control severe chronic pain, can lead to the neonatal abstinence syndrome after birth.

Transfusion Therapy

Empirical therapy with transfusion of erythrocytes has been used to support women with sickle-cell disease in pregnancy. A single randomized trial was done to determine the maternal and fetal benefits of an aggressive transfusion regimen (3). In this study, pregnant women with sickle-cell anemia, hemoglobin SC disease, and sickle-β-thalassemia were randomly assigned to 1) a program of "emergent" transfusions, given for acute severe anemia or complications during pregnancy, or 2) routine transfusion to prophylactically reduce the number of circulating sickle erythrocytes. Women in the emergent group had hemoglobin values throughout pregnancy as low as 6.0 g/dL; women in the prophylactic group maintained a hemoglobin concentration of 10 g/dL. Despite aggressive prophylactic transfusion, there was no significant reduction in obstetric complications and no improvement in fetal birthweight or incidence of IUGR. There was, however, a significant reduction in the number of pain episodes but not in the complications (such as acute chest syndrome) of these pain episodes (Table 8-20).

These data do not support a recommendation for prophylactic transfusion in most pregnant women with sickle-cell disease, unless the woman is already receiving such therapy for a previous sickle-cell complication. Recommended indications for transfusion during pregnancy are listed in Box 8-8. If there is an acute indication for transfusion and the hemoglobin concentration is below the patient's baseline, a simple transfusion of packed red blood cells can

Table 8-20   Sickle-Cell Complications (Percent) in Pregnant Women Treated
with "Prophylactic" Transfusion Therapy (PRO) and "Emergent"
Transfusion Therapy (PRN)

	PRO	PRN
One pain episode	14	50*
Acute chest syndrome	6	8
Splenic sequestration	0	3
Severe anemia	3	8
Urinary tract infection	3	17*
Pyelonephritis	3	3

*Statistically significant difference.

**Box 8-8 Recommended Indications for Transfusion in Pregnant Women
with Sickle-Cell Disease**

Preeclampsia

Severe anemia (drop of 30% below baseline or Hb < 5.0 g/dL)

Acute renal failure

Septicemia/bacteremia

Acute chest syndrome/hypoxia

Anticipated surgery including cesarean section

---

be given to restore the hemoglobin value to baseline. If a long-term prophylactic transfusion program is planned, a single unit of packed red blood cells can be given once weekly for several consecutive weeks; care must be taken to ensure that the patient's baseline hemoglobin value is not significantly exceeded. If acute transfusion is indicated but the hemoglobin concentration is at the patient's baseline (steady-state) value, an exchange transfusion must be considered. Transfusion to hemoglobin values above the baseline value can result in increased blood viscosity and worsening of the patient's condition unless the sickle erythrocytes are removed first. In an exchange transfusion, which can be done on an apheresis instrument, the patient's erythrocytes are replaced by normal erythrocytes, typically 6 to 8 units of packed red blood cells. This automated erythrocytapheresis has been safely used in pregnancy and is well tolerated by both mother and fetus (14, 15). Any transfusion should be discussed and planned with the help of a health care professional who is familiar with sickle-cell disease.

Other Issues

Some patients with sickle-cell disease develop chronic complications before pregnancy, including stroke, pulmonary hypertension with chronic restrictive lung disease, hepatic dysfunction associated with viral hepatitis or iron overload due to transfusion therapy, or chronic renal failure. Pregnancies in these patients may be complicated or even contraindicated by end-organ damage. In some patients, these complications are well controlled with chronic transfusion therapy, which suppresses the sickle-cell disease. Transfusion therapy should be continued in these patients throughout pregnancy. Patients with sickle-cell disease who are maintained on chronic transfusion therapy very often need chelation therapy with deferoxamine to treat or prevent hemosiderosis secondary to transfusion therapy. Deferoxamine is considered a category C drug and should be withheld, if possible, during pregnancy. Prenatal vitamins without iron should be prescribed to avoid further iron overload.

Hemoglobin C Disease

Hemoglobin C trait results in no clinical manifestations, has no effect on pregnancy, and is a genetic carrier state. Homozygous hemoglobin C disease occurs when both β-chain genes have a single point mutation ($\beta^{6(glu \cdot lys)}$). Erythrocytes that contain hemoglobin C appear as target cells on the peripheral smear, with occasional areas of crystallization (hemoglobin C crystals). The erythrocytes are relatively fragile, resulting in a moderate chronic hemolytic anemia with hemoglobin values of 10 to 11 g/dL in steady-state, and associated reticulocytosis. Splenomegaly also occurs. There are a few reports of pregnancies complicated by homozygous hemoglobin C disease, but most reports note few, if any, maternal or fetal complications (16). Concomitant iron and folate deficiency resulting in worsening anemia has been noted in some of these pregnancies, prompting the recommendation of prenatal vitamins, additional folate supplementation, and additional iron supplementation, if needed (17, 18).

Hemoglobin E Disease

Hemoglobin E results from a single point mutation in the β-globin gene ($\beta^{26(glu \cdot lys)}$). Hemoglobin E trait has no clinical manifestations, may result in a slightly low erythrocyte MCV without anemia, and has no recognizable effect on pregnancy. Homozygous hemoglobin E disease results in mild chronic hemolytic anemia with a low erythrocyte MCV but no clinical symptoms. When hemoglobin E is inherited with β-thalassemia (HbE-β-0-thalassemia or HbE-β-(+)-thalassemia), the severity of anemia and microcytosis (low MCV) is worsened and splenomegaly is present. In women with homozygous hemo-globin E disease, pregnancy seems to be well tolerated with minimal maternal or fetal complications (19). In contrast, several case reports of pregnancy in women with hemoglobin E-β-0-thalassemia suggest that fetal growth may be compromised and the likelihood of fetal death may be increased (20). On the basis of this limited experience, it is recommended that the mother be sup-ported throughout the pregnancy with transfusions sufficient to sustain a he-moglobin value of 10 g/dL and that fetal monitoring be frequent after 28 weeks of gestation.

Thalassemias

Types

In thalassemia, there is underproduction of a hemoglobin chain due to a vari-ety of mutations that result in poor or no function of the globin gene. In α-thalassemia, the α-globin chain is underproduced, often because of an absence of one or more of the four genes that control production. In β-tha-lassemia, the β-globin chain is underproduced, often because of point muta-tions that result in dysfunctional genes. The common types of thalassemia are described in Table 8-21.

Pathophysiology

The most common thalassemia defects result in the underproduction of ei-ther α- or β-globin chains. Because the hemoglobin molecule is made up of two α-globin chains and two β-globin chains, underproduction of one results in an unmatched excess of the other. For example, patients with β-tha-lassemia have a relative excess of α-globin chains. The consequence of under-production of hemoglobin is microcytosis and "target cell" morphologic findings. Excessive, unused globin chains cause membrane damage and in-creased erythrocyte fragility. The result of these effects is a chronic hemolytic anemia, with compensatory reticulocytosis, and splenomegaly. In the most severe form of the disease, Cooley anemia, the patient is transfusion depen-dent and has growth retardation and a high incidence of infertility. Unless the patient is compliant with chelation therapy, secondary hemosiderosis results in early death.

Pregnancy and Thalassemias

In women with α- or β-thalassemia trait, pregnancy is generally well toler-ated and has no recognized complications for mother or fetus. Because these women often have mild microcytic anemia at baseline, iron studies may need to be done to evaluate for iron deficiency, which can occur during pregnancy despite the increased iron absorption that characterizes thalassemia. Patients

Table 8-21 Common Types and Characteristics of β- and α-Thalassemias

Type of Thalassemia	Genetics	Degree of Anemia	Mean Corpuscular Volume	Splenomegaly	Transfusion Dependent?
β-thalassemia	Controlled by two genes (maternal/ paternal)				
Thalassemia minor (β-thalassemia trait)	1 normal gene, 1 abnormal gene	None or mild	Normal or slightly low	May be present	No
Thalassemia intermedia	2 mildly abnormal genes	Mild or moderate	Low	Present	Sometimes
Thalassemia major (Cooley anemia)	2 severely abnormal or absent genes	Severe	Low	Present	Always
α-thalassemia	Controlled by 4 genes (2 maternal, 2 paternal)				
α-thalassemia trait	3 normal genes, 1 missing gene	None	Normal	Absent	No
"2-gene minus"	2 normal genes, 2 missing genes	None or mild	Normal or slightly low	May be present	No
Hemoglobin H disease	1 normal gene, 3 missing genes	Moderate or severe	Low	Present	Sometimes
Hydrops fetalis with hemoglobin Bart's	4 genes missing	←——— Incompatible with life–death in utero ———→			

with Cooley anemia and β-thalassemia intermedia seem to have significant compromise in fertility, and few pregnancies have been reported in these women. Up to 50% of these pregnancies have been complicated by stillbirth, IUGR, and preterm delivery (21). Successful pregnancies have been reported with 1) transfusion support to maintain a hemoglobin value of 1.0 g/L during pregnancy and 2) careful maternal and fetal monitoring (22).

Prenatal Counseling

Because pregnancy is very well tolerated in women with minor thalassemia traits and is infrequent in women with severe β-thalassemia, the major obstetric focus is on prenatal testing. Prenatal detection of both α- and β-thalassemia is increasingly feasible as more of the common mutations are characterized with the use of DNA hybridization techniques from fetal cells obtained by amniocentesis, chorionic villus sampling, or percutaneous cord-blood sampling (10, 21). Early diagnosis may allow intervention (beyond elective termination), including in utero bone marrow transplantation for fetal hydrops.

High-Affinity Hemoglobins

Abnormal hemoglobin variants with a high affinity for oxygen result in a secondary polycythemia as a compensatory mechanism for poor release of oxygen to the tissues. There are few reports of pregnancy in women with high-affinity hemoglobins. In a small series of families with these variants, no evidence of increased spontaneous abortion, IUGR, or adverse maternal outcomes was seen (23). In these families, it is assumed that there is increased uterine or fetal blood flow, with potential for fetal polycythemia in response to hypoxia, resulting in normal fetal outcomes.

REFERENCES

1. **Rust OA, Perry KG.** Pregnancy complicated by sickle hemoglobinopathy. Clin Obstet Gynecol. 1995;38:472-84.

2. **Smith JA, Espeland M, Bellevue R, Bonds D, Brown AK, Koshy M.** Pregnancy in sickle cell disease: experience of the Cooperative Study of Sickle Cell Disease. Obstet Gynecol. 1996;87:199-204.

3. **Koshy M, Burd L, Wallace D, Moawad A, Baron J.** Prophylactic red-cell transfusions in pregnant patients with sickle cell disease: a randomized cooperative study. N Engl J Med. 1988;319:1447-52.

4. **Koshy M, Chisum D, Burd L, Orlina A, How H.** Management of sickle cell anemia and pregnancy. J Clin Apheresis. 1991;6:230-3.

5. **Powars DR, Sandhu M, Niland-Weiss J, Johnson C, Bruce S, Manning PR.** Pregnancy in sickle cell disease. Obstet Gynecol. 1986;67:217-28.

6. **Billett H, Langer O, Regan O, Anyaegbunam A.** Doppler velocimetry in pregnant patients with sickle cell anemia. Am J Hematol. 1993;42:305-8.

7. **Anyaegbuman A, Langer O, Brustman L, Whitty J, Merkatz I.** Third-trimester prediction of small-for-gestational-age infants in pregnant women with sickle cell disease: development of the ultradop index. J Reprod Med. 1991;36:577-80.

8. **Howard R, Tuck S, Pearson T.** Blood transfusion in pregnancies complicated by maternal sickle cell disease: effects on blood rheology and uteroplacental Doppler velocimetry. Clin Lab Haematol. 1994;16:253-9.

9. **Anyaegbunam A, Morel M, Merkatz I.** Antepartum fetal surveillance tests during sickle cell crisis. Am J Obstet Gynecol. 1991;165:1081-3.

10. **Fischel-Ghodsian N.** Prenatal diagnosis of hemoglobinopathies. Clin Perinatol. 1990;17:811-28.

11. **Rementeria J, Nuang N.** Narcotic withdrawal in pregnancy: stillbirth incidence with a case report. Am J Obstet Gynecol. 1973;116:1152-6.

12. **Koshy M, Burd L.** Management of pregnancy in sickle cell syndromes. Hematol Oncol Clin North Am. 1991;5:585-96.

13. **Rathmell J, Viscomi C, Ashburn M.** Management of nonobstetric pain during pregnancy and lactation. Anesth Analg. 1997;85:1074-87.

14. **Lee W, Werch R, Rokey J, Pivarnik J, Miller J.** Physiologic observations of pregnant women undergoing prophylactic erythrocytapheresis for sickle cell disease. Transfusion. 1991;31:59-62.

15. **Morrison J, Morrison F, Floyd R, Roberts W, Hess L, Wise W.** Use of continuous flow erythrocytapheresis in pregnant patients with sickle cell disease. J Clin Apheresis. 1991;6:224-9.

16. **Maberry M, Mason R, Cunningham G, Pritchard J.** Pregnancy complicated by hemoglobin CC and C-β-thalassemia disease. Obstet Gynecol. 1990;76:324-7.

17. **Anderson M, Bluestone R, Milner P.** Pregnancy and homozygous haemoglobin C disease. J Obstet Gynaecol Brit Cwlth. 1967;74:694-6.

18. **Kitay D, Perrin E.** Homozygous hemoglobin C disease and pregnancy. Obstet Gynecol. 1968;32:657-63.

19. **Ong H.** Maternal and fetal outcome associated with hemoglobin E trait and hemoglobin E disease. Obstet Gynecol. 1975;45:672-4.

20. **Ferguson J, O'Reilly R.** Hemoglobin E and pregnancy. Obstet Gynecol. 1985;66:136-40.

21. **Kilpatrick S, Laros R.** Thalassemia in pregnancy. Clin Obstet Gynecol. 1995;38:485-96.

22. **Morel N, Birkenfel A, Goldfarb A, Rachmilewitz E.** Successful full-term pregnancy in homozygous β-thalassemia major: case report and review of the literature. Obstet Gynecol. 1989;73:837-40.

23. **Charache S, Catalano P, Burns S, Jones R, Koler R, Rutstein R, Williams R.** Pregnancy in carriers of high-affinity hemoglobins. Blood. 1985;65:713-8.

VI. Maternal Isoimmunization
Erin Keely

Isoimmunization is the most common cause of hemolytic disease in the neonate and was a major cause of perinatal death until an effective treatment for it was established after the development of Rho(D) immune globulin in 1968. Although it may threaten the life of the fetus, isoimmunization has no consequences to the mother. Maternal antibodies form when the mother is exposed to antigens that she does not carry on her erythrocytes. Most cases of isoimmunization are due to Rh incompatibility (D antigen), although with the use of Rhogam prophylaxis, a greater percentage of cases is now due to other erythrocyte antigens, such as Kell, Duffy (Fy^a), and Kidd (Jk^a, Jk^b).

Maternal sensitization may occur during pregnancy or after an autologous blood transfusion. Because of careful screening of ABO and Rh status before blood transfusion, pregnancy is the most common reason for anti-D development; exposure to the other erythrocyte antigens more commonly results from transfusion. The fetus does not develop erythrocyte antigens until 35 days of gestation, so maternal sensitization does not occur before this point (1). The risk for sensitization increases as pregnancy progresses because of increasing maternal exposure to fetal antigens; sensitization is most common after 28 weeks of gestation. Maternal exposure to fetal antigens may also occur with first-trimester abortion, abruptio placenta, cordocentesis, amniocentesis, external cephalic version, and abdominal trauma during pregnancy. Approximately 3% to 10% of Rh-negative women become sensitized after a first pregnancy when no immune prophylaxis is given.

The consequences to the fetus range from mild hemolytic anemia to hydrops fetalis to death. Increased hematopoiesis in the liver leads to portal hypertension and to decreased production of hepatic proteins, including albumin, causing ascites and effusion. Bilirubin is released from the hemolyzed erythrocytes and can be measured in cord blood and amniotic fluid. High-output cardiac failure may develop when the fetal hematocrit decreases. The severity of fetal disease in the first affected pregnancy can be predicted somewhat by antibody titers, but obstetric history is more predictive of fetal outcome in subsequent pregnancies.

Screening for Isoimmunization

All women should be screened with a blood type test, an Rh status test, and an indirect Coombs test in the first trimester to determine whether they are at risk (Rh negative with no antibodies) or already sensitized. If an antibody is identified, the titer and the antigen against which it is directed must be determined. Antibodies against Lewis antigens do not cause fetal disease; all other antibodies are capable of causing severe anemia.

Prophylaxis in the Rh-Negative Mother

If the partner of an Rh-negative mother is heterozygous for RhD (most Rh-positive persons are), there is a 50% chance of an Rh-positive fetus. Prophylaxis is aimed at reducing maternal antibody production from exposure to Rh-positive fetal cells. Good evidence shows that routine antenatal anti-D prophylaxis reduces the risk for sensitization in pregnancy 2-fold to 16-fold (2, 3). The dose required depends on the amount of fetomaternal bleeding and thus is lower in first-trimester bleeding events. A Kleihauer test can estimate the amount of fetal blood present in the maternal circulation, but the role of this test in dose determination is controversial. Dosing recommendations vary internationally and depend on the product used. In general, 100 to 125 µg of anti-D immunoglobulin is used in first-trimester bleeding interventions and 300 µg is used at 28 weeks of gestation. If the neonate is Rh positive, 300 µg is given postpartum.

Treatment in a Previously Sensitized Mother

The risk to the fetus is dependent on the antigen status of the fetus, maternal antibody titers (risk is increased with titers >1:8 to 1:16), and previous obstetric history, and risk assessment will guide the degree of fetal surveillance. Fetal monitoring may include amniocentesis to measure bilirubin as evidence of fetal hemolysis (plotted on Liley curves), ultrasonography to seek evidence of hydrops, and cordocentesis with possible intrauterine infusion. Fetal Rh status can now be determined by amniocentesis or by typing fetal cells isolated from maternal serum (4). If the fetus is Rh negative, no further investigations or treatments are required throughout the pregnancy. Affected fetuses are treated with in utero blood transfusions and, in severe cases, occurs when there is lung maturity.

REFERENCES

1. **Gollin YG, Copel JA.** Management of the Rh-sensitized mother. Clin Perinatol. 1995:545-55.
2. **James D.** Anti-D prophylaxis in 1997: the Edinburgh consensus statement. Arch Dis Child. 1998:78;F161-3.
3. **Crowther CA, Keirse MJNC.** Anti-D administration in pregnancy. In: Neilson JP, Crowther CA, Hodnett ED, Hofmeyr GJ, Keirse MJNC, Renfrew MJ, eds. Pregnancy and Childbirth Module of the Cochrane Database of Systematic Reviews [Updated 6 June 1996].
4. **Lo YMD, Hjelm NM, Fidler C, Sargent IL, Murphy MF, Chamberlain PF, et al.** Prenatal diagnosis of fetal RhD status by molecular analysis of maternal plasma. N Engl J Med. 1998;339:1734-8.

CHAPTER 9

Rheumatologic Disorders and the Antiphospholipid Antibody Syndrome

I. Antiphospholipid Antibody Syndrome
Robert M. Silver, MD, and Susan Z. Cowchock, MD

II. Systemic Lupus Erythematosus
Karen Rosene-Montella, MD

III. Rheumatoid Arthritis
J. Lee Nelson, MD

IV. Scleroderma
Karen Rosene-Montella, MD

I. Antiphospholipid Antibody Syndrome
Robert M. Silver and Susan Z. Cowchock

Antiphospholipid antibodies (aPLs) are a heterogeneous group of autoantibodies that recognize negatively charged phospholipids, phospholipid-associated proteins, or a phospholipid–protein complex. Although several aPLs have been described, the two that are best characterized and most widely accepted for clinical use are lupus anticoagulant (LA) and anticardiolipin antibody (aCL). These antibodies have been associated with numerous clinical problems, including arterial and venous thrombosis, autoimmune thrombocy-

Key Values and Normal Physiologic Changes for Rheumatologic Disorders

	Direction of Change	Percentage Change or Normal Range for Pregnancy
Autoantibodies (e.g., ANA, RF, anti-DNA, SSA, SSB)	↔	
Complement levels	↑	
C3	↑	70 to 140 U/mL
C4	↑↑	40 to 100 U/mL
CH50	↑	>100 U/mL
Erythrocyte sedimentation rate	↑↑	20 to 100 mm/h
Immunoglobulins	↑	10% to 20% increase

↑ Increase
↓ Decrease
↔ No change

topenia (ITP), and recurrent pregnancy loss (1–4). Patients who have these clinical features in addition to specific aPL levels are considered to have the antiphospholipid syndrome (APS) (Box 9-1). Other autoimmune conditions, especially systemic lupus erythematosus (SLE), often coexist with APS. Patients with APS who have another autoimmune disease are considered to have secondary APS (2, 4). Primary APS occurs in persons who do not have SLE or other multisystem immune disorders (2, 3).

In addition to fetal loss, aPL and other thrombophilias have been associated with several obstetric disorders. Pregnancies that result in surviving infants in women with thrombophilias are often complicated by early severe preeclampsia, intrauterine growth restriction (IUGR), placental insufficiency, and preterm birth (5, 6). Pregnancy and the puerperium period may also pose increased risk for some of the medical complications associated with aPL. Because women with aPL often have other serious medical conditions, such as previous thromboembolism or SLE, they are frequently managed by multidisciplinary teams that include internists and obstetricians. This review focuses on the practical, clinical aspects of medical care for pregnant women with aPL. New developments and areas of controversy are emphasized. Other thrombophilias are discussed in Chapter 8.

Antiphospholipid Antibody Testing

Laboratory detection of aPL can be confusing to practicing clinicians. As a relatively new and evolving science, aPL testing has been hampered by unac-

---

Box 9-1 Suggested Clinical and Laboratory Criteria for Diagnosis of Antiphospholipid Syndrome*

Clinical criteria
 Pregnancy loss
  Recurrent spontaneous abortion[†]
  Unexplained fetal death
 Thrombosis
  Venous thrombosis
  Arterial thrombosis, stroke
 Autoimmune thrombocytopenia
 Other disorders
  Autoimmune hemolytic anemia
  Transient ischemic attacks
  Amaurosis fugax
  Chorea gravidarum
  Livedo reticularis
Laboratory criteria
 Lupus anticoagulant
 Anticardiolipin antibodies >15–20 GPL units[‡]

---

*Patients should meet at least one clinical and one laboratory criterion to receive a diagnosis of antiphospholipid syndrome.
[†]Three or more spontaneous abortions with no more than one live birth
[‡]See text for details.

---

ceptable interlaboratory variation, nonstandardized assays, and inadequate quality control (7, 8). In addition, controversy and uncertainty surround the true antigen specificity of clinically important aPL. Finally, new assays for aPL are continually being developed and are often widely marketed without proof of clinical usefulness. These issues are currently being resolved through ongoing studies and international workshops. Meanwhile, clinicians should recognize the limitations of available assays and should seek out a laboratory with interest and expertise in aPL testing.

Lupus Anticoagulant

Lupus anticoagulant is an unusual name for an antibody, and it is also a double misnomer: It is present in patients without SLE, and it usually predisposes to thrombosis rather than bleeding. It is detected indirectly, through its ability to interfere with the results of any of several in vitro phospholipid-dependent clotting assays (e.g., activated partial thromboplastin time, dilute Russell viper venom time, kaolin clotting time, Textarin time, plasma clotting time). In these assays, phospholipids serve as a template on which enzymes and cofactors of the clotting cascade interact. If it is present, LA binds to these phospholipids (or associated proteins) and interferes with the timely interaction of the clotting factors, prolonging the clotting time. This observation prompted the term *lupus anticoagulant*. The sensitivity and specificity of each test for LA are influenced by the type and concentration of phospholipids used and vary among laboratories. Thus, results from one laboratory may not apply in another, and the "best" test for LA may differ by institution.

Factors other than LA that can prolong clotting assay times include clotting factor deficiencies, anticoagulant medications, improperly processed specimens, and factor-specific inhibitors. Thus, plasma that is suspected to contain LA on the basis of a prolonged clotting time should undergo confirmatory testing in which the test is repeated after normal plasma has been added in a ratio of 1:2 or 1:1. If a clotting factor deficiency is present, the prolonged clotting time will correct toward normal because the deficient factor is provided by the normal plasma. In contrast, the assay time will remain prolonged in the presence of an inhibitor, such as LA. A second confirmatory test, such as the platelet neutralization procedure, is used to ensure that the inhibitor is phospholipid dependent. Regardless of the assays used, LA cannot be quantified and is simply reported as either present or absent.

Anticardiolipin Antibody

Anticardiolipin antibody is detected by immunoassays that use purified cardiolipin as the solid-phase antigen. Interlaboratory variation in these assays prompted the development of standard serum specimens, which are available from the Antiphospholipid Standardization Laboratory in Atlanta (9). Results from assays using these standard positive serum calibrators are consistent among laboratories and allow for determination of semiquantitative antibody levels. Standard serum specimens have been assigned numeric values, which are termed GPL (IgG aCL), MPL (IgM aCL), and APL (IgA aCL) units. Results are related to these units and reported as negative, low positive, medium positive, or high positive.

A finding of low-positive aCL or isolated IgM aCL (when tests for LA give negative results) has questionable clinical significance and should not be considered diagnostic of APS (10). In addition, the relevance of IgA aCL is uncertain. Low-positive aCL or isolated IgM aCL is present in at least 4% of healthy persons (11) and can be due to infection (12) or nonspecific binding. In contrast, medium-positive and high-positive IgG aCL and LA correlate best with the clinical disorders associated with aPL (1, 13, 14) and thus are a diagnostic criterion for APS (2, 4). Positive results on aPL tests can be transient and should be confirmed on two occasions several weeks apart (2, 14). Many persons with LA have aCL and vice versa, but the correlation between the two aPLs is imperfect (15). We recommend testing for both LA and aCL when APS is suspected because some patients with APS have either LA or aCL but not both.

Other Antiphospholipid Antibodies

The antibody responsible for false-positive serologic test results for syphilis was one of the first recognized aPLs. Although it is often seen in patients with LA or aCL, it correlates relatively poorly with the clinical problems associated with aPL. Thus, tests for this antibody are not recommended in the evaluation of suspected APS.

Several other aPLs can be detected with immunoassays directed against phospholipid antigens other than cardiolipin, such as phosphatidylserine, phosphatidylcholine, phosphatidylethanolamine, phosphatidylinositol, phosphatidylglycerol, and phosphatidic acid. These aPLs, especially antiphosphatidylserine antibodies, are sometimes present in patients with APS or clinical disorders associated with aPL (16, 17). Most patients with these antibodies, however, also have LA or IgG aCL (17). One problem is that assays for other aPLs have not been subjected to standardization and are still prone to interlaboratory variation. Finally, although tests for multiple aPLs may identify additional patients with APS, they also increase the cost of screening and the chance of a false-positive test result. When only two phospholipid antibody tests are considered (those for IgG aCL and LA), a survey of the literature found that the rate of positive results in patients with recurrent pregnancy loss was, at most, 20%. When considering laboratory performance, remember that the total rate of positive results should not be much higher in similar populations (18). Thus, although tests for aPLs other than LA and aCL may prove useful, it is uncertain whether they should be recommended for clinical use.

It is now apparent that aPLs probably bind either phospholipid-associated proteins or a phospholipid–protein complex rather than phospholipids themselves. In 1990, three groups independently showed that the plasma glycoprotein beta2-glycoprotein-1 (beta2-GP-1) greatly enhances the binding of aPL to phospholipid (19–21). Thus, beta2-GP-1 is considered to be a critical cofactor for aPL binding. Anticardiolipin antibody can be separated into beta2-GP-1–dependent and beta2-GP-1–independent antibodies (20, 22, 23). Moreover, beta2-GP-1–dependent antibodies correlate better with the clinical features of APS than beta2-GP-1–independent antibodies do (22, 23). Fortunately, the standard assay for aCL uses serum specimens containing beta2-GP-1 and consequently identifies beta2-GP-1–dependent aCL.

Substantial evidence indicates that beta2-GP-1 may be the major epitope recognized by aPL (24, 25). Antibodies binding to beta2-GP-1 in the absence of phospholipid can be directly measured and have been associated with many of the medical conditions associated with aPL (26–28). In fact, some studies in rheumatologic and hematologic populations have indicated that anti–beta-2-GP-1 is a more specific marker for the clinical manifestations of APS than aPL is (27–30). However, the association between anti–beta2-GP-1 and pregnancy loss is less clear (30–32). Assays for anti–beta2-GP-1 may prove to be more consistent than those for aCL because it is easier to work with proteins than with phospholipids. Conversely, anti–beta2-GP-1 strongly correlates with aCL, and testing for both antibodies may be more expensive and no better than testing for aCL alone. The assay has not yet been standardized; after standardization, the clinical usefulness and cost effectiveness of testing for anti–beta-2-GP-1 can be evaluated.

Indications for aPL testing are shown in Box 9-2. It is important to recall that aPL, especially low-titer and IgM isotypes, is present in normal persons. In the absence of pertinent clinical disorders, the presence of aPL is probably meaningless. Clinicians who test for aPL in patients without clinical features

---

Box 9-2 Indications for Antiphospholipid Antibody Testing

Recurrent spontaneous abortion*
Unexplained fetal death in the second or third trimester
Severe preeclampsia before 34 weeks of gestation
Unexplained venous thrombosis
Unexplained arterial thrombosis
Unexplained stroke
Unexplained transient ischemic attack or amaurosis fugax
Systemic lupus erythematosus or other connective tissue disease
Autoimmune thrombocytopenia
Autoimmune hemolytic anemia
Livedo reticularis
Chorea gravidarum
False-positive result on serologic test for syphilis
Unexplained prolongation in clotting assay
Unexplained severe intrauterine growth restriction

*Three or more spontaneous abortions with no more than one live birth.

of APS may be left with an uninterpretable result and a management dilemma. It is best to test only women with appropriate indications.

Obstetric Complications

The association between aPL and pregnancy loss has been recognized for decades and has been confirmed in numerous case series and retrospective cohorts (1, 33–35). In fact, the rate of pregnancy loss in untreated women with LA and previous fetal loss may be as high as 80% (5, 36). Prospective studies in unselected (37–40) and selected (5, 36, 41, 42) populations have confirmed the strong association between aPL and pregnancy loss.

A large proportion of pregnancy losses in patients with aPL are second- or third-trimester fetal deaths. Fetal deaths account for only a small percentage of all pregnancy losses in the general population (43), but 50% of pregnancy losses in a large cohort of women with APS were fetal deaths (44). Eighty percent of the women in this cohort had at least one fetal death.

In addition, aPL is associated with recurrent spontaneous abortion. Cohort–control studies have consistently shown a higher proportion of positive results on tests for aPL in women with recurrent early pregnancy loss (14, 16, 44–51). Most studies report positive test results for aPL in 5% to 20% of patients with recurrent spontaneous abortion (18). It is noteworthy that some of the positive results were of low titer and thus of questionable clinical significance. In contrast to recurrent pregnancy loss, sporadic early pregnancy loss is not associated with aPL (52). This is an expected observation given the many causes of individual pregnancy losses, especially spontaneous abortions, which are often due to genetic abnormalities. Some (53, 54) but not all (55) studies have indicated aPL in 10% to 15% of women with unselected fetal deaths.

In addition to frequently ending in fetal loss, pregnancies in women with APS are often complicated by obstetric disorders characterized by abnormal placentation, including preeclampsia, IUGR, and abnormal fetal testing. These conditions are all consequences of uteroplacental insufficiency and can result in fetal death if appropriate obstetric intervention is not provided. Preeclampsia occurs in 18% to 48% of patients with genuine APS (5, 6). In addition, aPL was reported to be a prospective risk factor for preeclampsia in two studies (39, 40) but not in a third (38). It is also present in a substantial proportion of women with preeclampsia, especially those who develop severe preeclampsia at less than 34 weeks of gestation (56–59). Intrauterine growth restriction has been associated with aPL, complicating 15% to 30% of pregnancies in women with APS (5, 6, 60, 61). Similarly, abnormal fetal heart rate tracings indicative of uteroplacental insufficiency occur in up to 50% of APS pregnancies (5, 6). Placental insufficiency can be evident in fetal heart rate tracings as early as the second trimester (62). Increased rates of preeclampsia, IUGR, and abnormal fetal heart rate tracings all contribute to an increased rate of preterm birth in women with APS. Preterm birth has been reported in 12% to 35% of women with aPL (5, 6, 40, 61). The risk for clinically significant preterm birth is greatest in patients who meet strict criteria for APS; about one third of these patients have clinically significant preterm birth (5).

Medical Complications

The most important medical complication associated with aPL is thrombosis; about 2% of patients with an episode of unexplained venous thrombosis are found to have aPL (63). The most common thrombosis associated with aPL is the most common thrombosis in all pregnant women: deep venous thrombosis of the leg (64). The second most common is pulmonary embolus secondary to deep venous thrombosis or pelvic thrombophlebitis. However, unlike the usual gravida, women with aPL may have thrombosis at unusual sites. The most frequently reported site is the cerebral circulation, including the retinal veins (64–67). Patients that have had previous thromboses have a risk for recurrence of thrombosis during pregnancy and the postpartum period of approximately 12% (68). The actual size of the increase in risk associated with aPL beyond the incidence of thrombosis associated with pregnancy is unknown because almost all women with the diagnosis of aPL receive some form of prophylactic anticoagulation throughout pregnancy and the postpartum period. The risk during pregnancy may parallel risks reported for nonpregnant patients with aPL in the absence of SLE: A meta-analysis estimated the odds ratio for venous thrombosis to be 3.2 (95% CI, 1.10 to 9.28) when only high titers of aCL were considered. For patients with LA, the odds ratio was 11.1 (95% CI, 3.8 to 32.3) (69).

Various neurologic conditions are associated with aPL (70). Although not limited to pregnancy, the ongoing process of cerebral arterial thrombosis of small vessels is underappreciated: Patients with lupus have vasculopathies that are not associated with aPL, so the role of aPL as a cause of central nervous system disease in patients with lupus is uncertain (71, 72). Again, LA was associated with a higher risk: Patients with SLE who were positive for LA were two to three times more likely than those who were LA negative to be identified as cognitively impaired on a test battery (72). Even patients with aPL whose only problem was mild headaches had focal areas of low perfusion on single-photon emission computed tomography of the brain (73). What must be impressed on pregnant women with high levels of aPL or LA is the need for ongoing surveillance after delivery, or even after the childbearing years, by physicians knowledgeable about this syndrome.

Other autoimmune disorders can first appear during pregnancy in association with aPL. Vasculitic, tender nodules may appear on palms and, less commonly, on the soles. Flares of lupus or lupus-like joint disease (like flares of most autoimmune diseases) tend to occur after delivery (74). A clinically significant low platelet count may be associated with APL alone, but after heparin-associated thrombocytopenia has been reasonably excluded the co-occurrence of aPL syndrome and ITP should be considered (75). Even after a short period of follow-up after diagnosis (mean, 3.2 years), new clinical events were common in women presenting with pregnancy loss and high APL levels. In addition to developing thrombosis, some developed autoimmune disorders such as SLE or ITP (76).

The catastrophic aPL syndrome—a serious, often fatal complication in patients with aPL—has been well characterized in Asherson's review of the literature (77). An inflammatory insult, such as surgery or sepsis, can trigger widespread platelet thrombi in the microvasculature and large vasculature. The syndrome is almost always associated with high aCL or LA levels. The postpartum occurrence of catastrophic aPL syndrome is described in several case reports (78–80).

Mechanisms of Thrombosis and Vascular Disease in Antiphospholipid Syndrome

The spectrum of antibody specificities and the expansion of our understanding of demonstrated and potential pathophysiologic mechanisms have given elegance to what was once considered a simple clotting abnormality. The aPLs are directed to complexes of phospholipids and phospholipid-binding proteins. The first physiologic effects of aPL to be described were 1) in vitro interference with the conversion of prothrombin to thrombin, which prolonged clotting times, and 2) the tendency of patients with aPL to have both arterial and venous thrombosis. Even then, it was noted that recurrent thromboses tended to be site specific (e.g., in a patient with arterial thrombosis, recurrence tended to be another arterial thrombosis) (81). The first protein epitope described was beta-2-GP-1. Although the autoantibodies detected through enzyme-linked immunosorbent assays for aCL are often directed to phospholipids conjugated to this protein, the role of this protein in the genesis of thrombosis is still unclear. Cross-linked anti–beta2-GP-1 complexes bind tightly to membranes and inhibit binding of other phospholipid-binding proteins (82). Some of these are naturally occurring anticoagulants (e.g., annexin V, which is expressed on endothelial cells and trophoblasts) (83). Other proteins, such as prothrombin itself, have been determined to be part of the antigen complex to which aPL is directed. Antibodies to protein C and protein S may inhibit the physiologically important protein C anticoagulant pathway.

All of these are potential and possibly interactive pathways that may lead to thrombosis and pregnancy loss.

Interactions among autoantibodies to phospholipid–protein complexes and endothelial cells and blood monocytes may be major causes of vascular and thrombotic disorders in patients with aPL. Beta2-GP-1 antibodies bind to endothelial cells and induce upregulation of adhesion molecules, such as E-selectin, vascular cell adhesion molecule-1, and intracellular adhesion molecule-1 (82). Synthesis of cytokines—specifically, interleukin-1beta—is also increased (84, 85). Antibodies to beta2-GP-1 also enhance monocyte adherence to endothelial cells. Tissue factor is a major initiator of normal and pathologic coagulation and can be induced by a variety of inflammatory stimuli. It has been shown that aPL increases monocyte tissue factor expression, and this expression is correlated with thrombosis (85). The veritable cascade of aPL-mediated or aPL-initiated effects on the blood and tissue coagulation systems that may lead to thrombosis and fetal death is shown in Figure 9-1.

Because APS is characterized by thrombosis and uteroplacental insufficiency, many believe that thromboses within the uteroplacental circulation cause fetal death. Annexin V may be an example of direct interactions between aPL and placental tissue; aPL may promote intervillous thrombosis by displacing this endogenous anticoagulant protein on the surface of trophoblast tissues (83). Pathology studies have shown intervillous thrombosis in placentas from patients with aPL (86).

Treatment of Pregnant
Women with Antiphospholipid Syndrome

Prompted by the high rate of fetal loss as well as the risk for thrombosis during pregnancy, clinicians have used a variety of drugs to treat women with aPL (68). Treatments are intended to suppress the immune system or prevent clotting. The use of corticosteroids is now limited to short-term management of coincident autoimmune disorders (87). Corticosteroid therapy not only increases maternal risk for such complications as gestational diabetes, hypertension, and osteoporosis but is associated with an unacceptable rate of preterm delivery when used in patients with APS.

Heparin anticoagulation is the mainstay of treatment. It is not certain whether the addition of low-dose aspirin improves outcomes for mother or infant, but aspirin (80 mg/d) does not seem to increase maternal risk for bleeding or to be associated with any significant fetal risk. However, studies evaluating fetal outcome have shown that heparin is the more effective anticoagulant (88, 89). Patients without active thrombosis need only prophylactic levels of heparin anticoagulation. A consensus from published studies is that

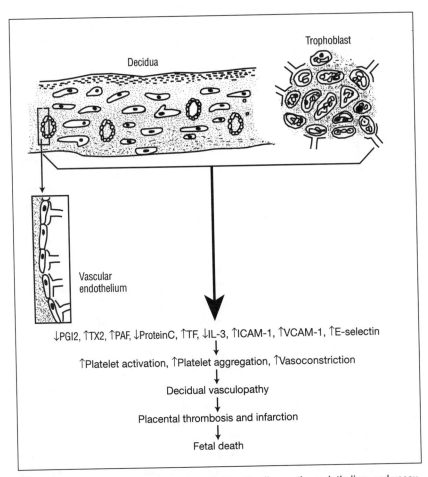

Figure 9-1 Multiple effects of antiphospholipid antibodies on the endothelium and vascular clotting systems. These effects tend to promote systemic and placental vascular thromboses and, ultimately, fetal death.

unfractionated heparin should be given for prophylaxis in doses equivalent to the 5000 U given subcutaneously every 12 hours to nonpregnant patients.

However, the dose of unfractionated heparin needed to achieve this level of anticoagulation during pregnancy is certainly higher, and doses may need to be given more often. The need for higher doses and the significant interpatient variability in dosage requirements during pregnancy mandate measurement of plasma heparin levels with assays based on inactivation of factor Xa. Dahlman and co-workers (90) first reported that higher doses of subcutaneous heparin were needed to achieve postinjection peak levels of 0.10 to 0.15 (the target level for nonpregnant patients). The average twice-daily dose for their patients was 8200 IU. Brancazio and colleagues (91) have reported on the pharmacokinetics of subcutaneous heparin early in the third trimester of pregnancy. Heparin is cleared much faster during pregnancy, and both peak level and the time to peak were significantly lower in pregnant women than in nonpregnant controls. The faster clearance of heparin during pregnancy means that three-times-daily dosing is sometimes required. Barbour and co-workers (92) also noted significant interpatient variability in dosage requirements; the variability was not related to weight. Activated partial thromboplastin times tend to vary greatly in pregnancy. Pregnant women who receive subcutaneous heparin in doses sufficient to reach a targeted peak level may still be unprotected during part of the day. In women who are considered high risk on the basis of medical or obstetric history, it may be necessary to measure preinjection heparin levels to determine the best dosing interval. Women at high risk include pregnant women with recent thrombosis and pregnant women with additional thrombophilic risk factors, such as the factor V Leiden mutation (93) (see Chapter 8).

Low-molecular-weight heparin (LMWH) is attractive because it may produce less risk for bleeding and a lower incidence of heparin-associated thrombocytopenia, according to studies in nonpregnant populations. Women receiving LMWH rather than standard heparin throughout pregnancy may have lower total bone density loss, but evidence is insufficient to allow estimation of the clinical significance of any difference in postpartum bone density after LMWH and after unfractionated heparin. Renal clearance is elevated during pregnancy, and LMWH is not bound to endothelial cells but remains in the plasma and is cleared by the kidneys. Clearance rates for LMWH are also faster during pregnancy, so higher doses and more frequent dosing may be required (94).

The role of intravenous infusions of gamma globulin for treatment of the aPL syndrome in pregnancy is uncertain. When pregnant women receiving heparin need to be treated for more than a few weeks, these infusions are the immunosuppressant of choice because the combination of prednisone and heparin is associated with rapid and severe osteopenia, including vertebral fracture. A classic example of the need for immunosuppression with anticoagulation is coincident ITP and aPL syndrome. Intravenous infusions of gamma globulin have been used for other indications, such as previous failure of heparin for the treatment of APS, severe placental insufficiency, and early-onset preeclampsia, but no evidence exists for or against efficacy in these circumstances (78).

Obstetric Management and Postpartum Counseling

Ideally, women with APS should have preconception counseling about their medical and obstetric risks. If the diagnosis of APS is uncertain, the presence of LA and IgG aCL should be confirmed. There is no proven benefit of serial testing for aPL during pregnancy once the diagnosis is certain or of titrating medical therapy to suppress antibody levels. Office visits during pregnancy should be frequent (e.g., every 2 weeks in the second trimester and every week in the third) to screen for preeclampsia, IUGR, and placental insufficiency. Nonstress testing or an equivalent form of antepartum testing should be initiated at 32 weeks of gestation. Fetal monitoring may be useful in selected cases (e.g., women with preeclampsia, IUGR, and previous midtrimester fetal death) as early as 24 to 25 weeks of gestation. The authors and others (62) have noted spontaneous decelerations of the fetal heart rate in the second trimester in APS pregnancies. Intervention with preterm delivery may improve outcome in severe cases. Serial ultrasonography should be used to evaluate fetal growth in cases of suspected IUGR. Finally, women with related conditions, such as SLE, renal disease, hypertension, thrombocytopenia, and thrombosis, may require additional specialized care as outlined elsewhere in this text.

After delivery, women with APS should be counseled about their risks for the development of nonobstetric disorders associated with aPL (76). Women with previous thromboses should receive long-term anticoagulation with coumarin (95). Because aPL can prolong prothrombin times as well as partial thromboplastin times, it can be difficult to use prothrombin times to monitor coumarin therapy. A baseline prothrombin time should be obtained before patients are switched from heparin to coumarins. It is uncertain whether patients with APS but no previous thromboses should receive thromboprophylaxis. Finally, estrogen-containing oral contraceptives are relatively contraindicated in women with APS.

REFERENCES

1. **Harris EN, Chan JK, Asherson RA, et al.** Thrombosis, recurrent fetal loss and thrombocytopenia. Arch Intern Med. 1986;146:2153-6.

2. **Harris EN.** Syndrome of the black swan. Br J Rheumatol. 1987;26:324-6.

3. **Asherson RA, Khamashta MA, Ordi-Ros J, et al.** The "primary" antiphospholipid syndrome: major clinical and serologic features. Medicine (Baltimore). 1989;68:366-74.

4. **Alarcon-Segovia D, Perez-Vasquez ME, Villa AR, Drenkard C, Cabiedes J.** Preliminary classification criteria for the antiphospholipid syndrome within systemic lupus erythematosus. Semin Arthritis Rheum. 1992;21:275-86.

5. **Branch DW, Silver RM, Blackwell JL, Reading JC, Scott JR.** Outcome of treated pregnancies in women with antiphospholipid syndrome: an update of the Utah experience. Obstet Gynecol. 1992;80:614-20.

6. **Lima F, Khamashta MA, Buchanan NMM, et al.** A study of sixty pregnancies in patients with the antiphospholipid syndrome. Clin Exp Rheumatol. 1996;14:131-6.

7. **Coulam CB, McIntyre JA, Wagenknecht D, Rote N.** Interlaboratory inconsistencies in detection of anticardiolipin antibodies. Lancet. 1990;335:865-6.

8. **Peaceman AM, Silver RK, MacGregor SN, Socol ML.** Interlaboratory variation in antiphospholipid antibody testing. Am J Obstet Gynecol. 1992;166:1780-7.

9. **Harris EN.** The Second International Anti-Cardiolipin Standardization Workshop/The Kingston Anti-Phospholipid Antibody Study (KAPS) group. Am J Clin Pathol. 1990; 94:476-84.

10. **Silver RM, Porter TF, van Leeuwen I, Jeng G, Scott JR, Branch DW.** Anticardiolipin antibodies: clinical consequences of "low titers." Obstet Gynecol. 1996;87:494-500.

11. **Harris EN, Spinnato JA.** Should anticardiolipin tests be performed in otherwise healthy pregnant women? Am J Obstet Gynecol. 1991;165:1272-7.

12. **Vaarala O, Paluso T, Kleemola M, et al.** Anticardiolipin response in acute infections. Clin Immunol Immunopathol. 1986;41:8-15.

13. **Lockshin MD.** Pregnancy does not cause systemic lupus erythematosus to worsen. Arthritis Rheum. 1989;32:665-70.

14. **Rai RS, Regan L, Clifford K, et al.** Antiphospholipid antibodies and beta2-glycoprotein-I in 500 women with recurrent miscarriage: results of a comprehensive screening approach. Hum Reprod. 1995;10:2001-5.

15. **Lockshin MD.** Antiphospholipid antibodies: babies, blood clots, biology. JAMA. 1997; 277:1549-51.

16. **Yetman DL, Kutteh WH.** Antiphospholipid antibody panels and recurrent pregnancy loss: prevalence of anticardiolipin antibodies compared with other antiphospholipid antibodies. Fertil Steril. 1996;66:540-6.

17. **Branch DW, Silver RM, Pierangeli SS, van Leeuwen I, Harris EN.** Antiphospholipid antibodies in women with recurrent pregnancy loss, fertile controls, and antiphospholipid syndrome. Obstet Gynecol. 1997;89:549-55.

18. **Branch DW, Silver RM.** Autoimmunity and pregnancy loss. Infertil Reprod Med Clin North Am. 1996;7:775-94.

19. **Galli M, Comfurius P, Maassen C, et al.** Anticardiolipin antibodies (ACA) directed not to cardiolipin but to a plasma protein cofactor. Lancet. 1990;335:1544-7.

20. **Matsuura E, Igarashi Y, Fujimoto M.** Anticardiolipin cofactor(s) and differential diagnosis of autoimmune disease. Lancet. 1990;336:177-8.

21. **McNeil HP, Simpson RJ, Chesterman CN, Krilis SA.** Antiphospholipid antibodies are directed against a complex antigen that includes a lipid binding inhibitor of aggregation: beta2-glycoprotein I (apolipoprotein H). Proc Natl Acad Sci U S A. 1990;87:4120-6.

22. **Hunt JE, Adelstein S, Krilis SA.** A phospholipid-beta2-glycoprotein I complex is an antigen for anticardiolipin antibodies occurring in autoimmune disease but not with infection. Lupus. 1992;1:83-90.

23. **Aoki K, Dudkiewicz AB, Matsuura E, Novotny M, Kaberlein G, Gleicher N.** Clinical significance of beta2-glycoprotein I-dependent anticardiolipin antibodies in the reproductive autoimmune failure syndrome: correlation with conventional antiphospholipid antibody detection systems. Am J Obstet Gynecol. 1995;172:926-31.

24. **Koike T, Matsuura E.** What is the "true" antigen for anticardiolipin antibodies? Lancet. 1991;337:671-2.

25. **Roubey RAS.** Autoantibodies to phospholipid-binding plasma proteins: a new view of lupus anticoagulants and other "antiphospholipid" autoantibodies. Blood. 1994;84: 2854-67.

26. **Viard JP, Amoura Z, Bach JF.** Association of anti-beta-2 glycoprotein I antibodies with lupus-type circulating anticoagulants and thrombosis in systemic lupus erythematosus. Am J Med. 1992;93:181-6.

27. **Cabiedes J, Cabral AR, Alarcon-Segovia D.** Clinical manifestations of the antiphospholipid syndrome in patients with systemic lupus erythematosus associate more

strongly with anti-beta2-glycoprotein-I than with antiphospholipid antibodies. J Rheumatol. 1995;22:1899-906.

28. **McNally T, Purdy G, Mackie IJ, Machin SJ, Isenberg DA.** The use of an anti-beta2-glycoprotein-I assay for discrimination between anticardiolipin antibodies associated with infection and increased risk of thrombosis. Br J Haematol. 1995;91:471-3.

29. **Roubey RAS, Maldonado MA, Byrd S.** Comparison of an enzyme-linked immunosorbent assay for antibodies to beta-2-glycoprotein-I and a conventional anticardiolipin immunoassay. Arthritis Rheum. 1996;39:1606-7.

30. **Tsutsumi A, Matsuura E, Ichikawa K, et al.** Antibodies to beta-2-glycoprotein-I and clinical manifestations in patients with systemic lupus erythematosus. Arthritis Rheum. 1996;39:1466-74.

31. **Martinuzzo ME, Forastiero RR, Carreras LO.** Anti-beta-2-glycoprotein-1 antibodies: detection and association with thrombosis. Br J Haematol. 1995;89:397-402.

32. **Teixido M, Font J, Reverter JC, et al.** Anti-beta-2-glycoprotein-I antibodies: a useful marker for the antiphospholipid syndrome. Br J Rheumatol. 1997;36:113-6.

33. **Reece EA, Romero R, Clyne LP, Kriz NS, Hobbins JC.** Lupus-like anticoagulant in pregnancy. Lancet. 1984;1:344.

34. **Branch DW, Scott JR, Kochenour NK, Hershgold E.** Obstetric complications associated with the lupus anticoagulant. N Engl J Med. 1985;313:1322-6.

35. **Lockshin MD, Druzin ML, Goei S, et al.** Antibody to cardiolipin as a predictor of fetal distress or death in pregnant patients with systemic lupus erythematosus. N Engl J Med. 1985;313:152-6.

36. **Rai RS, Clifford K, Cohen H, Regan L.** High prospective fetal loss rate in untreated pregnancies of women with recurrent miscarriage and antiphospholipid antibodies. Hum Reprod. 1995;10:3301-4.

37. **Lockwood CJ, Romero R, Feinberg RF, Clyne LP, Coster B, Hobbins JC.** The prevalence and biologic significance of lupus anticoagulant and anticardiolipin antibodies in a general obstetric population. Am J Obstet Gynecol. 1989;161:369-73.

38. **Lynch A, Marlar R, Murphy J, et al.** Antiphospholipid antibodies in predicting adverse pregnancy outcome. Ann Intern Med. 1994;120:470-5.

39. **Pattison NS, Chamley LW, McKay EJ, et al.** Antiphospholipid antibodies in pregnancy: prevalence and clinical associations. Br J Obstet Gynaecol. 1993;100:909-13.

40. **Yasuda M, Takakuwa K, Tokunaga A, Tanaka K.** Prospective studies of the association between anticardiolipin antibody and outcome of pregnancy. Obstet Gynecol. 1995; 86:555-9.

41. **Cowchock FS, Reece EA, Balaban D, Branch DW, Plouffe L.** Repeated fetal losses associated with antiphospholipid antibodies: a collaborative randomized trial comparing prednisone to low-dose heparin treatment. Am J Obstet Gynecol. 1992;166:1318-27.

42. **Out HJ, Bruinse HW, Godlieve CML, et al.** A prospective, controlled multicenter study on the obstetric risks of pregnant women with antiphospholipid antibodies. Am J Obstet Gynecol. 1992;167:26-32.

43. **Goldstein SR.** Embryonic death in early pregnancy: a new look at the first trimester. Obstet Gynecol. 1994;84:294-7.

44. **Oshiro BT, Silver RM, Scott JR, Yu H, Branch DW.** Antiphospholipid antibodies and fetal death. Obstet Gynecol. 1996;87:489-93.

45. **Petri M, Golbus M, Anderson R, Whiting-O'Keefe Q, Corash L, Hellmann D.** Antinuclear antibody, lupus anticoagulant, and anticardiolipin antibody in women with idiopathic habitual abortion. Arthritis Rheum. 1987;30:601-6.

46. **Barbui T, Cortelazzo S, Galli, et al.** Antiphospholipid antibodies in early repeated abortions: a case-controlled study. Fertil Steril. 1988;50:589-92.

47. **Parazzini F, Acaia B, Faden D, Lovotti M, Marelli G, Cortelazzo S.** Antiphospholipid antibodies and recurrent abortion. Obstet Gynecol. 1991;77:854-7.

48. **Parke AL, Wilson D, Maier D.** The prevalence of antiphospholipid antibodies in women with recurrent spontaneous abortion, women with successful pregnancies, and women who have never been pregnant. Arthritis Rheum. 1991;34:1231-5.

49. **Out HJ, Bruinse HW, Derksen RHWM.** Antiphospholipid antibodies and pregnancy loss. Hum Reprod. 1991;6:889-97.

50. **MacLean MA, Cumming GP, McCall F, Walker ID, Walker JJ.** The prevalence of lupus anticoagulant and anticardiolipin antibodies in women with a history of first trimester miscarriages. Br J Obstet Gynaecol. 1994;101:103-6.

51. **Balasch J, Creus M, Fabregues F, et al.** Antiphospholipid antibodies and human reproductive failure. Hum Reprod. 1996;11:2310-5.

52. **Infante-Rivard C, David M, Gauthier R, Rivard GE.** Lupus anticoagulants, anticardiolipin antibodies, and fetal loss: a case-control study. N Engl J Med. 1991;325:1063-6.

53. **Bocciolone L, Meroni P, Parazzini F, et al.** Antiphospholipid antibodies and risk of intrauterine late fetal death. Acta Obstet Gynecol Scand. 1994;73:389-92.

54. **Ahlenius I, Floberg J, Thomassen P.** Sixty-six cases of intrauterine fetal death: a prospective study with an extensive test protocol. Acta Obstet Gynecol Scand. 1995;74:109-17.

55. **Haddow JE, Rote NS, Dostal-Johnson D, Palomaki GE, Pulkkinen AJ, Knight GJ.** Lack of an association between late fetal death and antiphospholipid antibody measurements in the second trimester. Am J Obstet Gynecol. 1991;165:1308-12.

56. **Branch DW, Andres R, Digre KB, Rote NS, Scott JR.** The association of antiphospholipid antibodies with severe preeclampsia. Obstet Gynecol. 1989;73:541-5.

57. **Milliez J, Lelong F, Bayani N, et al.** The prevalence of autoantibodies during third trimester pregnancy complicated by hypertension or idiopathic fetal growth retardation. Am J Obstet Gynecol. 1991;165:51-6.

58. **Sletnes KE, Wislof F, Moe N, Dale PO.** Antiphospholipid antibodies in preeclamptic women: relation to growth retardation and neonatal outcome. Acta Obstet Gynecol Scand. 1992;71:112-7.

59. **Moodley J, Bhoola V, Duursma J, Pudfin D, Byrne S, Kenoyer DG.** The association of antiphospholipid antibodies with severe early onset preeclampsia. S Afr Med J. 1995;85:105-7.

60. **Caruso A, DeCarolis S, Ferrazzani S, et al.** Pregnancy outcome in relation to uterine artery flow velocimetry waveforms and clinical characteristics in women with antiphospholipid syndrome. Obstet Gynecol. 1993;82:970-7.

61. **Kutteh WH.** Antiphospholipid antibody associated recurrent pregnancy loss: treatment with heparin and low-dose aspirin is superior to low dose aspirin alone. Am J Obstet Gynecol. 1996;174:1584-9.

62. **Druzin ML, Lockshin M, Edersheim TG, Hutson JM, Krauss AL, Kogut E.** Second trimester fetal monitoring and preterm delivery in pregnancies with systemic lupus erythematosus and/or circulating anticoagulant. Am J Obstet Gynecol. 1987;157:1503-10.

63. **Badacarro MH, Vessey M.** Recurrence of venous thromboembolic disease and the use of oral contraceptives.

64. **Rosene-Montella K.** Hypercoagulable states in pregnancy. In: Current Obstetric Medicine. 1993;2:141-61.

65. **Schafer AI.** The hypercoagulable states. Ann Intern Med. 1985;102:814-28.

66. **Hughes GRV.** The antiphospholipid syndrome: ten years on. Lancet. 1993:342:341-4.

67. **Toubi E, Khamashta MA, Panarra A, Hughes GR.** Association of antiphospholipid antibodies with central nervous system disease in systemic lupus erythematosus. Am J Med. 1995:99:397-401.

68. **Branch DW, Silver RM, Blackwell JL, Reading JC, Scott JR.** Outcome of treated pregnancies in women with antiphospholipid syndrome: an update of the Utah experience. Obstet Gynecol. 1992;80:614-20.

69. **Wahl DG, Guillemin F, de Maistre E, et al.** Meta-analysis of the risk of venous thrombosis in individuals with antiphospholipid antibodies without underlying autoimmune disease or previous thrombosis. Lupus. 1998;7:15-22.

70. **Levine SR, Deegan MJ, Futrell N, Welch KM.** Cerebrovascular and neurologic disease associated with antiphospholipid antibodies: 48 cases. Neurology. 1990:40:1181-9.

71. **Haculla E, Michon-Pasturel U, Leys D, et al.** Cerebral magnetic resonance imaging in patients with or without antiphospholipid antibodies. Lupus. 1998;124-31.

72. **Denburg SD, Carbotte RM, Ginsberg JS, Denburg JA.** The relationship of antiphospholipid antibodies to cognitive function in patients with systemic lupus erythematosus. J Int Neuropsychol Soc. 1997;3:377-86.

73. **Kato T, Morita A, Matsumoto Y.** Hypoperfusion of brain single photon emission computerized tomography in patients with antiphospholipid antibodies. J Dermatol Sci. 1997:14:200-28.

74. **Laskin CA, Amin S, Teoh TG.** Medical and obstetric considerations in the management of women with systemic lupus erythematosus. In: Current Obstetric Medicine. 1996;4:273-303.

75. **Leuzzi RA, Davis GH, Cowchock FS, Murphy S, Vernick JJ.** Management of immune thrombocytopenic purpura associated with the antiphospholipid antibody syndrome. Clin Exp Rheumatol. 1997;15:197-200.

76. **Silver RM, Draper ML, Scott JR, Lyon JL, Reading J, Branch DW.** Clinical consequences of antiphospholipid antibodies: an historic cohort study. Obstet Gynecol. 1994;83:372-7.

77. **Asherson RA.** The catastrophic antiphospholipid syndrome. J Rheumatol. 1992;19: 508-12.

78. **Kochenour NK, Branch DW, Rote NS, Scott JR.** A new postpartum syndrome associated with antiphospholipid antibodies. Obstet Gynecol. 1987;69:460-8.

79. **Hochfeld M, Druzin ML, Maia D, et al.** Maternal-fetal catastrophe: fulminant and fatal thrombosis in pregnancy complicated by primary antiphospholipid syndrome. Obstet Gynecol. 1994;83:804-5.

80. **Kupferminc MJ, Lee MJ, Green D, et al.** Severe postpartum pulmonary, cardiac, and renal syndrome associated with antiphospholipid antibodies. Obstet Gynecol. 1994;83: 806-7.

81. **Rosove MH, Brewer PM.** Antiphospholipid thrombosis: clinical course after first thrombotic event. Ann Intern Med. 1992;117:303-8.

82. **Rouby RAS, Hoffman M.** From antiphospholipid syndrome to antibody-mediated thrombosis. Lancet. 1997;350:1491-3.

83. **Rand JH, Wu XX, Andree HAM, et al.** Pregnancy loss in the antiphospholipid antibody syndrome—a possible thrombogenic mechanism. N Engl J Med. 1997;337:154-60.

84. **Simantov R, LaSala JM, Lo SK, Gharavi AE, Sammaritano LR, Salmon JE, Silverstein RL.** Activation of cultured vascular endothelial cells by antiphospholipid antibodies. J Clin Invest. 1995;96:2211-9.

85. **Cuadrado MJ, Lopez-Pedrera C, Khamashta MA, et al.** Thrombosis in primary antiphospholipid syndrome: a pivotal role for monocyte tissue factor expression. Arthritis Rheum. 1997;40:834-41.

86. **Salafia CM, Cowchock FS.** Placental pathology and antiphospholipid antibodies: a descriptive study. Am J Perinatol. 1997;14:435-41.

87. **Cowchock S.** Prevention of fetal death in the antiphospholipid antibody syndrome. Lupus. 1996;5:467-72.

88. **Rai R, Cohen H, Dave M, Regan L.** Randomised controlled trial of aspirin and aspirin plus heparin in pregnant women with recurrent miscarriage associated with phospholipid antibodies (or antiphospholipid antibodies). BMJ. 1997;314:253-7.

89. **Kutteh WH.** Antiphospholipid antibody associated recurrent pregnancy loss: treatment with heparin and low-dose aspirin is superior to low dose aspirin alone. Am J Obstet Gynecol. 1996;174:1584-9.

90. **Dahlman TC, Hellgren MSE, Blomback M.** Thrombosis prophylaxis in pregnancy with use of subcutaneous heparin adjusted by monitoring heparin concentration in plasma. Am J Obstet Gynecol. 1989;161:420-5.

91. **Brancazio LR, Roperti KA, Stierer R, Laifer SA.** Pharmacokinetics and pharmacodynamics of subcutaneous heparin during the early third trimester of pregnancy. Am J Obstet Gynecol. 1995;173:1240-5.

92. **Barbour LA, Smith JM, Marlar RA.** Heparin levels to guide thromboembolism prophylaxis during pregnancy. Am J Obstet Gynecol. 1995;173:1869-73.

93. **Preston FE, Rosendaal FR, Walker ID, et al.** Increased fetal loss in women with heritable thrombophilia. Lancet. 1996;348:913-6.

94. **Frydman A.** Low-molecular weight heparins: an overview of their pharmacodynamics, pharmacokinetics, and metabolism in humans. Haemostasis. 1996;26(Suppl 2):24-38.

95. **Khamashta MA, Cuadrado MJ, Mujic F, Taub NA, Hunt BJ, Hughes GRV.** The management of thrombosis in the antiphospholipid-antibody syndrome. N Engl J Med. 1995;332:993-7.

II. Systemic Lupus Erythematosus
Karen Rosene-Montella

Systemic lupus erythematosus is a multisystem disease characterized by exacerbations and remissions of uncertain cause. Like most autoimmune diseases, it is more prevalent in women than in men (cases in females outnumber cases in males 10 to 1). It occurs in 1/700 women. The peak incidence of SLE is seen at about age 30 years, and SLE complicates 1/5000 pregnancies (some recent studies report a higher incidence). Fertility is not altered by SLE unless there is premature ovarian failure as a result of immunosuppressive therapy. Systemic lupus erythematosus is a fascinating paradigm for the study of the fetal effects of maternal disease because autoantibodies in the maternal circulation cross the placenta and are directly responsible for fetal and neonatal complications.

Effect of Pregnancy on Systemic Lupus Erythematosus

The clinical course of SLE is variable during pregnancy, and the frequency of flares has been a source of major controversy. Earlier studies probably overestimated the incidence of flares because strict criteria for the exclusion of pregnancy-related illnesses that can masquerade as lupus were not applied. Modifications made to treatment regimens because of pregnancy may also have contributed to flares. A universal finding was an increase in the occurrence of new-onset proteinuria and thrombocytopenia in pregnant women compared with nonpregnant controls, although this condition was not distinguished from preeclampsia. Variations in enrollment criteria and a lack of matched controls make earlier studies difficult to interpret. More recent studies that include controls suggest that there is little difference between flare rates in pregnant patients and in properly matched nonpregnant controls (Tables 9-1 and 9-2). There is a clear consensus that when SLE is in remission at the time of conception, the lowest flare rates (10% to 20%) are seen during

Table 9-1 Effect of Pregnancy on Systemic Lupus Erythematosus: Case Control Studies on Risk for Flare

Authors	No. of Patients	No. of Pregnancies	Control	Risk for Flare
Zulman (1980)	23	24	Before pregnancy	Increased
Lockshin (1984)	28	33	Matched, not pregnant	No change
Meehan (1987)	18	22	Matched, not pregnant	No change
Petri (1991)	36	39	After pregnancy, not pregnant	Increased

Adapted from Petri M. Hopkins Lupus Pregnancy Center: 1987 to 1996. Rheumatol Dis Clin North Am. 1997;23:1-13.

Table 9-2 Effect of Pregnancy on Systemic Lupus Erythematosus: Flares by Trimester (Number/Percent)

Author	1st Trimester	2nd Trimester	3rd Trimester	Postpartum
Fraga (1974)	0 (0)	3 (43)	2 (29)	2 (29)
Zulman (1980)	3 (13)	3 (13)	12 (52)	5 (22)
Mintz (1986)	30 (57)	7 (13)	7 (13)	9 (17)
Petri (1991)	6 (18)	16 (47)	5 (15)	7 (21)

Adapted from Petri M. Hopkins Lupus Pregnancy Center: 1987 to 1996. Rheumatol Dis Clin North Am. 1997;23:1-13.

pregnancy. If SLE is active at conception, the flare rate increases in some studies to as much as 30% to 50%. The presence of lupus nephritis may further increase the flare rate; some authors report flare rates of 70% and worsening of nephropathy in up to 30% of patients (1–4).

Effect of Systemic Lupus Erythematosus on Pregnancy

Fetal and Neonatal Complications

The effect of SLE on pregnancy is somewhat clearer (Box 9-3). Fetal complications include increased perinatal morbidity and mortality and the neonatal lupus syndromes. There is an increase in the incidence of miscarriage, intrauterine fetal demise, growth restriction, and prematurity. Not only are mean gestational age and birthweight likely to be lower in patients with established SLE but it was also found in neonates of women who later developed the disease. This suggests that the perinatal risk has an immune cause.

Although the complications mentioned above occur in the presence of SLE alone, they are three times more likely to occur with the coexistence of SLE and aPLs (Table 9-3). Pregnancy outcome is best when SLE is in remission for 6 to 12 months before conception. The prognosis is worst in patients whose SLE was active at the time of conception and in patients with lupus

---

Box 9-3 Effects of Systemic Lupus Erythematosus on Pregnancy

Fetal/neonatal effects
  Intrauterine fetal demise
  Stillbirth
  Intrauterine growth restriction
  Prematurity
  Neonatal lupus
    Cutaneous events (rash, thrombocytopenia)
    Complete heart block
  Subsequent learning difficulties
Maternal effects
  SLE flare
  Superimposed preeclampsia
  Thrombosis

nephropathy; complication rates exceed 50% once the serum creatinine level exceeds 1.6 mg/dL.

Neonatal lupus (NLE) is a rare syndrome seen in the infants of mothers with anti-Ro (SSA) or anti-La (SSB) antibodies, which are present in about one third of patients with SLE and may occur in mothers without SLE. The syndrome can occur in the absence of SLE, but 100% of offspring with NLE are born to mothers with anti-Ro (SSA), anti-La (SSB), or both. Direct deposition of antibody in the fetal myocardium and in cutaneous tissues has been reported. Cutaneous NLE occurs in about 25% of the children of mothers with SSA or SSB antibodies and is characterized by rash with or without associated hepatosplenomegaly or thrombocytopenia. Congenital complete heart block (CCHB), a less common but more serious complication of maternal antibody deposition, is associated with a 31% fetal–neonatal mortality rate. It is not possible to predict which neonates of mothers with SSA or SSB antibodies will develop cutaneous NLE, but there is more specificity in the antibodies responsible for CCHB. It occurs almost exclusively in infants of mothers who have antibodies to both the Ro/SSA 52-kd antigens and the La/SSB 48-kd antigens. Infants of mothers who are anti-La/SSB—negative or in whom the SSA is directed at the 60-kd and not the 52-kd antigen seem to have low risk (5).

Congenital complete heart block is thought to be preceded by an inflammatory myocarditis that may present as fetal arrhythmia or intermittent heart block at 18 to 30 weeks of gestation. This stage is followed by fibrosis with irreversible damage to the fetal cardiac conduction system, resulting in CCHB. Congestive heart failure is common, and the need for neonatal pacing may require delivery in a center where neonatal cardiac surgery is available. Trials of early intervention with steroids, plasmapheresis, or maternal intravenous immunoglobulin therapy to reduce levels of antibody to which the fetus will be exposed by transplacental passage have had mixed results. Theoretically, prevention through maternal treatment early in the inflammatory process could prevent progression to permanent fibrosis, but data are insufficient to support specific recommendations.

Table 9-3 Complications in Patients with Systemic Lupus Erythematosus with and without Antiphospholipid Antibodies (Including Lupus Anticoagulant)

	SLE and aPLs Present (%)	SLE Present/aPLs Absent (%)
Thrombosis	42	13
Fetal loss	59	20
Thrombocytopenia	37	10

From McNeil HP, Chesterman CN, Krilis SA. Immunology and clinical importance of antiphospholipid autoantibodies. Adv Immunol. 1991;49:193-280; with permission.

Long-term outcomes have shown that children of mothers with SLE, especially male children, have more evidence of developmental difficulties, immune-related disorders, and non-righthandedness. It seems that maternal immunoreactivity, as seen in women with SLE, may be a special risk factor for subsequent learning difficulties in offspring, especially male offspring.

Maternal Complications

Maternal complications of SLE during pregnancy include flares, for which the greatest risk factor is active SLE at the time of conception; superimposed preeclampsia (or hypertension, proteinuria, or thrombocytopenia not defined as preeclampsia); and thrombosis. Although thrombosis is much more likely in the presence of aPL or the nephrotic syndrome, some evidence indicates that SLE alone may be a risk factor for maternal thrombosis. Pregnant patients with SLE have increased levels of von Willebrand factor antigen and anti-endothelial cell antibodies that are not seen in normal pregnant controls. This suggests a possible cause of SLE-related hypercoagulability.

The single most difficult dilemma in a woman with SLE is having to differentiate between an SLE flare and preeclampsia. Hypertension, proteinuria, thrombocytopenia, hemolytic anemia, and abnormalities of serum renal and liver function tests are common in both conditions, and both conditions may be complicated by seizures or pulmonary edema. Decreasing complement levels, particularly alternative pathway (CH50); other clinical stigmata of SLE, such as rash or arthritis; urinary erythrocyte casts; or increasing titers of anti-dsDNA suggest SLE, whereas the abrupt onset of proteinuria is more likely in preeclampsia. The presence of active lupus nephritis or preeclampsia increases risk for preterm delivery and fetal death. In a patient with active, demonstrable SLE nephritis in whom hypertension, proteinuria, and renal function may be worsening, it may be impossible to exclude superimposed preeclampsia. In some cases, it may be necessary to treat both diseases with steroids, antihypertensive agents, and consideration of delivery as soon as possible. Renal biopsy when disease worsens remote from term (24 to 28 weeks of gestation) may be indicated to clarify the diagnosis.

Diagnosis and Management

Diagnosis of SLE in pregnancy is essentially the same as diagnosis of SLE in the nonpregnant state and relies on the ARA criteria outlined in Table 9-4. Care must be taken not to interpret normal pregnancy findings, such as palmar and facial erythema, fatigue, and nonspecific musculoskeletal problems, as suggestive of SLE. Once normal pregnancy-related findings (mild anemia,

Table 9-4 ARA Criteria for Diagnosis of Systemic Lupus Erythematosus

Criterion	Definition
Malar rash	Fixed erythema, flat or raised, over the malar eminences, tending to spare the nasolabial folds
Discoid rash	Erythematous raised patches with adherent keratonic scaling and follicular plugging; atrophic scarring may occur in older lesions
Photosensitivity	Skin rash as a result of unusual reaction to sunlight, by patient history or physician observation
Oral ulcers	Oral or nasopharyngeal ulceration, usually painless, noted by physician
Arthritis	Nonerosive arthritis involving two or more peripheral joints and characterized by tenderness, swelling, or effusion
Serositis	*Pleuritis* – convincing history of pleuritic pain, or rub heard by physician, or evidence of pleural effusion; *or* *Pericarditis* – documented by electrocardiogram or rub, or evidence of pericardial effusion
Renal disorder	*Persistent proteinuria* >0.5 g/day or >3+ if quantitation not performed; *or* *Cellular casts* – may be red cell, hemoglobin, granular, tubular, or mixed
Neurologic disorder	*Seizures* – in the absence of offending drugs or known metabolic derangements (e.g., uremia, ketoacidosis, electrolyte imbalance); *or* *Psychosis* – in the absence of offending drugs or known metabolic derangements (e.g., uremia, ketoacidosis, electrolyte imbalance)
Hematologic disorder	*Hemolytic anemia* with reticulocytosis; *or* *Leukopenia* – <4000 mm^3 on two or more occasions; *or* *Lymphopenia* – <1500 mm^3 on two or more occasions; *or* *Thrombocytopenia* – <100,000/mm^3 in the absence of offending drugs
Immunologic disorder	Positive LE cell preparation; *or* Antibody to native DNA in abnormal titer; *or* Presence of antibody to Sm nuclear antigen; *or* False positive result on serologic test for syphilis know to be positive for at least 6 months and confirmed by *Treponema pallidum* immobilization or fluorescent treponemal antibody absorption test
Antinuclear antibody	An abnormal titer of antinuclear antibody by immunofluorescence or an equivalent assay at any time and in the presence of drugs known to be associated with "drug-induced lupus" syndrome

*From Arthritis Foundation. Bull Rheum Dis. 1997;46:4; with permission.

elevated erythrocyte sedimentation rate and complement levels, and increasing proteinuria) are taken into consideration, pregnancy (in the absence of preeclampsia) should not alter the clinical presentation or the frequency of laboratory findings in patients with SLE (Table 9-5).

Table 9-5 Laboratory Findings in Patients with Systemic Lupus Erythematosus*

Autoantibodies	Frequency (%)
Antinuclear	>79
Anti–double-stranded-DNA	>80
Anti-SM	30
Anti-Ro/(SSA)	25
Anti-La/(SSB)	20
Anti-RNP	20
Rheumatoid factor	25
Anticardiolipin (ACA)	40
Lupus anticoagulant (LAC)	20

*Other findings include thrombocytopenia, hemolytic anemia, decreased complement levels (C3, C4, CH50); elevated BUN, creatinine levels; and urinary protein, red blood cell casts.

Pregnancy management should begin with a baseline assessment of function and disease markers, both to assess prognosis and to ensure that changes from baseline can be detected later. At the first visit or during preconception counseling, baseline laboratory studies should include complete blood count; platelet count; measurement of uric acid, aspartate aminotransferase, alanine aminotransferase, blood urea nitrogen, and creatinine; 24-hour urine collection for evaluation of protein and creatinine clearance; and microscopic urinalysis to evaluate urinary sediment. Serologic markers, ANA, anti-dsDNA, anti-Ro/SSA, anti-La/SSB, anti-RNP, anti-Smith, serum complement levels (C3, C4, and CH50), LA, and aPL should also be measured. Pregnancy may increase complement levels, so decreasing titers, even in the normal range, may be an early clue to an SLE flare. Similarly, increasing ANA or anti-dsDNA titers may precede clinical exacerbations, especially in lupus nephritis, and should be followed closely. We recommend the management strategy outlined in Box 9-4.

Treatment of SLE during pregnancy requires vigilance for early diagnosis and a commitment to not withhold treatment from a patient for fear of damage to the fetus. A serious exacerbation of maternal disease carries the most significant fetal risk.

The safety of maternal steroid therapy for the fetus is well established and is discussed elsewhere in this text. Complications of glucocorticoid therapy are similar in pregnant and nonpregnant women and include fluid retention, bone demineralization, gastrointestinal disease, and glucose intolerance. H_2-blockers can help prevent gastric irritation. Glucose intolerance can result in gestational diabetes, so close monitoring of blood glucose is important.

Steroids are given for the same indications in pregnant and nonpregnant persons; these indications include arthritis, arthralgias, mild renal disease, neurovascular disease, and cardiopulmonary and hematologic complications.

Box 9-4 Management of the Pregnant Patient with Systemic Lupus Erythematosus

---

1. At initial visit:
   Baseline CBC, platelet count, BUN, creatinine, uric acid, AST
   Urinalysis, 24-h urine for protein, creatinine clearance
   Anticardiolipin antibody
   Lupus anticoagulant
   Anti-Ro, Anti-La antibodies (SSA, SSB)
   Complement levels (C3, C4, CH50)
2. Monthly:
   Platelet count, urine sediment, creatinine measurement
3. Each trimester and with symptoms:
   24-h urine creatinine clearance
   24-h urine protein if proteinuria present
   Complement levels (C3, C4, CH50)
   Anti-DNA antibody
4. Fetal monitoring for growth, activity per OB, NSTs
5. Repeat CBC, platelet count, BUN, creatinine, uric acid, AST and all
   trimester tests with any symptoms or signs of SLE or preeclampsia

---

Adapted from Rosene K. SLE in pregnancy. Journal SOGC. 1992 (Aug); 51-9.

If platelet counts decrease to less than 50,000 and delivery is anticipated within 1 week, steroids should be administered to prevent severe thrombocytopenia during surgical delivery. If thrombocytopenia is severe and delivery is imminent, intravenous immunoglobulin may have a more immediate effect; it is acceptable for use in pregnancy.

The leading causes of death in patients with SLE are renal disease, infectious complications, and the effects of cardiopulmonary and neurovascular manifestations. Coronary artery disease has emerged as an important cause of death, accounting for 30% of all deaths in one series.

Immunosuppressive drugs that include cytotoxic agents have been shown to be more efficacious than prednisone alone in controlling clinical signs of active nephritis (6), in preventing renal scarring, and, ultimately, in reducing risk for end-stage renal disease, but they have not been shown to reduce risk for death (7, 8). Intermittent-pulse cyclophosphamide therapy seems to have the best therapeutic profile and continues to be the first-choice regimen for patients with diffuse proliferative or severe focal proliferative glomerulonephritis. In the presence of biopsy-proven worsening nephritis, this treatment recommendation should not be altered by pregnancy.

Prophylaxis for infections, including antibiotics for invasive dental and genitourinary procedures and immunization with influenza and pneumococcal vaccines, is generally recommended in patients with SLE and should be recommended for these patients during pregnancy.

Careful control of cardiac and renal risk factors, especially hypertension, is essential and should not be altered because of pregnancy. The only necessary change in management is that the antihypertensive agent chosen should not include an angiotensin-converting enzyme (ACE) inhibitor. Patients with substantial proteinuria should have antithrombin III levels measured to assess the need for thrombosis prophylaxis.

Antimalarial agents and nonsteroidal anti-inflammatory drugs (NSAIDs) are discussed elsewhere and may be used with the modifications and monitoring suggested in the section on rheumatoid arthritis. Thalidomide and retinoids, both of which are known teratogens, are now used for cutaneous lupus. They should be avoided in women who are pregnant or contemplating pregnancy. The drugs used for SLE and other rheumatic diseases and their effects on pregnancy are listed in the Drug Table at the end of this chapter.

REFERENCES

1. **Whiting-O'Keefe Q, Henke JE, Shearn MA, Hopper J Jr, Biava CG, Epstein WV.** The information content from renal biopsy in systemic lupus erythematosus. Ann Intern Med. 1982;96:718-23.

2. **Magil AB, Puterman ML, Ballon HS, Chan V, Lirenman DS, Rae A, et al.** Prognostic factors in diffuse proliferative lupus glomerulonephritis. Kidney Int. 1988;34:511-7.

3. **Austin HA 3d, Antonovych TT, MacKay K, Boumpas DT, Balow JE.** NIH conference. Membranous nephropathy. Ann Intern Med. 1992;116:672-82.

4. **Coritsidis G, Rifici V, Gupta S, Rie J, Shan ZH, Neugarten J, Schlondorff D.** Preferential binding of oxidized LDL to rat glomeruli in vivo and cultured mesangial cells in vitro. Kidney Int. 1991;39:858-66.

5. **Buyon JP, Winchester RJ, Slade SG, Arnett F, Copel J, Friedman D, Lockshin MD.** Identification of mothers at risk for congenital heart block and other neonatal lupus syndromes in their children: comparison of enzyme-linked immunosorbent assay and immunoblot for measurement of anti-SS-A/Ro and anti-SS-B/La antibodies. Arthritis Rheum. 1993;20:1263-73.

6. **Donadio JV Jr, Holley KE, Ferguson RH, Ilstrup DM.** Treatment of diffuse proliferative lupus nephritis with prednisone and combined prednisone and cyclophosphamide. N Engl J Med. 1978;299:1151-5.

7. **Balow JE, Austin HA 3d, Muenz LRT, Joyce KM, Antonovych TT, Klippel JH, et al.** Effect of treatment on the evolution of renal abnormalities in lupus nephritis. N Engl J Med. 1984;311:491-5.

8. **Steinberg AD, Steinberg SC.** Long-term preservation of renal function in patients with lupus nephritis receiving treatment that includes cyclophosphamide versus those treated with prednisone only. Arthritis Rheum. 1991;34:945-50.

III. Rheumatoid Arthritis
J. Lee Nelson

Rheumatoid arthritis (RA) is a systemic autoimmune disease; its hallmark is symmetrical polyarthritis. In addition to having joint involvement, patients with RA sometimes experience lung disease, pericarditis, neuropathy, and vasculitis. The spectrum of RA is wide and includes mild episodes of arthritis that resolve spontaneously, severe progressive joint destruction, and disease involving internal organs. The autoantibody rheumatoid factor is detected in 80% to 90% of patients with RA but is also found in patients with other diseases and in some normal persons. Rheumatoid factor titers do not correlate with disease activity. Rheumatoid arthritis affects women at least three to four times as often as men, and the incidence of RA in women continues to increase with age at least into the seventh or eighth decade of life (1). However, RA can occur at any age and, because it is relatively common, primary care practitioners, obstetricians, obstetric internists, and rheumatologists can expect to encounter patients with RA who are pregnant or planning pregnancies.

Effect of Pregnancy on Maternal Rheumatoid Arthritis

Alleviation of the symptoms and signs of RA during pregnancy was first described more than 60 years ago. Presence or absence of rheumatoid factor, duration of disease, patient age, and functional class (degree of disability) have not been found to predict the experience during pregnancy. For most women, improvement begins in the first trimester, and further relief is often experienced as pregnancy progresses. About 75% of women have some alleviation during pregnancy, and more than half of this 75% have complete remission and are able to discontinue all medication with freedom from all signs and symptoms of RA (2).

Physicians who care for patients with RA are often asked whether a woman should discontinue use of arthritis medications before becoming pregnant.

Possible Explanations for the
Pregnancy-Induced Alleviation of Rheumatoid Arthritis

Research into the cause of remission of RA during pregnancy contributed to the eventual discovery of cortisone. Despite the importance of this discovery, subsequent studies indicated that increased serum cortisol concentrations in pregnancy did not explain the alleviation of RA seen in pregnancy. Support for other proposed explanations, including elevated levels of sex hormones or of a serum factor pregnancy-associated beta2-globulin, was not forthcoming. It has been proposed that neuroendocrine changes (3) and pregnancy-induced changes in the percentage of IgG immunoglobulins that lack the terminal galactose units in the oligosaccharide chains attached to CH2 regions may play a role (4). The HLA antigens are known to be important in immune responses and in discrimination of self from nonself. In other studies, child–mother pairs were examined for HLA antigens, and pregnancies in which arthritis was alleviated or remitted were compared with those in which arthritis was active. Fetal–maternal disparity in the HLA class II antigens DR and DQ was found to correlate significantly with alleviation of RA during pregnancy (5). Several mechanisms may account for this finding. First, the maternal antibody response to paternal HLA antigens mediates a beneficial effect on the mother's arthritis. Second, pregnancy induces regulatory T cells that suppress maternal autoimmune responses. Third, the beneficial effect of fetal (paternal) HLA disparity is mediated by an effect of fetal HLA peptides on the maternal T-cell repertoire. In addition to presenting foreign antigens, HLA molecules also present self-peptides derived from other HLA molecules, and some investigators propose that RA occurs when one HLA molecule presents a peptide derived from another (self) HLA molecule. According to this model, autoimmunity in patients with RA results from a defect in the recognition or presentation of an HLA class II self-peptide. It is now known that fetal cells cross into the maternal circulation early in most normal pregnancies. Thus, such an effect could be mediated by fetal cells or, alternatively, by HLA peptides derived from fetal cells. Finally, the explanation for this intriguing biological phenomenon is probably multifactorial, and changes in sex hormones and shifts in cytokine production from Th1 to Th2 during pregnancy may contribute.

Discontinuation of Medication Use Before Pregnancy

Patients with RA often use NSAIDs for symptoms and sometimes take other medications that are collectively referred to as *disease-modifying drugs* (DMARDs). Cessation of use of salicylates and NSAIDs such as ibuprofen, indomethacin, naproxen, piroxicam, fenoprofen, ketoprofen, diclofenac, and mefenamic acid before pregnancy is not necessary; these medications are not known to be teratogenic in humans (6).

Little specific information is available on the issue of discontinuing DMARD use before pregnancy in patients with RA. However, guidelines have been established as a result of experience with some of these drugs in other conditions. In one suggested approach, sulfasalazine can be continued during pregnancy (and breastfeeding). Sulfasalazine has been used during pregnancy without harmful effects in many patients with inflammatory bowel disease. The use of hydroxychloroquine during pregnancy is debated. It can be continued during pregnancy if it is strictly necessary; there is little indication of adverse fetal effects.

No evidence suggests that gold causes an increase in neonatal malformations, although transplacental passage of gold does occur. One approach in patients who are receiving parenteral gold is to administer the monthly injection on the first day of menses so that gold therapy can be discontinued as soon as pregnancy is recognized. Potential effects of penicillamine are less clear, and whether this medication can act as a human teratogen is debated. Some physicians recommend prophylactic withdrawal before pregnancy; others recommend tapering and withdrawal once pregnancy is achieved.

Use of the cytostatic drugs methotrexate, chlorambucil, and cyclophosphamide should always be discontinued at least 3 months before a woman tries to conceive. It is well known that methotrexate increases risk for congenital malformations. In contrast, the experience with azathioprine in renal transplant recipients is extensive, and this drug is not known to be teratogenic in humans. For more information, the reader is referred to a recent review of antirheumatic drug treatment during pregnancy (7).

Medications During Pregnancy and Lactation

Because patients with RA often have alleviation or remission of RA with pregnancy, therapeutic intervention is often obviated. When a patient has active arthritis in one or a few joints, intra-articular steroid injections can be used. Prednisone is often recommended if medication is needed for active RA during pregnancy. Prednisone is used instead of other corticosteroids because fetal plasma levels of the active metabolite, prenisolone, are almost ten-fold lower than maternal levels. Patients with RA rarely require more than modest doses of prednisone (5 to 15 mg/d). Studies in animals have shown that corticosteroid use is associated with neonatal malformations, particularly cleft palate, but extensive experience with prednisone has not shown an increased risk for malformations in humans (8). The neonate of a woman using prednisone should be monitored for possible adrenal suppression (although this is rare) as well as gestational diabetes. Stress doses of corticosteroids are given for labor and delivery in women who use corticosteroids during pregnancy. Low-dose prednisone (<20 mg) is also considered to be safe during breast-feeding (9).

NSAIDs can inhibit prostaglandin synthesis in the fetus. Ibuprofen, indomethacin, and ketoprofen have been found to reduce fetal renal output and decrease the volume of amniotic fluid, and the same is expected to occur with other NSAIDs that are inhibitors of prostaglandin synthesis. Evidence suggests that after drug withdrawal, renal function in the fetus quickly recovers. NSAIDs can constrict the ductus arteriosus (10). The constriction has been shown to resolve with discontinuation of the therapy. Use of aspirin and NSAIDs is always discontinued in the third trimester because of the increased risk for neonatal bleeding at delivery, including central nervous system hemorrhage, and because of the potential constrictive effect on the ductus arteriosus. A recent study (11) compared 49 patients with rheumatic disease who used standard doses of NSAIDs with 45 nonusers for an average of 15 weeks during gestation. Use of NSAIDs was discontinued at least 6 weeks before term in all cases, and no adverse maternal or neonatal effects were seen in NSAID users. A study of almost 15,000 women (12) showed no increase in the rate of congenital malformations in the children of women who used moderate doses of aspirin during pregnancy.

Effect of Rheumatoid Arthritis on Pregnancy Complications and Delivery

Patients with RA do not seem to have an increased frequency of preeclampsia or an increase in premature labor. Vaginal delivery can be impeded by hip disease, particularly in women who have had joint replacement, although hip disease or joint replacement does not preclude normal vaginal delivery. If a patient with RA needs anesthesia and intubation, precautions must be taken to ensure cervical stability because RA can affect the cervical spine and cause instability, particularly at the C1, C2 articulation.

Effect of Rheumatoid Arthritis on Fetal Outcome

Women with RA do not seem to have an increase in spontaneous abortions or premature infants or a significant decrease in neonatal birthweight. Thus, no increase in any adverse pregnancy outcome is seen in patients with RA (2). A report that suggested an increased rate of spontaneous abortion in patients with RA before disease was not confirmed in subsequent studies, nor was a report suggesting an increase of stillbirths in women with RA before disease onset. Thus, there is no indication that an adverse pregnancy outcome predisposes to development of RA.

Postpartum Disease Activity and Long-Term Prognosis

Rheumatoid arthritis is characteristically active in the postpartum period, both in women who have experienced gestational remission and in those who have not. Recurrence is seen within 3 to 4 months after delivery in more than 95% of women. The return of RA is unrelated to resumption of menstruation or lactation. Flares of RA can also occur after spontaneous or induced abortion. Although pregnancy often results in an alleviation of RA, active disease predictably occurs postpartum. Is the overall effect of pregnancy positive or negative with respect to long-term disability from RA? Studies are in progress to address this question, but the answer is currently unknown.

Fecundity and Fertility: Risk for New-Onset Rheumatoid Arthritis During Pregnancy and Postpartum

There is some suggestion that fecundity may be subtly decreased in patients with RA. In other words, time to conception may be delayed. However, this information is derived largely from studies of pregnancy history before disease onset, and there is no indication of an increase of infertility in women with RA.

Numerous studies have shown that women who have had at least one term pregnancy have a decreased risk for RA. Studies have also shown that there is a reduced likelihood that a woman will first develop RA during pregnancy. In contrast, there is an increased risk for RA in the first year postpartum. It should be noted that observations about risk for new-onset RA are partly analogous to the experience of women who have RA before pregnancy, but they also differ. The decreased risk for new-onset RA during pregnancy and the increased risk for new-onset RA seen in the year after delivery in women who have never had RA may be considered analogous to pregnancy-induced remission and postpartum flare in women who had RA before becoming pregnant. However, the risk for developing RA 1 to 2 years postpartum is reduced by about 40% relative to women who have never had a term pregnancy.

REFERENCES

1. **Silman AJ, Hochberg MC.** Rheumatoid arthritis. In: Silman AJ, Hochberg MC, eds. Epidemiology of the Rheumatic Diseases. New York: Oxford Medical Publications; 1993:7-68.
2. **Nelson JL, Ostensen ME.** Pregnancy and rheumatoid arthritis. Rheum Dis Clin North Am. 1997;23:195-212.
3. **Wilder RL.** Neuroendocrine-immune system interactions and autoimmunity. Annu Rev Immunol. 1995;13:307-38.
4. **Rook G, Steele J, Brealey R, Whyte A, Isenberg D, Sumar N, et al.** Changes in IgG glycoform levels may be relevant to remission of arthritis during pregnancy. J Autoimmun. 1991;4:779-94.
5. **Nelson JL, Hughes KA, Smith AG, Nisperos BB, Branchaud AB, Hansen JA.** Maternal-fetal disparity in HLA class II alloantigens and the pregnancy-induced amelioration of rheumatoid arthritis. N Engl J Med. 1993;329:466-71.

6. **Brooks PM, Needs CJ.** The use of antirheumatic medication during pregnancy and in the puerperium. Rheum Dis Clin North Am. 1989;15:789-806.
7. **Ostensen M.** Optimization of anti-rheumatic drug treatment in pregnancy. Clin Pharmacokinet. 1994;27:486-503.
8. **Fraser FC, Sajoo A.** Teratogenic potential of corticosteroids in humans. Teratology. 1995;51:45-6.
9. **Committee on Drugs, American Academy of Pediatrics.** The transfer of drugs and other chemicals into human breast milk. Pediatrics. 1989;84:924-36.
10. **Moise KJ Jr, Huhta JC, Sharif DS, et al.** Indomethacin in the treatment of preterm labor: effects on the fetal ductus arteriosus. N Engl J Med. 1988;319:327-31.
11. **Ostensen M, Ostensen H.** Safety of nonsteroidal anti-inflammatory drugs in pregnant patients with rheumatic disease. J Rheumatol. 1996;23:1045-9.
12. **Slone D, Siskind V, Heinonen OP, Monson RR, Kaufman DW, Shapiro.** Aspirin and congenital malformations. Lancet. 1976;1:1373-5.

IV. Scleroderma
Karen Rosene-Montella

Systemic sclerosis, or scleroderma, is an autoimmune disease that is three to five times more common in women than in men. Overall, the mean age at presentation is 40 years, but the pattern of presentation differs in women and men. In women, the incidence of scleroderma begins to increase sharply in the 20s, increases further throughout the 30s and 40s, and then clearly declines. It is thought that because the years of high incidence are the years that follow childbearing, this pattern of presentation in women may result from maternal exposure to fetal cells during pregnancy.

Fetal cells have been detected in maternal peripheral blood in most normal pregnancies, and the influx of fetal cells into the maternal circulation increases with parturition. Recently, it was found that fetal progenitor cells persist in the maternal peripheral blood for decades after childbirth (1). The implication of this finding for the effect of pregnancy on susceptibility to autoimmune disease, especially scleroderma, is of great interest. As noted, scleroderma has a strong female preponderance, and its incidence increases steeply after the childbearing years. Contributing to this theory is the repeated observation of the marked clinical similarity of scleroderma to chronic graft-versus-host disease after allogeneic bone marrow transplantation (Table 9-6) (2).

Effect of Scleroderma on Pregnancy

The effect of scleroderma on fertility and pregnancy seems to be less than previously thought. Recent studies have found no decrease in overall fertility in

Table 9-6   Clinical Similarity of Scleroderma to Chronic Graft-Versus-Host Disease

Feature	Scleroderma	Chronic Graft-Versus-Host Disease
Hallmark skin disease with:		
Induration	+++	+++
Sclerosis	+++	+++
Contractures	+++	+++
Ulcerations	+++	+++
Atrophy	+++	+++
Hair loss	+++	+++
Myositis	++	+
Sicca syndrome	++	++
Gastrointestinal events	II	+
Pulmonary events	++	+
Renal events	+	0/+
Raynaud phenomenon	+++	0/+

From Nelson JL. Pregnancy immunology and autoimmune disease. J Reprod Med. 1998;43:335-40; with permission.

patients with scleroderma. When patients with scleroderma were compared with patients with RA and with normal controls, no difference in fertility rates or in the percentage of women with at least a 1-year delay in conception was seen. Men with scleroderma have a high incidence of erectile dysfunction (12% to 60%), probably because of decreased penile blood flow, and thus may have difficulty impregnating their partners. If future fertility is an issue, these men should be encouraged to store sperm in case impotence appears.

In most recent case-control studies, the incidence of adverse pregnancy outcome is increased in patients with scleroderma, but to a lesser extent than previously thought (Table 9-7). A slight increase was seen in rates of miscarriage, prematurity, and term babies that were small for gestational age (3). Higher rates of loss were seen in patients who had diffuse rather than limited disease (Table 9-8).

Effect of Pregnancy on Scleroderma

Most reports on the overall effects of pregnancy on scleroderma disease activity and progression have concluded that disease status does not change during pregnancy (Table 9-9). Unfortunately, it is difficult to assign cause to symptoms such as reflux, which may worsen during pregnancy even in the absence of scleroderma. All earlier reports of the devastating consequences of pregnancy on scleroderma were in patients with renal disease or pulmonary

Table 9-7 Maternal and Pregnancy Outcomes in Women with Scleroderma

Source	Scleroderma Worsened/ Pregnancies	Miscarriage	Premature Birth No.	Neonatal Death	Maternal Death	Adverse Outcome in Scleroderma Patients (%)	Adverse Outcomes in Controls (%)
Individual case reports	36/42	ND	ND	12	14	50	
Series							
Johnson	ND/36	3	ND	1	0	11	
Slate	6/17	13	0	2	1	88	
Donaldson	ND/17	1	4	0	2	41	
Weiner	14/30	1	4	2	0	20	
Black	15/21	4	ND	1	1	29	
Case-control studies			%→				
Giordano[+]	80/299	17	ND	0	0	17	10
Siamopoulou-Mavridou[#]	14/36	22	0	0	0	22*	12
Silman[#]	115/ND	29	ND	ND	0	29*	17
Englert[#]	204/331	15	ND	2.4	0	15	13
Steen[†]	48/133	15	11	4	2	32	21
Steel[||]	214/498	12	9	3.5	1	30	27

* Adverse outcome analyzed was miscarriage.
[+] Disease status at time of pregnancy unknown.
[#] Only pregnancies before onset of scleroderma
[†] Only women with one pregnancy during scleroderma.
[||] All pregnancies before or after onset of scleroderma.
From Steen VD. Scleroderma and pregnancy. Rheum Dis Clin North Am. 1997;23:133–47; with permission.

Table 9-8 Prospective Pregnancy Outcomes in Women with Scleroderma Based on Severity of Maternal Disease

	All Patients with Scleroderma	Early Limited/Late Limited	All Limited	Early Diffuse/Late Diffuse	All Diffuse	Retrospective Controls
No. of patients	60	9/15	24	10/16	26	48
No. of pregnancies (PG)	67*	11/22	33	10/24	34	158†
Miscarriage (% PGs)	18	9/14	12	10/29	24	13
Premature infant (% PGs)	26	18/23	21	40/25	29	5
Full-term birth (% PGs)	55	73/59	63	50/46	47	67

*Mean baby weight 8.3 lb, mean pregnancy duration 37.5 weeks (all live births).
†Mean baby weight 7.3 lb, mean pregnancy duration 39.5 weeks (all live births).
From Steen VD. Scleroderma and pregnancy. Rheum Dis Clin North Am. 1997;23:133–47; with permission.

Table 9-9 Effects of Pregnancy in Women with Scleroderma

Scleroderma Involvement	Change During Pregnancy
Overall	Disease generally stable
Skin	Can have onset during pregnancy; some patients with diffuse scleroderma have progression of skin disease postpartum
Joints	More arthralgias; similar to nonscleroderma pregnancy
Gastrointestinal	More reflux; similar to nonscleroderma pregnancy
Cardiopulmonary	Shortness of breath and changes that may occur in pregnancy as in any other disease
Kidney	Renal crisis during early diffuse scleroderma with or without pregnancy
Raynaud phenomenon	Improved during; worse after or during complicated deliveries

From Steen VD. Scleroderma and pregnancy. Rheum Dis Clin North Am. 1997;23:133-47; with permission.

hypertension. Scleroderma renal crisis may be difficult to differentiate from preeclampsia because both conditions may be characterized by severe hypertension and proteinuria and this group has a significant risk for superimposed preeclampsia. Renal crisis is the most critical complication of nonpregnant scleroderma and the most common cause of maternal death in association with pregnancy. Maternal and fetal survival rates have improved dramatically with the use of ACE inhibitors. Scleroderma renal crisis is the only time in pregnancy when the benefit of an ACE inhibitor outweighs the risks of its use.

Management of Scleroderma in Pregnancy

The most important determinants of maternal and fetal outcome of patients with scleroderma are the extent and severity of the underlying visceral disease (4). Patients with early, diffuse disease and antitopoisomerase antibodies are more likely to have severe, aggressive disease than are patients with anticentromere antibodies and disease of long duration (Box 9-5). A serious degree of visceral involvement, particularly with cardiomyopathy, restrictive lung disease, or renal failure, will necessitate careful consideration of the mother's longevity and her ability to care for a child should she have a successful pregnancy. Too often, the emphasis in these discussions is on the pregnancy itself and on the need for fetal monitoring rather than on the fundamental and tragic issue of maternal survival.

Management of scleroderma in pregnancy (Box 9-6) involves early baseline assessment and adjustment of medications (5, 6). It is important to note that

---

Box 9-5 Scleroderma Patients at Highest Risk During Pregnancy

Diffuse disease
Diffuse cutaneous scleroderma
Antitopoisomerase antibody
Severe visceral involvement
  Cardiac EF < 30%
  Pulmonary: FVC < 50% predicted
  G: extensive malabsorption
  Renal:Creatine > 2.0

---

corticosteroids have been found to increase risk for renal crisis during pregnancy, and probably in scleroderma in general, and their use should be avoided. Beta-adrenergic agents, because of risk for myocardial ischemia and pulmonary edema, should also be avoided. When a pharmacologic agent is used for preterm labor, nifedipine may be preferred in patients with scleroderma because it provides added vascular benefit.

At delivery, epidural anesthesia is an excellent choice because it may improve skin perfusion as a result of peripheral vasodilatation. The skin changes of systemic sclerosis and localized morphea do not interfere with normal vaginal delivery or the healing of obstetric incisions. Smaller-than-usual doses of regional anesthesia may be required because patients with scleroderma may have prolonged sensory and motor blockade at delivery.

No evidence suggests the existence of a neonatal scleroderma syndrome, and there is no increased risk for scleroderma in the offspring of patients with scleroderma (see section on Systemic Lupus Erythematosus for a discussion of SSA/SSB antibodies that may be present in scleroderma).

Summary

Patients with scleroderma may expect relatively good pregnancy outcomes if they have limited disease. Women with diffuse disease are at greatest risk for serious cardiac, pulmonary or renal problems in the first few years of the disease and should consider delaying pregnancy until the disease has stabilized. The high risk for preterm labor, small babies, and superimposed preeclampsia necessitates careful fetal monitoring. Finally, unlike any other form of hypertension in pregnancy, renal crisis in pregnant women with scleroderma requires prompt institution of therapy with ACE inhibitors.

Box 9-6 Management of Scleroderma in Pregnancy

First visit
  Baseline evaluation
    Antibody status
    Visceral involvement
    Cardiac, renal, pulmonary function
  Discontinue teratogenic disease-remitting drugs (e.g., penicillamine)
  Arrange for care in high-risk setting
  Avoid corticosteroids (increased risk for renal crisis possible)
Ongoing care
  Frequent maternal monitoring
    Blood pressure, home monitoring
    Urinalysis
    Renal function
    Cardiac, pulmonary status
  Frequent fetal monitoring
    Growth
    Amniotic fluid volume
    Uterine activity
  Aggressive treatment
    Hypertension: ACE inhibitors
    GERD: H_2-blockers, antacids, antireflux measure, proton-pump inhibitors/
      Reglan if disease interferes with maternal nutrition
    Vascular symptoms: calcium-channel blockers
Peripartum period
  Avoid use of beta-adrenergic-agonists for preterm labor
  Epidural anesthesia preferred
  Special warming of delivery room, IV fluids, patient
  Venous access established before delivery (may be difficult due to thickened
    skin)
  Reinstitute medication use immediately postpartum
  Aggressive treatment of hypertension with ACE inhibitors

REFERENCES

1. **Nelson JL.** Pregnancy, persistent microchimerism, and autoimmune disease. J Am Med Wom Assoc. 1998;53:31-47.
2. **Nelson JL.** Pregnancy immunology and autoimmune disease. J Reprod Med. 1998;43 :335-40.
3. **Steen VD.** Scleroderma and pregnancy. Rheum Dis Clin North Am. 1997;23:133-47.

4. **Buyon JP, Nelson JL, Lockshin MD.** Short analytical review: the effects of pregnancy on autoimmune diseases. Clin Immunol Immunopathol. 1996;78:99-104.

5. **Ostensen M, Ostensen H.** Safety of nonsteroidal antiinflammatory drugs in pregnant patients with rheumatic disease. J Rheumatol. 1996;23:1045-9.

6. **Brooks PM, Needs CJ.** The use of antirheumatic medication during pregnancy and in the puerperium. Rheum Dis Clin North Am. 1989;15:789-806.

APPENDIX: DRUGS FOR RHEUMATOLOGIC DISORDERS

The drug table on page 544 is for reference when there is a clinical indication for treatment with one of the medications listed. Decisions about medication use in pregnancy should be made on the basis of a benefit-to-risk ratio, avoiding unnecessary treatment of symptoms but with consideration of the fact that fetal well-being depends on maternal well-being. Because the U.S. Food and Drug Administration is working on a new classification system of medications used in pregnancy, we have classified medications as follows:

Data Suggest Drug Use May Be Justified When Indicated
When data and/or experience supports the safety of the drug.

Data Suggest Drug Use May Be Justified in Some Circumstances
When less extensive or desirable data are reported, but the drug is reasonable as a second-line therapy or may be used on the basis of the severity of maternal illness.

Data Suggest Drug Use Is Rarely Justified
Use drug only when alternatives supported by more experience and/or a better safety profile are not available.

Pregnancy pharmacokinetics may necessitate a significant increase in dose or dosing frequency, and dosing recommendations may require modification according to individual circumstances.

Drugs for Rheumatologic Disorders

Drug	Use May Be Justified When Indicated	Use May Be Justified in Some Circumstances	Use Is Rarely Justified	Comments/Dose Adjustment
Antimalarial agents (e.g., hydroxy-chloroquin)	√			
Aspirin		√		High dose (325 mg) may increase maternal/neo-natal bleeding risk at term
Azathioprine (<2 mg/kg/d)		√		Large experience with renal transplant recipients indi-cates no immediate danger to offspring at maternal doses ≤2 mg/kg/d; high doses may induce neona-tal immune suppression
Chlorambucil			√	Teratogenic first trimester
Chloroquine		√		
Corticosteroids*	√			Prednisone, hydrocorti-sone, and methylpred-nisolone preferred
Cyclophosphamide			√	Teratogenic, abortifacient
Heparin*	√			Does not cross placenta; preferred agent for APS
IV IgG	√			Crosses placenta later in gestation
Low-dose aspirin (80 mg)*	√			
Methotrexate			√	Teratogenic, abortifacient, induces myelosuppres-sion in newborn
Narcotic analgesics	√ 2nd & 3rd trimester	√ close to term		Neonatal withdrawal syndromes
NSAIDS (2nd and 3rd trimesters)		√		Monitor amniotic fluid vol-ume; possible premature closure or narrowing of PDA; prolongation of labor
NSAIDS (1st trimester) Indomethacin Ibuprofen Naproxen Ketoprofen	√			

*Preferred drug in class.

CHAPTER 10

Gastrointestinal and Liver Disease

I. Hyperemesis Gravidarum and Total Parenteral Nutrition
Catherine Nelson-Piercy, MA

II. Hepatitis
Linda J. Scully, MD

III. Gestational Liver Disease
Caroline A. Riely, MD

IV. Gastrointestinal Disorders
Malcolm C. Champion, MD

I. Hyperemesis Gravidarum and Total Parenteral Nutrition
Catherine Nelson-Piercy

Nausea and vomiting are common in pregnancy, affecting 70% and 60% of pregnant women, respectively. They form part of the normal spectrum of first-trimester symptoms and usually resolve by 12 to 16 weeks of gestation. Although the nausea and vomiting associated with pregnancy are colloquially called "morning sickness," they may occur at any time of day or may be constant throughout the day. Most women who have nausea and vomiting during pregnancy can continue to eat and drink enough to avoid hospitalization, intravenous fluid therapy, or antiemetic treatment.

Key Values and Normal Physiologic Changes for Gastrointestinal and Liver Disease

	Direction of Change	Percentage Change or Normal Range for Pregnancy
Albumin	↓	3.0 to 3.5 g/dL
Alkaline phosphate	↑↑ (produced by placenta)	>100 U/L
ALT	↔	Values unchanged by pregnancy
Amylase	↔	50 to 125 U/L
AST	↔	10 to 35 U/L
Gall bladder	↓ emptying	↑ size
GGTP	↔	1 to 70 U/L
GI motility	↓	Delayed gastric emptying, ↓ LES tone, ↓ peristalsis
Lipase	↔	3 to 20 U/dL
Total protein	↔ or ↓	6 to 8 g/dL
Urinary lipase	↑	

↑ Increase
↓ Decrease
↔ No change

Hyperemesis gravidarum affects 0.5 to 10 per 1000 pregnancies (1). It can be defined as persistent nausea and vomiting so severe that adequate hydration, electrolyte balance, or nutritional status cannot be maintained. Unlike "morning sickness," which is generally considered a benign and physiologic condition, hyperemesis may have severe consequences for both mother and fetus. Severe hyperemesis that is refractory to conventional management with intravenous fluids and antiemetic agents is rare and disabling. It is associated with multiple hospital admissions, time away from work and family, and psychological morbidity. In extreme cases, women may request—or their obstetricians may recommend—termination of the pregnancy. If inadequately or inappropriately treated, hyperemesis may cause Wernicke encephalopathy, central pontine myelinolysis, and death (2). The differential diagnosis of hyperemesis gravidarum is given in Box 10-1.

Clinical Features

Hyperemesis is a diagnosis of exclusion because we have no single confirmatory test for it. Onset is always in the first trimester, usually at weeks 6 to 8 of gestation. Vomiting beginning after the 12th week of amenorrhea should not be attributed to hyperemesis; other causes of nausea and vomiting should be

---

Box 10-1 Differential Diagnosis of Hyperemesis Gravidarum

Genitourinary conditions
  Urinary tract infection
  Uremia
Endocrine conditions
  Thyrotoxicosis
  Diabetic ketoacidosis
  Addison disease
  Hypercalcemia
Gastrointestinal conditions
  Gastritis
  Peptic ulcer
  Pancreatitis
  Bowel obstruction
  Hepatitis
Central nervous system or vestibular disease
Drug-induced vomiting (especially by iron supplements)

---

considered. Hyperemesis tends to recur in subsequent pregnancies, so a history of hyperemesis makes the diagnosis more likely.

In addition to nausea and vomiting, ptyalism and spitting may be seen. There is usually evidence of weight loss, and muscle wasting may occur (Box 10-2). Signs of dehydration, postural hypotension and tachycardia, and ketosis are common at presentation. Abdominal pain is unusual, but the patient may have dyspepsia and retrosternal discomfort related to reflux esophagitis or repeated vomiting.

Ultrasonography of the uterus should be done to confirm gestational age, diagnose multiple gestations, and exclude hydatidiform mole. Both multiple gestations and hydatidiform mole are associated with an increased incidence of hyperemesis.

Investigation

Laboratory studies usually show hyponatremia, hypokalemia, a low serum urea concentration, and ketonuria (Table 10-1). Metabolic hypochloremic alkalosis is seen unless the condition is very severe, in which case acidemia may be found. The hematocrit and specific gravity of the urine are increased. Ab-

---

Box 10-2 Clinical Features of Hyperemesis Gravidarum

Nausea*
Vomiting*
Ptyalism
Weight loss
Ketonuria
Dehydration
Muscle wasting

*Onset in first trimester

Table 10-1 Laboratory Investigations in Hyperemesis Gravidarum

Area of Investigation	Usual Findings
Urea and electrolytes	Hyponatremia
	Hypokalemia
	Low urea level (unless extremely dehydrated)
	Low chloride level
	Elevated bicarbonate level
Liver function	Aminotransferase level elevated three-fold
Thyroid function	Suppressed TSH
	Elevated free T_4
Blood	Raised hematocrit with or without increased hemoglobin concentration
Urine	Specific gravity increased
	Ketonuria

normal results on thyroid function tests appear in two thirds of patients with hyperemesis (3). The picture is that of a "biochemical thyrotoxicosis" with an increased free thyroxine level or a suppressed thyroid-stimulating hormone level. An increased incidence of gestational thyrotoxicosis has been shown in Asians compared with Europeans. Women with hyperemesis are clinically euthyroid without thyroid antibodies, except in the very rare case of autoimmune thyrotoxicosis coincidentally presenting early in pregnancy. The abnormal thyroid function test results resolve as hyperemesis is alleviated. Antithyroid drug treatment is inappropriate and unnecessary.

Abnormal liver function test results are found in 25% to 40% of patients with hyperemesis (4). The most usual abnormalities are a moderate increase in aminotransferase levels (above the normal range but <200 U). The bilirubin level may be slightly increased, but jaundice is uncommon. Mildly elevated serum amylase levels can be seen. Significantly elevated aminotransferase levels, especially in the presence of jaundice, should prompt a search for viral hepatitis or other conditions. As the patient with hyperemesis improves spontaneously or is treated, liver function abnormalities resolve.

Pathogenesis

The pathophysiology of hyperemesis is poorly understood. Various hormonal, mechanical, and psychological factors have been implicated. Studies have shown direct relationships between the severity of hyperemesis (defined by disturbances in serum electrolyte levels and liver function test results) and the degree of biochemical hyperthyroidism, the human chorionic gonadotropin (hCG) level, and estriol levels (5). It is likely that hCG, which shares a common alpha subunit with thyroid-stimulating hormone, acts as a thyroid stimulator in patients with hyperemesis. The positive correlation between severity of hyperemesis and hCG levels explains the increased incidence of this condition in multiple gestations and hydatidiform mole. The theory is also supported by the fact that the peak in hCG levels, at 6 to 12 weeks of gestation, coincides with the presentation of hyperemesis.

The pregnancy-associated decrease in lower esophageal sphincter pressure, decrease in gastric peristalsis, and delayed gastric emptying may exacerbate the symptoms of hyperemesis but are unlikely to be causative in isolation (6). Hyperemesis often has a psychological component, but it is very difficult to establish causation because hyperemesis itself can cause extreme psychological morbidity. Psychological factors may play a role in some cases, and this may be revealed by rapid improvement after hospitalization as a result of removal from a stressful home environment.

Complications

Maternal Complications

Since the advent of routine intravenous fluid and electrolyte supplementation, rates of maternal death due to hyperemesis have decreased dramatically (1). In the 1970s and 1980s, no deaths from hyperemesis were reported in the Confidential Enquiries into Maternal Deaths in the United Kingdom. However, between 1991 and 1993, three maternal deaths occurred. Two were probably the result of Wernicke encephalopathy, and one resulted from aspiration of vomitus.

Serious morbidity may result if hyperemesis is inadequately or inappropriately treated (Box 10-3). Wernicke encephalopathy due to thiamine (vitamin B$_1$) deficiency is characterized by diplopia, abnormal ocular movements, ataxia, and confusion. Wernicke encephalopathy may develop in any condition causing prolonged vomiting and inadequate nutrition, but it is most often seen in alcoholic patients. It may be precipitated by ingestion of carbohydrate-rich foods and intravenous dextrose or glucose, particularly in the context of intravenous hyperalimentation in the presence of inadequate thiamine stores. Abnormal liver function test results are more common in hyperemesis complicated by Wernicke encephalopathy (47%) than in hyperemesis in general (25%) (4). As in alcoholic patients, the abnormally functioning liver may participate in the development of Wernicke encephalopathy through the decreased conversion of thiamine to its active metabolite, thiamine pyrophosphate, and through its decreased capacity to store thiamine (4). Although the institution of thiamine replacement may alleviate the symptoms of Wernicke encephalopathy, residual impairment is not uncommon (7). If retrograde amnesia, impaired ability to learn, and confabulation (Korsakoff psychosis) have supervened, the recovery rate is only about 50%.

Hyponatremia (plasma sodium concentration <120 mmol/L), lethargy, seizures, and respiratory arrest have been reported. Both severe hyponatremia and its rapid reversal may precipitate central pontine myelinolysis (the osmotic demyelination syndrome). This is associated with symmetrical destruction of myelin at the center of the basal pons and causes pyramidal tract signs, spastic quadraparesis, pseudobulbar palsy, and impaired consciousness. Central pontine myelinolysis and Wernicke encephalopathy may coexist dur-

---

Box 10-3 Maternal Complications of Hyperemesis

Protein or calorie malnutrition

Anemia

Vitamin deficiencies

Wernicke encephalopathy

Central pontine myelinolysis

Mallory-Weiss tears

Aspiration pneumonia

Death

Iatrogenic complications (e.g., oculogyric crises or extrapyramidal effects secondary to antiemetics, infection related to venous cannulation)

Psychological problems (e.g., problems related to separation from family and prolonged hospital admission)

ing pregnancy, although no reported cases have been associated with a recorded serum sodium concentration less than 126 mmol/L and some have suggested that thiamine deficiency may render the myelin sheaths of the central pons more sensitive to changes in serum sodium concentrations (2).

Other vitamin deficiencies that occur in hyperemesis include cyanocobalamin (vitamin B_{12}) and pyridoxine (vitamin B_6) depletion causing anemia and peripheral neuropathy. A recent study from South Africa (8) found suboptimal biochemical status of thiamine, riboflavin (vitamin B_2), pyridoxine (vitamin B_6), and vitamin A in more than 60% of patients with hyperemesis.

Prolonged vomiting may lead to Mallory-Weiss tears of the esophagus and episodes of hematemesis. Protein and calorie malnutrition result in weight loss, which may be profound (10% to 20%), and muscle wasting with consequent weakness.

Certain psychological problems may predate the onset of hyperemesis, but others result from the condition itself. The latter problems relate to separation from family, inability to work, and anger over feeling neither "blooming" nor even well. Guilt may ensue when anger is turned inward toward the fetus and resentment of the pregnancy results. Requests for termination of pregnancy should not be assumed to indicate or confirm that the pregnancy is unwanted but should be taken as an indication of the degree of desperation felt by the patient.

Iatrogenic maternal complications in hyperemesis include 1) the problems of central venous cannulation associated with total parenteral nutrition (TPN) and 2) sepsis from long-term central or peripheral venous cannulation. Oculogyric crises, extrapyramidal side effects, or, rarely, the neuroleptic malignant syndrome may complicate antiemetic treatment. Problems related to inadequate or inappropriate fluid and electrolyte replacement may also be seen.

Fetal Complications

It has traditionally been thought that vomiting during pregnancy is not associated with adverse fetal outcomes and may even predict successful outcome. Pregnancies associated with mild-to-moderate nausea and vomiting are less likely to end in miscarriage, preterm delivery, or stillbirth. The risk for congenital malformations is not increased. However, it has been shown that infants of mothers with *severe* hyperemesis associated with repeated admissions to the hospital, abnormal biochemistry findings, and weight loss exceeding 5% have significantly lower birthweights and birthweight percentiles compared with infants of mothers with mild hyperemesis or uncomplicated pregnancies (9). Other recent studies dispute this association, and the discrepancy probably relates to the criteria used to define severity of hyperemesis. Hyperemesis causing Wernicke encephalopathy is associated with fetal death in 40% of cases (4).

Management

Conventional management of nausea and vomiting in pregnancy avoids the use of antiemetic drugs before 12 to 14 weeks of gestation. Pregnant women and their physicians fear the possibility that these drugs will affect fetal development. These concerns stem principally from the thalidomide tragedy of the early 1960s. After that event, a scare led to the withdrawal of Debendox/Bendectin (doxylamine, dicyclomine, and pyridoxine) from the market in 1983 even though use of the drug in 33 million pregnancies provided no evidence to substantiate claims of teratogenicity. After the withdrawal of Bendectin, hospital admissions for hyperemesis increased by 50% in Canada and similar trends were seen in the United States (10).

The potential maternal and fetal complications of hyperemesis discussed above argue for early and aggressive treatment of nausea and vomiting in pregnancy. The natural history of hyperemesis includes gradual improvement as pregnancy progresses, but this is not a reason to withhold antiemetic agents. A more relaxed attitude toward the outpatient prescription of drugs that have been shown to be safe in pregnancy and are often prescribed to inpatients may prevent some hospital admissions and decrease morbidity.

Any woman who is ketotic and unable to maintain adequate hydration should be hospitalized. Iron supplementation should be temporarily discontinued because it causes nausea and vomiting in some women. Women with hyperemesis should be weighed at least weekly.

Intravenous Fluids

Adequate and appropriate fluid and electrolyte replacement are the most important components of management. Infusion of dextrose-containing fluids (dextrose saline, 5% dextrose, and 10% dextrose) is thought by some to be a good way to provide calories, but this assumption is erroneous and dangerous. First, as discussed above, Wernicke encephalopathy may be precipitated by the use of intravenous dextrose (2). Second, the hyponatremia seen with hyperemesis necessitates the infusion of sodium-containing fluids (dextrose saline contains only 30 mmol/L of Na^+, and 5% dextrose contains no Na^+). Normal saline (sodium chloride, 0.9%; Na^+, 150 mmol/L) or Hartmann solution (sodium chloride, 0.6%; Na^+, 131 mmol/L) are appropriate solutions. Potassium chloride is added to the infusion bags as needed. The use of double-strength saline ($2N$ saline) has no place even in cases of severe hyponatremia because it results in excessively rapid correction of serum sodium concentrations with the risk for central pontine myelinolysis. Fluid and electrolyte regimens must be adapted daily and titrated in response to daily serum sodium and potassium measurements and fluid balance charts.

Thiamine

Routine thiamine supplementation should be given to all women hospitalized with prolonged vomiting. Thiamine requirements increase during pregnancy (2). If a woman can tolerate tablets, she can receive thiamine as thiamine hydrochloride tablets 25 to 50 mg three times daily. If she cannot tolerate tablets and intravenous treatment is required, 100 mg of thiamine is diluted in 100 mL of normal saline and infused over 30 to 60 minutes (6). The intravenous preparation is required only weekly.

Pyridoxine

The theoretical benefit of pyridoxine for nausea and vomiting in pregnancy relates to a possible pyridoxine deficiency. Pyridoxine was one of the components of Debendox and was shown to significantly reduce nausea in a randomized, placebo-controlled trial of 342 women with nausea during pregnancy in Thailand (11). However, it did not significantly alleviate vomiting. Another study (12) suggested that pyridoxine may be useful for patients with severe nausea but that it was no better than placebo for women with mild or moderate nausea. The widespread use of Debendox before its withdrawal from the market suggests that pyridoxine is safe in pregnancy, but pyridoxine was probably not the active antinausea agent in Debendox (10).

Antiemetic Agents

Pharmacologic antiemetic treatment should be offered to women who do not respond to intravenous fluids and electrolytes alone. Anxiety in the wake of the thalidomide tragedy of the 1960s has resulted in an understandable reluctance to prescribe antiemetic agents for hyperemesis, but extensive data show a lack of teratogenesis with dopamine antagonists (metoclopramide and domperidone) (13), phenothiazines (chlorpromazine and prochlorperazine) (14), and antihistamines (promethazine and cyclizine) (15). A meta-analysis (15) of 24 studies including more than 200,000 women exposed to antihistamines (H_1 blockers), used mainly for morning sickness in the first trimester, concluded that no increased teratogenic risk existed; the odds ratio of 0.76 even suggested a protective effect. A recent study from California (16) showed the efficacy of continuous droperidol infusions and boluses of intravenous diphenhydramine in the management of hyperemesis.

Antiemetic drugs are listed in the Drug Table at the end of this chapter. If one drug is ineffective, a second or third should be tried because different women respond to different classes of drug. Side effects of antiemetic agents include drowsiness (particularly with phenothiazines) and extrapyramidal effects and oculogyric crises (particularly with metoclopramide and phenothiazines). Ironically, the best data on fetal safety are available for Debendox/Benectin/Diclectin, and Diclectin is still available in Canada as a slow-release preparation of 10 mg of doxylamine (an antihistamine) and 10 mg of pyridoxine (10). In Australia, promethazine (Avomine) is the medication most frequently prescribed in the outpatient setting for nausea and vomiting in pregnancy (17).

Histamine-receptor blockers (ranitidine and cimetidine) and the proton-pump inhibitor (PPI) omeprazole have been used in some cases. More recently, the successful use of ondansetron, a highly selective HT3-receptor antagonist that is used with dramatic effect for postoperative and chemotherapy-induced nausea and vomiting, was reported in three cases of intractable hyperemesis. Since then, a U.S. group (18) has compared intravenous ondansetron 10 mg with intravenous promethazine 50 mg in 30 women with severe hyperemesis. Both agents were given as a stat dose followed by 8 hourly doses only if required. No benefit of ondansetron over promethazine could be shown for relief of nausea, weight gain, days of hospitalization, or total doses of medication. Although this study claimed to study women with severe hyperemesis, it enrolled patients at the time of admission and the minimal amount of medication needed to effect a clinical response in both groups (approximately three total doses) was notable. The authors comment that the intravenous hydration alone may have led to improvement.

Alternative Therapies

Attempts to avoid conventional pharmacologic agents in pregnancy have prompted studies of the efficacy of alternative therapies. Powdered ginger root given to 30 women in a double-blind, randomized, crossover trial was significantly better than placebo in diminishing or eliminating the symptoms of hyperemesis gravidarum (19). A systematic review of published controlled trials in which the P6 acupuncture point was stimulated for treatment of nausea or vomiting associated with pregnancy found that symptoms were often significantly alleviated (20). However, nausea rather than the severity or frequency of vomiting was primarily affected.

Corticosteroids

Uncontrolled data support a beneficial effect of corticosteroids in women with severe hyperemesis. The successful use of oral prednisolone (40 to 60 mg/d) or intravenous hydrocortisone (50 to 100 mg twice daily) has been reported in studies (21, 22) in which steroids were given only to women who had persistent nausea and vomiting despite adequate intravenous fluid replacement, thiamine supplementation, and regular antiemetic therapy. All women had refractory hyperemesis with multiple admissions and weight loss, and some had terminated previous pregnancies because of hyperemesis. Some were requesting termination of their current pregnancy, and at least four had been receiving TPN. The response to steroids was dramatic, rapid, and complete in all patients, but the studies were not controlled. An n-of-1 trial suggested that prednisolone (50 mg/d) was no more effective than ascorbic acid (100 mg/d) (23). In patients who do respond to steroid therapy the dose must be reduced slowly, and one study (22) showed that prednisolone in dosages exceeding 15 mg per day was required for 10.6 ± 4.7 weeks (range, 6 to 20 weeks). In some extreme cases, prednisolone use cannot be discontinued until delivery. It is usually possible to taper the dose of prednisolone to a maintenance dose less than 20 mg, but screening for the complications of steroid treatment in pregnancy, particularly an increased risk for urinary tract infection and gestational diabetes, is recommended in patients who need long-term therapy (24). Safari and colleagues (25) reported a 94% response rate to 48 mg of methylprednisone in 18 patients with refractory hyperemesis.

Prednisolone is metabolized by the placenta and transfer across the placenta is slow, so very little active drug reaches the fetus. The concentration of active compound in fetal blood is 10% of that in the mother. Although hydrocortisone (cortisol) crosses the placenta rapidly, most of it is quickly converted to inactive cortisone by fetal enzymes. Studies examining the use of corticosteroids for asthma in pregnancy have shown no congenital malformations or adverse fetal effects attributable to maternal steroid therapy (26).

Because steroids are effective in the treatment of chemotherapy-induced vomiting, it is thought that they may also be of use in other conditions (such as hyperemesis) in which vomiting is thought to have a central origin involving the chemoreceptor trigger zone. Pilot data support a beneficial role for corticosteroids in the treatment of severe hyperemesis gravidarum, and intramuscular adrenocorticotropic hormone has been shown to be no more effective than placebo in the treatment of hyperemesis (27). A randomized, double-blind study comparing methylprednisone with promethazine found a lower readmission rate in the steroid group, although no difference was seen in the numbers of patients in each group who did not stop vomiting in 2 days (28). Nelson-Piercy and co-workers (29) recently reported the results of a randomized, double-blind, placebo-controlled trial of steroids for severe hyperemesis. They showed no significant benefit of steroids with respect to nausea, vomiting, or dependence on intravenous fluids, but the study was not large enough to exclude such benefit.

Resistant Cases

In extremely severe cases of hyperemesis, termination of pregnancy may be appropriate. Experience with use of TPN for treatment and supportive management in severe hyperemesis gravidarum is increasing.

Psychological Support

All patients with hyperemesis require emotional support, including frequent reassurance and encouragement from nursing and medical staff. Psychiatric referral may be appropriate in some cases. Psychotherapy, hypnotherapy, and behavior therapy have been reported to aid in the treatment of hyperemesis.

Total Parenteral and Enteral Nutrition

Long-term maternal malnutrition may have adverse effects on fetal well being. In cases of severe maternal starvation, decreased protein intake may lead to reduced plasma volume expansion, causing insufficient placental perfusion and fetal compromise (30). Prolonged calorie deprivation and use of fatty acids as an energy source results in ketosis, which also adversely affects the fetus (30). Infant birthweight is influenced by maternal prepregnancy weight and weight gain during pregnancy. Infants of underweight mothers with inadequate weight gain during pregnancy are at increased risk for low birthweight, perinatal morbidity, and death. Compromised maternal nutrition may result in a growth-restricted fetus because of decreased maternal glucose levels, hepatic glycogen levels, and adipose tissue.

Indications for Total Parenteral Nutrition

The indications for TPN in pregnancy include any condition in which the mother cannot tolerate oral intake to the degree that maternal protein or calorie malnutrition results. Experience with TPN in pregnancy is growing as TPN is recognized to be a safe and effective method of nutritional support. Examples of conditions for which TPN has been used in pregnancy are given in Box 10-4 (31).

As well as serving as necessary supportive therapy in very severe cases of hyperemesis, TPN has been shown to have a rapid therapeutic effect in some patients (32). Possible criteria for the institution of TPN include persisting ketosis, maternal weight loss exceeding 1 kg per week for 4 consecutive weeks, and total maternal weight loss of 6 kg.

Total parenteral nutrition is not recommended for hyperemesis before optimal rehydration, antiemetic therapy, and a trial of corticosteroids or on-

---

Box 10-4 Indications for Total Parenteral Nutrition During Pregnancy

Severe protracted hyperemesis gravidarum
Diabetic gastroenteropathy
Inflammatory bowel disease
Severe pancreatitis
Massive gut resection, jejunoileal bypass, short-bowel syndrome
Bowel obstruction, esophageal stricture
Radiation enteritis
Corrosive burns to gastrointestinal tract
Prolonged postoperative ileus
Neuromuscular disease
Anorexia nervosa
Neoplastic disease
Cystic fibrosis

---

dansetron fail to cause improvement. If TPN is used, it is vital to coadminister thiamine.

Complications of Total Parenteral Nutrition in Pregnancy

The outcome of pregnancies in which TPN is used relates to the condition for which TPN is required. Thus, better pregnancy outcomes have been reported in conditions that are self-limited, such as hyperemesis or acute exacerbations of inflammatory bowel disease (IBD). Poor outcome is more common in cases of progressive systemic disease, such as diabetes with associated nephropathy and autonomic neuropathy or neoplasia (30). Similarly, earlier concerns about a possible association between TPN and preterm labor have been shown to relate to underlying medical or obstetric conditions associated with preterm labor rather than TPN itself (30, 33). There was concern that lipid infusions may initiate uterine contractions. The purported explanation was that increased levels of fatty acid precursors, such as linoleic acid, increase levels of arachidonic acid which, in turn, are a precursor for prostaglandins that may initiate preterm labor (34). However, a literature review of 73 cases of lipid-containing parenteral nutrition during pregnancy from 1984 to 1990 showed no increase in idiopathic preterm labor. In the past, there was concern from animal work that parenteral lipid emulsions may damage the placenta, but lipid emboli have not been found in human placentae after the administration of solutions containing up to 50% lipid emulsions (33).

Metabolic and infectious complications are a risk with TPN, and strict protocols and careful monitoring are obligatory. Use of TPN in pregnancy is still relatively rare, and it may be appropriate for pregnant women who need TPN to be transferred to centers that regularly use TPN and have the necessary nursing, pharmacy, and physician support (31).

The central venous catheter may be inserted into a central vein or a peripheral vein. The peripherally inserted catheter eliminates the complications related to central venous access, such as pneumothorax and cardiac tamponade. It may also reduce the risk for infectious complications from chronically indwelling catheters. Whichever route is chosen, insertion of the catheter must be done under strict aseptic technique. Reported infectious complications of TPN in pregnancy include localized bacterial infection, candidal fungemia, *Klebsiella* pneumonia, and other catheter infections resulting in bacteremia and necessitating line removal (31). The catheter site must be inspected regularly for signs of infection or thrombus.

Phlebitis and thrombosis are other recognized complications of TPN. Catheter-related endothelial disruption may provoke thrombosis, but the direct endothelial injury secondary to a hyperosmolar infusate is also likely to contribute. The hypercoagulability of pregnancy and dehydration related to the underlying need for TPN may further increase the risks, and right atrial thrombus as a complication of TPN for persistent hyperemesis has been reported (35).

Some have expressed concern that continuous infusion of high concentrations of glucose may be hazardous to the fetus, much as conditions in the diabetic mother are. However, with the addition of insulin to the TPN plus strict glucose monitoring, levels can be maintained within the normal range (30).

Constituents of Total Parenteral Nutrition

Total parenteral nutrition solutions contain variable amounts of essential amino acids (4.5% to 6%) for the formation of body protein and dextrose (15% to 25%) as an easily usable calorie source (Box 10-5). When prolonged TPN is used, lipid emulsion or intralipids (10% to 20%) should be included to supply essential fatty acids necessary to prevent fatty acid deficiency in mother and fetus. Fatty acid deficiency may adversely affect placental growth and production of surfactants. Fatty acids can be given weekly or daily, but no more than 30% to 35% of daily total nonprotein calories should be supplied by fats (30).

If a woman is taking nothing orally, she normally requires about 3 L of fluid per day, although this amount should be adjusted depending on the individual situation. For example, women with vomiting or diarrhea require more fluids, and those with renal impairment, preeclampsia, or heart failure re-

---

Box 10-5 Constituents of Total Parenteral Nutrition

Amino acids

Dextrose

Lipid emulsion

Water and electrolytes

Water-soluble vitamins, including thiamine and vitamin K

Fat-soluble vitamins

Folic acid and iron

Trace elements

---

quire less. Electrolyte requirements do not increase in pregnancy but may increase as a result of the condition for which TPN is given. These include sodium, potassium, magnesium, calcium, and phosphorus. Vitamins are usually given in a multivitamin solution, but additional vitamins A, E, and B_6 may be required. Thiamine supplementation is mandatory if TPN is used in patients with hyperemesis or any condition with pre-existing malnutrition; otherwise, the use of high concentrations of glucose may precipitate acute thiamine deficiency syndromes (2). Folic acid and vitamin B_{12} should be given daily to meet the demands of increased erythropoiesis in pregnancy, and iron may be given either in the TPN solution or intramuscularly. Folate and iron demands increase in pregnancy, and folate supplementation is especially important before conception and in the first trimester to prevent neural tube and other congenital defects. Vitamin K and trace elements, such as selenium, manganese, chromium, and zinc, are added to the TPN solution (30). Zinc deficiency has been reported to cause fetal growth retardation and is a particular concern in women with gastrointestinal disorders such as Crohn disease. Hyperglycemia may result from the increased glucose load, and varying amounts of insulin are added to the TPN solution to maintain euglycemia.

The optimal daily requirements of calories, nitrogen, trace elements, and vitamins in pregnancy are unknown and, until recently, few guidelines were available. Advice from nutritionists and dietitians who understand the nutritional demands of pregnancy should be solicited which give specific guidelines for calculating requirements. Their recommendations are based on a total caloric requirement derived from the basal energy expenditure (dependent on weight, height, and age) with an allowance for the increased nutritional demands of pregnancy and the stress of hyperalimentation. An additional 300 kcal per day accounts for the usual increase in maternal caloric intake and weight gain during pregnancy. The total daily caloric requirements for most women will be 2000 to 2500 kcal. Protein requirements are also higher in pregnancy (approximately 1.0 to 1.5 g per kg of body weight per day) (30).

Total parenteral nutrition can be given by continuous intravenous infusion or in a cyclic fashion to allow mobility and, if appropriate, oral intake of food and fluid during the day. Compared with continuous infusion of hypertonic dextrose, cycled TPN decreases the duration of hyperinsulinemia and hepatic lipogenesis and improves liver function. Cyclic TPN may not be appropriate for diabetic patients who require insulin.

Monitoring During Use of Total Parenteral Nutrition

When TPN is first initiated, daily measurements of electrolytes and glucose are necessary. During refeeding, hypokalemia, hypophosphatemia and hypomagnesemia may develop (30). Glycosuria is not a reliable indicator of hyperglycemia in pregnancy because of the decreased renal threshold for glucose in pregnancy, and blood glucose level is the only reliable indicator of the need for exogenous insulin. Careful monitoring of maternal liver function test results, cholesterol, and renal function test results are also mandatory, and these must be interpreted in the light of the normal ranges for pregnancy. Adequacy of protein supplementation may be assessed with serum levels (although, in cases of diabetic nephropathy, the baseline may be altered) and with nitrogen balance estimations. Periodic measurement of trace elements and hematologic indices should also be undertaken.

All pregnant women who require TPN should have fetal growth assessed regularly, and maternal weight gain must be checked weekly to ensure that calculated caloric requirements are accurate (30).

Enteral Feeding in Pregnancy

When the gastrointestinal tract is intact and usable, enteral hyperalimentation is preferable for the treatment of malnutrition (31). Use of the gastrointestinal tract provides physiologic benefits. Nutrition delivered enterally is better used. It prevents gut mucosal atrophy; maintains barrier function, normal gut flora, and immunocompetence; and better supports hepatic protein synthesis. Many studies comparing enteral and parenteral feeding have shown a decrease in septic complications with enteral feeding. Enteral hyperalimentation may be poorly tolerated because of nausea and vomiting and may even be contraindicated because of the risk for aspiration or the inability of the gut to absorb nutrients. Frequent tube displacement may also be a problem. Esophageal problems or poor tolerance of a nasogastric tube can be bypassed by use of a gastrostomy feeding tube. To minimize risk for aspiration, the feeding tube may be placed beyond the pylorus, but this necessitates radiation exposure for correct positioning of the tube. Enteral feeding costs considerably less than TPN (36).

The principles for calculating nutritional requirements and the addition of vitamins and trace elements in enteral feeding are similar to those in TPN. The stomach should be aspirated periodically to prevent gastric retention and decrease the risk for aspiration. Iso-osmotic solutions are recommended to facilitate absorption, and low volumes of formula are used initially and are gradually increased until the desired rate of infusion to meet daily requirements is reached. Blood glucose levels must be monitored as they are in TPN.

A recent report (37) has described the successful use of enteral feeding through a nasogastric tube in seven patients with hyperemesis that did not respond to antiemetics. Nausea and vomiting improved within 1 day of continuous infusion, and patients were discharged within 8 days, although enteral feeding was maintained for a mean of 6 weeks. All of these women had meal-related nausea and vomiting only. The reported experience in hyperemesis and diabetes shows enteral nutrition to be well tolerated and safe, provided that stabilization of hydration and electrolyte balance has been achieved. However, in women with severe hyperemesis and symptoms of nausea and vomiting that are not limited to the consumption of food, less success may be seen with the enteral route.

Because of the aforementioned advantages, enteral feeding may be attempted before TPN in women with functioning gastrointestinal tracts.

REFERENCES

1. **Hod M, Orvieto R, Kaplan B, Friedman S, Ovadia J.** Hyperemesis gravidarum: a review. J Reprod Med. 1994;39:605-12.

2. **Bergin PS, Harvey P.** Wernicke's encephalopathy and central pontine myelinolysis associated with hyperemesis gravidarum. BMJ. 1992;305:517-8.

3. **Goodwin TM, Montero M, Mestman JH.** Transient hyperthyroidism and hyperemesis gravidarum: clinical aspects. Am J Obstet Gynecol. 1992;167:648-52.

4. **Rotman P, Hassin D, Mouallem M, Barkai G, Farfel Z.** Wernicke's encephalopathy in hyperemesis gravidarum: association with abnormal liver function. Isr J Med Sci. 1994;30:225-8.

5. **Goodwin TM, Montero M, Mestman JH, Pekary AE, Hershman JM.** The role of chorionic gonadotropin in transient hyperthyroidism of hyperemesis gravidarum. J Clin Endocrinol Metab. 1992;75:1333-7.

6. **Nelson-Piercy C.** Hyperemesis gravidarum. Curr Obstet Gynaecol. 1997;7:98-103.

7. **Selvaraj S.** Wernicke's encephalopathy as a complication of hyperemesis gravidarum. J Obstet Gynaecol. 1997;17:365.

8. **van Stuijvenberg ME, Schabort I, Labadarios D, Nel JT.** The nutritional status and treatment of patients with hyperemesis gravidarum. Am J Obstet Gynecol. 1995; 172:1585-91.

9. **Godsey RK, Newman RB.** Hyperemesis gravidarum: a comparison of single and multiple admissions. J Reprod Med. 1991;36:287-90.

10. **Pastuszak A.** Doxylamine/pyridoxine for nausea and vomiting of pregnancy. Canadian Pharmaceutical Journal. 1995;128:39-42.

11. **Vutyavanich T, Wongrangan S, Ruangsri R.** Pyridoxine for nausea and vomiting of pregnancy: a randomized, double-blind, placebo-controlled trial. Am J Obstet Gynecol. 1995;173:881-4.

12. **Sahakian V, Rouse D, Sipes, et al.** Vitamin B6 is effective therapy for nausea and vomiting of pregnancy: a randomized, double-blind placebo controlled study. Obstet Gynecol. 1991;78:33-6.

13. **Milkovich L, Van Den Berg BJ.** An evaluation of the teratogenicity of certain antinauseant drugs. Am J Obstet Gynecol. 1976;125:244-8.

14. **Godet PF, Marie-Cardine M.** Neuroleptics, schizophrenia and pregnancy: an epidemiological and teratologic study. Encephale. 1991;17:543-7.

15. **Seto A, Einarson T, Koren G.** Pregnancy outcome following first trimester exposure to antihistamines—meta analysis. Am J Perinatol. 1997;14:119-24.

16. **Nageotte MP, Briggs GG, Towers CV, et al.** Droperidol and diphenhydramine in the management of hyperemesis gravidarum. Am J Obstet Gynecol. 1996;174:1801-5.

17. **Abraham S.** Nausea and vomiting in pregnancy. Current Therapeutics. 1996;37:41-8.

18. **Sullivan CA, Johnson CA, Roach H, Martin RW, Stewart DK, Morrison JC.** A pilot study of intravenous ondansetron for hyperemesis gravidarum. Am J Obstet Gynecol. 1996;174:1565-8.

19. **Fischer-Rasmussen W, Kjaer SK, Dahl C, Asping U.** Ginger treatment of hyperemesis gravidarum. Eur J Obstet Gynecol Reprod Biol. 1991;38:19-24.

20. **Murphy PA.** Alternative therapies for nausea and vomiting of pregnancy. Obstet Gynecol. 1998;91:149-55.

21. **Nelson-Piercy C, de Swiet M.** Corticosteroids for the treatment of hyperemesis gravidarum. Br J Obstet Gynaecol. 1994;101:1013-5.

22. **Taylor R.** Successful management of hyperemesis gravidarum using steroid therapy. Q J Med. 1996;89:103-7.

23. **Magee LA, Redman CWG.** An N-of-1 trial for the treatment of hyperemesis gravidarum. Br J Obstet Gynaecol. 1996;103:478-80.

24. **Nelson-Piercy C.** Handbook of Obstetric Medicine. Oxford: Isis Medical Media; 1997.

25. **Safari HR, Alsulyman OM, Gherman RB, Goodwin TM.** Experience with oral methylprednisolone in the treatment of refractory hyperemesis gravidarum. Am J Obstet Gynecol. 1998;178:1054-8.

26. **Fitzsimons R, Greenberger PA, Patterson R.** Outcome of pregnancy in women requiring corticosteroids for severe asthma. J Allergy Clin Immunol. 1986;78:349-53.

27. **Ylikorkala O, Kauppila A, Ollanketo ML.** Intramuscular ACTH or placebo in the treatment of hyperemesis gravidarum. Acta Obstet Gynecol Scand. 1979;58:453-5.

28. **Safari HR, Fassett MJ, Souter IC, Alsulyman OM, Goodwin TM.** The efficacy of methylprednisolone in the treatment of hyperemesis gravidarum: a randomized, double-blind, controlled study. Am J Obstet Gynecol. 1998;179:921-4.

29. **Nelson-Piercy C, Fayers P, de Swiet M.** Randomized, double-blind, placebo-controlled trial of corticosteroids for the treatment of hyperemesis gravidarum. Br J Obstet Gynaecol. In press.

30. **Badgett T, Feingold M.** Total parenteral nutrition in pregnancy: case review and guidelines for calculating requirements. J Matern Fetal Med. 1997;6:215-7.

31. **Lee RV, Rodgers BD, Young C, Eddy E, Cardinal J.** Total parenteral nutrition during pregnancy. Obstet Gynecol. 1986;68:563-71.

32. **Charlin V, Borghesi L, Hasbun J, Von-Mulenbrock R, Moreno MI.** Parenteral nutrition in hyperemesis gravidarum. Nutrition. 1993;9:29-32.

33. **Levine MG, Esser D.** Total parenteral nutrition for the treatment of severe hyperemesis gravidarum: maternal nutritional effects and fetal outcome. Obstet Gynecol. 1988;72:102-7.

34. **Greenspoon JS, Safarik RH, Hayashi JT, Rosen DJD.** Parenteral nutrition during pregnancy: lack of association with idiopathic preterm labor or preeclampsia. J Reprod Med. 1994;39:87-91.

35. **Turrentine MA, Smalling RW, Parisi VM.** Right atrial thrombus as a complication of total parenteral nutrition in pregnancy. Obstet Gynecol. 1994;84:675-7.

36. **van de Ven CJM.** Nasogastric enteral feeding in hyperemesis gravidarum. Lancet. 1997;349:445.

37. **Hsu JJ, Clark-Glena R, Nelson DK, Kim CH.** Naso-gastric enteral feeding in the management of hyperemesis gravidarum. Obstet Gynecol. 1996;88:343-6.

II. Hepatitis
Linda J. Scully

Several conditions specifically affect the liver during pregnancy, but viral hepatitis is the most common cause of hepatic dysfunction and jaundice in pregnant women (1). This is especially true in less developed countries, where crowding and poor sanitation permit several types of viral hepatitis to flourish. Six distinct causes of viral hepatitis have been described: the hepatitis A, B, C, D, E, and G viruses. These viruses are genetically unrelated, but they all have a propensity to infect the liver. Cytomegalovirus, Epstein-Barr virus, and herpes simplex virus (HSV) usually cause more systemic illnesses but occasionally produce significant liver involvement. With the exception of hepatitis E and HSV infection, the clinical symptoms and prognosis of the various hepatitis virus infections are unaffected by pregnancy. Here, we describe the clinical features of, serologic testing for, and management of viral hepatitis in pregnancy. An approach to viral hepatitis in pregnancy is presented in Table 10-2.

Hepatitis A

Hepatitis A is caused by the hepatitis A virus (HAV), an RNA virus that is usually acquired through close contact with an infected person. It accounts for

25% of cases of acute symptomatic hepatitis in the United States. In children, HAV infection is seldom symptomatic and rarely causes jaundice. Adults have a more severe clinical course, and 20% to 40% of adults develop overt jaundice. Most persons in North America who are older than 60 years of age are immune to HAV, whereas less than 15% of young North American adults are protected (2). Therefore, younger persons are at risk for HAV infection, especially if they travel to countries where hepatitis A is endemic. Similar declining immunity to HAV is being detected worldwide. This changing epidemiology will put more persons at risk for HAV infection in local outbreaks, such as the one recently seen in Tennessee (3).

The hepatitis A virus is spread by the fecal–oral route. When infectious, it is present at high levels in the stool. Box 10-6 outlines common sources of infection. The virus is shed in the stool before symptoms occur, and patients are most infectious before clinical disease develops. Viremia is relatively short-

Table 10-2 Acute Hepatitis in Pregnancy

Risk Factors	Physical Findings	Laboratory Investigations
Intravenous drug use	No stigmata of chronic liver	CBC
Sexual contact	disease	AST, ALT, Alk Phos
Contact with person with	Tender hepatomegaly	Albumin, INR
known hepatitis	Jaundice	Hep A IgM
Travel to countries where	Skin lesions (e.g., associated	HBsAg, anti-HBc
hepatitis is prevalent	with herpes or Hepatitis B)	Hepatitis C Ab
Blood transfusion (rare)		CMV IgM
Drug-induced hepatitis may		EBV IgM
mimic acute viral hepatitis		HSV IgM
		HEV Ab if high-risk area visited
		Consider ceruloplasmin, ANA,
		anti–smooth muscle Ab

Box 10-6 Sources of Hepatitis A Virus Infection

Formites (e.g., water taps and door handles)

Water supplies contaminated with fecal matter

Food (from infected food handler with poor hygiene)

Shellfish from contaminated water

Intravenous drug user (probably secondary to gastrointestinal carriage of drugs)

lived, although the polymerase chain reaction (PCR) has detected HAV RNA in serum up to 7 days after peak elevations in liver enzyme concentrations (4).

For the most part, HAV infection in adults results in an acute self-limited illness that has nausea, anorexia, loss of taste for cigarettes, fatigue, and right upper-quadrant discomfort as prodromal symptoms. Approximately one third of infected adults develop obvious jaundice. The incubation period after infection is 15 to 50 days (mean, 28 days). Peak serum aminotransferase levels are often up to 500 times greater than normal and usually improve dramatically within weeks. Acute HAV infection is diagnosed by the detection of IgM anti-HAV antibodies in serum. These antibodies are almost always detectable by the time the patient is symptomatic, and they disappear within 3 to 6 months, during which time the IgG anti-HAV antibodies develop. The IgG anti-HAV antibodies usually persist for life, protect against re-infection, and can be used to determine whether a traveler or someone in a high-risk profession is at risk for HAV infection and requires vaccination.

Almost all patients with acute HAV infection completely recover within 3 to 6 months, although postviral fatigue and depression have been reported, as has relapse in the convalescent period. Fulminant hepatitis is rare, occurring in less than 1 in 1000 cases of HAV infection. Only one case of chronic HAV infection has been reported, and chronic carriers as a continuing source of infection are therefore not a problem (5).

Excellent live attenuated vaccines for HAV are now available (6, 7). They produce high-level protective antibodies and are well tolerated. Combinations of HAV and hepatitis B virus (HBV) vaccines have recently been developed and produce antibody response rates similar to those seen when the vaccines are administered separately.

The symptoms and prognosis of acute HAV infection are unaffected by pregnancy. In a hepatitis A outbreak in Shanghai, 34 pregnant women with acute HAV infection were studied, and no increase in morbidity or mortality rates was seen in the mothers or neonates. The study noted no maternal–fetal transmission of HAV, although this may be partly due to the immune serum globulin (ISG) that was given to the infants at birth (8).

There is one recent report of prenatal transmission of HAV to a fetus (9). The mother recovered completely, but ultrasonography at 27 weeks of gestation showed fetal ascites. Fundipuncture revealed normal aminotransferase levels in the fetus and positivity for IgM anti-HAV antibodies. It is conceivable that intrauterine transmission of HAV takes place more often than we realize and that HAV usually causes milder disease. Maternal–fetal transmission may occur through maternal blood containing HAV or through fecal contact at delivery (10).

Outbreaks of HAV infection in neonatal units have been described, but in most cases the initial infection was attributed to a contaminated blood product given to one infant (11). The suggestion that neonates may have prolonged shedding of HAV has been offered as a possible explanation for the number of outbreaks reported in neonatal units (12). However, the high rate of contact with stool and, occasionally, poor infection control practices on the part of the staff play a significant role. Neonates clear HAV infection normally, and no long-term sequelae have been seen. Table 10-3 compares neonatal transmission from all viral hepatidites.

If a mother receives a diagnosis of acute HAV infection at term, the infant should be isolated and the staff must take precautions to prevent spread of HAV. The infant should receive an ISG injection at birth (13).

Hepatitis B

The hepatitis B virus is a double-stranded DNA virus that can infect only humans and chimpanzees. It is estimated that there are more than 200 million carriers of HBV worldwide; in endemic areas, most of these persons were infected at birth. It is estimated that in the United States alone, more than 20,000 infants each year are born to mothers who are positive for the hepatitis B surface antigen (HBsAg). Hepatitis B virus causes significant liver disease and results in cirrhosis or hepatocellular carcinoma in up to 20% of persons with chronic infection (14).

For unknown reasons, only 5% to 10% of older children or adults with acute HBV infection develop chronic infection, and the remaining 90% to 95% clear HBV spontaneously after a short illness (15). In contrast, 90% to 95% of neonates infected at the time of birth become chronic carriers of HBV

Table 10-3 Hepatitis and Neonatal Viral Transmission

Virus	Diagnostic Tests	Neonatal Transmission	Prevention of Transmission
Hepatitis A	IgM anti-HAV	Occasional	ISG at birth
Hepatitis B	HBsAg IgM anti-HBV	90%	HBIg Hepatitis B vaccine
Hepatitis C	Anti-HCV HCV RNA	<5%	None available
Hepatitis D	HBsAg Anti-HDV	Rare	HBIg Hepatitis B vaccine
Hepatitis E	Anti-HEV	Occasional	None available
Herpes simplex	Anti-HSV Presence of skin lesions Liver biopsy?	Common	Acyclovir

(16). It is perinatal infection that is responsible for most cases of the chronic carrier state worldwide, especially in regions where HBV infection is endemic, such as Southeast Asia (17). It is therefore essential that we identify all infected mothers at the time of delivery and take appropriate measures to prevent transmission to the neonate. Fortunately, hepatitis B immune globulin (HBIg) and the HBV vaccine, when administered at birth, successfully prevent HBV infection and development of the chronic carrier state in more than 90% of these infants (18–20). If routine immunization of all neonates, along with injection of HBIg in neonates of mothers known to be HBsAg positive, were to be implemented globally, HBV infection could be almost eliminated within a few decades.

When present, HBV is found in large quantities in blood and at lower levels in other body fluids, such as saliva, semen, tears, and synovial fluid. The complete HBV virion consists of a core structure that contains the viral DNA polymerase required for viral replication. This core protein is surrounded by the surface coat known as HBsAg. The hepatitis B virus is unique in that it produces a vast excess of this surface protein, which is easily detected directly in the blood by radioimmunoassay or enzyme-linked immunosorbent assay. It is the only virus for which routine testing detects a viral antigen rather than an antibody response. Anyone with HBsAg in the blood should be considered infectious, although there are exceptions to this rule.

For safety's sake, all HBsAg-positive persons should be treated as infectious. However, the current gold standard for determining HBV infectivity is detection of HBV DNA in the serum with the highly sensitive and specific PCR assay (21). Studies using this assay have shown that HBV DNA is present in most but not all HBsAg-positive persons (22). When present in serum, the hepatitis B e antigen (HBeAg), a derivative of the core protein, indicates active viral replication, high-level infectivity, and high levels of viral DNA (23). However, the absence of HBeAg may indicate clearance of the replicating virus (24) or, as recently described, the development of a genetic mutation in one gene of the virus so that the virus continues to replicate but cannot produce the HBeAg protein (25).

In adults in North America, HBV is spread most often by sexual transmission or blood-to-blood contact, such as that which may occur during intravenous drug use (26). In 20% of persons, no risk factor for HBV can be identified and inapparent parenteral or percutaneous transmission is assumed. The virus is not spread by infected food or water.

Acute HBV infection is symptomatic in only 50% of infected adults. A small proportion of persons may develop urticaria, arthralgia, and frank arthritis, which are rare in other forms of acute hepatitis and are therefore helpful in diagnosis. The incubation period before the onset of symptoms and abnormal aminotransferase levels is 6 to 12 weeks, although HBsAg is detectable in blood within a few weeks of infection (27). Normal symptoms include nausea, fatigue, and right upper-quadrant discomfort, as seen in patients with any form of acute hepatitis. Only 10% of infected persons develop jaundice. The vast majority of asymptomatic persons found to be HBsAg positive are chronic carriers. Most patients with acute HBV infection have markedly elevated aminotransferase levels, often more than 500 times greater than normal. These levels can rapidly decline toward normal, and the single most useful diagnostic test for proving that the infection is recent is a test for IgM anti–hepatitis B core antibody. This antibody is not present in most chronic carriers of HBV.

More than 90% of acutely infected adults have a minor illness, clear the virus and HBsAg from the serum, and develop protective anti-HBs antibodies. Less than 1% of infected persons develop fulminant hepatitis, which is thought to be due to an overexuberant immune response to HBV (28). Five percent to 10% of acutely infected adults develop chronic infection, with liver damage varying from none to minimal inflammation to chronic active hepatitis and, ultimately, cirrhosis. It is patients with cirrhosis that are at risk for hepatocellular carcinoma but usually after 30 to 40 years of infection. Interferon therapy is the only effective treatment for HBV infection, but it eradicates HBV in only 40% of those treated and is not very helpful in persons who have been infected for many years or persons who were infected at birth (29). Fortunately, lamivudine, which has been widely used in the treatment of HIV infection, is showing promise in the treatment of HBV infection.

Acute Hepatitis B Virus Infection in Pregnancy

The clinical course of acute HBV infection in pregnancy does not seem to pose any specific risk to the pregnancy or the mother and is similar to the clinical course of acute HBV infection in nonpregnant patients. However, the timing of the acute infection determines the risk for transmission of HBV to the neonate (30). Acute HBV infection is diagnosed by the constellation of appropriate symptoms, markedly elevated aminotransferase levels, and the detection of HBsAg and IgM anti–hepatitis B core antibody in serum. The risk for transmission to the neonate is greatest if the acute infection appears during the third trimester or the puerperium. One study (30) reported transmission rates of 0%, 6%, 61%, and 100% in the first trimester, second trimester, third trimester, and puerperium, respectively. However, all infants born to mothers with acute HBV infection during pregnancy should receive HBIg and vaccine at birth, even if the mother has cleared HBsAg by the time of delivery. Low levels of HBV DNA can still be detected in the serum of some persons for months after the apparent clearance of HBV, and it is not clear whether these persons are infectious (31). Aggressive preventive measures should be taken because the outcome of persons who acquire HBV infection in the neonatal period is ultimately poor.

Chronic Hepatitis B Virus Infection in Pregnancy

Almost every country in the world recommends testing all pregnant women for HBsAg. Testing only persons from high-risk groups would miss 50% of those who are found to be positive on routine testing. The vast majority of HBsAg-positive women identified on routine testing are previously unrecognized chronic carriers of HBV. This is especially true in high-risk regions, such as Southeast Asia and Africa. The HBsAg-carrier rate in pregnant women varies; it is 0.15% in white women, 0.6% in black women born in the United States, 2.0% in Asian women born in the United States, 5% in black women born outside of the United States, and 8.9% in Asian women born outside of the United States (26). These HBsAg-positive persons may have normal or mildly to moderately elevated aminotransferase levels (usually less than five times greater than normal). As mentioned above, anyone with detectable HBsAg should be considered infectious, although patients who are HBeAg positive have especially high levels of viremia and are much more likely to transmit HBV to their offspring (32–34). Several studies have indicated that without intervention, 90% to 95% of infants born to HBeAg-positive mothers compared with 10% of infants born to HBeAg-negative mothers will become chronic carriers. This perinatal transmission probably accounts for the vast majority of chronic HBV carriers in some areas.

Chronic HBV infection per se has little effect on the pregnancy itself. Female HBV carriers tend to have less liver inflammation than male carriers and are much less likely, over the long term, to develop cirrhosis or hepatocellular carcinoma. Therefore, most female HBV carriers have relatively healthy livers, especially during their childbearing years, and rarely have severe hepatic dysfunction or complications (such as portal hypertension) to complicate pregnancy or delivery. In addition, pregnancy has no observed effects on the activity of the HBV-induced liver disease, and no dramatic changes in aminotransferase levels have been reported. Interferon therapy is not used in pregnancy for the chronic carrier state.

Prevention of Perinatal Transmission of Hepatitis B Virus

The vast majority of HBV-infected infants are asymptomatic, have slightly elevated aminotransferase levels, and become HBsAg positive between 4 and 6 weeks postpartum. The timing of HBsAg positivity indicates infection at the time of birth rather than in utero. It is assumed that the neonate is infected by blood or other secretions with which it comes into contact during delivery.

Occasionally, HBsAg is detectable in the infant at birth; this indicates transplacental infection (32). The HBV vaccine and HBIg are not effective in the latter group of infants, and chronic hepatitis almost always develops, resulting in the 5% failure rate of this preventive regimen seen in most studies. A state of immune tolerance to the viral antigens has been postulated (35). In contrast, HBIg and vaccine given within the first few days of life is 95% effective in preventing the development of chronic HBV infection in the infant infected at the time of birth (18–20).

Numerous studies of the prevention of perinatal HBV transmission have been done using a variety of doses and regimens of HBV vaccine, usually in conjunction with HBIg (36–39). Most studies have shown that infection in the neonate is prevented in more than 89% of cases. It has also been shown that the response in preterm infants is almost as good as that in full-term infants (20), that the addition of HBIg does not blunt immune response to the vaccine (34), and that booster vaccines are not required and long-term protection is provided by immunization at birth (36, 37).

Only a few studies of the HBV vaccine alone have been done in infants born to HBsAg-positive mothers, and these studies have had somewhat conflicting results. In the study by Poovarawan and associates (40), it seems that the vaccine alone was more than 85% successful in preventing infection of the neonate. Similarly, Yao and colleagues (41) showed excellent results with a combined intramuscular–intradermal HBV vaccination schedule. In Malaysia, investigators immunized infants in their homes within 1 week of birth without knowing maternal HBsAg status (42). At 1 year, the prevalence of HBsAg was 1.4% in infants who received three doses of vaccine; the baseline prevalence was 6.2%. If these results are confirmed in larger studies, one could conceivably forego testing mothers for HBsAg and just immunize all infants. This would be especially helpful in poorer areas of the world where medical facilities are scarce and HBsAg testing and HBIg are not readily available.

It is currently recommended that all pregnant women be screened for HBsAg. All infants born to HBsAg-positive mothers should receive HBIg at birth and one of the two available vaccines at day 1, month 1, and month 6 after birth (43). Both vaccines currently licensed in North America (Engerix-B, SmithKline Beecham; and Recombivax HB, Merck) are equally protective. Both are very safe; side effects are rare and include transient poor feeding, irritability, mild fever, and redness and soreness at the injection site.

In 1991, the Centers for Disease Control and Prevention (CDC) endorsed a recommendation for the universal vaccination of all infants against HBV infection. This practice has been adopted in most areas of the United States. By the end of 1993, two thirds of infants who were being vaccinated against normal childhood infections were also receiving the HBV vaccine. Forty-seven percent of U.S. hospitals were offering HBV vaccines to all newborns; this rate was much higher than the rate seen in 1989 (44). It has also been shown that if a mother is HBsAg negative, the HBV vaccine can be given to the child later (with other routine immunizations) with no detrimental effect on the immune response to HBV or the other antigens given; this may improve vaccination rates (45).

Some states and Canadian provinces have adopted the routine immunization of all infants against HBV infection. Unfortunately, others—influenced by cost-effectiveness analyses that may have been flawed—have chosen to immunize only infants born to HBsAg-positive mothers and to immunize all other offspring in early adolescence (46). It is hoped that the data on long-term immune response to the neonatal vaccination regimen and the ease of administering HBV vaccines with other routine immunization will change this situation. With increased emigration of persons from countries endemic for HBV, increased use of day care facilities, and subsequent increased exposure of children to HBV, the routine vaccination of all infants should be strongly encouraged.

Problems with Hepatitis B Prophylaxis for Neonates

Even though the CDC in 1991 recommended screening for HBsAg in all pregnant women, a significant percentage of HBsAg-positive mothers is not being detected and the infants born to these women are not receiving appropriate prophylaxis for HBV infection. The reasons for these failures are multiple. In the United States, 16% of 3982 infants born after March 1993 were born to mothers who had not received the recommended HBsAg testing (47). Of 183 hospitals surveyed, 75% had maternal HBsAg screening policies but only 56% had standing orders for the testing of pregnant women who present without previous serologic test results. Mothers with continued high-risk behaviors during pregnancy, such as intravenous drug use, and mothers with many sexual partners should ideally be retested during the puerperium to detect recently acquired infection. The results of HBsAg testing must be available quickly enough that HBIg and the HBV vaccine can be administered in a timely manner.

Another problem with current protocols is the lack of reliable transmission of HBsAg test results to the clinicians caring for the infants involved. As a result, some infants do not receive the complete vaccination schedule. Only about 30% of 732 U.S. pediatricians surveyed thought that they reliably received prenatal HBsAg test results (48).

More education is required to encourage physicians who care for pregnant women and infants to offer HBV vaccine to all infants at birth. In 1993, 18% of California pediatricians did not agree with the recommendation for universal HBV immunization and did not plan to implement the recommended approaches in their practices (49).

Another rare but well-described complication of the HBIg–HBV vaccine regimen is the development of mutations in the HBsAg gene. These mutations allow HBV to replicate and to evade the anti-HBs response (50). This event is rare enough that it should not be a deterrent to universal HBV vaccination.

Mothers Positive for Hepatitis B Surface Antigen

All body fluids of HBsAg-positive persons may be infectious, and bloodstained drapes and towels should be identified and handled properly to prevent infection of housekeeping staff, laundry workers, and other staff persons. All obstetricians and delivery room staff should be vaccinated against HBV. The mother and infant should be cared for in a single room if bleeding or staining continues. Patients who are positive for HBsAg or anti-HBs antibodies can certainly share a room without risk.

Breastfeeding by HBsAg-positive mothers is not contraindicated as long as the infant has received HBIg and HBV vaccine. The benefits of breastfeeding are thought to outweigh the risk for HBV transmission by this route, although HBsAg has occasionally been detected in breast milk (51).

Hepatitis C

The hepatitis C virus (HCV), a unique RNA virus, causes more than 95% of cases of what was previously termed non-A, non-B hepatitis. It is the etiologic agent in almost all cases of post-transfusion hepatitis (52). A diagnostic test for HCV became routinely available in 1990 (53). In a short period of time, an incredible amount of information has appeared on the epidemiology of HCV infection and, specifically, on the risk for neonatal transmission of HCV.

Hepatitis C Virus Infection

Acute HCV infection is symptomatic in less than 30% of persons, and symptoms often consist only of mild, flu-like problems. Studies of post-transfusion hepatitis indicate that the mean incubation period is 7.8 weeks when HCV is acquired through transfusion, but the incubation period for non–parenterally acquired infection is unknown. With acute HCV infection, aminotransferase levels are more than 15 times greater than normal in 75% of patients.

One of the most important characteristics of HCV is its propensity to cause chronic infection (54). It is estimated that 80% to 85% of persons with acute infection will develop chronic infection and that 50% to 60% will develop chronic hepatitis. Over a 20-year period, 20% of the infected group will develop cirrhosis, and some will develop associated hepatocellular carcinoma (55). Approximately 20% of all HCV-infected persons ultimately develop life-threatening complications of HCV infection. However, the disease may be milder in North Americans and in persons who acquired infection from sources other than transfusion, such as intravenous drug use. Many of these persons are asymptomatic, and stigmata of chronic liver disease are unusual.

The hepatitis C virus is essentially spread by blood-to-blood contact, and the vast majority of HCV infections are caused by intravenous drug use or transfusions of blood or blood products (56, 57). Sexual transmission is much less common.

In some high-risk groups, HCV infection is very common. Studies have shown that 60% to 85% of intravenous drug users, 50% to 60% of persons with hemophilia, and 20% of hemodialysis recipients have HCV infection (58). In contrast, the rate of HCV infection in healthy blood donors is less than 0.5% in most North American centers (59, 60). The highest prevalence is in persons 30 to 49 years of age. Although the number of new cases of HCV infection is declining, the current number of persons with chronic infection indicates that HCV may surpass alcohol as the most common cause of cirrhosis and need for liver transplantation in the decades to come (61).

Diagnostic Tests

A diagnosis of HCV infection is made by the detection of antibodies to various regions of the hepatitis C virus (62, 63). These antibodies, like antibodies to HIV, indicate ongoing infection rather than immunity (64). The enzyme immunoassay, although sensitive, has a 40% to 50% false-positive rate in healthy blood donors and other low-risk persons, such as pregnant women. Therefore, a supplementary recombinant immunoblot assay (RIBA) is required to confirm the diagnosis in low-risk persons (65). However, 90% to 95% of all persons with risk factors (such as intravenous drug use) and elevated serum aminotransferase levels are truly positive for HCV and will have this confirmed by RIBA. Positivity on RIBA is highly associated with infectivity (65). It is important to note that there is a long "window period" after an acute infection during which the patient is negative for anti-HCV antibodies. On average, it takes 8 weeks to (rarely) 1 year to develop detectable HCV antibody levels, and a negative test result does not rule out HCV infection in the acute setting (66). Immunosuppressed patients may have a minimal or delayed anti-HCV response.

The gold standard for the detection of HCV is the PCR assay. This assay can detect very low-level viremia by specifically amplifying HCV RNA. The test is not without its pitfalls, however, and is very costly and operator dependent (67).

Acute Hepatitis C Virus Infection and Pregnancy

Multiple studies of HCV infection in pregnant women and their offspring indicate that chronic HCV infection itself has little influence on pregnancy. There are few data on acute HCV infection in pregnancy, but nothing suggests that the severity, course, or prognosis of this infection is altered by pregnancy (30).

In a few recent case reports of acute HCV infection in pregnancy, PCR data have been available for both mother and infant. In one report (68), two infants born to mothers who had acute hepatitis C in the last trimester were reported to be positive for HCV on PCR during follow-up. However, in another report (69), an infant in a similar situation was not infected. Acute HCV infection is so rarely diagnosed that data on the subject are difficult to obtain.

Chronic Hepatitis C Virus Infection and Pregnancy

Since HCV testing was introduced, large studies of HCV infection in pregnant women have been undertaken (70). Available data indicate that HCV infection in the mother does not adversely affect the pregnancy (71). Most of the mothers in whom these data were collected were probably not infected for a prolonged period and probably did not have significant liver synthetic dysfunction. No data suggest that pregnancy adversely affects the severity of hepatitis and, in one study (72), 27 of 29 HCV-positive mothers had normal aminotransferase levels that remained normal during pregnancy and for 6 months postpartum.

Perinatal Transmission of Hepatitis C Virus

Because of our knowledge of the high risk for neonatal transmission of HBV and HIV, perinatal transmission of HCV was one of the first topics to be investigated when HCV serologic testing became routinely available in 1990. Numerous published studies have shown that, in the absence of HIV co-infection, perinatal transmission of HCV is uncommon; it occurs in approximately 5% of infants of infectious mothers (73). The title of one review, "Hepatitis C: You Cannot Blame It on Your Mother," accurately describes the state of our current knowledge (74).

Studies of neonatal HCV transmission require PCR for the detection of virus because HCV antibody testing alone in neonates reflects the passive transfer of maternal antibody. Up to 50% of neonates born to infected mothers have detectable HCV antibodies that usually disappear by 6 to 7 months postpartum, although antibodies occasionally persist for up to 1 year (75, 76). Very high levels or increasing titers, however, usually indicate true infection as shown by positivity on PCR (77).

Co-infection with HIV and HCV is associated with a slightly increased risk for acquiring HCV infection at birth (78–82) (Table 10-4). This is mainly attributed to the increased HCV viremia found in HIV-infected persons, secondary to immunosuppression. Sexual transmission from co-infected persons is also more common, presumably for the same reasons.

Hepatitis C Virus and Breastfeeding

Few studies have directly addressed the possibility of HCV transmission through breastmilk, and the results of these studies are somewhat contradictory. More prospective studies are required, but it is likely that some mothers with high-level viremia have detectable HCV in breastmilk (83). Given the numerous studies indicating that the vast majority of offspring are HCV negative at one year, the available data indicate that transmission through breastfeeding is very rare. The recommendation by the recent National Institutes of Health Consensus Conference on Hepatitis C (84) is that breastfeeding is not contraindicated in HCV-positive women. Mothers should be advised that a very small, undefined risk exists but that the benefits probably outweigh the disadvantages.

Prevention of Perinatal Hepatitis C Virus Transmission

Vaccines for HCV infection have not been developed but are currently under active investigation and may aid in the prevention of perinatal infection. Studies previously used ISG to prevent post-transfusion non-A, non-B hepatitis, with equivocal results. Given the lack of anti-HCV antibodies in North American ISG products and the low rate of HCV neonatal transmission, one cannot recommend the routine administration of ISG to infants of HCV-positive mothers.

The data suggest that the method of delivery—vaginal delivery or cesarean section—has no significant effect on the rate of neonatal infection. Given the low rate of HCV transmission, other potential confounding variables (such as viral load), and the numbers required to definitively answer this question, it is

Table 10-4 Hepatitis C Virus Transmission Related to HIV Status

Study	HIV and HCV Infection	HCV Infection Only
Granovsky et al. (78)	4/83	2/40
Zucotti et al. (81)	5/13	2/8
Tovo et al. (80)	3/80	25/165
Zanetti et al. (79)	8/22	0/94
Total	20/198	29/307

unlikely that we will ever be able to ascribe a particular risk to a particular delivery route.

Neonatally Acquired Hepatitis C Virus Infection

There are no accepted guidelines on the management of infants born to HCV-positive mothers. Fifty percent of neonates born to infectious mothers have passively acquired HCV antibodies, and these often persist for 6 to 7 months or even 1 year. If infants are tested in this period and found to be antibody positive, most will subsequently be negative on PCR, but the studies themselves will generate unnecessary anxiety in the parents. Even some PCR-positive infants will clear HCV in the first year of life. In addition, if the infant does have a true infection, the infection seldom has clinical significance at this stage. Treatment with interferon and ribavirin would certainly not be considered in an infant, especially one with mild disease. Given our current therapies and the evidence for lack of household transmission, early diagnosis has little advantage.

Early information, although limited, indicates that the severity of hepatitis C in infants and children seems mild, and some infants and children have normal aminotransferase levels despite RNA positivity. Longer-term prospective trials are needed to assess the clinical significance of perinatally acquired HCV infection. If our therapy for HCV dramatically improves, recommendations for early diagnosis and monitoring may change significantly.

A recent study by Badizadegan and co-workers (85) has shown more significant liver damage in children who had biopsy, on average, 6.8 years after HCV infection. In two thirds of patients with cirrhosis, the infection was vertically acquired; this indicates that perinatally acquired HCV infection is not always benign. We eagerly await the results of ongoing large, prospective trials on the natural history of neonatally acquired HCV infection.

Hepatitis C Virus in the Delivery Room

Without a doubt, obstetricians and case-room staff are exposed to large quantities of blood and body fluids and therefore are frequently exposed to HCV. Infection with HCV is uncommon in hospital workers (86, 87), probably because HCV, when present, circulates at low levels in the blood and blood-to-blood contact is required for efficient transmission. The available data suggest that the risk for acquiring HCV from patients is low; the possible exceptions are persons who regularly perform invasive procedures on persons at high risk for HCV infection.

Studies of HCV transmission resulting from needlestick injuries have reported transmission rates of 0% to 10.3% (88–90). Overall, the risk for transmission of HCV by such occupational exposure seems to be low and, if infection occurs, the resulting disease seems to be relatively benign. It is hoped that an effective vaccine will become available to reduce risk even further.

Hepatitis D

Hepatitis delta virus (HDV, or hepatitis D), an incomplete RNA virus, requires HBsAg for packaging and entry into hepatocytes and is therefore found only in HBsAg-positive persons. In North America, HDV is predominantly found in intravenous drug users (91), but in some parts of Europe (such as southern Italy) HDV infection is endemic and the mode of HDV transmission is unclear (92). In all studies, HDV infection is rare in children; this constitutes circumstantial evidence that perinatal transmission of HDV is uncommon. Infection with HDV is also rare in pregnant women in most parts of the world that have been tested.

There are two scenarios of HDV infection. The virus can be acquired simultaneously with HBV (co-infection), in which case the ultimate outcome of the HDV infection is determined by response to the HBV infection. If HBV is cleared normally, as it is in 90% of adults, HBsAg is also cleared and HDV cannot persist. The more usual scenario is the superinfection of an already HBsAg-positive person with HDV, which is usually acquired through intravenous drug use. Chronic HDV infection results in liver disease that is more severe than that caused by HBV alone (93). An HDV infection is diagnosed by detection of anti-HDV antibody.

No specific data are available on acute HDV and pregnancy. However, in some geographic regions where HDV is endemic, no increased severity with pregnancy has been documented. Vertical transmission of HDV is uncommon (94).

As noted above, HDV requires HBsAg to persist. Therefore, if one prevents HBV infection, one also prevents HDV infection. If perinatal HBV vaccination strategies were to be introduced globally, both HDV and HBV infection could be almost eradicated.

Hepatitis E

The hepatitis E virus (HEV) is responsible for the vast majority of cases of what was formerly called *enterically transmitted non-A, non-B hepatitis* (95). This virus is spread by the fecal–oral route and by contaminated water supplies. It has not been described in North America except in a few travelers returning from places where HEV is endemic, including Nepal, Burma, India, and Ethiopia. Acute HEV infection is diagnosed by the presence of anti-HEV antibody (IgG and IgM) on an assay that is now routinely available in most centers.

Infection with HEV is unique in that it is associated with a very high mortality rate in pregnant women, especially if acquired in the third trimester (95, 96). In countries where HEV is endemic, it may be difficult to clinically differentiate between severe HEV infection in pregnancy and acute fatty liver of pregnancy (AFLP). The reason for this is unknown. Tsega and associates in Ethiopia (97) reported that 8 of 19 pregnant women with acute HEV infection, 0 of 10 men with acute HEV infection, and 0 of 7 nonpregnant women with acute HEV infection died. Infection with HEV is not only more severe in pregnant women but has a predilection for these women; HEV caused the hepatitis seen in 19 of 32 pregnant women (59%), 7 of 34 nonpregnant women (21%), and 7 of 18 (38%) of adult males. However, these data may be influenced by the fact that the severity of HEV infection is worse during pregnancy and increases the likelihood that patients will seek medical attention. Poor fetal outcomes have been reported. In the study by Tsega and associates, four premature deliveries, five in utero deaths, and one postpartum death were reported. These poor fetal outcomes may be related more to the severity of maternal illness than to a direct effect of HEV.

The hepatitis E virus has been reported to be transmitted to neonates, although the exact route of transmission is unknown. Of eight women infected with HEV in the third trimester, six had infants who were shown to be positive for HEV RNA in cord blood on PCR. Two of these infants died of hepatic failure (98). No therapy is available to interrupt this vertical transmission, although the search for an effective vaccine is ongoing.

Hepatitis G

Hepatitis G virus (HGV) is a newly described hepatitis virus that appears in the same patient populations and has some of the same risk factors for transmission as HCV. Transmission during blood transfusion is well documented, as is transmission resulting from intravenous drug use. However, unlike HCV, HGV has not been documented to cause any significant liver disease, even with chronic infection (99). However, rare cases of fulminant hepatic failure have been attributed to HGV infection.

The hepatitis G virus is efficiently transmitted from mother to infant. In one study (100), transmission of GBV-C to offspring took place in 21 of 34 infants (62%), resulting in minimal transaminitis. No infants developed jaundice or severe liver disease. Transmission of HCV in the same group occurred in only 5% of infants, indicating that GBV-C is more easily transmitted by this route. The importance, if any, of this finding is unknown. Current understanding is that HGV infection, even long-term HGV infection, does not cause significant liver disease. It has been referred to as "an infection looking for a disease."

Herpes Simplex Hepatitis

Hepatitis secondary to disseminated HSV infection is rare in immunocompetent persons. However, there are numerous case reports of fulminant hepatitis secondary to HSV infection in pregnant women, with a high mortality rate. Approximately half of cases of disseminated HSV infection reported in healthy persons have occurred in pregnant women, especially in the third trimester (101, 102). The vast majority of patients have a prodromal illness with fever, and most are initially misdiagnosed with a presumptive bacterial infection and are treated with antibiotics. Most but not all persons have a primary HSV infection with oropharyngeal or vulvar lesions. In some persons, however, these lesions are very subtle or appear after the hepatitis. In most reported cases, patients have markedly elevated aminotransferase levels (>2000 U/L) and severe coagulopathy but little if any elevation of bilirubin levels.

Liver biopsy is most helpful in making the diagnosis. Herpes simplex virus IgG and IgM antibodies can be measured in the serum, but this often takes too long to be clinically helpful. Most severe infections have been attributed to HSV II.

The current therapy for disseminated HSV infection is acyclovir. Only a few reports on acyclovir therapy in pregnant women are available, but these are very encouraging. Of 14 pregnant women with HSV hepatitis whose case reports were published before 1991, 6 died. Four of 5 patients treated with acyclovir and 2 of 3 patients treated with vidarabine survived. Acyclovir therapy of the infant also seems to aid in preventing transmission to the neonate. Because treatment can be successful, it is essential to be aware of the association between fulminant herpes hepatitis and pregnancy.

REFERENCES

1. **Friedlaender P, Osler M.** Icterus and pregnancy. Am J Obstet Gynecol. 1967;97:894-900.
2. **Szmuness W, Deinstag JL, Purcell RH, et al.** Distribution of antibody to hepatitis A in urban adult populations. N Engl J Med. 1976;295:755-9.
3. **Willner IR, Uhl MD, Howard SC, et al.** Serious hepatitis A: an analysis of patients hospitalized during an urban epidemic in the United States. Ann Intern Med. 1998;128:111-4.

4. **Yotsuyangi H, Iino S, Koike K, et al.** Duration of viraemia in human hepatitis A viral infection as determined by polymerase chain reaction. J Med Virol. 1993;40:35-8.

5. **McDonald GSA, Courtney MG, Shatrock AG, et al.** Prolonged IgM antibodies and histopathological evidence of chronicity in hepatitis A. Liver. 1989;9:223-8.

6. **Horng YC, Chang MH, Lee CY, et al.** Safety and immunogenicity of hepatitis A vaccine in healthy children. Pediatr Infect Dis J. 1993;12:359-62.

7. **Sjogren MH.** The success of hepatitis A vaccine. Gastroenterology. 1993;104:1214-6.

8. **Zhang RH, Zeng JS, Zhang HZ.** Survey of 34 pregnant women with hepatitis A and their neonates. Chin Med J Peking. 1990;103:552-5.

9. **Leikin E, Lysikewicz A, Garry D, Tejani N.** Intrauterine transmission of hepatitis A virus. Obstet Gynecol. 1996;88:690-1.

10. **Watson JC, Fleming DW, Borella AJ, et al.** Vertical transmission of hepatitis A resulting in an outbreak in a neonatal intensive care unit. J Infect Dis. 1993;167:567-71.

11. **Azimi PH, Roberto RR, Guralnik J, et al.** Transfusion acquired hepatitis A in a premature infant with secondary spread in an intensive care nursery. Am J Dis Child. 1986;140:23-7.

12. **Rosenblum LS, Villarino ME, Nainan OV, et al.** Hepatitis A outbreak in a neonatal intensive care unit: risk factors for transmission and evidence of prolonged viral excretion among preterm infants. J Infect Dis. 1991;164:476-82.

13. **Krugman S, Ward R, Giles JP, et al.** Infectious hepatitis: studies on the effect of gamma globulin on the incidence of unapparent infection. JAMA. 1960;174:823-7.

14. **Beasley RP, Hwang LY, Lin CC, et al.** Hepatocellular carcinoma and hepatitis B virus: a prospective study of 22,707 men in Taiwan. Lancet. 1981;1:1129-33.

15. **McMahon BJ, Alward WLM, Hall DB, et al.** Acute hepatitis B virus infection: relation of age to the clinical expression of disease and subsequent development of the carrier state. J Infect Dis. 1985;151:599-603.

16. **Stevens CE, Neurath RA, Beasley RP, et al.** HBeAg and anti-HBe detection by radioimmunoassay: correlation with vertical transmission of hepatitis B virus in Taiwan. J Med Virol. 1979;3:237-41.

17. **Lok ASF.** Natural history and control of perinatally acquired hepatitis B virus infection. Dig Dis. 1992;10:46-52.

18. **Beasley RP, Hwang LY, Lee GC, et al.** Prevention of perinatally transmitted hepatitis B virus infection with hepatitis B immune globulin and hepatitis B vaccine. Lancet. 1983;2:1099-102.

19. **Stevens CE, Taylor PE, Tong MJ, et al.** Yeast-recombinant hepatitis B vaccine: efficacy with hepatitis B immune globulin in the prevention of perinatal hepatitis B virus transmission. JAMA. 1987;257:2612-6.

20. **Hadler SC, Margolis HS.** Hepatitis B immunization. Curr Clin Top Infect Dis. 1992;12:282-308.

21. **Brechot C.** Polymerase chain reaction for the diagnosis of viral hepatitis B and C. Gut. 1993;34:S39-44.

22. **Kaneko S, Miller RH, Di Bisceglie AM, et al.** Detection of hepatitis B virus DNA in serum by polymerase chain reaction. Gastroenterology. 1990;99:799-804.

23. **Shikata T, Karasawa T, Abe K, et al.** Hepatitis B e antigen and infectivity of hepatitis B virus. J Infect Dis. 1977;136:571-6.

24. **Realdi G, Alberti A, Rugge M, et al.** Seroconversion from hepatitis B e antigen to anti-HBe in chronic hepatitis B virus infection. Gastroenterology. 1980;79:195-9.

25. **Carman WF, Hadziyannis S, McGarvey MJ, et al.** Mutation preventing formation of hepatitis B e antigen in patients with chronic hepatitis B infection. Lancet. 1989;2: 588-91.

26. **Margolis HS, Alter MJ, Hadler SC.** Hepatitis B: evolving epidemiology and implications for control. Semin Liver Dis. 1991;11:84-92.

27. **Hoofnagle JH, Di Bisceglie AM.** Serologic diagnosis of acute and chronic viral hepatitis. Semin Liver Dis. 1991;11:73-83.

28. **Woolf IL, El-Sheikh N, Cullens H, et al.** Enhanced HBsAb production in pathogenesis of fulminant viral hepatitis type B. BMJ. 1976;2:669-71.

29. **Thomas HC, Scully LJ.** Antiviral therapy in hepatitis B infection. Br Med Bull. 1985;41:374-80.

30. **Tong MJ, Thursby M, Rakela J, et al.** Studies on the maternal-infant transmission of the viruses which cause acute hepatitis. Gastroenterology. 1981;80:999-1004.

31. **Michalak TI, Pasquinelli C, Guilhot S, et al.** Hepatitis B virus persistence after recovery from acute hepatitis. J Clin Invest. 1994;93:230-9.

32. **Beasley RP, Trepo C, Stevens CE, et al.** The e antigen and vertical transmission of hepatitis B surface antigen. Am J Epidemiol. 1977;105:94-9.

33. **Badur S, Lazizi Y, Ugurlu M, et al.** Transplacental passage of hepatitis B virus DNA from hepatitis B e antigen negative mothers and delayed immune response in newborns. J Infect Dis. 1994;169:704-6.

34. **Ip HMH, Lelie PN, Wong VCW, et al.** Prevention of hepatitis B virus carrier state in infants according to maternal serum levels of HBV DNA. Lancet. 1989;1:406-10.

35. **Milich DR, Jones JE, Hughes JL, et al.** Is a function of the secreted hepatitis B e antigen to induce immunologic tolerance in utero? PNAS USA. 1990;87:6599-603.

36. **Lo KJ, Lee SD, Tsai YT, et al.** Long-term immunogenicity and efficacy of hepatitis B vaccine in infants born to HBeAg positive HBsAg-carrier mothers. Hepatology. 1988;8: 1647-50.

37. **Delage G, Remy-Prince S, Montplaisir S.** Combined active-passive immunization against the hepatitis B virus: five-year follow-up of children born to hepatitis B surface antigen-positive mothers. Pediatr Infect Dis J. 1993;12:126-30.

38. **Sehgal A, Gupta I, Sehgal R, et al.** Hepatitis B vaccine alone or in combination with anti-HBs immunoglobulin in the perinatal prophylaxis of babies born to HBsAg carrier mothers. Acta Virol. 1992;36:359-66.

39. **Belloni C, Chirico G, Pistorio A, et al.** Immunogenicity of hepatitis B vaccine in term and preterm infants. Acta Paediatr. 1998;87:336-8.

40. **Poovarawan Y, Sampavat S, Pongpunlert W, et al.** Comparison of a recombinant DNA hepatitis B vaccine alone or in combination with hepatitis B immune globulin for the prevention of perinatal acquisition of hepatitis B carriage. Vaccine. 1990;8:S56-9.

41. **Yao FB, Li XX, Du YX, Ye SL.** Combined intramuscular-intradermal protocol of universal neonate hepatitis B vaccination irrespective of mother's status of HBsAg. Vaccine. 1998;16:586-9.

42. **Ruff TA, Gertie DM, Otto BF, et al.** Lombok Hepatitis B Model Immunization Project: toward universal infant hepatitis B immunization in Indonesia. J Infect Dis. 1995;17: 290-6.

43. **American Academy of Pediatrics, Committee on Infectious Diseases.** Universal hepatitis B immunization. Pediatrics. 1992;89:795-800.

44. **Woodruff BA, Stevenson J, Yusuf H, et al.** Progress toward integrating hepatitis B vaccine into routine infant immunization schedules in the United States, 1991 through 1994. Connecticut Hepatitis B Project Group. Pediatrics. 1996;97:798-803.

45. **Giammanco G, Moiraghi A, Zotti C, et al.** Safety and immunogenicity of a combined diptheria-tetanus-acellular pertussis-hepatitis B vaccine administered according to two different primary vaccination schedules. Multicenter Working Group. Vaccine. 1998;16:722-6.

46. **Bloom BS, Hillman AL, Fendrick AM, et al.** A reappraisal of hepatitis B virus vaccination strategies using cost-effectiveness analysis. Ann Intern Med. 1993;118:298-306.

47. **Yusuf HR, Mahoney FJ, Shapiro CN, Mast EE, Polish L.** Hospital-based evaluation of programs to prevent perinatal hepatitis B virus transmission. Arch Pediatr Adolesc Med. 1996;150:593-7.

48. **Rosenthal P, Wood DL, Greenspoon JS, Pereyra M.** Hepatitis B virus serology in pregnant women: transmittal of results from obstetricians to pediatricians in California. Pediatr Infect Dis J. 1995;14:927-31.

49. **Wood DL, Rosenthal P, Scarlata D.** California pediatricians' knowledge of and response to recommendations for universal infant hepatitis B immunization. Arch Pediatr Adolesc Med. 1995;149:769-73.

50. **Hsu HY, Chang MH, Ni YH, et al.** Surface gene mutants of hepatitis B virus in infants who develop acute or chronic infections despite immunoprophylaxis. Hepatology. 1997;26:786-91.

51. **Lin HH, Hsu HY, Chang MH, et al.** Hepatitis B virus in the colostra of HBeAg-positive carrier mothers. J Pediatr Gastroenterol Nutr. 1993;17:207-10.

52. **Choo QL, Kuo G, Weiner AJ, et al.** Isolation of a cDNA clone from a blood-borne non-A, non-B viral hepatitis genome. Science. 1989;244:359-62.

53. **Alter HJ, Purcell RH, Shih JW, et al.** Detection of antibody to hepatitis C virus in prospectively followed transfusion recipients with acute and chronic non-A, non-B hepatitis. N Engl J Med. 1989;32:1494-500.

54. **Farci P, Alter HJ, Wong D, et al.** A long-term study of hepatitis C virus replication in non-A, non-B hepatitis. N Engl J Med. 1991;325:98-104.

55. **Di Bisceglie AM, Goodman ZD, Ishak KG, et al.** Long-term clinical and histopathological follow-up of chronic post-transfusion hepatitis. Hepatology. 1991;14:969-74.

56. **Scully LJ, Mitchell S, Gill P.** Clinical and epidemiologic characteristics of hepatitis C in a gastroenterology/hepatology practice in Ottawa. Can Med Assoc J. 1993;148:1173-7.

57. **Alter MJ, Hadler SC, Judson FN, et al.** Risk factors for acute non-A, non-B hepatitis in the United States and association with hepatitis C infection. JAMA. 1990;264:2231-5.

58. **McHutchison JG, Person JL, Govindarajan S, et al.** Improved detection of hepatitis C antibodies in high-risk populations. Hepatology. 1992;15:19-25.

59. **Dawson GJ, Leseniewski RR, Stewart KM, et al.** Detection of antibodies to hepatitis C in US blood donors. J Clin Microbiol. 1991;29:551-6.

60. **Stevens CE, Taylor PE, Pindych J, et al.** Epidemiology of hepatitis C virus: a preliminary study in volunteer blood donors. JAMA. 1990:49-53.

61. **Lee WM.** The silent epidemic of hepatitis C. Gastroenterology. 1993;104:661-2.

62. **Mimms L, Vallari D, Ducharme L, et al.** Specificity of anti-HCV ELISA assessed by reactivity to the three immunodominant HCV regions. Lancet. 1990;336:1590-1.

63. van der Poel CL, Cuypers HTM, Reesink HW, et al. Confirmation of hepatitis C virus infection by new four antigen recombinant immunoblot assay. Lancet. 1991;337:317-9.

64. Esteban JI, Lopez-Talavera JC, Genesca J, et al. High rate of infectivity and liver disease in blood donors with antibodies to hepatitis C virus. Ann Intern Med. 1991; 115:443-9.

65. Alter HJ, Tegtmeier GE, Jett BW, et al. The use of a recombinant immunoblot assay in the interpretation of anti-hepatitis C virus reactivity among prospectively followed patients, implicated donors and random donors. Transfusion. 1991;31:771-6.

66. Barrera J, Prancis B, Ercilla G, et al. Improved detection of anti-HCV in post-transfusion hepatitis by a third generation ELISA. Vox Sang. 1995;68:15-8.

67. Zaaijer HL, Cuypers HTM, Reesink HW, et al. Reliability of polymerase chain reaction for detection of hepatitis C virus. Lancet. 1993;341:722-4.

68. Hunt CM, Carson KL, Sharara AI. Hepatitis C in pregnancy. Obstet Gynecol. 1997; 89:883-90.

69. Zuckerman MA, Aitken C, Whitby K, et al. Acute hepatitis C viral infection during pregnancy: failure of mother to infant transmission. J Med Virol. 1997;52:161-3.

70. Ohto H, Terazawa S, Sasaki N, et al. Transmission of hepatitis C virus from mothers to infants. N Engl J Med. 1994;330:744-50.

71. Silverman NS, Jenkin BK, Wu C, et al. Hepatitis C virus in pregnancy: seroprevalence and risk factors for infection. Am J Obstet Gynecol. 1993;169:583-7.

72. Floreani A, Paternoster D, Zappala F, et al. Hepatitis C virus infection in pregnancy. Br J Obstet Gynaecol. 1996;103:325-9.

73. Wejstal R, Widell A, Mansson AS, et al. Mother-to-infant transmission of hepatitis C virus. Ann Intern Med. 1992;117:887-90.

74. Lomas R. Hepatitis C: you cannot blame it on your mother. AJG. 1993;88:1972-3.

75. Tanzi M, Bellelli E, Benaglia G, et al. The prevalence of HCV infection in a cohort of pregnant women, the related risk factors and possibility of vertical transmission. Eur J Epidemiol. 1997;13:517-21.

76. Ni YH, Lin HH, Chen PJ, et al. Temporal profile of hepatitis C virus antibody and genome in infants born to mothers infected with hepatitis C virus but without human immunodeficiency coinfection. J Hepatol. 1994;20:641-5.

77. Thaler MM, Park CK, Landers DV, et al. Vertical transmission of hepatitis C virus. Lancet. 1991;338:17-8.

78. Granovsky MO, Minkoff HL, Tess BH, et al. Hepatitis C infection in the mothers and infants cohort study. Pediatrics. 1998;102:355-9.

79. Zanetti AR, Tanzi E, Paccagnini S, et al. Mother-to-infant transmission of hepatitis C virus. Lancet. 1995;345:289-91.

80. Tovo PA, Palomba E, Ferraris G, et al. Increased risk of maternal-infant hepatitis C virus transmission for women coinfected with human immunodeficiency virus type 1. Italian Study Group for HCV Infection in Children. Clin Infect Dis. 1997;25:1121-4.

81. Zucotti GV, Ribero ML, Giovannini M, et al. Effect of hepatitis C genotype on mother-to-infant transmission of virus. J Pediatr. 1995;127:278-80.

82. Novati R, Thiers V, Monforte AD, et al. Mother-to-infant transmission of hepatitis C virus detected by nested polymerase chain reaction. J Infect Dis. 1992;165:720-3.

83. Ogesawara S, Kage M, Kosai KI, et al. Hepatitis C virus RNA in saliva and breastmilk of hepatitis C carrier mothers. Lancet. 1993;341:561.

84. NIH Consensus Development Conference on Management of Hepatitis C; 1997.

85. **Badizadegan K, Jones MM, Ott MJ, et al.** Histopathology of the liver in children with chronic hepatitis C viral infection. Hepatology. 1998;28:1416-23.

86. **Hofmann H, Kunz C.** Low risk of health care workers for infection with hepatitis C virus. Infection. 1990;18:286-8.

87. **Thomas DL, Factor SH, Kelen GD, et al.** Viral hepatitis in health care personnel at the Johns Hopkins Hospital: the seroprevalence of and risk factors for hepatitis B virus and hepatitis C virus infection. Arch Intern Med. 1993;153:1705-12.

88. **Mitsui T, Iwanok K, Masuko K, et al.** Hepatitis C virus infection in medical personnel after needle stick accident. Hepatology. 1992;16:1109-14.

89. **Kiyosawa K, Sodeyama T, Tanak E, et al.** Hepatitis C in hospital employees with needle stick injuries. Ann Intern Med. 1991;115:367-9.

90. **Hernandez ME, Bruguera M, Puyuelo T, et al.** Risk of needle stick injuries in the transmission of hepatitis C virus in hospital personnel. J Hepatol. 1992;16:56-8.

91. **DeCock KM, Govindarajan S, Chin KP, et al.** Delta hepatitis in the Los Angeles area: a report of 126 cases. Ann Intern Med. 1986;105:108-14.

92. **Ponzetto A, Forzani B, Parravicini PP, et al.** Epidemiology of hepatitis delta virus infection. Eur J Epidemiol. 1986;1:257-63.

93. **Rizzetto M, Verme G, Recchia S, et al.** Chronic HBsAg positive hepatitis with intrahepatic expression of delta antigen: an active and progressive disease unresponsive to immunosuppressive treatment. Ann Intern Med. 1983;98:437-41.

94. **Zanetti RA, Tanzi E, Ferroni P, et al.** Vertical transmission of the HBV-associated delta agent. In: Viral Hepatitis and Delta Infection. New York: Alan R. Liss; 1983.

95. **Bradley DW, Andjaparadze A, Cooke H, et al.** Aetiological agent of enterically transmitted non-A, non-B hepatitis. J Gen Virol. 1988;68:731-8.

96. **Khuroo MS, Duermeyer SA, Zargar MA, et al.** Acute sporadic non-A, non-B hepatitis in India. Am J Epidemiol. 1983;118:360-4.

97. **Tsega E, Hansson BG, Krawczynski K, et al.** Acute sporadic viral hepatitis in Ethiopia: causes, risk factors and effects on pregnancy. Clin Infect Dis. 1992;14:961-5.

98. **Khuroo MS, Kamili S, Jameel S.** Vertical transmission of hepatitis E virus. Lancet. 1995;345:1025-6.

99. **Feucht HH, Zollner B, Polywka S, et al.** Distribution of hepatitis G viraemia and antibody response to recombinant proteins with special regard to risk factors in 709 patients. Hepatology. 1997;26:491-4.

100. **Zanetti AR, Tanzi E, Romano L, et al.** Multicenter trial on mother-to-infant transmission of GBV-C virus. The Lombardy Study Group on Vertical/Perinatal Hepatitis Viruses Transmission. J Med Virol. 1998;54:107-12.

101. **Klein NA, Mabie WC, Shaver DC, et al.** Herpes simplex virus hepatitis in pregnancy: two patients successfully treated with acyclovir. Gastroenterology. 1991;100:239-44.

102. **Mudido P, Marshall GS, Howell RS, et al.** Disseminated herpes simplex virus infection during pregnancy: a case report. J Reprod Med. 1993;38:964-8.

III. Gestational Liver Disease
Caroline A. Riely

Liver disease is never welcome, but it is particularly feared in the pregnant woman, and rightly so. It can have an ominous prognosis for both the mother and her unborn child. But pregnant women are, for the most part, young and healthy, and with timely diagnosis and management, pregnant patients with even the most serious liver disease should return to full health with no sequelae. The challenge is to recognize the disorder, often on clinical grounds alone. The aim of this section is to familiarize the practitioner with the clinical hallmarks and management of 1) the liver diseases unique to pregnancy, 2) the routine liver diseases that can be exacerbated or precipitated by pregnancy, and 3) the chronic liver diseases during which pregnancy can occur. The internist's valued partner in the management of these conditions is the obstetrician, often an expert in maternal–fetal medicine.

Liver Diseases Unique to Pregnancy

Liver diseases that occur only in pregnant women have no animal models, are of unclear pathogenesis, and are unfamiliar to the practitioner. They are diagrammed in Figure 10-1 with their usual trimester of onset and their primary clinical hallmark.

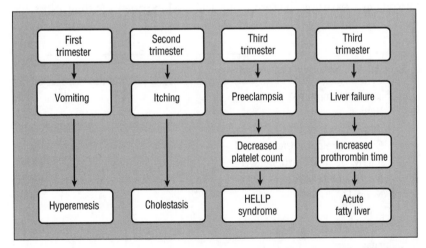

Figure 10-1 Liver diseases unique to pregnancy. This simplified schema presents the four liver diseases unique to pregnancy (*bottom line*), the signs or symptoms that should suggest each diagnosis (*middle lines*), and the trimester when each disorder has its onset (*top line*).

Cholestasis of Pregnancy

Cholestasis of pregnancy usually begins in the second trimester but can start in the third or, rarely, at the end of the first (Box 10-7). Its hallmark is pruritus (worse at night) of the palms and soles that may progress to an intolerable degree, causing the patient to beg for delivery or threaten suicide. Many affected patients are referred first to a dermatologist. Laboratory evaluation shows elevations in the results of "hepatic" as opposed to "cholestatic" tests, with aspartate aminotransferase (AST) and alanine aminotransferase (ALT) levels that can reach 1000 U. The serum bilirubin level is elevated only in the most severe cases, but tests for bilirubin in urine may be positive more often. Levels of serum bile acids, which may be tested by using the cholyglycine level, are elevated. Of note, the gamma glutamyl transpeptidase (GGTP) level, which is elevated in most forms of cholestasis, is normal or close to normal (1). Steatorrhea occurs, but the prothrombin time is usually normal. Liver biopsy is rarely indicated. When liver biopsy is done, it shows bland cholestasis without inflammation (2).

The clinical course is usually progressive, with worsening pruritus that remits—along with the liver test abnormalities—shortly after delivery. Some women have a fluctuating course with episodic alleviation of pruritus and improvement in liver test results before delivery (3). The fetus is at risk, and studies show small but significant increases in rates of stillbirth and prematurity (4).

Management starts with recognition of the condition. This is done most directly by measuring the serum bile acid level in patients with pruritus and

---

Box 10-7 Cholestasis of Pregnancy

Signs and symptoms
  Itching
Laboratory test results
  Elevated aminotransferase level
  Rarely, elevated bilirubin level
  Increased bile acids
  Normal GGTP level
Concerns
  Increased fetal wastage
Management
  Ursodeoxycholic acid (possibly)
  Delivery

abnormal aminotransferase levels. The risk for unappreciated steatorrhea is real, and patients should receive parenteral vitamin K supplementation before delivery. In moderately severe cases, the risk for intrauterine death may prompt consideration of early delivery, by 38 weeks in moderate cases and after 36 weeks in severe cases. Unfortunately, in one small study (4), fetal monitoring did not successfully predict intrauterine deaths.

Alleviating pruritus before delivery is not easy. Antipruritic agents, such as hydroxyzine, may provide some relief. The bile acid–binding resin cholestyramine has been used, but it is not very effective and it aggravates steatorrhea and fat malabsorption. Ursodeoxycholic acid alleviates the liver test abnormalities and the pruritus in primary biliary cirrhosis, another cholestatic disorder, and has been shown to be useful in cholestasis of pregnancy in small studies (5). No reports of ill effects on the fetus are available, but until use of the bile acid in pregnancy is more thoroughly studied, it should be restricted to severe cases.

The pathogenesis of cholestasis of pregnancy remains elusive. Progestational hormones, either endogenous or exogenously administered, may play a role (1, 5). The concentration of the condition in certain ethnic groups, especially in Chile and Scandinavia, suggests genetic or environmental contributions. A rare cholestatic syndrome of children, a form of progressive intrahepatic cholestasis, shares with cholestasis of pregnancy the unusual characteristic of a normal GGTP level in the face of profound cholestasis. The mother of an affected child with a newly described genetic defect leading to progressive intrahepatic cholestasis was reported to have cholestasis of pregnancy; this suggests that at least some affected women may be heterozygous for a defect in bile formation (6). Until we better understand the pathogenesis of cholestasis in pregnancy, management of this condition will primarily address symptoms.

Preeclamptic Liver Disease

It has long been known that women dying of preeclampsia have a unique liver lesion: hemorrhage and fibrin deposition most prominent in the zone immediately adjacent to the portal triads. But it was only in the early 1980s that the HELLP syndrome was defined (7). Patients with preeclampsia or eclampsia who have *hemolysis*, usually modest in extent with burr cells and schistocytes seen on peripheral smear; *elevated liver* enzyme levels, primarily with respect to the aminotransferases; and *low platelet* counts (<100 000/cm) are defined as having the HELLP syndrome (Box 10-8). When sought, the syndrome is found in up to 20% of patients with severe preeclampsia (8).

Affected patients may present with severe abdominal pain that is midepigastric or in the right upper quadrant and chest. They may have signs of

---

Box 10-8 HELLP Syndrome

Signs and symptoms
  Abdominal pain
  Preeclampsia
Laboratory tests
  Hemolysis-burr cells and schistocytes
  Platelet count <100,000
  Elevated AST level (>70, usually <1000, mean 250 U)
Concerns
  Prematurity
  Progression to hepatic rupture
Management
  Delivery
  Treatment of preeclampsia

---

preeclampsia, such as headache and excessive thirst. Or patients may be asymptomatic and, on routine laboratory screening of patients with preeclampsia, found to be thrombocytopenic and to have elevated aminotransferase levels. As many as 30% of affected patients present, or are diagnosed, after delivery (8). Diagnosis is made on clinical grounds; liver biopsy shows the typical findings of preeclampsia but usually is not necessary for the diagnosis (9).

As is true of patients with other complications of preeclampsia, patients with the HELLP syndrome usually have a progressive course, with worsening until delivery. In patients diagnosed after delivery, steady improvement is to be anticipated. Some patients stabilize before delivery and can be tided over until more fetal maturity is gained. Rare patients progress to hepatic hematoma, rupture, or infarction.

Management is largely supportive and primarily consists of prompt delivery. Temporizing may be successful in some patients (10). The thrombocytopenia may suggest thrombotic thrombocytopenia purpura (TTP), but patients with the HELLP syndrome are not febrile as a rule and patients with TTP do not have liver disease. As in TTP, plasmapheresis has been advocated (11). The HELLP syndrome may recur in subsequent pregnancies (12). The risk to the fetus is that of prematurity; liver disease or thrombocytopenia is not found in babies born to women with the HELLP syndrome (13).

Hepatic hematoma that may lead to rupture of the liver is rare; it occurs in women with preeclampsia and is presumably related to underlying HELLP syndrome (Table 10-5). Affected women tend to be older and multigravid.

Table 10-5 Comparison of HELLP Syndrome, Rupture, and Infarction in Preeclampsia

Variable	HELLP Syndrome	Rupture	Infarction
Signs and symptoms	None, abdominal pain	Abdominal swelling, shock	Fever, pain
Laboratory value	Decreased platelet count	Anemia	Anemia, very high AST level
Associations	Common	Rare Multigravida	Rare Abdominal CT scan

They present with abdominal pain and, if rupture has occurred, with abdominal distention and shock. Magnetic resonance imaging and computed tomography are useful in assessing the nature and extent of injury (14). Management is surgical and best done by those with expertise in trauma. At surgery, the hematoma below the Glisson capsule around the liver is found to have lifted the capsule up, leaving the underlying liver bleeding from multiple tears. Occasionally, patients have been managed with liver transplantation (15, 16). Like the HELLP syndrome, hepatic hematoma has been reported to recur in subsequent pregnancies (17).

Occasionally, patients with preeclampsia have intrahepatic hemorrhage or infarction. Such patients have abdominal pain and fever and may have a decreased hematocrit (18). Imaging shows geographic infarctions within the liver. Biopsy shows necrosis, with periportal hemorrhage and leukocyte infiltration in the periphery of the lesions. The aminotransferase levels may be very high, greater than 4000 U. Despite clinical and computed tomographic findings, patients have resolution of the condition without specific therapy. In some of these patients, the condition may be related to thrombosis of the hepatic vein draining the affected area (19, 20).

The pathogenesis of the HELLP syndrome remains, like the pathogenesis of preeclampsia itself, elusive. Hepatic hematoma and infarction presumably result when the periportal hemorrhage coalesces just under the surface of the liver or deep in the parenchyma.

Acute Fatty Liver of Pregnancy

Acute fatty liver of pregnancy is a form of hepatic failure unique to pregnancy. This rare but feared condition has been an enigma, but recent work suggests a fascinating explanation for at least some cases of AFLP.

Patients with AFLP present in the third trimester with symptoms and signs that vary widely (Box 10-9) (21, 22). Many are clinically ill, with

---

Box 10-9 Acute Fatty Liver of Pregnancy

Signs and symptoms
 Nausea, vomiting, lethargy, jaundice, or none
Laboratory test results
 Elevated aminotransferases level but <1000 U
 Increased prothrombin time
 Decreased fibrinogen level
Concerns
 Potentially lethal to both mother and fetus (DNA testing of family indicated)
Management
 Prompt delivery
 Maximal support

---

malaise, nausea, vomiting, and jaundice. In severe cases, there may be worsening mental status with hyperammonemia, hypoglycemia, and coagulopathy with frank bleeding. Many affected patients have preeclampsia, although with hepatic failure, blood pressure is low because of a marked decrease in systemic vascular resistance. The clinical hallmark is coagulopathy with a prolonged prothrombin time and a low fibrinogen level, which is especially striking because fibrinogen levels are usually high during pregnancy. There are probably patients with subclinical AFLP, and reports of patients without jaundice exist (21). Aminotransferase levels are elevated but are usually less than 1000 U. Patients with AFLP and severe hepatic failure have disseminated intravascular coagulation with thrombocytopenia and may meet the diagnostic criteria for the HELLP syndrome. However, most investigators believe that the HELLP syndrome and AFLP are distinct both clinically and pathologically. Like the HELLP syndrome, AFLP can present in the postpartum period. Liver biopsy specimens from patients with AFLP show microvesicular fatty infiltration that is most prominent in the central region. Fat may be seen in the biopsy specimens of patients with the HELLP syndrome, but it is not microvesicular and is not restricted to the centrilobular areas (9).

The course of AFLP may be marked by descent into coma and death. With early diagnosis and prompt treatment (that is, delivery), death should be the exception, not the rule. Improvement begins with delivery and is reflected in improvements in the prothrombin time. But with severe injury, the patient needs maximum support as the liver recovers and may have a variety of complications, including acute respiratory failure, renal failure, gastrointestinal hemorrhage, or acute pancreatitis. The bilirubin level often increases even as the patient begins to improve clinically. The course may be complicated by nephrogenic diabetes insipidus (23). Fetal demise is common. Surviving patients return to full health with no hepatic sequelae. Many well-documented patients have had recurrent AFLP in subsequent pregnancies, but most patients have uncomplicated gestations after an affected one (24, 25). Liver transplantation has been done for patients with AFLP, but prompt recognition of AFLP should make transplantation unnecessary (26).

The pathogenesis of AFLP has been an enigma. The microvesicular fat seen in biopsy specimens is similar to that seen in the Reye syndrome and in Jamaican vomiting sickness, disorders known to result from poisoning of mitochondrial function. Recent reports show that at least some women with AFLP are heterozygous carriers for a defect in long-chain 3-hydroxyl-acyl CoA dehydrogenase (LCHAD), one of the enzymes governing intramitochondrial beta oxidation of fatty acids (27). Such women are asymptomatic except when they are pregnant with homozygous, affected infants who may be well but cause AFLP during gestation. The gene defects that result in LCHAD deficiency are known, and DNA testing for them is available (28). Affected women, their partners, and their baby can be tested. This is particularly important for the infant because LCHAD deficiency can result in a Reye-like syndrome with death in nonketotic hypoglycemia after stress (29) and for the mother should she choose to have subsequent pregnancies. The possible role that preeclampsia (which is seen in 50% or more of patients with AFLP) may play in pathogenesis is unclear. Preeclampsia may precipitate AFLP in LCHAD-deficient women or other, as yet unsuspected pathogenic mechanisms may exist.

Liver Diseases Exacerbated by Pregnancy

For the most part, common liver diseases are no worse when they occur in women who happen to be pregnant than when they occur in the non-pregnant population. Good examples are hepatitis B or hepatitis C. Some diseases, however, are worse when they occur during pregnancy or can occur in anyone but are precipitated by the normal physiologic changes of pregnancy.

Hepatitis E and Herpes Simplex Hepatitis

Infection with HEV or HSV is more prone to follow a fulminant course in the pregnant woman (particularly in the third trimester) than in the nonpregnant patient (Box 10-10). Thus, something about pregnancy—presumably some partial immunodeficiency—renders pregnant women prey to HEV and HSV, both of which are otherwise usually benign.

Box 10-10 Hepatitis E and Herpes Simplex Hepatitis

Signs and symptoms
  Acute hepatic failure (anicteric)
Laboratory test results
  Positive results on serologic testing
  Increased prothrombin time
  Very high aminotransferase level
Concerns
  Transmission to infant
Management
  Acyclovir for herpes simplex hepatitis

Infection with HEV (an RNA virus), like infection with HAV, is spread by the fecal–oral route and occurs in epidemics associated with contaminated water supplies, typically during natural disasters such as floods. Luckily, it has not occurred in the United States, with one possible exception. It is very common in densely populated parts of the developing world, such as Africa, India, and Mexico. In this setting, up to 20% of women who develop hepatitis E in the third trimester die in fulminant failure (30). The hepatitis E virus can spread to the fetus in utero, resulting in symptomatic hepatitis in the newborn (31). The physician should bear this risk in mind when counseling pregnant patients about international travel.

During primary infection with HSV, there is systemic spread and hepatitis may occur. This hepatitis is usually mild and subclinical, although both Epstein-Barr virus and cytomegalovirus can cause clinically significant hepatitis in immunosuppressed patients, such as liver transplant recipients. There are many reports of HSV hepatitis in immunosuppressed patients, but this hepatitis also occurs in otherwise healthy women who are pregnant. And, like hepatitis E, HSV hepatitis is more likely to be a clinical problem, associated with fulminant hepatitis, during the third trimester of pregnancy (32). Affected patients have very high aminotransferase levels and prolongation of the prothrombin time, but they are usually anicteric and have a bilirubin level of 3 mg/dL or less. Encephalopathy may occur as a result of either liver failure or encephalitis. A vesicular rash helps suggest the correct diagnosis but may be subtle, limited to the perineum or even to the uterine cervix. Thus, it may be difficult to distinguish HSV hepatitis from AFLP. Herpes simplex virus serologic tests are helpful but are usually not available on an emergent basis. The liver biopsy specimen is diagnostic, showing punched-out areas with typical inclusion bodies, but biopsy is not usually done. Patients respond promptly to acyclovir, and delivery is not necessary. Care should be taken with the infant at delivery, although acyclovir given to the mother should also treat the fetus.

Budd-Chiari Syndrome

Spontaneous thrombi of the major hepatic veins returning the splanchnic flow to the heart is catastrophic and occurs more frequently in late pregnancy or the immediate postpartum period. Although pregnancy represents a hypercoagulable state (33), many patients who develop the Budd-Chiari syndrome with pregnancy have a second risk factor for thrombosis, such as deficiency of protein C or S or the presence of an anticardiolipin antibody (34). Treatment is similar to that of the Budd-Chiari syndrome outside of pregnancy and includes systemic anticoagulation and sometimes liver transplantation (35).

Malignancy

Although rare, metastases to the liver may be present in pregnancy, and the modest immunosuppression of pregnancy may promote tumor growth. Possible primary sites include the colon, pancreas, and breast (36).

Pregnancy in Patients with Chronic Liver Disease

Chronic liver disease is associated with ovulatory failure, amenorrhea, and infertility. As a result, most women with cirrhosis and hepatic decompensation do not become pregnant. But pregnancy can occur in women with portal hypertension without cirrhosis or in women with some successfully treated chronic liver diseases. Such pregnancies present special problems for both patient and clinician (Table 10-6).

Portal Hypertension

Portal hypertension can occur in the absence of cirrhosis—for example, in patients with portal vein thrombosis, hepatoportal sclerosis, or congenital hepatic fibrosis. Such patients retain fertility but have severe portal hypertension that can be associated with the usual complications of variceal hemorrhage or ascites formation. Often, the patient is unaware of the underlying pathology. During gestation, with its associated increase in blood volume, the esophageal varices (37) or a splenic artery aneurysm (38) may rupture. Shunt surgery has been successful in this setting, as has sclerotherapy (39).

Table 10-6 Pregnancy in Patients with Chronic Liver Disease

Disorder	Concern or Management Approach
Portal hypertension	Possible variceal hemorrhage
	Increased risk for prematurity and stillbirth
Autoimmune liver disease:	
Autoimmune hepatitis	Continue immunosuppression
Primary biliary cirrhosis	Use of ursodeoxycholic acid
Wilson disease	Continue chelation
Hepatic masses (adenoma, focal nodular	Hemorrhage into mass with rupture
hyperplasia, hemoangina)	
Liver transplantation	Monitor immunosuppression
	Increased risk for prematurity and maternal
	complications

Women with inactive cirrhosis but significant portal hypertension (for example, from alcoholic liver disease or chronic hepatitis) can conceive. Deterioration of their liver disease may occur, or the gestation may be uneventful. Such patients may have an increased risk for premature birth or intrauterine death (37). Prospectively acquired data on pregnancy in chronic liver disease are not available.

When faced with a woman with chronic liver disease who wishes to become pregnant, what should the clinician advise? The patient should be told about her own increased risk for complications of liver disease, especially variceal hemorrhage, and of the increased risk for intrauterine death of her baby. Upper endoscopy may be advisable to determine whether varices are present and to identify their severity and extent. The women may benefit from beta-blocker therapy and should be monitored during pregnancy by an expert in maternal–fetal medicine.

Autoimmune Hepatitis and Primary Biliary Cirrhosis

Autoimmune diseases are more common in women than in men, and clinicians may encounter fertile women with autoimmune conditions of the liver, either autoimmune hepatitis or primary biliary cirrhosis. Autoimmune hepatitis improves dramatically with immunosuppression, usually with prednisone and azathioprine, and affected women regain fertility. Immunosuppression should be continued because relapse is associated with progression of the liver disease. The low doses of azathioprine used are not known to be teratogenic. Obstetric complications such as prematurity are increased in these patients, and referral to an expert in maternal–fetal medicine is warranted (40). The disease may flare with the return of normal immunity after the pregnancy ends, and patients should be followed with care for the first 4 to 6 months after delivery.

Patients with primary biliary cirrhosis may weather pregnancy with no ill effects. Ursodeoxycholic acid has been successfully used to treat this cholestatic condition, and in one small series, no detriment during pregnancy was seen with this treatment (41).

Wilson Disease

Like women with autoimmune hepatitis, women successfully treated for Wilson disease (with copper chelation and either penicillamine or trientine) can regain fertility and have successful pregnancies. Chelation should be continued throughout pregnancy because discontinuation can lead to sudden copper release, fulminant hepatic failure, and death (42).

Hepatic Masses

Women with known masses in the liver may seek advice about whether to become pregnant. Or, a mass may be discovered during pregnancy, often on ultrasonography. These masses are usually benign neoplasms, adenomas, focal nodular hyperplasias, hemangiomas, or cystic parasites such as echinocochleal cysts. Adenoma is a known complication of prolonged use of oral contraceptives, and hemorrhage into the adenoma, possibly with rupture into the abdomen, is a reported complication of pregnancy. Focal nodular hyperplasia and hemangiomas can also hemorrhage during pregnancy (43). There are few prospectively acquired data about the course of these tumors during gestation. If a tumor is large or symptomatic, pregnancy should be started with caution. If possible, the tumor should be removed before conception. But if the tumor is discovered during gestation and the patient is asymptomatic, watchful waiting, perhaps with serial ultrasonography to measure tumor size and look for hemorrhage into the mass, is advisable.

Liver Transplantation

More and more survivors of liver transplantation are becoming pregnant. These women must continue immunosuppressive therapy with heightened surveillance, and no teratogenicity has been reported in this setting (44). But maternal complications, primarily elevated blood pressure and preterm delivery, are common, and these women should be under the care of an expert in maternal–fetal medicine (45).

REFERENCES

1. **Bacq Y, Sapey T, Brechot M, et al.** Intrahepatic cholestasis of pregnancy: a French prospective study. Hepatology. 1997;26:358-64.
2. **Rolfes DB, Ishak KG.** Liver disease in pregnancy. Histopathology. 1986;10:555-70.
3. **Reyes H.** The enigma of intrahepatic cholestasis of pregnancy: lessons from Chile. Hepatology. 1982;2:87-96.
4. **Rioseco A, Ivankovic M, Manzur A, et al.** Intrahepatic cholestasis of pregnancy: a retrospective case control of perinatal outcome. Am J Obstet Gynecol. 1994;170:890-5.
5. **Meng L, Reyes H, Axelson M, et al.** Progesterone metabolites and bile acids in serum of patients with intrahepatic cholestasis of pregnancy: effect of ursodeoxycholic acid therapy. Hepatology. 1997;26:1573-9.
6. **Devree J, Jacquemin E, Sturm E, et al.** Mutations in the MDR3 gene cause progressive familial intrahepatic cholestasis. Proc Natl Acad Sci U S A. 1998;95:282-7.
7. **Weinstein L.** Syndrome of hemolysis, elevated liver enzymes, and low platelet count: a severe consequence of hypertension in pregnancy. Am J Obstet Gynecol. 1982;142:159-67.
8. **Sibai B, Ramadan M, Usta I, et al.** Maternal morbidity and mortality in 442 pregnancies with hemolysis, elevated liver enzymes, and low platelets (HELLP syndrome). Am J Obstet Gynecol. 1993;169:1000-6.
9. **Barton J, Riely C, Adamec T, et al.** Hepatic histopathologic condition does not correlate with laboratory abnormalities in HELLP syndrome (hemolysis, elevated liver enzymes, and low platelet count). Am J Obstet Gynecol. 1992;167:1538-43.
10. **Visser W, Wallenburg H.** Temporising management of severe pre-eclampsia with and without the HELLP syndrome. Br J Obstet Gynaecol. 1995;102:111-7.
11. **Martin J, Files J, Blake P, et al.** Postpartum plasma exchange for atypical preeclampsia-eclampsia as HELLP syndrome. Am J Obstet Gynecol. 1995;172:1107-25.
12. **Sullivan C, Magaan E, Perry KJ, et al.** The recurrence risk of the syndrome of hemolysis, elevated liver enzymes, and low platelets (HELLP) in subsequent gestations. Am J Obstet Gynecol. 1994;171:940-3.
13. **Harms K, Rath W, Herting E, Kuhn W.** Maternal hemolysis, elevated liver enzymes, and low platelet count, and neonatal outcome. Am J Perinatol. 1995;12:1-6.
14. **Barton J, Sibai B.** Hepatic imaging in HELLP syndrome (hemolysis, elevated liver enzymes, and low platelet count). Am J Obstet Gynecol. 1996;174:1820-5.
15. **Erhard J, Lange R, Niebel W, et al.** Acute liver necrosis in the HELLP syndrome: successful outcome after orthopedic liver transplantation. A case report. Transpl Int. 1993;6:179-81.
16. **Hunter S, Martin M, Benda J, Zlatnik F.** Liver transplant after massive spontaneous hepatic rupture in pregnancy complicated by preeclampsia. Liver Transplant. 1995;85:819-22.
17. **Greenstein D, Henderson J, Boyer T.** Liver hemorrhage: recurrent episodes during pregnancy complicated by preeclampsia. Gastroenterology. 1994;106:1668-71.
18. **Krueger K, Hoffman B, Lee W.** Hepatic infarction associated with eclampsia. Am J Gastroenterol. 1990;85:588-92.
19. **Ilbery M, Jones A, Sampson J.** Lupus anticoagulant and HELLP syndrome complicated by placental abruption, hepatic, dermal and adrenal infarction. Aust N Z J Obstet Gynaecol. 1995;35:215-7.

20. **Alsulyman O, Castro M, Zuckerman E, et al.** Preeclampsia and liver infarction in early pregnancy associated with the antiphospholipid syndrome. Obstet Gynecol. 1996;88:644-6.

21. **Riely C, Latham P, Romero R, Duffy T.** Acute fatty liver of pregnancy: a reassessment based on observations in nine patients. Ann Intern Med. 1987;106:703-6.

22. **Reyes H, Sandoval L, Wainstein A, et al.** Acute fatty liver of pregnancy: a clinical study of 12 episodes in 11 patients. Gut. 1994;35:101-6.

23. **Cammu H, Velkeniers B, Charels K, et al.** Idiopathic acute fatty liver of pregnancy associated with transient diabetes insipidus: case report. Br J Obstet Gynecol. 1987; 94:173-8.

24. **Barton J, Sibai B, Mabie W, Shanklin D.** Recurrent fatty liver of pregnancy. Am J Obstet Gynecol. 1990;163:534-8.

25. **Schoeman MN, Batey RG, Wicken B.** Recurrent acute fatty liver of pregnancy associated with a fatty-acid oxidation defect in the offspring. Gastroenterology. 1992;100: 544-8.

26. **Ockner SA, Brunt EM, Cohn SM, Krul ES.** Fulminant hepatic failure caused by acute fatty liver of pregnancy treated by orthotopic liver transplantation. Hepatology. 1990; 11:59-64.

27. **Treem W, Shroup M, Hale D, et al.** Acute fatty liver of pregnancy, hemolysis, elevated liver enzymes, and low platelets syndrome, and long chain 3-hydroxyacyl-coenzyme A dehydrogenase deficiency. Am J Gastroenterol. 1996;91:2293-300.

28. **Sims H, Brackett J, Powell C, et al.** The molecular basis of pediatric long chain 3-hydroxyacyl-coA dehydrogenase deficiency associated with maternal acute fatty liver of pregnancy. Proc Natl Acad Sci U S A. 1995;92:841-5.

29. **Wilcken B, Leung KC, Hammond J, et al.** Pregnancy and fetal long chain 3-hydroxyacyl-coenzyme A dehydrogenase deficiency. Lancet. 1993;341:407-8.

30. **Hamid S, Jafri S, Khan H, et al.** Fulminant hepatic failure in pregnant women: acute fatty liver or acute viral hepatitis. J Hepatol. 1996;25:20-7.

31. **Rab M, Bile M, Mubarik M, et al.** Water-borne hepatitis E virus epidemic in Islamabad, Pakistan: a common source outbreak traced to the malfunction of a modern water treatment plant. Am J Trop Med. 1997;57:151-7.

32. **Klein N, Mabie W, Latham P, et al.** Herpes simplex virus hepatitis in pregnancy. Gastroenterology. 1991;100:239-44.

33. **Deitcher S, Gardner J.** Physiologic changes in coagulation and fibrinolysis during normal pregnancy. In: Reily C, ed. Clinic in Liver Disease, v. 3. Philadelphia: WB Saunders; 1999:83-96.

34. **Ouwendijk R, Koster J, Wilson J, et al.** Budd-Chiari syndrome in a young patient with anticardiolipin antibodies: need for prolonged anticoagulant treatment. Gut. 1994;35:1004-6.

35. **Fickert P, Ramschak H, Kenner L, et al.** Acute Budd-Chiari syndrome with fulminant hepatic failure in a pregnant woman with factor V Leiden mutation. Gastroenterology. 1996; 111:1670-3.

36. **Maeta M, Yamashiro H, Oka A, et al.** Gastric cancer in the young patient with special reference to 14 pregnancy-associated cases: analysis based on 2,325 consecutive cases of gastric cancer. J Surg Oncol. 1995;58:191-5.

37. **Schreyer P, Caspi E, El-Hindi J, Eschar J.** Cirrhosis-pregnancy and delivery: a review. Obstet Gynecol Surv. 1982;37:304-12.

38. **Hillemanns P, Knitza R, Muller-Hocker J.** Rupture of splenic artery aneurysm in a pregnant patient with portal hypertension. Am J Obstet Gynecol. 1996;174:1665-6.

39. **Iwase H, Morise K, Kawase T, Horiuchi Y.** Endoscopic injection sclerotherapy for esophageal varices during pregnancy. J Clin Gastroenterol. 1994;18:80-3.

40. **Steven MM, Buckley J, Mackay I.** Pregnancy in chronic active hepatitis. Q J Med. 1979;48:519-31.

41. **Chazouilleres O, Poupon R, Bonnand A, Poupon R.** Pregnancy and ursodeoxycholic acid (UDCA) treatment induce remission of primary biliary cirrhosis (PBC). Hepatology. 1998;28:545A.

42. **Walshe J.** The management of pregnancy in Wilson's disease treated with trientine. Q J Med. 1986;58:81-7.

43. **Athanassiou A, Craigo S.** Liver masses in pregnancy. Semin Perinatol. 1998;22:166-77.

44. **Jain A, Venkataramanan R, Fung J, et al.** Pregnancy after liver transplantation under tacrolimus. Transplantation. 1997;64:559-65.

45. **Radomski J, Moritz M, Munoz S, et al.** National transplantation pregnancy registry: analysis of pregnancy outcomes in female liver transplant recipients. Liver Transplant Surg. 1995;1:281-4.

IV. Gastrointestinal Disorders
Malcolm C. Champion

The most common gastrointestinal symptoms in pregnancy are nausea, vomiting, heartburn, indigestion (dyspepsia), and constipation. The most frequent reasons for the upper gastrointestinal symptoms are morning sickness and gastroesophageal reflux disease (GERD). Management of morning sickness, hyperemesis gravidarum, and liver disease has been discussed earlier in this chapter. The common gastrointestinal problems in pregnancy discussed in this section are GERD, peptic ulcer disease (PUD), gastroparesis, cholelithiasis/cholecystitis, pancreatitis, appendicitis, IBD, and constipation. Drugs for the treatment of gastrointestinal disorders are reviewed in the Drug Table at the end of the chapter.

Gastrointestinal Motility

Many gastrointestinal problems in pregnancy are related to the decreased gastrointestinal motility and lower esophageal sphincter pressure (LESP) found in pregnant women. The motility changes seen in pregnancy have many causes but are broadly due to altered levels of hormones (e.g., estrogen and progesterone) and to mechanical factors (e.g., increased intra-abdominal pressure and displacement of the gastrointestinal organs by the uterus). The reader is referred to a more detailed review of motility changes in pregnancy (1).

Gastroesophageal Reflux Disease

Heartburn, regurgitation, and nausea are common symptoms in GERD. Heartburn during pregnancy is common, occurring in 30% to 50% of all pregnancies (2). The symptoms usually increase during the last trimester, but most women first have symptoms of GERD by the fifth month of pregnancy (3). The incidence of heartburn does not differ in primiparous and multigravid women. The diagnosis of heartburn can normally be made by a careful medical history, and heartburn can be distinguished from other types of chest pain by the retrosternal burning character of pain normally brought on by eating, lying recumbent, or bending over. Partial or complete relief is achieved with antacids. Other symptoms associated with heartburn include regurgitation, nausea, and, in severe cases, dysphagia and vomiting. There may also be symptoms of altered upper gastrointestinal motility with early satiety, postprandial epigastric discomfort, bloating, and vomiting. The symptoms of GERD can be very mild with only occasional heartburn or can progress to severe disease with complications of ulceration and stricture formation. These severe symptoms and complications are very rare in pregnant patients without pre-existing GERD.

Investigation

Investigation is rarely necessary for patients who present with mild symptoms of gastroesophageal reflux. Atypical presentations of GERD during pregnancy, including atypical chest pain, excessive coughing, or wheezing, may require further study. Endoscopy is safe and is the most useful diagnostic tool in GERD (3–5). Twenty-four hour ambulatory pH monitoring may also be useful, although no trimester-specific data are available for the normal range of reflux and esophageal acid contact time in the pregnant patient.

Treatment

The management of the pregnant patient with GERD can be divided into three phases (Figure 10-2). The author's proposed management approach (top diagram), which has been previously published (6), is here compared with that of a recent consensus conference on guidelines for the treatment of GERD in nonpregnant patients (bottom diagram) (7).

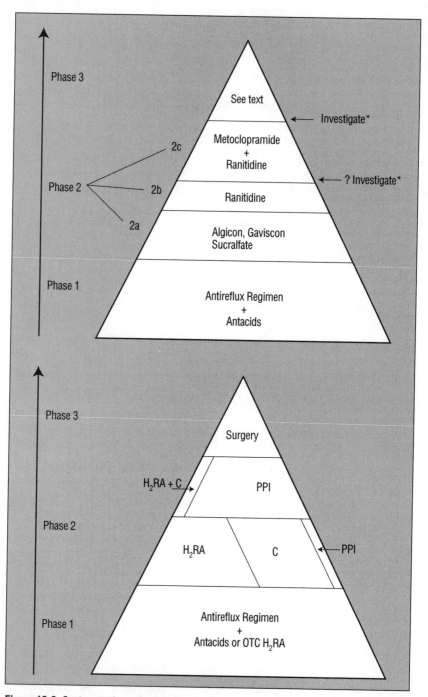

Figure 10-2 Gastroesophageal reflux disease. Proposed treatment in pregnant patients (*top*) and traditional treatment in nonpregnant patients (*bottom*). Investigations (*) include upper gastrointestinal endoscopy with or without 24-hour ambulatory pH monitoring. C = cisapride; H_2RA = H_2-receptor antagonist; OTC = over-the-counter; PPI = proton-pump inhibitor.

Phase 1

Simple lifestyle changes together with antacid use at bedtime and as needed can play a major role in the treatment of GERD. Phase 1 effects relief in up to 60% of nonpregnant patients who present to general practitioners with symptoms of gastroesophageal reflux, and it should be equally effective in pregnant patients.

Antireflux measures should include dietary changes, smoking cessation, medication review, avoidance of lying down after meals, elevation of the head during sleep, and use of antacids at bedtime.

1. *Diet*—A diet low in fatty foods and foods that decrease LESP (such as chocolate, peppermint, and coffee) and small, frequent meals are beneficial. Patients do not need a rigid, bland diet but should avoid foods that cause heartburn. Table 10-7 lists foods and other agents that may exacerbate GERD by decreasing LESP or delaying gastric emptying.
2. *Smoking*—Nicotine is a potent relaxer of the LESP, and its use should be stopped if at all possible.
3. *Medication Review*—Many commonly used drugs decrease LESP or slow gastric emptying, and the use of these drugs should be discontinued if at all possible in patients with symptoms of GERD (see Table 10-7).
4. Patients with GERD should avoid lying down soon after meals because reflux is greatly increased immediately after eating.
5. Patients with GERD should be advised to sleep with the head of the bed elevated 6 to 8 inches; this decreases acid contact time at night. This may be difficult to do as pregnancy develops, but even a minimal elevation of the head will decrease acid contact time.
6. Patients should be advised to take antacids 1) at bedtime, to neutralize any gastric acids before lying recumbent, and 2) as needed, whenever they have heartburn. Liquid antacids are more effective than tablets, although patients may find it more convenient to carry packets of tablets during the day and to use liquids at home and at night. Antacids with a calcium base (such as Tums and Rolaids) should be avoided because calcium stimulates acid production.

Table 10-7 Agents That Decrease Lower Esophageal Sphincter Pressure and/or Slow Gastric Emptying

Foods	Drugs	Hormones and Miscellaneous Agents
Fat	Anticholinergic agents	Progesterones
Chocolate	Nitrates	Estrogen
Coffee	Theophyllines	Cholecystokinin
Peppermint	Nicotine (smoking)	Somatostatin
	Alpha-blockers	Beta-antagonists
	Calcium-channel blockers	Prostaglandins
	Levodopa	
	Narcotics	

Phase 2

If the first phase of therapy does not relieve symptoms, further intervention may be considered. Phase 2 therapy can be divided into the three categories listed below. Upper gastrointestinal medications are reviewed in the Drug Table at the end of this chapter.

    1. *Nonsystemic Agents* that offer esophageal mucosal protection, namely the so-called RAFT agents and sucralfate—The antacids alginate (Algicon) and alginic acid (Gaviscon), when combined with saliva, form a viscous antacid film barrier that floats on the stomach contents and protects the esophagus against reflux of gastric contents. These agents have not been shown to be superior to placebo in the relief of symptoms related to GERD (8), but many patients report alleviation of their symptoms of gastroesophageal reflux, particularly heartburn, with use of these medications. Liquid sucralfate (carafate and sucrate) was studied in a randomized trial of 66 patients treated for heartburn associated with pregnancy. Forty-two women were given sucralfate 1 g three times daily, and 24 women were given only an antireflux regimen (phase 1 treatment). The sucralfate group had significant alleviation of both heartburn and regurgitation after 15 and 30 days (9).

    2. *Acid-Suppressing Agents*, comprising the H_2-receptor antagonists (cimetidine, ranitidine, famotidine, and nizatidine) and proton-pump inhibitors (PPIs) (omeprazole, lanzoprazole, and pantoprazole)—If clinically necessary, short-term ranitidine (Zantac) therapy may be used during pregnancy (10). The known antiandrogen effects of cimetidine make it the least desirable drug in pregnancy because of theoretical concern about male sexual development. The clinician should consider using ranitidine 150 mg twice daily for 2 to 4 weeks and then trying to discontinue or taper use of the medication to an HS dose only. Neither omeprazole nor pantoprazole is recommended in pregnancy because of concern about toxicity affecting fetal and postnatal development. If a PPI must be used, the drug of choice is lanzoprazole, which has not been shown to have any fetal toxicity in animal studies. The PPIs should be used only if the benefits outweigh the risk to both patient and fetus. They are effective in prophylaxis against acid aspiration pneumonitis (the Mendelson syndrome) as well.

    3. *Prokinetic Agents* (such as metoclopramide, domperidone, and cisapride*) that improve gastrointestinal motility mainly by increasing LESP, increasing esophageal peristalsis, and stimulating gastric emptying—Metoclopramide has been studied in late pregnancy as prophylaxis against acid aspiration pneumonitis. Intravenous metoclopramide has been shown to increase LESP in pregnant women (6). Domperidone gave similar results (6). We have no data on the use of metoclopramide, domperidone, or cisapride in the management of GERD in pregnancy. Because of the lack of data on dom-

---

*Cisapride is no longer available in the United States because of its association with serious ventricular arrhythmias (torsades de pointes).

peridone and cisapride and the potential side effects of metoclopramide, the preferred initial drug is ranitidine unless vomiting is a significant component of the patient's symptom complex. If vomiting is significant, a short-term course of metoclopramide 5 to 10 mg four times daily with concomitant ranitidine therapy is indicated.

Phase 3

If Phase 3 is reached and the patient does not improve while receiving a combination of ranitidine and metoclopramide, endoscopy and possibly 24-hour ambulatory pH monitoring must be considered to confirm the diagnosis. More aggressive therapy for GERD would then include higher doses of ranitidine or possibly a PPI (preferably lanzoprazole) when the benefits of use outweigh the risks. As we gain more experience with lanzoprazole in pregnancy, we will probably use lanzoprazole rather than ranitidine and metoclopramide to treat pregnant patients with severe GERD, just as we do with nonpregnant patients.

Peptic Ulcer Disease

Peptic ulcer disease is common in persons 20 to 40 years of age, but its incidence in pregnancy is unknown. Furthermore, the symptoms of PUD—dyspepsia, heartburn, nausea, and vomiting—are common symptoms during pregnancy.

Pathophysiology

Most gastric and duodenal ulcers are caused by *Helicobacter pylori* or the use of nonsteroidal anti-inflammatory drugs (NSAIDs). In patients not using NSAIDs, the incidence of *H. pylori* infection of the stomach is approximately 95% for patients with duodenal ulcer and 65% for patients with gastric ulcer. The other significant risk factor for PUD is smoking. Less convincing risk factors for PUD include family history, stress, socioeconomic status, and heavy alcohol use (11).

Symptoms

As mentioned above, the symptoms of PUD overlap considerably with symptoms commonly found in pregnancy. If nausea and vomiting develop later in pregnancy or continue beyond the first trimester or if pain is severe, diagnoses other than pregnancy-associated morning sickness or GERD should be considered.

Investigations

Endoscopy, if indicated, is safe in pregnancy and is the study of choice if PUD is being considered (3–5). If an ulcer is found, biopsy can be done at the same time to look for *H. pylori*, particularly if the patient is not receiving an NSAID.

Management of Peptic Ulcer Disease in Pregnancy

Patient with Peptic Ulcer Disease Before Pregnancy

Patients with a history of PUD, particularly those whose disease is unrelated to NSAID use, should be studied with endoscopy. Biopsy can be done at the time of endoscopy to establish the presence or absence of *H. pylori*, or *H. pylori* serologic tests should be done. If *H. pylori* is present, it should be eradicated before conception. Therapy for *H. pylori* is rapidly evolving, and the physician should consult a gastroenterologist about the most appropriate eradication regimen.

The regimens most often used to eradicate *H. pylori* in nonpregnant patients are 1) a PPI twice daily, clarithromycin 500 mg twice daily, and metronidazole 500 mg twice daily; or 2) a PPI twice daily, clarithromycin 500 mg twice daily, and amoxicillin 1 g twice daily. Both of these regimens are used for 7 to 14 days (11).

Noncomplicated Peptic Ulcers in Pregnancy

In pregnant patients who present with severe nausea and vomiting with or without epigastric pain, particularly after the first trimester, endoscopy to rule out PUD should be considered. In nonpregnant patients, approximately 30% of peptic ulcers may be silent, and patients may present with no pain but with other upper gastrointestinal symptoms, particularly nausea and vomiting. If PUD is diagnosed by endoscopy, biopsy can be done to evaluate *H. pylori* status. If *H. pylori* is present, an appropriate regimen for eradicating it should be considered in the postpartum period but not during pregnancy. Unfortunately, several of the drugs now used to eradicate *H. pylori* (PPIs, bismuth, and clarithromycin) are relatively contraindicated in pregnancy.

Treatment

Diet plays no specific role in the management of PUD. Patients should be encouraged to eat small, frequent meals and to avoid foods that produce indigestion (often, spicy or fatty foods).

High-dose antacid therapy alone has been shown to be effective for duodenal ulcer. However, this therapy has a high incidence of side effects, and its safety in pregnancy has not been studied. Antacids should be used as needed for the treatment of symptoms that have not resolved with the use of other medication. There are two choices for the medical treatment of proven peptic ulcer during pregnancy: sucralfate or histamine-receptor antagonist. Sucralfate, a nonabsorbable drug, has been shown to be an effective treatment for both duodenal and gastric ulcer at dosages of 1 g four times daily or 2 g twice daily. The preferred histamine-receptor antagonist is ranitidine 150 mg twice daily. Both of these regimens should ideally be continued for 6 to 8 weeks. In patients who do not respond to these regimens, a PPI (preferably, lanzoprazole) may be considered.

Upper Gastrointestinal Bleeding in Pregnancy

The management of upper gastrointestinal bleeding is the same in pregnant and nonpregnant patients. Patients should be hospitalized and should receive intravenous fluid resuscitation and, if necessary, blood transfusion. For severe bleeding, endoscopy should be considered not only to confirm the diagnosis but to assure that diathermy or injection therapy can be done for the bleeding ulcer if necessary. At the same time, there is the opportunity to biopsy to look for *H. pylori*. Therapy for the ulcer is essentially the same as that discussed above, although acid suppression with ranitidine is the preferred treatment for a bleeding ulcer in pregnant patients.

Gastroparesis

The combination of gastroparesis and pregnancy is generally found only in patients with diabetes mellitus. The main symptoms of gastroparesis are similar to the symptoms of morning sickness—principally, nausea and vomiting. There may be early satiety, epigastric pain, anorexia, heartburn, or regurgitation. Patients may vomit undigested food that was eaten several hours earlier.

Diabetic Patients with Established Gastroparesis Who Are Pregnant or Wish To Become Pregnant

Diabetic patients with established gastroparesis are already taking a gastric prokinetic agent (metoclopramide, domperidone, or cisapride) that is controlling the symptoms of gastroparesis. If these patients wish to become pregnant, the physician has two choices. First, use of the prokinetic agent can be discontinued and can be restarted if the symptoms of gastroparesis become prominent or problematic as pregnancy develops. Second, if the gastroparesis is severe, the physician can counsel the patient on the risks and benefits of continuing to use the prokinetic drug throughout pregnancy and can prescribe the lowest possible effective dose.

Gastroparesis Developing During Pregnancy

Gastroparesis in pregnancy can be difficult to diagnose because the patient may be thought to have prolonged or severe morning sickness. The initial presentation of gastroparesis in the diabetic patient is unusual in pregnancy. This diagnosis should be considered in all patients who have had longstanding diabetes, particularly those with other complications of diabetes, such as peripheral neuropathy.

Treatment

There is no special diet for the treatment of gastroparesis. Patients should avoid high-fat foods and leguminous vegetables, which are emptied from the stomach with difficulty. Patients should be advised to eat small, frequent meals and to space their meals throughout the day.

Prokinetic agents should ideally be taken half an hour before meals and at bedtime. The bedtime dose is important because it restores a more normal migratory motor complex that is important in evacuating indigestible material from the stomach in the fasting state and minimizes the risk for retained food or bezoa formation in the stomach. None of the prokinetic agents now available in North America (metoclopramide, domperidone, and cisapride) is approved for use during pregnancy. Metoclopramide is the only prokinetic agent approved for the treatment of gastroparesis in the United States (12). In Canada, metoclopramide (12), domperidone (13), and cisapride (14) are all approved for the treatment of gastroparesis. The longest experience is with metoclopramide, and this drug seems to be safe in pregnancy when used in the short term. However, when metoclopramide is not well tolerated, cisapride may be used for long-term treatment during pregnancy. Even though cisapride is no longer available in the United States, it is approved for the treatment of gastroparesis in Canada. Very limited data exist on the efficacy and safety of cisapride use in pregnancy (15).

Cholelithiasis/Cholecystitis

The incidence of gallstones is increased in pregnancy and seems directly related to the number of pregnancies that a woman has had (16). With this increased risk for gallstones comes the potential for an increased risk for cholecystitis, biliary colic, and pancreatitis. Because gallstone disease is a common condition in females in this age group, it is unclear whether pregnancy itself is a risk factor for gallstone formation. Patients with known cholelithiasis do not require cholecystectomy before conception because the pregnant patient does not seem to have any increased risk for complications related to previously documented cholelithiasis (17).

Acute cholecystitis in relation to pregnancy may be more common postpartum than antepartum (18). The classic location—the right upper quadrant with radiation to the back—may be different in pregnancy because the gastrointestinal organs are displaced by the gravid uterus. Patients usually complain of fatty food intolerance associated with epigastric or right upper-quadrant pain that may or may not radiate to the back or right shoulder. True biliary colic normally lasts at least 1 hour and may last for several hours, and it is constant with some degree of colic. Other symptoms include nausea, vomiting, and, if cholangitis is present, fever and chills. The differential diagnosis of this presentation in the pregnant patient includes hepatitis, PUD, pancreatitis, appendicitis, right lower lobe pneumonia, and pulmonary embolism, all of which may present with right upper-quadrant pain.

Investigation

Investigation is similar to that done in nonpregnant patients. Clinical examination may show right upper-quadrant tenderness (the Murphy sign), leukocytosis may be present, and, in biliary colic, there may be an increase in bilirubin, gamma glutamyl transferase (GGT), and alkaline phosphatase levels. Minimal elevation of the AST and ALT levels may also be seen. Abdominal ultrasonography should show gallstones and may be helpful in defining any evidence of cholecystitis or common bile duct dilatation. If the symptoms are suggestive and the results of the above investigations are normal, it is worthwhile to perform sequential blood work for 3 days after a pain episode because it can take time for the bilirubin, alkaline phosphatase, and GGT levels to increase after an acute episode of biliary colic.

Treatment

The causes of acute cholecystitis are similar in pregnant and nonpregnant patients, and this condition does not seem to pose an increased risk to the fetus unless significant infection is present.

Because cholecystitis normally subsides within 1 to 2 days of conservative therapy, this therapy is the preferred initial approach. Conservative therapy involves bowel rest with nasogastric suction if there is significant vomiting, intravenous fluid rehydration, and antibiotics (17, 18). If necessary, emergency cholecystectomy can be done by an open laparotomy or laparoscopically, depending on the duration of the pregnancy and the experience of the surgeon. Surgery is reserved for patients with recurrent attacks, sepsis, or complications. Surgery must also be considered when a patient does not improve after 24 to 48 hours of medical therapy or, alternatively, has symptomatic common bile duct stones. Laparascopic cholecystectomy has been done in pregnant patients but is not generally recommended. The performance of cholecystectomy during pregnancy is unusual and has been reported in less than 0.1% of cases (17). Surgery in the first trimester has been shown to increase risk for abortion, and surgery later in gestation may contribute to preterm labor.

Many authorities recommend the following scenario (18):

- *First Trimester*—Medical therapy; elective cholecystectomy in the second trimester if indicated
- *Second Trimester*—Medical therapy; cholecystectomy if indicated
- *Third Trimester*—Medical therapy; cholecystectomy in postpartum period

Symptomatic common bile duct stones require endoscopic retrograde cholangiopancreatography (ERCP) with papillotomy and stone retrieval. This procedure can be done with limited radiation to the fetus and avoids the risks associated with general anesthesia and laparotomy. Pancreatitis associated with common bile duct stones may be alleviated with conservative therapy, but ERCP and papillotomy are invariably required to remove any common bile duct stones. Failure to remove stones endoscopically necessitates a surgical approach.

Pancreatitis

The most common causes of pancreatitis in the western world are alcohol use and gallstones; these account for at least 90% of cases. Other causes to consider in pregnancy include drugs, trauma, hypercalcemia, and hypertriglyceridemia, which may be related to pregnancy. Acute pancreatitis in pregnancy has an incidence of 0.09% to 0.009% and is normally due to cholelithiasis.

Acute pancreatitis has the same clinical presentation in pregnant and nonpregnant women. In pregnant women, it most often occurs in the third trimester. Fortunately, most attacks of pancreatitis in pregnancy are mild. The most common symptom is constant epigastric pain, which may be severe and may radiate to the back. Severe pancreatitis can be associated with pseudocyst, abscess, fistula, jaundice, and ileus (19).

Differential Diagnosis

The differential diagnosis of constant epigastric pain includes acute cholecystitis, intestinal perforation (ulcer disease), ischemia, preeclampsia, and ruptured ectopic pregnancy. The serum amylase level is often increased, and an increased serum lipase level was recently shown to be a more sensitive test for pancreatitis (20). The serum amylase level can also be increased in a variety of other conditions, including diabetic ketoacidosis, renal dysfunction, and other intra-abdominal catastrophes. The severity of the pancreatitis can be determined by using clinical outcome criteria, the most common of which are the Ranson criteria (21).

Investigation

Patients with pancreatitis require acute monitoring in an intensive care unit and regular evaluation for the development of severe pancreatitis and its complications. Patients should be studied with abdominal ultrasonography.

Treatment

Most patients with acute pancreatitis have resolution with bowel rest, intravenous fluids, and analgesics. Nasogastric suction should be used only in patients with persistent vomiting or evidence of significant ileus or bowel obstruction. Rarely, patients can progress to necrotic pancreatitis, which is a serious and life-threatening condition even in nonpregnant patients.

Appendicitis

Appendicitis is common in this age group, and its presentation in the pregnant patient may be atypical. The progression of nonspecific abdominal pain to localized peritonitis in the right lower quadrant is the same in the first and second trimesters as it is in nonpregnant patients. In the third trimester, the appendix can rotate deep into the right upper quadrant as the uterus expands. For this reason, tenderness may be difficult to localize and the pain may be principally in the right upper quadrant. Anorexia, nausea, and even vomiting are relatively common and nonspecific in pregnancy and are found with appendicitis. Pregnancy is associated with leukocytosis, and it has been suggested that fever and tachycardia are less common because of the increased steroid levels seen in pregnancy. In addition, because of the proximity of the appendix to the kidney, pyuria can occur in up to 20% of pregnant patients with appendicitis (22). The differential diagnosis of right lower-quadrant pain in early pregnancy includes ectopic pregnancy and ovarian cystic disease. Up to 25% of ovarian cysts can rupture during pregnancy, and patients with such rupture can present with localized peritoneal irritation. These patients lack evidence of inflammation (fever or leukocytosis), and their pain normally subsides rather than increasing as it does in appendicitis. Ovarian torsion can occur in pregnancy and can present with sudden onset of severe right lower-quadrant pain with no evidence of inflammation. The differential diagnosis for right upper-quadrant pain is discussed above in the section on cholecystitis.

Investigation

Ultrasonography can be useful in early pregnancy, but its applications are more limited in the third trimester. It is helpful in delineating other possible differential diagnoses. Laparoscopy may become useful in this clinical setting (23).

Treatment

Appendectomy in pregnancy is safe if clinically indicated. Morbidity from appendicitis in pregnancy most often results from a delay in diagnosis. Reluctance to perform surgery and diagnostic difficulty seem to contribute to the 30% perforation rate found in late pregnancy (22, 23).

Inflammatory Bowel Disease

The principal symptoms of IBD are diarrhea and abdominal pain. Bloody diarrhea is more prominent in ulcerative colitis, and pain is more common in Crohn disease. The diagnosis of either of these conditions during pregnancy is unusual because most patients with IBD are diagnosed before they become pregnant. The management of the pregnant patient with IBD can be divided into several areas and was recently extensively reviewed (24).

Oral Contraceptives and the Development of Inflammatory Bowel Disease

Whether the use of oral contraceptives is associated with an increased risk for ulcerative colitis and Crohn disease remains controversial. The slight increase seen in risk for IBD has never reached statistical significance. The data do suggest that a subset of patients who present with IBD while using oral contraceptives may have a pill-related colitis that resolves on discontinuation of contraceptive use. This discontinuation should be considered in patients with IBD who are using oral contraceptives and are not responding to medical therapy.

Fertility

Women
Fertility does not seem to be impaired in women with ulcerative colitis and does not differ in these women compared with the normal population (25).

However, fertility in women with Crohn disease can be impaired (26); this is influenced by the severity of disease and impaired ovulation due to disease or associated cachexia. Fallopian tube blockage may be due to the IBD, and dispareunia related to the inflammation (particularly perianal disease), the fear of going through a pregnancy with IBD, or the avoidance of pregnancy on medical advice (24) all contribute to decreased fertility.

Men

In men, IBD does not cause infertility, but sulfasalazine has been shown to reduce total sperm count and sperm motility. These effects reverse with discontinuation of sulfasalazine therapy. This problem is not found with the 5-aminosalicylic acid preparations (Asacol and Pentasa) and therefore seems to be due to the sulfapyridine component of sulfasalazine.

Risk for Inheriting Inflammatory Bowel Disease

The chance of having a child who will develop IBD is difficult to define. The previously suggested figure of 30% seems to be incorrect. Recent data show that approximately 10% to 15% of patients with IBD have a family history of IBD. There is now considerable interest in the genetic predisposition to IBD. Data suggest that Crohn disease and ulcerative colitis are related complex genetic diseases. That is, several genes seem to be involved in this genetic predisposition (27).

Effect of Inflammatory Bowel Disease on Pregnancy

Ulcerative Colitis

Ulcerative colitis during pregnancy seems to have a minimal effect with respect to low birthweight and fetal abnormalities, and most patients have normal full-term babies (28). The incidence of spontaneous abortion (8%), congenital abnormalities (1%), and stillbirths (1%) is similar to that seen in the healthy normal population (25). Patients with asymptomatic ulcerative colitis who become pregnant rarely have exacerbations of their disease during pregnancy or in the postpartum period. Patients with more active disease are likely to have exacerbation of symptoms during the first trimester. Symptoms often subside in the second trimester, possibly because cortisol levels increase as pregnancy develops. The previously hypothesized increased incidence of relapse of ulcerative colitis in the postpartum period has not been substantiated.

Crohn Disease

The data on normal healthy pregnancy and full-term delivery in Crohn disease is similar to that in ulcerative colitis, but clinical experience indicates that patients with Crohn disease are more likely than patients with ulcerative colitis to have problems during pregnancy. The incidence of spontaneous abortion, congenital abnormalities, and stillbirth has been shown to be similar to that expected in the general population (29). Patients who have active Crohn disease at the time of conception seem to have poorer fetal outcomes than do patients with inactive disease. Ideally, patients with Crohn disease should be symptom-free at conception. Seventy percent of those who are will remain symptom free during pregnancy and the postpartum period. The overall prospects for pregnancy in Crohn disease are good, and pregnancy is not contraindicated. However, patients should be advised that conception while the disease is inactive is preferred. Some data suggest that previous pregnancies in patients with Crohn disease, but not patients with ulcerative colitis, are associated with a decreased exacerbation rate and a lower rate of surgical intervention. This was found in both patients with ileal Crohn disease and patients with colonic Crohn disease. The postpartum period seems to represent a high-risk time for flares of disease.

Surgical Treatment During Pregnancy

If absolutely necessary, patients can undergo surgery for IBD during pregnancy. Anesthesia is associated with an increased risk for spontaneous abortion. No large series have been published on the effect of surgery for IBD in pregnancy. Patients with a rectal–vaginal fistula or previous surgery for this fistula may wish to consider cesarean section to avoid exacerbation of the fistula (23) with vaginal delivery.

Pregnancy in Patients with Ileostomy

In 119 pregnant patients with an ileostomy, fetal outcome was similar to that expected in the general population. There were 18 stoma problems, including intestinal obstructions (50%) and stomal prolapses (30%) (30). Patients with ileo-anal pouches can have successful pregnancies and vaginal delivery.

Drug Treatment for Inflammatory Bowel Disease During Pregnancy

Sulfasalazine and Prednisone
Sulfasalazine and prednisone seem to be safe and to have no significant adverse effects for the fetus (26). The 5-aminosalicylic acid preparations also seem to be safe for both fetus and mother during pregnancy (31, 32).

Metronizadole
Metronizadole for the treatment of IBD in pregnancy has not been closely studied. However, metronizadole used during pregnancy for *Trichomonas*

vaginalis infection seems to have no negative effect on the fetus. This drug is not commonly used in the management of IBD, except for perianal disease.

Immunosuppressive Therapy

Immunosuppressive therapy with azathioprine or 6-mercaptopurine should be avoided if possible in pregnant patients with IBD. Most of the data available on the use of immunosuppressive therapy in pregnancy are on the use of azathioprine after renal and liver transplantation (24). These data suggest that immunosuppressive therapy is relatively safe in pregnancy, particularly with the lower dose used in patients with IBD. Retrospective studies in patients with IBD who become pregnant while receiving immunosuppressive therapy confirm that there is minimal or no drug risk to the fetus (24).

Breastfeeding

Previous concerns about sulfasalazine use as a risk factor for kernicterus have not been borne out. The 5-aminosalicylic acid compounds are not secreted in large amounts in breast milk, and their use is considered compatible with breastfeeding.

Approach to Patients with Inflammatory Bowel Disease Who Wish To Become Pregnant

In patients with ulcerative colitis, maintenance therapy (with sulfasalazine, Asacol, or Pentasa) should use the lowest effective dose. The risks of maintenance therapy seem to be minimal, but the patient and the attending physician must decide together whether to continue maintenance therapy throughout the pregnancy. Patients with active disease should be advised not to become pregnant until their colitis has been in remission and they are no longer using prednisone (ideally, they should have not have used prednisone for at least 3 months).

Maintenance therapy in Crohn disease is more controversial. Again, it involves a joint decision by the patient and the attending physician. If the patient has not had an exacerbation of Crohn disease for 1 to 2 years, it is reasonable to consider stopping the maintenance therapy and observing the patient for 3 months. Patients with active Crohn disease who become pregnant have poorer fetal outcomes, and patients with this disease should be advised against becoming pregnant until their disease has been in remission (with no prednisone therapy) for at least 3 months.

Finally, a simple but often overlooked recommendation is that the attending physician and the obstetrician should work in the same hospital. This facilitates easy communication and clinical care, particularly if the patient has to be admitted.

Constipation

Constipation can be defined as 1) a decreased frequency of bowel movements or 2) difficulty in evacuation of the bowel, normally because the stool is hard or scyballous. Constipation is common in pregnancy; it has been reported to occur in 11% to 40% of pregnant patients (33). The mechanism of constipation in pregnancy is poorly understood but is related to the effect of progesterone on intestinal smooth muscle and to pressure on the sigmoid colon by the enlarging uterus. Other factors include increased absorption of electrolytes and water that is not compensated for by appropriate fluid intake (34). Iron supplements can also contribute to constipation in pregnancy.

Investigation

Pregnant patients with constipation do not require investigation unless they develop symptoms of obstruction. If any clinical suspicion exists, hypothyroidism should be excluded as a cause of constipation.

Treatment

Simple dietary changes and increased fluid intake are effective in most patients. Patients should be encouraged to eat 1 to 2 heaping tablespoons of natural bran powder per day (15 to 30 g of bran) and to drink at least 6 to 8 glasses of fluids per day. For patients who do not tolerate the natural bran powder, psyllium bulk-forming agents, such as Metamucil, are effective if taken in the same quantity. The diet should be high in fiber and should focus on leguminous vegetables, salads, and whole-grain breads and cereals. Stool softeners, such as Docusate, are often used in pregnancy, although few data indicate that they have any benefit as a laxative in either pregnant or nonpregnant patients. The stimulant laxatives Bisacodyl, Dulcolax, and senna (Senokot) are commonly used and seem to be safe during pregnancy, particularly if they are used only over the short term. Long-term use may damage the colonic enteric nervous system. These laxatives should not be used during breastfeeding. The safest and most effective laxative during pregnancy is lactulose 30 cc once or twice daily. Patients with continued difficulty in evacuation may benefit from a glycerine suppository.

Summary

This section has reviewed the common gastrointestinal problems found in pregnancy. An initial conservative approach that avoids the use of systemic medication is often effective in the management of the two most common problems, GERD and constipation. The management of pregnancy in patients with IBD is challenging and requires a joint effort by the obstetrician and the attending physician.

Acknowledgments—The author thanks Karyn Curtis for her assistance in preparing this section.

REFERENCES

1. **Baron TM, Ramirez B, Richter JE.** Gastrointestinal motility disorders during pregnancy. Ann Intern Med. 1993;118:366-75.

2. **Bassey O.** Pregnancy and heartburn in pregnancy. J Obstet Gynaecol Brit Empire. 1958;65:1019.

3. **Castro L de P.** Reflux esophagitis as the cause of heartburn in pregnancy. Am J Obstet Gynecol. 1967;98:1-10.

4. **Cappell MS, Colon VJ, Sidhom OA.** A study of eight medical centers of the safety and clinical efficacy of esophagogastroduodenoscopy in 83 pregnant females with follow-up of fetal outcome in comparison to control groups. Am J Gastroenterol. 1996;91:348-54.

5. **Cappell MS.** The safety and efficacy of gastrointestinal endoscopy during pregnancy. Gastroenterol Clin North Am. 1998;27:37-71.

6. **Champion MC.** Upper gastrointestinal disorders during pregnancy. Curr Obstet Med. 1996;4:209-45.

7. **Beck IT, Champion MC, Thomson ABR, et al.** The Second Canadian Consensus Conference on the Management of Patients with Gastroesophageal Reflux Disease. Can J Gastroenterol. 1997;11(Suppl B):7B-20B.

8. **McCallum RW, Champion MC.** Physiology, diagnosis and treatment of gastroesophageal reflux disease. In: McCallum RW, Champion MC, eds. Gastrointestinal Motility Disorders: Diagnosis and Treatment. Philadelphia: Williams & Wilkins; 1989: 135-62.

9. **Ranchet G, Gangemi O, Pretone M.** Sucralfate in the treatment of gavidic pyrosis. Giornale Italiano di Ostrecia e Ginecologia. 1990;22:1-16.

10. **Larson JD, Patatanian E, Miner PB Jr, Rayburn WF, Robinson MG.** Double blind, placebo controlled study of ranitidine for gastroesophageal reflux symptoms during pregnancy. Obstet Gynecol. 1997;90:83-7.

11. **Louw JA, Solly Marks IN.** The treatment of peptic ulcer disease. Curr Opin Gastroenterol. 1997;13:457-64.

12. **Albibi R, McCallum RW.** Metoclopramide pharmacology and clinical application. Ann Intern Med. 1982;98:86-95.

13. **Champion MC, Yen M, Hartnett M.** Domperidone—pharmacology and review of the literature. Can Med Assoc J. 1986;135:457-61.

14. **Champion MC.** Treatment of gastroparesis. In: Champion MC, Orr WC, eds. Evolving Concepts in Gastrointestinal Motility. New York: Blackwell Science; 1996:108-47.

15. **Bailey B, Addis A, Lee A, Sanghvi K, et al.** Cisapride use during human pregnancy: a prospective, controlled multicenter study. Dig Dis Sci. 1997;42:1848-51.

16. **Sama B, Morselli C, Labate AM, et al.** A population study on the prevalence of gallstone disease. The Sirmione Study. Hepatology. 1987;7:913-7.

17. **Glenn F, McSherry CK.** Gallstones and pregnancy among 300 young women treated by cholecystectomy. Surg Gynecol Obstet. 1968;127:1067.

18. **Dixon NP, Faddis DM, Silberman H.** Aggressive management of cholecystitis during pregnancy. Am J Surg. 1987;154:292-4.

19. **Mayer IE, Hussain H.** Abdominal pain during pregnancy. Gastroenterol Clin North Am. 1998;27:1-36.

20. **Strickland DM, Hauth JC, Widish J, et al.** Amylase and isoamylase activities in serum of pregnant women. Obstet Gynecol. 1984;63:389.

21. **Glazer G, Mann DV.** United Kingdom guidelines for the management of acute pancreatitis. Gut. 1998;42(Suppl 2):S1-13.

22. **Weingold AB.** Appendicitis in pregnancy. Clin Obstet Gynecol. 1983;26:801.

23. **Firstenberg MS, Malangoni MA.** Gastrointestinal surgery during pregnancy. Gastroenterol Clin North Am. 1998;27:73-88.

24. **Korelitz B.** Inflammatory bowel disease and pregnancy. Gastroenterol Clin North Am. 1998;27:221.

25. **Willoughby CP, Truelove SC.** Ulcerative colitis and pregnancy. Gut. 1980;21:469-74.

26. **Baiocco PJ, Korelitz BI.** The influence of inflammatory bowel disease and its treatment on pregnancy and fetal outcome. Gastroenterol Clin North Am. 1998;27:213-24.

27. **Cho JH, Brant SR.** Genetics and genetic markers in inflammatory bowel disease. Curr Opin Gastroenterol. 1998;14:283-8.

28. **Willoughby CP.** Fertility, pregnancy and inflammatory bowel disease. In: Allan RN, Keighley MRB, Hawkins CF, Alexander-Williams J, eds. Inflammatory Bowel Diseases, 2d ed. New York: Churchill-Livingstone; 1990;547-58.

29. **Woolfson K, Cohen Z, McLeod RS.** Crohn's disease and pregnancy. Dis Colon Rectum. 1990;33:869-73.

30. **Neilson OH, Andreasson B, Bondesen S, Jacobson O, Jarnum S.** Pregnancy in Crohn's disease. Scand J Gastroenterol. 1984;19:724-32.

31. **Habal FM, Hui G, Greenberg GR.** Oral 5-aminosalicylic acid for inflammatory bowel disease in pregnancy: safety and clinical course. Gastroenterology. 1993;105:1057-60.

32. **Diav-Citrin O, Park YH, Veerasuntharam G, et al.** The safety of mesalamine in human pregnancy: a prospective controlled cohort study. Gastroenterology. 1998;114:23-8.

33. **Anderson AS.** Constipation during pregnancy: incidents and methods used in its treatment in a group of Cambridgeshire women. Health Visitor. 1984;12:363.]

34. **Bonapace ES Jr, Fisher FS.** Constipation and diarrhea in pregnancy. Gastroenterol Clin North Am. 1998;27:197-211.

APPENDIX: DRUGS FOR GASTROINTESTINAL DISORDERS

The drug table on page 618 is for reference when there is a clinical indication for treatment with one of the medications listed. Decisions about medication use in pregnancy should be made on the basis of a benefit-to-risk ratio, avoiding unnecessary treatment of symptoms but with consideration of the fact that fetal well-being depends on maternal well-being. Because the U.S. Food and Drug Administration is working on a new classification system of medications used in pregnancy, we have classified medications as follows:

Data Suggest Drug Use May Be Justified When Indicated

When data and/or experience supports the safety of the drug.

Data Suggest Drug Use May Be Justified in Some Circumstances

When less extensive or desirable data are reported, but the drug is reasonable as a second-line therapy or may be used on the basis of the severity of maternal illness.

Data Suggest Drug Use Is Rarely Justified

Use drug only when alternatives supported by more experience and/or a better safety profile are not available.

Pregnancy pharmacokinetics may necessitate a significant increase in dose or dosing frequency, and dosing recommendations may require modification according to individual circumstances.

Drugs for Gastrointestinal Disorders

Drug	Use May Be Justified When Indicated	Use May Be Justified in Some Circumstances	Use Is Rarely Justified	Comments/Dose Adjustments
Antacids	√			May decrease iron absorption
Asacol, Pentasa (5-ASA compounds)	√			Use for inflammatory bowel disease
Azathioprine		√		See Chapter 9 Drug Table (p 544)
Bisacodyl (Dulcolax)	√			
Chlorpromazine	√			Use as antiemetic; may cause dystolic reactions
Cisapride*			√	Very limited data
Corticosteroids	√			Use in inflammatory bowel disease for same indications as for non-pregnant patients
Dimenhydrinate	√			
Diphenoxylate/ atropine (Lomotil)	√			
Docusate (Colace)	√			
Famotidine, nizatidine, cimetidine, ranitidine	√			Randitidine preferred H_2-blocker
Lansoprazole		√		Limited human data; teratogenic in animals
Loperamide (Imodium)	√			
Metoclopramide	√			Preferred promotility agent
Misoprostol			√	May induce uterine bleeding and contractions; very limited data
MOM	√			May cause sodium retention
Odansteran (Zofran)		√		
Omerperazine		√		Limited human data; teratogenic in animals
Prochlorperazine	√			
Promethrine	√			Use as antiemetic
Psyllium	√			
Pyridoxine (B_6)	√			Efficacy demonstrated by randomized trial
Sucralfate	√			
Sulfasalazine		√		Theoretic risk of neonatal hyperbilirubinemia

*Unavailable in the United States.

CHAPTER 11

Oncology

I. Chemotherapeutic Agents
Robert D. Legare, MD

II. Abnormal Papanicolaou Smears
Donald Schmidt, MD

III. Hematologic Malignancies
Isabelle Bence-Bruckler, MD

IV. Breast Cancer
Kimberly K. Leslie, MD

I. Chemotherapeutic Agents
Robert D. Legare

Cancer is the leading cause of death in women 35 to 54 years of age, accounting for approximately 41% of deaths in this age group. It is also a leading cause of nonaccidental death in women 15 to 34 years of age, accounting for approximately 19% of such deaths (1). Cancer complicates approximately 1 in 1000 pregnancies (2), resulting in an estimated 3500 cases annually. Cervical cancer is the most common cancer encountered during pregnancy, followed by breast cancer, melanoma, ovarian cancer, thyroid cancer, leukemia, lymphoma, and colorectal carcinoma (3). Because the incidence of cancer typically increases with age (4), the diagnosis of cancer during pregnancy will probably become more common as women increasingly delay childbearing until the fourth and fifth decades of life.

Few situations in medicine are as challenging as cancer in pregnancy, and few have such seemingly antithetical medical, ethical, philosophical, and spiritual features. Legal issues, such as the rights of the fetus, occasionally arise, especially when maternal treatments threaten fetal viability or health (5, 6). Care for the woman who receives a diagnosis of cancer during pregnancy is multidisciplinary and involves a team that includes an obstetrician, a surgical oncologist, a medical oncologist, a social worker, clergy, and family. Communication, education, counseling, and support must be optimal to empower a woman to make the most informed decision about treatment options.

Because chemotherapy is integral to the treatment of lymphoma, leukemia, and breast and ovarian carcinoma, decisions must be made about the timing of chemotherapy, the chemotherapeutic agents to be used, and the continuation of pregnancy. In the nonpregnant state, decisions about therapy for a particular cancer are made on the basis of outcome data from prospective, randomized clinical trials. In the pregnant state, these decisions are influenced by pregnancy-associated physiologic changes in the mother and the potential deleterious effects of chemotherapy in the developing fetus. (The table at the end of this chapter provides specific information on chemotherapeutic agents.)

Most chemotherapeutic agents ultimately kill cancer cells by altering cell cycle kinetics. Cancer cells are particularly susceptible to these agents not because they are dividing faster than normal cells but because the proportion of malignant cells that are dividing is greater than the proportion of normal cells that are dividing (Table 11-1). The means by which apoptotic cell death is accomplished vary, depending on the mechanisms of action of the individual agents (3, 7, 8).

Pharmacokinetics comprises drug absorption, distribution, metabolism, and excretion and may be altered during pregnancy as a result of physiologic adaptation (3, 9). Pregnancy is associated with an increase in plasma volume, an alteration in the volume of distribution, an increase in the glomerular filtration rate, and a change in the serum protein concentration, and it may affect hepatic function (10). It also creates a physiologic third space—amniotic fluid—that can potentially act as a pharmacologic third space (11). These changes can alter toxicity, optimal dose, and the efficacy of an administered dose. For instance, the increased glomerular filtration rate and plasma volume expansion seen in pregnancy may lead to a reduction of the area-under-the-concentration-versus-time curve, diminishing the tumoricidal effect of agents that are principally excreted renally. Alternatively, the increased volume of distribution and, in some cases, impaired hepatic function may result in more sustained drug levels and increased toxicity (10). In addition, changes

Table 11-1 Classification of Chemotherapeutic Agents

Agent	Mechanism of Action*
Alkylating agents Cyclophosphamide Thiotepa Chlorambucil Melphalan Busulfan Isophamide BCNU Decarbazine Cisplatin, carboplatin	Covalent adduction formation on cellular DNA leads to a lethal interaction with DNA
Antimetabolites Aminopterin MTX 5-FU and its analogues	Inhibit cellular reactions necessary for synthesis of the building blocks of DNA, RNA, and protein
Nucleoside analogues Cytarabine Gemcitabine Fludarabine 2-CDA	Incorporated into DNA and RNA, leading to inhibition of DNA, RNA, and protein synthesis
Topoisomerase I inhibitors Topotecan Irinotecan	Interact with enzyme DNA complex and lead to single-strand DNA breaks that are lethal to cells undergoing DNA synthesis

Topoisomerase II inhibitors
Etoposide
Anthracyclines
  Doxorubicin
  Davnorubicin
  Idarubicin
	Inhibit regulation of DNA cleaved by topoisomerase II, including protein-linked breaks in DNA

Other antibiotics Dactinomycin Bleomycin	Intercalation and DNA break Free-radical formation DNA strand breaks
Vinca Alkaloids Vincristine Vinblastine Vinorelbine	Disruption of microtubules, especially those in the mitotic spindle
Taxanes Paclitaxele Taxotera	Disruption of mitosis by binding to tubules

*How agents cause cell death.

in gastric motility associated with pregnancy may alter the absorption of orally administered agents. Unfortunately, we have no clear recommendations on dosing modification during pregnancy because we have few or no pharmacokinetic data for individual antineoplastic agents. Currently, the dosing of chemotherapeutic agents should be similar in pregnant and nonpregnant patients.

The placenta may be a biological barrier to some antineoplastic agents, although most antineoplastic agents seem to readily traverse it (12–14) and would be expected to do so because they typically have low molecular weight and high lipid solubility and are bound loosely to maternal plasma proteins (15). Information on the effects of chemotherapeutic agents on the developing embryo is derived primarily from reports describing teratogenic and mutagenic effects in animal experiments and from case reports describing the outcome of pregnancies complicated by cancer (16). The extent of fetal malformation varies widely in these reports. Doll and colleagues (11) reported that 24 of 139 children (17%) who received chemotherapy in utero developed fetal malformations. However, they presented no data on maternal status and the familial incidence of congenital abnormalities. In addition, some children received radiation therapy in utero and it is difficult to determine the exact incidence of congenital malformations that are secondary only to chemotherapy (17). The antimetabolite aminopterin, formerly used as an abortifacient, may be the most studied teratogenic agent associated with central nervous system (CNS) anomalies (18). In 1952, Thiersch (19) noted hydrocephalus, hair lip, and cleft palate in two infants when 2 of 12 women for whom aminopterin was prescribed did not have abortion. Several comprehensive reviews have been published in the past 40 years (17, 18, 20–26). Nicholson's 1968 report (18) is heavily quoted in the literature, and observations made at the time this report was published have been reinforced by more recent analyses (17, 21, 24). Chemotherapy given in the first trimester, at the time of organogenesis, is associated with a significant risk for spontaneous abortion and major birth defects. Chemotherapy in the second and third trimesters may be associated with low birthweight due to both significantly lower gestational age and substantial intrauterine growth restriction, but it is not associated with a significant risk for fetal malformation. However, exposure in the second and third trimesters may have nonteratogenic effects on the CNS, which develops throughout pregnancy.

In 1985, the National Cancer Institute established a registry for in utero exposure to chemotherapeutic agents. In the first 210 cases studied, there were 29 abnormal outcomes with a total of 52 anomalies. Of the 29 abnormal cases, 27 resulted from first-trimester exposure. Most patients had been treated for leukemia and lymphoma. Because data are voluntarily reported to this registry, bias toward and against abnormal outcomes may have been introduced (27). Nevertheless, this database may be crucial to our understanding of 1) the immediate effect of chemotherapy on fetal outcome and 2) long-term complications in persons exposed to chemotherapy in utero.

The long-term effects of chemotherapy given during childhood have begun to be reported only recently. For example, daunorubicin therapy, in the absence of radiation, has been associated with late echocardiographic abnormalities in 65% of survivors of childhood leukemia. These abnormalities may be progressive and may result in congestive heart failure (28, 29). As Garber (26) suggests, the experience of cancer survivors exposed to chemotherapy in childhood indicates several areas in which late manifestations of in utero exposure to chemotherapy may appear; these areas include physical growth, intellectual and neurologic function, gonadal function and reproductive capacity, transplacental mutagenesis of germ-line tissue, and transplacental carcinogenesis. Unfortunately, the delayed effects of chemotherapy in utero are essentially unknown. Avilés and co-workers (17) reported on 43 children 3 to 19 years of age; 19 of the 43 had received chemotherapy during the first trimester. The children were evaluated by history, physical examination, complete blood count (CBC), renal and hepatic tests, chromosome analysis, school visits, teacher evaluations, Wechsler intelligence tests, and Bender-Gestalt tests. All mothers had hematologic cancer: Eighteen had non-Hodgkin lymphoma (NHL), 14 had Hodgkin disease, 7 had acute leukemia, and 4 had chronic myelogenous leukemia. Alkylating agents, antimetabolites, anthracyclines, and vinca alkaloids were included in many treatment regimens. A control group of 25 nonrelated children with similar ages and environmental backgrounds was also evaluated. In all of the children studied, physical, neurologic, psychological, hematologic, immune function, and cytogenetic variables were normal. Another report, by Reynoso and associates (30), offers little further insight. Current data are insufficient to allow any meaningful comment on the late effects of exposure to chemotherapy in utero.

When chemotherapy is given during pregnancy, typical toxicities, including myelosuppression, will occur. Neutropenia in the mother will increase risk for maternal and fetal infection. The use of growth factors during pregnancy has not been documented. Exacerbation of the anemia of pregnancy may profoundly affect maternal well being and may have adverse hemodynamic effects. Significant thrombocytopenia will place the mother at risk for bleeding. Any of these complications, if they occur during delivery, can seriously complicate delivery; bleeding and infection in the mother and fetus are the most critical complications. Because myelosuppression is most manifest approximately 10 to 14 days after the administration of most chemotherapy regimens, it is recommended that chemotherapy not be given later than 21 days before delivery. In an unexpected delivery, erythrocyte and platelet support may be indicated.

Severe myelosuppression from exposure to chemotherapy in utero has been documented in newborns (17, 31, 32). Blood counts should therefore be checked and monitored in the early postpartum period. Many chemotherapeutic agents have been found in breastmilk, and breastfeeding is therefore contraindicated in women receiving chemotherapy (33–35). If a child has been exposed to chemotherapy in utero, his or her pediatrician should be alerted. Although no specific surveillance program can be recommended, knowledge of this exposure may guide evaluation of any abnormalities in physical, intellectual, or psychological development.

The decision to use chemotherapy during pregnancy is a highly personal one. It is made by the patient after extensive education and counseling done in a multidisciplinary setting according to the informed consent paradigm. Ideally, the management of cancers diagnosed during pregnancy is similar to the management of cancers diagnosed in the nonpregnant state. When possible, however, chemotherapy should be avoided during the first trimester, given the high risk for fetal malformation and spontaneous abortion associated with first-trimester use. For cancers diagnosed in the third trimester, chemotherapy may sometimes be deferred until after delivery without a decrease in efficacy, especially if the cancers are solid tumors that present in the last 2 months of pregnancy. Chemotherapy given in the second and third trimesters is not associated with a significant risk for fetal malformation, but we currently lack an understanding of the long-term effects of exposure to chemotherapy in utero. The National Cancer Institute maintains a registry of children exposed in utero to chemotherapy given for maternal cancer. To permit the systematic long-term follow-up of exposed persons and an accurate assessment of the incidence and nature of late complications of exposure, contributions to the registry are encouraged. The registry is maintained at the Oklahoma University Health Science Center, Children's Hospital Genetics Center, and one may register a case by calling 405-271-8685.

REFERENCES

1. **Antonelli NM, Dotters DJ, Katz VL, Kuller JA.** Cancer in pregnancy: a review of the literature. Part I. Obstetrical and gynecological survey. 1996;51:125-34.

2. **Potter JF, Schoeneman M.** Metastasis of maternal cancer to the placenta and fetus. Cancer. 1970;25:380-8.

3. **Buekers TE, Lallas TA.** Chemotherapy in pregnancy. Obstet Gynecol Clin North Am. 1998;25:323-9.

4. **Ries LAG, Kosary CL, Hankey BF, Miller BA, Harras A, Edwards BK, eds.** SEER Cancer Statistics Review, 1973-1994. Bethesda, MD: National Cancer Institute; 1997: NIH publication no. 97-2789.

5. **Shaw MW.** Conditional prospective rights of the fetus. J Leg Med. 1984;5:65-106.

6. Grodin v. Grodin. 102 Mich App. 396, 30 N.W. 2d, 1980; p869.

7. **DeVita VT Jr, Hellman S, Rosenberg SA.** The cell cycle, drug resistance, and the p53 tumor suppressor gene pathway. Cancer: Principles & Practice of Oncology, 5th ed. Philadelphia: Lippincott Williams & Wilkins; 1997;1:338-42.

8. **DeVita VT Jr, Hellman S, Rosenberg SA.** Pharmacology and cancer chemotherapy. Cancer: Principles & Practice of Oncology, 5th ed. Philadelphia: Lippincott Williams & Wilkins; 1997;1:405-83.

9. Cunningham FG, MacDonald PC, Gant NF, et al. Neoplastic diseases. In: Williams' Obstetrics, 19th ed. Norwalk, CT: Appleton & Lange; 1993;1267-9.

10. Falkenberry SS. Cancer in pregnancy. Surg Oncol Clin North Am. 1998;7:375-97.

11. Doll DC, Ringenberg S, Yarbro DW. Management of cancer during pregnancy. Arch Intern Med. 1988;148:2058.

12. Petrek JA. Breast cancer during pregnancy. Cancer. 1994;74:518-27.

13. Roboz J, Gleicher N, Wu K, Chahinian P, Kerenyi T, Holland J. Does doxorubicin cross the placenta? Lancet. 1979;2:1382.

14. Williamson RA, Karp LE. Azathioprine teratogenicity: review of the literature and case report. Obstet Gynecol. 1981;58:247-50.

15. Redmond GP. Effect of drugs on intrauterine growth. Clin Perinatol. 1979;6:5-19.

16. Turchi JJ, Villasis C. Anthracyclines in the treatment of malignancy in pregnancy. Cancer. 1988;61:435-40.

17. Avilés A, Diaz-Maqueo JC, Talavera A, Guzman R, Garcia EL. Growth and development of children of 16. mothers treated with chemotherapy during pregnancy: 17. current status of 43 children. Am J Hematol. 1991;36:243-8.

18. Nicholson HO. Cytotoxic drugs in pregnancy. J Obstet Gynaecol Br Cwlth. 1968;75:307-12.

19. Thiersch JB. Therapeutic abortions with a folic acid antagonist, 4-aminopteroylglutamic acid (4-amino PGA) administered by oral route. Am J Obstet Gynecol. 1952;63:1298-304.

20. Sokal JE, Lessmann EM. Effects of cancer chemotherapeutic agents on the human fetus. JAMA. 1960;172:151-7.

21. Sweet DL, Kinzie J. Consequences of radiotherapy and antineoplastic therapy for the fetus. J Reprod Med. 1976;17:241-6.

22. Sieber SM, Adamson RH. Toxicity of antineoplastic agents in man: chromosomal aberrations, antifertility effects, congenital malformations, and carcinogenic potential. Adv Cancer Res. 1975;22:57-155.

23. Gililland J, Weinstein L. The effects of cancer chemotherapeutic agents on the developing fetus. Obstet Gynecol. 1983;38:6-13.

24. Zemlickis D, Lishner M, Degendorfer P, Panzarella T, Sutcliffe SB, Koren G. Fetal outcome after in utero exposure to cancer chemotherapy. Arch Intern Med. 1992;152:573-6.

25. Barnicle MM. Chemotherapy and pregnancy. Semin Oncol Nurs. 1992;8:124-32.

26. Garber JE. Long-term follow-up of children exposed in utero to antineoplastic agents. Semin Oncol. 1989;16:437-44.

27. Randall T. National registry seeks scarce data on pregnancy outcomes during chemotherapy. JAMA. 1993;269:323.

28. Lipschultz SE, Colan SD, Gelber RD, Perez-Atayde AR, Sallan SE, Sanders SP. Late cardiac effects of doxorubicin therapy for acute lymphoblastic leukemia in childhood. N Engl J Med. 1991;324:808-15.

29. Lipschultz SE, Colan SD. The use of echocardiography and Holter monitoring in the assessment of anthracycline-treated patients. In: Green DM, D'Angio GJ, eds. Cardiac Toxicity after Treatment for Childhood Cancer. New York: Wiley-Liss; 1993:54-62.

30. Reynoso E, Sheperd FA, Messner HA, Fargharson HA, Garvey MB, Baker MA. Acute leukemia during pregnancy: the Toronto Leukemia Study Group experience with long-term follow-up of children exposed in utero to chemotherapeutic agents. J Clin Oncol. 1987;5:1098.

31. **Murray NA, Acolet D, Deave M, Price J, Roberts IA.** Fetal marrow suppression after maternal chemotherapy for leukemia. Arch Dis Child. 1994;71:F209-10.
32. **Raffles A, Williams J, Costeloe K, Clark P.** Transplacental effects of maternal cancer chemotherapy: case report. Br J Obstet Gynaecol. 1989;96:1099-100.
33. **Ben-Baruch G, Menczer J, Goshen R, Kaufman B, Gorodetsky R.** Cisplatin excretion in human milk. J Natl Cancer Inst. 1992;84:451-2.
34. **Egan PC, Costanza ME, Dodion P, Egorin MJ, Bachur NR.** Doxorubicin and cisplatin excretion into human breast milk. Cancer Treat Rep. 1985;69:1387-9.
35. **Briggs GG, Freeman RK, Yaffe SJ.** Drugs in Pregnancy and Lactation: A Reference Guide to Fetal and Neonatal Risk, 5th ed. Philadelphia: Lippincott/Williams & Wilkins; 1998; 722-6.

II. Abnormal Papanicolaou Smears
Donald Schmidt

Abnormal Papanicolaou (Pap) smears are common during pregnancy. In most cases, they result from benign abnormalities for which definitive treatment may be postponed until after delivery. However, in some patients, an abnormal Pap smear indicates the presence of a lesion that requires immediate assessment and treatment. A general understanding of abnormal Pap smears by all physicians who care for pregnant women is useful in coordinating patient care.

This discussion is intended as a brief summary to give the generalist or internist a basic understanding of the classification of Pap smears, the conditions that warrant concern, and the differences in treatment in pregnant and nonpregnant patients. It is not intended as a definitive source of treatment guidelines.

Cervical Carcinoma

Cervical carcinoma is the most common gynecologic cancer occurring in pregnancy. It is estimated to occur in approximately 1 in 2200 pregnancies (1) and is the eighth most common cancer in women. In theory, all cervical carcinomas can be prevented with early detection and simple treatment procedures.

The most common presenting symptom of cervical carcinoma is bleeding, although bleeding in pregnancy is more often associated with benign conditions, such as polyps, miscarriage, or placental separation. Despite this, bleeding in pregnancy should always alert the physician to check the Pap smear and review the patient's risk factors for cervical neoplasia.

Abnormal Pap Smears

With a few exceptions, assessment and treatment of the cause of an abnormal Pap smear are similar in pregnant and nonpregnant patients. The choice of a method and the timing of treatment during pregnancy should be individualized in each patient and may be altered by gestational age. In noninvasive lesions, definitive treatment might be postponed until after delivery. Treatment of reactive and benign changes is similar to that in nonpregnant patients. In the presence of low-grade or high-grade squamous intraepithelial lesions (LSILs or HSILs), colposcopy and directed biopsy are indicated. When colposcopic assessment is inadequate, cold-knife conization is preferred for excisional biopsy and pathologic examination; cryotherapy and endocervical curettage are contraindicated in pregnancy.

Origin of Abnormal Cervical Cells

In 85% of cases, cervical carcinoma is of the squamous cell variety; adenocarcinomas make up the remaining 15%. These two cell types make up the epithelial layer of the cervix and endocervical canal. Most abnormal cells originate from the squamocolumnar interface of the cervix (transformation zone), where squamous cells are actively replacing the columnar cells by squamous metaplasia. The active division of this area (which is increased during pregnancy) combined with exposure to bacteria, human papillomaviruses (HPVs), and other irritants provides the conditions that result in abnormal cells. Three other, rare types of cervical carcinoma exist: clear cell carcinoma, which is usually associated with DES exposure in utero, sarcoma, and lymphoma.

Infection with HPV has been associated with the presence of abnormal cervical cells and cervical dysplasia, and the likelihood of HPV infection increases with the severity of the dysplasia. In addition, some HPV types are associated with low-grade cervical dysplasia that is unlikely to progress to carcinoma and other types indicate a high risk for progression to carcinoma. Types 6, 11, 42, and 44 are considered low risk and have not been associated with carcinoma; types 16, 18, 31, and 33 are considered high risk (2) and have been associated with carcinoma. Clinical testing for HPV type may inform the physician and patient of the potential risk for cervical dysplasia and carcinoma, but this testing cannot be used as a way to determine treatment. Patients may carry more than one HPV type, and a single test may not show all of the types that are present. Patients may also contract additional HPV types after being tested. Because no treatment is available for HPV infection, HPV testing provides limited benefit and is currently used primarily as a research tool or an adjunct to Pap smear and biopsy.

Sampling Technique

The Pap smear is considered to be the most effective and simplest screening tool for cervical carcinoma, but the test has significant false-positive and false-negative rates. Ten percent to 25% of patients may have a false-negative Pap smear result in the presence of abnormal cells; this result may be related to both sampling and reading techniques. Proper sampling technique is very important in obtaining accurate results. Endocervical cell sampling tools, such as the Cytobrush, have been shown to be safe and effective during pregnancy (3). Patients should be warned about minimal bleeding after use of this type of sampling tool.

Another reason why a Pap smear may show false-positive or false-negative results is the test's inability to identify abnormal cells among large populations of normal or atypical squamous cells of undetermined significance (ASCUS cells). Computerized cell-analyzing systems now being studied will locate rare suspicious cells in large populations of normal and ASCUS cells and present them to the cytologist for more critical review. These systems are likely to increase the rate of early detection of premalignant cells. However, Pap smears reviewed by these systems will be more expensive, and these systems now offer only limited improvement in patient care. Currently, these systems are investigational and are not the standard of care.

Pap smear cell sampling must be directed to the transformation zone and endocervical canal and any area of suspicious appearance. One should remember that Pap smears are intended for screening in cervices of normal appearance and that any area of suspicious appearance requires biopsy. Inability to visualize the entire transformation zone may be an indication for cone biopsy. To facilitate cell sampling, the American College of Obstetrics and Gynecology (4) and others have offered the following suggestions:

1. Before doing a Pap smear, remove any vaginal or cervical discharge that may interfere with sampling.
2. The entire portio should be visualized and sampled first, then endocervical sampling should be done. In DES-exposed patients, the upper two thirds of the vagina may also be sampled. Endocervical brushes may be

used to increase the yield of endocervical cells, but the patient should be advised that spotting may occur.

3. Avoid contamination of cell specimens with lubricant, and test for sexually transmitted diseases after taking the Pap smear.

4. Do the bimanual examination after Pap smear sampling. Concentrate on ruling out any suspicious masses.

The Pap Smear Report and the Bethesda System

The standard Pap smear report describes the status of cytologic normality or abnormality and the status of the cervix with respect to inflammation and infection. Varying degrees of cytologic atypia, inflammation, infection, minimal changes of cervical neoplasia, and HPV effects are noted. The degree of cervical dysplasia is described.

Compared with the older, "class" method for reporting Pap smear results, the Bethesda System (5) has expanded descriptions in each category (Box 11-1). It is important to remember that cells from all potentially premalignant lesions should be included as ASCUS, LSILs, and HSILs. Normal cytologic findings include benign, reactive, or reparative changes. Abnormalities associated with bacterial, fungal, parasitic, or viral infection (such as herpes infection) are included in this group. The designation ASCUS includes cells that are not normal or are atypical in appearance but that do not meet the criteria for LSIL or HSIL. The ASCUS category contains cells that truly have undetermined significance and require close attention or diagnostic testing. Most are benign, but a few may contain premalignant cells. Usually, no more than 5% of Pap smears are reported as ASCUS. Koilocytosis is now included in the LSILs. The HSILs suggest the presence of moderate or severe dysplasia or carcinoma in situ.

Treatment

The management of pregnant and nonpregnant patients whose Pap smears have cells in the benign reactive, inflammatory, or infectious category is similar. Cervical and vaginal cultures are usually obtained at the first prenatal visit and can be correlated with Pap smear findings. Antibiotic therapy is based on the type of bacteria found on culture. No definitive evidence indicates that the use of metronidazole to treat *Trichomonas* species infection in the first trimester is harmful to the fetus, despite earlier concerns. Metronidazole is thought to be safe in the second and third trimesters as well. In addition to treating the cause of the Pap smear abnormalities, antibiotics may

Box 11-1 The Bethesda System for Reporting Cervical and Vaginal Cytologic Diagnoses

Format of the Report
1. A statement on Adequacy of the Specimen for Evaluation
2. A General Categorization that may be used to assist with clerical triage (optional)
3. Descriptive Diagnosis

Adequacy of the Specimen for Evaluation
Satisfactory for evaluation
Satisfactory for evaluation but limited by . . . (specify reason)
Unsatisfactory for evaluation . . . (specify reason)

General Categorization (Optional)
Within normal limits
Benign cellular changes: see descriptive diagnosis
Epithelial cell abnormality: see descriptive diagnosis

Descriptive Diagnosis
Benign cellular changes
  Infection
    Trichomonas vaginalis
    Fungal organisms morphologically consistent with *Candida* species
    Predominance of coccobacilli consistent with shift in vaginal flora
    Bacteria morphologically consistent with *Actinomyces* species
    Cellular changes associated with herpes simplex virus
    Other
Reactive changes
  Reactive cellular changes associated with:
    Inflammation (includes typical repair)
    Atrophy with inflammation ("atrophic vaginits")
    Radiation
    Intrauterine contraceptive device
    Other
  Squamous cell
    Atypical squamous cells of undetermined significance: qualify*
    Low-grade squamous intraepithelial lesion encompassing:†
      HPV
      Mild dysplasia/CIN 1
    High-grade squamous intraepithelial lesion encompassing:
      Moderate and severe dysplasia
      CIS/CIN 2 and CIN 3
    Squamous cell carcinomia

Box 11-1 The Bethesda System (*continued*)

Descriptive Diagnosis (*continued*)
Reactive changes (*continued*)
  Glandular cell
        Endometrial cells, cytologically benign, in a postmenopausal woman
        Atypical glandular cells of undetermined significance: qualify*
        Endocervical adenocarcinoma
        Endometrial adenocarcinoma
        Extrauterine adenocarcinoma
        Adenocarcinoma, not otherwise specified
  Other malignant neoplasms: specify
  Hormonal evaluation (applied to vaginal smears only)
      Hormonal pattern compatible with age and history
      Hormonal pattern incompatible with age and history: specify
      Hormonal evaluation not possible due to: specify

---

*Atypical squamous or glandular cells of undetermined significance should be further qualified as to whether a reactive or a premalignant/malignant process is favored.
†Cellular changes of human papillomavirus—previously termed *koilocytosis atypia* or *condylomatous atypia*—are included in the category of low-grade squamous intraepithelial lesion.
From National Cancer Institute Workshop. JAMA. 1989; 262:931-4.

---

prevent premature labor that is thought to be associated with certain types of bacterial vaginal infections. For optimal treatment of bacterial vaginosis in pregnancies at risk for premature labor, the combination of oral metronidazole and erythromycin provides the most complete bacterial-spectrum coverage.

If the Pap smear is the first with an ASCUS designation and no other abnormal findings (such as bleeding or an area of the cervix that has a suspicious appearance on visual examination) are present, a repeated Pap smear in 3 to 6 months is usually adequate "treatment." Seventy percent of ASCUS abnormalities are histologically benign. The risk for finding a cervical intraepithelial neoplasia (CIN) lesion with LSIL or HSIL after ASCUS is about 30%. The risk for invasive carcinoma is approximately 1 in 1000. Patient who have ASCUS on two consecutive Pap smears show LSIL or HSIL by colposcopy in 40% to 60% of cases. Because of concern that early lesions may be missed with ASCUS, many gynecologists use colposcopy and biopsy as part of the evaluation and treatment of ASCUS reports.

Patients with LSILs should have Pap smears at least every 4 to 6 months. Approximately 60% of LSILs regress spontaneously, and 15% progress to a greater level of abnormality (6). Any report of HSILs warrants colposcopy and biopsy. In nonpregnant women, 1% to 3% of excisional biopsies show a more severe category of dysplasia than that found on colposcopic biopsy. In pregnant patients whose suspicious lesions are not well documented or are not easy to follow with colposcopy, conization of the cervix or excisional biopsy may be warranted. A meta-analysis (7) combining data from several previous studies on the natural history and progression of cervical squamous intraepithelial lesions estimated the rates for progression to a worse category after 24 months of observation to be between 7.13% (for ASCUS) and 20.81% (for LSILs). The rate of progression to invasive cancer after 24 months of observation was highest for HSILs (1.44%) and lowest for LSILs (0.15%). Regression rates were highest for ASCUS (68.19%) and lowest for HSILs (35.03%).

Aggressive treatment of all patients with abnormal Pap smears would result in too many procedures and an excessively high cost of care because much of this treatment would be unnecessary. In addition, aggressive treatment that includes conization of the cervix can cause pregnancy complications. In pregnancy, conization of the cervix is usually reserved for more suspicious or dysplastic lesions when 1) colposcopic biopsy is inadequate or 2) a lesion of higher-level dysplasia is suspected and diagnosis and treatment are required before delivery. If done carefully and early, removal of dysplastic lesions by conization can be both diagnostic and therapeutic and can allow the pregnancy to continue its normal course.

Close observation with biopsy of premalignant lesions usually allows time for vaginal delivery, and definitive treatment may be given postpartum. If the biopsy specimen is consistent with invasive carcinoma, treatment of the cancer requires alteration of the duration of the pregnancy. First-trimester pregnancies may need to be terminated so that appropriate therapy can be initiated as soon as possible. In the second and third trimesters, early delivery to facilitate treatment might be appropriate. The timing of the delivery would depend on many factors, including the type and aggressiveness of the carcinoma; the likelihood of metastasis; the surgical, radiation, and chemotherapy options available; and the facilities of the intensive care nursery for premature infants.

Delivery might be indicated at the time of fetal lung maturity, as documented by amniocentesis. This maturity often occurs as early as 34 weeks of gestation, but it is unpredictable and may not occur until 38 to 39 weeks of gestation. In more critical cases, and if a high level of care is available in the nursery, delivery at 30 to 32 weeks of gestation may avoid the most serious newborn complications of intraventricular CNS hemorrhage and may allow the mother to be treated 8 to 10 weeks earlier. Figure 11-1 shows an algorithm for management of an abnormal Pap smear (8).

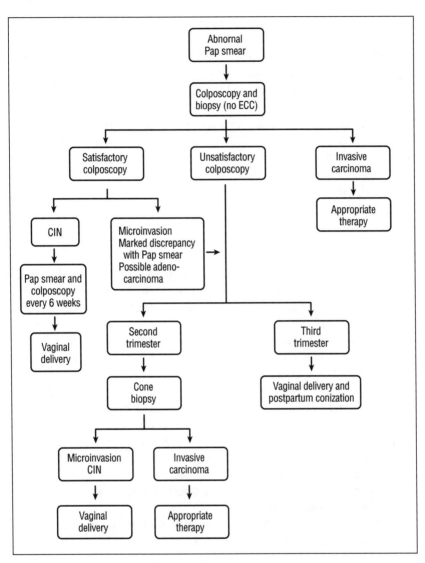

Figure 11-1 Algorithm for management of an abnormal Pap smear.

Human Immunodeficiency Virus Infection

It is known that women with immunosuppression, such as organ transplant recipients, or who have cancer or who are chronic corticosteroid users, are at increased risk for abnormal Pap smears and CIN. Consistent with this, HIV-infected women are more likely than HIV-negative women to have abnormal Pap smears (9). Rates of cervical dysplasia have been reported to be as high as

60% in HIV-infected women. After treatment, HIV-infected women are also more likely to have CIN recurrence; recurrence rates are as high as 62% in HIV-infected women compared with 18% in non–HIV-infected women (10). Although the Pap smear is thought to be an effective way to screen HIV-infected women for cervical abnormalities, many gynecologists proceed directly to colposcopic examination of the cervix in these patients. There is also a relation between the CD4+ T-lymphocyte count and the risk for CIN in HIV-positive women. Women with a CD4+ T-lymphocyte count less than 200 cells/mL have the greatest risk (11). In these patients, risks for recurrence of CIN of 87% have been reported. Progression to a higher-grade neoplasia is more likely in HIV-infected women.

Summary

1. Intervals for Pap smear screening and the treatment of vaginitis or benign findings are similar in pregnant and nonpregnant patients.
2. Bleeding is common in pregnancy but may be an early sign of dysplasia or carcinoma.
3. Pregnancy may accelerate growth of some types of carcinoma.
4. Colposcopy may allow diagnosis and close monitoring of atypical cells and CIN during pregnancy.
5. When colposcopic examination of the transformation zone is unsatisfactory, cold-knife conization is the preferred method for biopsy or complete excision of the transformation zone.
6. Electrocautery and cryotherapy are contraindicated in pregnancy.
7. Immunocompromised patients and patients with HIV infection may have accelerated cell growth and dysplasia.
8. If a preinvasive lesion is monitored closely, definitive treatment may be delayed until after delivery.
9. In the presence of invasive lesions, early termination of pregnancy or preterm delivery must be considered.

REFERENCES

1. **DiSaia PJ, Creasman WT, eds.** Preinvasive disease of the cervix, vagina and vulva. In: Clinical Gynecologic Oncology, 3d ed. St. Louis: Mosby; 1989:536-43.
2. **Ter Harmsel B, Smedts F.** Relationship between human papilloma virus type 16 in the cervix and intraepithelial neoplasia. Obstet Gynecol. 1999;93:46-50.
3. **Orr JW Jr, Barrett JM, Orr PF, Holloway RW, Holimon JL.** The efficacy and safety of the Cytobrush during pregnancy. Gynecol Oncol. 1992;44:260-2.
4. ACOG Technical Bulletin Number 183. Cervical Cytology: Evaluation and Management of Abnormalities. August 1993.

5. **National Cancer Institute Workshop.** The 1988 Bethesda system for reporting cervical/vaginal cytological diagnoses. JAMA. 1989;262:931-4.

6. **Montz FJ, Monk BJ, Fowler JM, Nguyen L.** Natural history of the minimally abnormal Papanicolaou smear. Obstet Gynecol. 1992;80:385-8.

7. **Melnikow J, Nuovo J, et al.** Natural history of cervical squamous intraepithelial lesions: a meta-analysis. Obstet Gynecol. 1998;92:727-35.

8. **Hacker NF, Berek JS, et al.** Carcinoma of the cervix associated with pregnancy. Obstet Gynecol. 1982;59:735.

9. **Maiman M, Fruchter RG, Serur E, Remy JC, Feuer G, Boyce J.** Human immunodeficiency virus infection and cervical neoplasia. Gynecol Oncol. 1990;38:377-82.

10. **Fruchter, RG, Maiman M, Sedlis A, et al.** Multiple recurrences of cervical intraepithelial neoplasia in women with the human immunodeficiency virus. Obstet Gynecol. 1996;87:338-44.

11. **Wright TC Jr, Ellerbrock TV, et al.** Cervical intraepithelial neoplasia in women infected with human immunodeficiency virus: prevalence, risk factors, and validity of Papanicolaou smears. Obstet Gynecol. 1994;84:591-7.

III. Hematologic Malignancies
Isabelle Bence-Bruckler

Fortunately, cancer during pregnancy is rare; cancer is estimated to complicate 1 in 1000 pregnancies (1). Leukemias and lymphomas are among the most common cancers in persons of reproductive age. Data on the management of such patients are limited to case reports and retrospective case series, making it impossible to formulate absolute guidelines. Each new case is a unique situation for both the hematologist–oncologist and the obstetrician. Management is complicated by restrictions in radiologic staging investigations and by the reluctance to initiate chemotherapy and radiation therapy during pregnancy. The health care team must ensure that an accurate diagnosis is made and must guide the patient and her family in making therapeutic decisions that will result in the best possible outcome for both mother and fetus.

The use of chemotherapy and radiation therapy in pregnancy raises obvious concerns. Much of the data on the teratogenicity of these therapies are derived from animal studies, the results of which can be difficult to extrapolate to humans. Similarly, interpretation of the literature must be done with caution because there may be a bias toward the reporting of specific outcomes. A few general statements, however, can be made.

The first concerns the risk for fetal malformation. Given a baseline rate of major congenital anomalies of 3% in the general population, chemotherapy does not seem to increase risk as long as it is not given during the first trimester (1–3). Many authors recommend therapeutic abortion if chemotherapy is required in the first trimester, but this is a complex issue and must be considered on an individual basis. An increased likelihood of spontaneous abortion and congenital anomalies is reported when chemotherapy is given in the first trimester; specifically, exposure to antimetabolites and alkylating agents seems to carry a risk for malformations of more than 25% (1, 2, 4). However, several cases with normal outcomes have been reported (2, 3). In support of this, a 1.3% incidence of fetal malformations was reported in a series of 150 patients undergoing chemotherapy in the second and third trimesters (1).

Compared with historical controls, an increase has been found in both intrauterine growth restriction and lower gestational age, resulting in lower-birthweight infants (2). There also seems to be an increased incidence of stillbirth, primarily in patients who have myelosuppressive chemotherapy for acute leukemia (5). Radiation to the abdominal and pelvic regions should not be given, and radiation that results in internal scatter and gives the fetus an exposure of more than 10 rads, particularly in the first trimester, should be avoided (6).

Delivery should be timed, when possible, to occur when blood counts have recovered from the effects of chemotherapy and the fetus is sufficiently mature. All newborns should undergo hematologic evaluation because pancytopenia can result from chemotherapy. Breastfeeding during chemotherapy is contraindicated because some agents cross into breastmilk.

The outcomes of children exposed to chemotherapy in utero are favorable; a review of 43 children (7), 19 of whom were treated during the first trimester, revealed normal growth and development and no childhood cancer.

The effect of pregnancy itself on leukemia and lymphoma has been addressed in several papers. Pregnancy involves a state of immune tolerance to prevent rejection of the fetus, so it is possible that cancers can behave more aggressively in this immunosuppressed milieu. In the case of lymphomas, no evidence supports an adverse effect of pregnancy on prognosis, as determined by case series comparing expected with observed survival (3, 8, 9). Survival is similar in pregnant and nonpregnant women with acute leukemia or chronic myeloid leukemia (CML) (5, 10, 11).

In the following discussion, specific issues in acute leukemia, CML, and the lymphomas are addressed.

Acute Leukemia

Acute leukemia is estimated to complicate fewer than 1 in 100,000 pregnancies (10, 11). When diagnosed, it presents a significant challenge to both the hematologist–oncologist and the obstetrician. If it is left untreated, median survival is less than 2 months. Therefore, it is necessary to rapidly formulate a comprehensive treatment plan, taking into account the complex medical, personal, ethical, and religious issues involved.

Acute leukemia, a cancer of immature marrow progenitor cells, is diagnosed when the bone marrow contains an increased number of blasts and the blasts make up more than 30% of the nucleated cells. Acute lymphoblastic leukemia (ALL) is common in childhood and has a lower incidence in adults; acute myeloid leukemia (AML) is rare in children and its incidence increases with age. There are several subtypes of AML and ALL (Table 11-2), and each subtype can have prognostic and therapeutic implications. A specific diagnosis is made with a combination of morphologic, cytochemical, immunophenotypic, and cytogenetic criteria.

In most cases, the cause of acute leukemia is unknown. Chemotherapy itself (specifically, the alkylating agents and the epipodophyllotoxins) can induce secondary AML. Radiation therapy and ionizing radiation have been linked to secondary leukemias. The adult T-cell leukemia–lymphoma virus, a retrovirus endemic in Japan and parts of the Caribbean region, is the etiologic agent of some T-cell cancers. Certain inherited conditions, such as ataxia telangectasia, common variable immunodeficiency, and Down syndrome, are also associated with an increased risk for hematologic cancers (mostly lymphomas).

The English-language literature contains more than 350 reports of leukemia during pregnancy (5, 11). In a review of 64 cases of acute leukemia diagnosed during pregnancy, there were 44 cases of AML and 20 cases of ALL (10). Most diagnoses were made in the later stages of pregnancy: Sixteen patients presented in the first trimester, 26 presented in the second trimester, and 30 presented in the third trimester. Of these 64 patients, 58 received chemotherapy during pregnancy: 13 in the first trimester, 22 in the second trimester, and 23 in the third trimester. There were 23 full-term births (43%) and 31 premature births (53%). Of the premature births, 5 were stillbirths. In addition, two elective and two spontaneous abortions were reported. There was only one congenital anomaly: an ocular abnormality occurring in a pa-

Table 11-2 Acute Leukemia*

Acute Myeloid Leukemia		Acute Lymphoblastic Leukemia	
Subtype	Description	Subtype	Description
M_0	Undifferentiated	L_1	Blast cells small, uniform, high nuclear cell to cytoplasmic cell ratio
M_1	Without maturation		
M_2	With granulocytic maturation	L_2	Blast cells larger, heterogeneous, lower nuclear cell to cytoplasmic cell ratio
M_3	Acute promyelocytic		
M_4	Granulocytic and monocytic maturation	L_3	Vacuolated blasts, basophilic cytoplasm
M_5	Monoblastic or monocytic		
M_6	Erythroleukemia		
M_7	Megakaryoblastic		

*French–American–British (FAB) classification.

tient who was not treated during the first trimester. Other case series report similar findings (3, 5).

Patients can present with symptoms of pancytopenia: fatigue from anemia, infection from neutropenia, and bleeding from thrombocytopenia. They can also have symptoms of headache, visual blurring, other neurologic deficits, pulmonary symptoms from hyperleukocytosis (blood blast count >100 $\times$ 10^9/L), and bone pain from marrow expansion.

Treatment involves multiagent myelosuppressive chemotherapy and results in prolonged hospitalization for pancytopenia, febrile neutropenia, bleeding, and transfusions. Standard therapy for AML is the combination of an anthracycline and cytarabine. This regimen induces marrow aplasia for a period of several weeks. About 75% of young patients will have a complete remission. Postremission therapy involves further consolidative chemotherapy; certain patients may undergo bone marrow transplantation. Patients who receive chemotherapy alone are seldom cured (median survival, 2 years). Young patients with chemosensitive AML who have transplantation during their first remission have a 50% rate of long-term disease-free survival (12). Transplantations done in second or subsequent remissions offer the possibility of cure, albeit at lower rates.

Standard induction therapy for ALL has historically involved vincristine, daunorubicin, prednisone, and L-asparaginase. Current protocols may include other active agents, such as cytarabine, methotrexate, etoposide, teniposide, 6-mercaptopurine, and cyclophosphamide, added either in the induction phase or the consolidation phase. Generally, these therapies are less myelosuppressive than AML treatment. Central nervous system prophylaxis is required and should include intrathecal chemotherapy and, in most cases, cranial radiation. Most protocols consist of many months of systemic chemotherapy followed by a maintenance phase. Adults can undergo transplantation during a first remission with results similar to those seen in AML. In adults, cure with chemotherapy alone is seen in less than 30% of patients; greater success is seen in the pediatric population, where 70% of patients can expect to be cured (13).

Although patients may become amenorrheic during therapy, most young women resume menses after completion of therapy. On the basis of a retrospective cohort study (14), women who receive standard chemotherapy in childhood and adolescence have no apparent decrease in fertility. Bone marrow transplantation, on the other hand, confers permanent infertility, with only a few exceptions (15–17).

Chronic Myeloid Leukemia

Chronic myeloid leukemia is a clonal stem-cell disorder that is classified as one of the myeloproliferative syndromes. It is characterized by a proliferation and accumulation of granulocytes resulting in peripheral leukocytosis with a left shift (bands, myelocytes, metamyelocytes), often with accompanying thrombocytosis. It is associated with the presence of the Philadelphia chromosome, a balanced translocation between chromosomes 9 and 22, which results in the formation of a chimeric *bcr-abl* gene. The presence of the Philadelphia chromosome or the *bcr-abl* transcript in a patient with leukocytosis is diagnostic of CML.

Patients with CML may be asymptomatic at diagnosis but more often present with fatigue, weight loss, and left upper-quadrant discomfort related to splenomegaly. The leukocyte count may be high and often exceeds 100×10^9/L.

The clinical course of CML begins with a chronic phase and proceeds to an accelerated phase, which transforms into a blast crisis. The chronic phase can last months to years (median duration, 4 years). The accelerated phase is characterized by a rapidly increasing leukocyte count along with increasing splenomegaly and hypermetabolic symptoms. In this phase, blood counts become more difficult to control. This phase transforms into a blast crisis, which is characterized by an increasing number of blasts in the marrow and blood and is, in effect, an acute leukemia. Median survival at this point is 6 months.

Treatment during the chronic phase consists of oral hydroxyurea, an antimetabolite, which normalizes blood counts but does not induce cytogenetic remission (Philadelphia chromosome–negative state). Busulphan, an oral alkylating agent, was used extensively in the past to treat CML. Its current role is limited because it has been shown to result in inferior survival compared with hydroxyurea (18). Interferon-alpha at high doses has the ability to convert a minority of patients (20%) to cytogenetic remission, which translates into a prolongation of survival (19). Up to 70% of patients with CML who have a matched sibling donor can be cured with bone marrow transplantation done early in the chronic phase (20).

In a pregnant patient in whom CML is diagnosed, two main issues arise. The first is the management of CML during the pregnancy; the second relates to definitive management of the CML, generally postpartum.

It may be possible to delay treatment until delivery if the patient is asymptomatic and the leukocyte count is not too high. Generally, one would not expect symptoms unless the count exceeds 50×10^9/L. Leukopheresis has been used successfully in some settings (21), although the decrease in the leukocyte count may last for only a few days. The use of hydroxyurea in pregnancy has been reported in five cases (22–25). In four of these cases, conception occurred during hydroxyurea therapy and the therapy was continued throughout pregnancy. Four women delivered healthy infants; the fifth developed eclampsia at 26 weeks and delivered a stillborn fetus that was phenotypically normal. There are four case reports of interferon-alpha use for CML in pregnancy (22, 26–28). Three patients conceived while receiving interferon, one initiated use of the drug in the first trimester, and one used the drug in the third trimester alone. All patients delivered healthy term infants. Additional data on the use of interferon in pregnancy come primarily from patients with essential thrombocythemia, another myeloproliferative syndrome seen in women of childbearing age. This disorder has been associated with an increased incidence of spontaneous abortion, intrauterine fetal death, and miscarriage, mainly on the basis of placental infarction from thrombosis. There are several reports of interferon use during pregnancy in this setting, all with good outcomes (29–35).

In summary, chronic-phase CML is relatively indolent and has the potential to be controlled during pregnancy. Definitive therapy, such as transplantation, can potentially be delayed to allow pregnancy to occur. This is particularly important because transplantation induces permanent infertility in almost all cases (15–17).

Lymphoma

The lymphomas are classified as Hodgkin lymphoma and NHL. Hodgkin lymphoma has an increased incidence in young adults and is therefore the lymphoma most often seen during pregnancy.

Hodgkin Lymphoma

Hodgkin lymphoma is a disease of young adults (mean age at diagnosis, 32 years), and this makes it the lymphoma most often diagnosed during pregnancy. It is divided into four histologic subtypes: nodular sclerosing, lymphocyte predominant, mixed cellularity, and lymphocyte depleted. Lymph node biopsy specimens contain the characteristic Reed-Sternberg cell, a Bilobed, multinucleated cell with nucleoli. Lymphocyte-predominant Hodgkin disease carries the most favorable prognosis, followed by nodular sclerosing, which is often seen in young adults and presents as limited-stage disease. Mixed-cellularity Hodgkin disease has a poorer prognosis and more often presents in an advanced stage.

The cause of Hodgkin lymphoma is not clear. The bimodal age distribution, with a peak in young adults and a second peak after age 55 years, suggests an infectious cause in young patients and an environmental cause in the elderly. The Epstein-Barr virus has been implicated, and Epstein-Barr virus DNA is detected in 20% to 80% of tumor specimens (36).

Patients most often present with painless cervical adenopathy; mediastinal adenopathy is the next most common presentation. Unexplained fever, night sweats, and weight loss are the "B symptoms" of Hodgkin lymphomas (and NHLs) and imply advanced-stage disease (stage III or IV). Pruritus can accompany the disease. On examination, the nodes are rubbery and nontender. Splenomegaly is rare.

Patients are staged in accordance with the Ann Arbor classification (Table 11-3), beginning with a detailed history and physical examination. Necessary studies include a CBC and serum biochemistry tests for renal and hepatic function, calcium, lactate dehydrogenase (LDH), and albumin (Box 11-2). Mild anemia is the most common hematologic abnormality, although the results of bone marrow examination are usually normal. Plain chest radiography, computed tomography (CT) of the thorax, abdomen, and pelvis, and bone marrow biopsy are required in nonpregnant patients. In pregnancy, chest ra-

Table 11-3   Ann Arbor Staging Classification for Hodgkin Lymphoma*

Stage	Definition
I	Involvement of a single lymph node region (I) or of a single extralymphatic organ or site (I_E)
II	Involvement of two or more lymph node regions on the same side of the diaphragm (II) or localized involvement of an extralymphatic organ or site and of one or more lymph node regions on the same side of the diaphragm (II_E)
III	Involvement of the lymph node regions on both sides of the diaphragm (III), which may be accompanied by involvement of the spleen (III_S) or by localized involvement of an extra lymphatic organ or site (III_E) or both (III_{SE})
IV	Diffuse or disseminated involvement of one or more extralymphatic organs or tissues, with or without associated lymph node involvement

*The absence or presence of fever, night sweats, and unexplained loss of 10% or more of body weight in the 6 months before admission are to be denoted in all cases by the suffix letters A (absence) or B (presence).

Box 11-2 Recommended Staging Evaluation for Hodgkin Lymphoma in Pregnancy

History and physical examination, including search for B symptoms
Complete blood count
Liver enzymes
BUN, creatinine, LDH, albumin, calcium
Erythrocyte sedimentation rate
Plain chest radiography (with abdominal shielding)
Ultrasonography of abdomen and pelvis*
Bipedial lymphangiography (if abdominal imaging negative)
Bilateral bone marrow aspiration and biopsy

*Consider MRI if abdominal disease is suspected.

diography should be done with abdominal shielding. To image the abdomen and pelvis, ultrasonography is useful if it reveals adenopathy or organomegaly. However, a normal result on ultrasonography does not exclude the presence of disease. Magnetic resonance imaging can be used instead of CT and does not expose the fetus to ionizing radiation. Bipedal lymphangiography, done more often in the past, is only useful if a positive result upgrades stage IIA disease to stage III disease, making the appropriate therapy combination chemotherapy rather than radiation therapy. In pregnancy, the use of bipedal lymphangiography should be limited to this setting. Similarly, staging laparotomy with splenectomy, which was used extensively in the past, is done less frequently. The reason for its use was to document occult abdominal disease in patients with normal abdominal imaging results. It is known that more than 50% of patients with clinical stage IIB disease have positive results on staging laparotomy, and most such patients receive combination chemotherapy protocols without laparotomy. Also arguing against staging laparotomy is the fact that highly effective salvage regimens exist for clinically staged stage I and IIA disease in patients in whom initial radiation therapy protocols fail.

Therapy is based on extent of disease. Patients with favorable early-stage disease may receive radiation alone; however, recent treatment strategies often include short-course chemotherapy combined with a less extensive radiation field. This results in long-term disease-free survival rates of 80% to 90%. Combination chemotherapy is used for stage III and IV disease, for stage IIB disease if the likelihood that staging laparotomy will reveal advanced-stage disease is high, and as part of combined-modality therapy in early-stage disease with bulky mediastinal masses. The combination chemotherapy regimen ABVD (adriamycin, bleomycin, vinblastine, and dacarbazine) results in complete remission in 70% to 80% of patients, much as MOPP (nitrogen mustard, vinblastine, procarbazine, and prednisone), used more frequently in the past, does (37, 38). Of responders, up to 30% will have relapse, and one third of those who have relapse become long-term disease-free survivors after salvage therapy or autologous bone marrow transplantation (39). Therefore, current therapy should cure about 70% of all patients with advanced-stage disease.

When Hodgkin lymphoma is diagnosed in pregnancy, it is important to stage the patient as accurately and safely as possible. In stage IA or IIA disease, radiation therapy can be given above the diaphragm with abdominal shielding until late in the third trimester. The inverted Y field cannot be used during pregnancy.

If the patient clearly has stage III or IV disease, chemotherapy is required. In selected cases, treatment may be deferred until after delivery (8), although this is done with some trepidation in patients with advanced-stage disease. Combination chemotherapy in the first trimester has been associated with an increased incidence of malformations and spontaneous abortion (1), although case reports of successful pregnancy outcomes in this setting do exist (3, 8). Specifically, alkylating agents and folic acid antagonists should be avoided because they lead to a 15% to 25% incidence of malformations (1, 4). Vinblastine as a single agent has been used with success for Hodgkin lymphoma during the first trimester (40). In a review of 14 patients treated with vinblastine in the first trimester, one congenital anomaly occurred (1). The risk for fetal malformations from chemotherapy in the second and third trimesters seems to be minimal (3).

Radiation therapy and chemotherapy can induce gonadal failure. Inverted Y radiation therapy generally involves the ovaries; in the past, when staging laparotomy was performed, oophoropexy was often done to avoid this. Most women remain fertile after standard ABVD chemotherapy for Hodgkin lymphoma; only 5% become amenorrheic (37). This is in contrast to the infertility rate of more than 50% seen in women older than 30 years of age who were treated with the MOPP regimen (41). Women who wish to become pregnant are counseled to delay conception until 2 years after treatment because most relapses will occur in those 2 years. Most patients who undergo autologous bone marrow transplantation for lymphoma relapse, however, are rendered permanently infertile (15–17).

Non-Hodgkin Lymphoma

Compared with Hodgkin lymphomas, NHLs present less often during pregnancy, are generally more aggressive, and generally have a poorer outcome (8, 42, 43). Some Hodgkin lymphomas are indolent, allowing therapy to be delayed until after delivery, but this is rarely the case with NHLs.

The NHLs are a heterogeneous group of diseases. Eighty-five percent arise from B cells and 15% arise from T cells. Numerous classification systems have been used. The most common in North America, the Working Formulation (44), was recently replaced by the Revised European-American Lymphoma (REAL) classification (Box 11-3) (45).

Most NHLs diagnosed in young patients are aggressive. The most common subtype is diffuse large-cell NHL, which often presents as advanced-stage disease. At diagnosis, most patients have painless adenopathy, and patients with advanced-stage disease can have fever, night sweats, and weight loss. Bone marrow involvement with advanced-stage disease is not uncommon. The staging classification for NHL is similar to that for Hodgkin lymphoma (see Table 11-3).

For patients with localized (stage I and II) aggressive NHL, an abbreviated course of CHOP (cyclophosphamide, doxorubicin, vincristine, prednisone) chemotherapy followed by involved-field radiation therapy has been proven to

---

Box 11-3   Revised European-American Lymphoma (REAL) Classification for Non-Hodgkin Lymphoma

---

Precursor B-lymphoblastic lymphoma or leukemia
B-cell chronic lymphocytic leukemia, prolymphocytic leukemia, or small lymphocytic leukemia
Lymphoplasmacytoid lymphoma
Mantle cell lymphoma
Follicular center cell lymphoma
   Grade I
   Grade II
   Grade III
   Diffuse, small cell
Extranodal marginal zone B-cell lymphoma (low-grade B-cell lymphoma of MALT type)
Nodal marginal zone B-cell lymphoma
Splenic marginal zone B-cell lymphoma
Hairy cell leukemia
Plasmacytoma or myeloma
Primary mediastinal large B-cell lymphoma
Burkitt lymphoma
High-grade B-cell lymphoma (Burkitt-like)
Precursor T-lymphoblastic lymphoma or leukemia
T-cell chronic lymphocytic leukemia
   T-cell type
   NK-cell type
Mycosis fungoides or Sézary syndrome
Peripheral T-cell lymphomas (unspecified)
Hepatosplenic γ-δ T-cell lymphoma
Angioimmunoblastic T-cell lymphoma

---

be superior to chemotherapy alone, resulting in a 5-year relapse-free survival rate of 77% (46). For patients with advanced-stage disease, CHOP has become standard therapy; 75% of patients achieve remission with a 5-year relapse-free survival rate of 45% (47). In cases of relapse of chemosensitive, aggressive NHL, high-dose therapy followed by autologous bone marrow transplantation cures 30% to 40% of patients and is superior to salvage chemotherapy alone (48).

At diagnosis, it is possible to predict the outcome of individual patients with aggressive NHL by using the International Prognostic Factors Index;

this model assigns scores for the adverse prognostic factors of age greater than 60 years, disease stage III or IV, elevated LDH level, two or more extranodal sites of involvement, and poor performance status (49). Patients are subdivided into four risk categories; 5-year survival rates range from 26% for the highest-risk group to 73% for the lowest-risk group. This is important because several studies are now addressing whether dose intensification (with autologous bone marrow transplantation) at diagnosis could improve survival in patients with poor prognosis.

Lymphoblastic and Burkitt lymphomas are very rare, are usually at an advanced stage at presentation, and require both intensive systemic therapy and CNS prophylaxis. Although remission can be achieved, many patients have poor prognostic features that keep relapse rates high; many current treatment strategies involve bone marrow transplantation as consolidative therapy.

Follicular or centrocytic lymphomas are rare in young patients. They are indolent diseases with a median survival of 8 to 10 years, but they remain incurable. Treatment is symptomatic; thus, if diagnosis occurs during pregnancy, therapy may be delayed until the postpartum period.

The literature currently contains more than 100 reports of NHL during pregnancy. Most women present with aggressive and advanced-stage disease (8, 42, 43) and require rapid treatment decisions. As in Hodgkin lymphoma, staging investigations are limited by the pregnancy. It is recommended that in this setting the following be done: complete history and physical examination, documentation of B symptoms, CBC, full biochemical profile including measurement of LDH, chest radiography with abdominal shielding, ultrasonography of the abdomen and pelvis, and bone marrow biopsy.

Although several reports of adverse maternal and fetal outcomes exist, many patients have been treated successfully (3, 8, 42, 43, 50–53). In a review of 19 women with NHL in pregnancy (43), 3 mothers (and their fetuses) died. The other 16 women underwent treatment; 8 of the 16 received chemotherapy during the first trimester. All 16 women delivered healthy infants with no malformations. The chemotherapies used were multiagent combinations of cyclophosphamide, doxorubicin, vincristine, prednisone, cytarabine, bleomycin, and methotrexate. Supradiaphragmatic radiation therapy with abdominal shielding has also been used for localized control of NHL in pregnancy. Although there is no safe dose of radiation during pregnancy, it is generally accepted that a fetal exposure of less than 10 rads is probably safe (6). There have been at least four reports of placental metastasis from NHL (54–57).

In summary, most NHLs in pregnancy are aggressive and present in an advanced stage. Chemotherapy should not be delayed because delay will compromise maternal and therefore fetal outcome. Combination chemotherapy has been given with success in this setting, particularly when initiated early in the course of disease.

Women treated for NHL are not likely to be rendered permanently infertile with standard chemotherapy. Autologous bone marrow transplantation, however, usually results in infertility, although case reports of subsequent pregnancy do exist (15–17).

REFERENCES

1. **Doll DC, Ringenberg QS, Yarbro JW.** Antineoplastic agents and pregnancy. Semin Hematol. 1989;16:337-46.

2. **Zemlickis D, Lishner M, Degendorfer P, et al.** Fetal outcome after in utero exposure to cancer chemotherapy. Arch Intern Med. 1992;152:573-6.

3. **Zuazu J, Julia A, Sierra J, et al.** Pregnancy outcome in hematologic malignancies. Cancer. 1991;67:703-9.

4. **Ebert U, Loffler H, Kirch W.** Cytotoxic therapy and pregnancy. Pharmacol Ther. 1997;74:207-20.

5. **Reynoso EE, Shepherd FA, Messner HA, et al.** Acute leukemia during pregnancy: the Toronto Leukemia Study Group experience with long-term follow-up of children exposed in utero to chemotherapeutic agents. J Clin Oncol. 1987;5:1098-106.

6. **Sutcliffe SB.** Treatment of neoplastic disease during pregnancy: maternal and fetal effects. Clin Invest Med. 19;8:333-8.

7. **Aviles A, Diaz-Maqueo JC, Talavera A, et al.** Growth and development of children of mothers treated with chemotherapy during pregnancy: current status of 43 children. Am J Hematol. 1991;36:243-8.

8. **Gelb AB, van de Rijn M, Warnke RA, et al.** Pregnancy-associated lymphomas. Cancer. 1996;78:304-10.

9. **Rodriguez J, Haggag M.** VACOP-B Chemotherapy for high grade non-Hodgkin's lymphoma in pregnancy. Clin Oncol. 1995;1995:445-54.

10. **Caligiuri MA, Mayer RJ.** Pregnancy and leukemia. Semin Oncol. 1989;16:388.

11. **McLain CR.** Leukaemia in pregnancy. Clin Obstet Gynecol. 1974;17:185-94.

12. **Clift R, Buckner C, Thomas E, et al.** The treatment of acute non-lymphoblastic leukemia by allogeneic marrow transplantation. Bone Marrow Transplant. 1987;1987:243-58.

13. **Rivera GK, Pinkel D, Simone JV, et al.** Treatment of acute lymphoblastic leukemia: 30 years' experience at St. Jude Children's Research Hospital. N Engl J Med. 1993;329:1289-95.

14. **Byrne J, Mulvihill J, Myers M, et al.** Effects of treatment on fertility in long term survivors of childhood or adolescent cancer. N Engl J Med. 1987;1987:1315-21.

15. **Lipton J, Derzko C, Fyles G, et al.** Pregnancy after BMT: three case reports. Bone Marrow Transplant. 1993;1993:415-8.

16. **Jackson GH, Wood A, Penelope R, et al.** Early high dose chemotherapy intensification with autologous bone marrow transplantation in lymphoma associated with retention of fertility and normal pregnancies in females. Leuk Lymphoma. 1997;28:127-32.

17. **Sanders J, Hawley J, Levy W, et al.** Pregnancies following high-dose cyclophosphamide with or without high-dose busulphan or total-body irradiation and bone marrow transplantation. Blood. 1996;1996:3045-6052.

18. **Hehlmann R, Heimpel H, Hasford J, et al.** Randomized comparison of busulfan and hydroxyurea in chronic myelogenous leukemia: prolongation of survival by hydroxyurea. Blood. 1993;82:398-407.

19. **Kantarjian HM, Smith TL, O'Brien S, et al.** Prolonged survival in chronic myelogenous leukemia after cytogenetic response to interferon-alpha therapy. Ann Intern Med. 1995;122:254-61.

20. **Champlin R, McGlave P.** Allogeneic bone marrow transplantation for chronic myeloid leukemia. In: Bone Marrow Transplantation. Boston: Blackwell Scientific Publications; 1994: 595-606.

21. **Fitzgerald JM, McCann SR.** Case report: the combination of hydroxyurea and leukapheresis in the treatment of chronic myeloid leukaemia in pregnancy. Clin Lab Haematol. 1993;15:63-5.

22. **Delmier A, Rio B, Bauduer F, et al.** Pregnancy during myelosuppressive treatment of chronic myelogenous leukaemia. Br J Haematol 1992;82:783-4.

23. **Tertian G, Tchernia G, Papiernik E, et al.** Hydroxyurea and pregnancy. Am J Obstet Gynecol. 1992;166:1868.

24. **Patel M, Dukes IAF, Hull JC.** Use of hydroxyurea in chronic myeloid leukemia during pregnancy: a case report. Am J Obstet Gynecol. 1991;165:565-6.

25. **Jackson N, Shukri A, Ali K.** Hydroxyurea treatment for chronic myeloid leukaemia during pregnancy. Br J Haematol. 1993;85:203-4.

26. **Baer MR, Ozer H, Foon KA.** Interferon-alpha therapy during pregnancy in chronic myelogenous leukaemia and hairy cell leukaemia. Br J Haematol. 1992;81:167-9.

27. **Crump M, Wang XH, Sermer M, et al.** Successful pregnancy and delivery during a-interferon therapy for chronic myeloid leukemia. Am J Hematol. 1992;40:238-43.

28. **Reichel RP, Linkesch W, Schetitska D.** Therapy with recombinant interferon alpha-2b during unexpected pregnancy in a patient with chronic myeloid leukaemia. Br J Haematol. 1992;82:472-3.

29. **Griesshammer M, Heimpel H, Pearson TC.** Essential thrombocythemia and pregnancy. Leuk Lymphoma. 1996;22:57-63.

30. **Vianelli N, Gugliotta L, Tura S, et al.** Interferon-alpha 2b treatment in pregnant woman with essential thrombocythemia. Blood. 1994;83:874-5.

31. **Petit JJ, Callis M, Fernandez de Sevilla A.** Normal pregnancy in a patient with essential thrombocythemia treated with interferon-alpha 2b. Am J Hematol. 1992;40:80.

32. **Pardini S, Dore F, Murineddu M, et al.** Alpha 2b-interferon therapy and pregnancy. Am J Hematol. 1993;43:78-9.

33. **Thornley S, Mancharan A.** Successful treatment of essential thrombocythemia with alpha interferon during pregnancy. Eur J Haematol. 1994;52:63-4.

34. **Williams JM, Schlesinger PE, Gray AG.** Successful treatment of essential thrombocythaemia and recurrent abortion with alpha interferon. Br J Haematol. 1994;88:647-8.

35. **Delage R, Demers C, Cantin G, et al.** Treatment of essential thrombocythemia during pregnancy with interferon-alpha. Obstet Gynecol. 1996;87:814-7.

36. **Pallesen G, Hamilton-Dutoit SJ, Rowe M, et al.** Expression of Epstein-Barr virus latent gene products in tumor cells of Hodgkin's disease. Lancet. 1991;337:320-2.

37. **Bonadonna G.** Modern treatment of malignant lymphomas: a multidisciplinary approach? Ann Oncol. 1994;5:5.

38. **Canellos GP, Anderson JR, Propert KJ, et al.** Chemotherapy of advanced Hodgkin's disease with MOPP, ABVD, or MOPP alternating with ABVD. N Engl J Med. 1992; 327:1478-84.

39. **Reece DE, Connors JM, Spinelli JJ, et al.** Intensive therapy with cyclophosphamide, carmustine, etoposide (cisplatin, and autologous bone marrow transplantation for

Hodgkin's disease in first relapse after combination chemotherapy. Blood. 1994;83: 1193.

40. **Peleg D, Ben-Ami M.** Lymphoma and leukemia complicating pregnancy. Obstet Gynecol Clin North Am. 1998;25:365-83.

41. **Schilsky R, Sherins RJ, Hubbard SM, et al.** Long-term follow-up of ovarian function in women treated with MOPP chemotherapy for Hodgkin's disease. Am J Med. 1981; 71:552-6.

42. **Ward FT, Weiss RB.** Lymphoma and pregnancy. Semin Oncol. 1989;16:397-409.

43. **Aviles A, Diaz-Maqueo JC, Torres V, et al.** Non-Hodgkin's lymphomas and pregnancy: presentation of 16 cases. Gynecol Oncol. 1990;37:335-7.

44. National Cancer Institute sponsored study of classifications of non-Hodgkin's lymphomas: the Non-Hodgkin's Lymphoma Classification Project. Cancer. 1982;49:2112-35.

45. **Harris NL, Jaffe ES, Stein H ea.** A revised European-American classification of lymphoid neoplasms: a proposal from the International Lymphoma Study Group. Blood. 1994;84:1361-92.

46. **Miller TP, Dahlberg S, Cassady JR, et al.** Chemotherapy alone compared with chemotherapy plus radiotherapy for localized intermediate- and high-grade non-Hodgkin's lymphoma. N Engl J Med. 1998;339:21-6.

47. **Fisher RI, Gaynor E, Dahlberg S, et al.** Comparison of a standard regimen (CHOP) with three intensive chemotherapy regimens for advanced non-Hodgkin's lymphoma. N Engl J Med. 1993;328:1002-6.

48. **Philip T, Gugliemi C, Hagenbeek A, et al.** Autologous bone marrow transplantation as compared with salvage chemotherapy in relapses of chemotherapy-sensitive non-Hodgkin's lymphoma. N Engl J Med. 1995;1995:1540-5.

49. **The International Non-Hodgkin's Lymphoma Prognostic Factors Project.** A predictive model for aggressive non-Hodgkin's lymphoma. N Engl J Med. 1993;329:987-94.

50. **Lishner M, Zemlickis D, Sutcliffe SB, et al.** Non-Hodgkin's lymphoma and pregnancy. Leuk Lymphoma. 1993;14:411-3.

51. **Nantel S, Parboosingh J, Poon MC.** Treatment of an aggressive non-Hodgkin's lymphoma during pregnancy with MACOP-B chemotherapy. Med Pediatr Oncol. 1990;18: 143-5.

52. **Lambert J, Wijermans PW, Dekker GA, et al.** Chemotherapy in non-Hodgkin's lymphoma during pregnancy. Neth J Med. 1991;38:80-5.

53. **Mavrommatis CG, Daskalakis GJ, Papageorgiou IS, et al.** Non-Hodgkin's lymphoma during pregnancy—case report. Eur J Obstet Gynecol Reprod Biol. 1998;79:95-7.

54. **Tsujimura T, Matsumoto K, Aozasa K.** Placental involvement by maternal non-Hodgkin's lymphoma. Arch Pathol Lab Med. 1993;117:325-7.

55. **Dildy GA 3d, Moise KJ Jr, Carpenter RJ Jr, et al.** Maternal malignancy metastatic to the products of conception: a review. Obstet Gynecol Surv. 1989;44:535-40.

56. **Kurtin PJ, Gaffey TA, Habermann TM.** Peripheral T-cell lymphoma involving the placenta. Cancer. 1992;70:2963-8.

57. **Pollack RN, Sklarin NT, Rao S, et al.** Metastatic placental lymphoma associated with maternal human immunodeficiency virus infection. Obstet Gynecol. 1993;81:856-7.

IV. Breast Cancer
Kimberly K. Leslie

This section addresses one of the most challenging diagnostic and treatment problems encountered in the care of pregnant women: breast cancer. The treatment of breast cancer is significantly affected by an ongoing pregnancy and results in an increased risk for poor outcome in the mother, often despite the best efforts of the care providers. This section reviews the definition, incidence, diagnosis, and treatment of breast cancer associated with pregnancy as well as normal physiologic changes that occur in the breast during pregnancy and contribute to the difficulty of diagnosing and treating breast cancer. The first question addressed is: How does pregnancy affect the incidence, treatment, and prognosis of breast cancer? The second question is: After a patient has been treated for breast cancer, what effect do subsequent pregnancies have on the disease? As a corollary: What effect does pregnancy have on a woman's lifetime risk for breast cancer? The available literature is often insufficient to definitively answer these questions, but current recommendations are discussed.

Incidence and Definition

The lifetime probability of developing breast cancer, assuming a lifespan of 85 years, is 13% for white women and 9% for black women (1). Most tumors occur in older women, but a subset of persons develop breast cancer early in life, during the childbearing years. Primarily because of the larger numbers of young women in the population, the number of premenopausal women with breast cancer is on the rise, and breast cancer is distinctly different in premenopausal and postmenopausal women. Specifically, younger women have worse survival outcome when matched with similarly-staged older women. Young women more often have positive lymph nodes, larger tumors, negative steroid hormone receptors, and a higher S-phase fraction (the percentage of cells in the DNA-synthesis stage of the cell cycle) (2). Why does breast cancer in younger women seem to be more aggressive than breast cancer in postmenopausal women? At least two factors play a role. First, more of the tumors in young women represent a form of familial cancer that occurs at an earlier age and is more aggressive in nature. Second, premenopausal women are more likely to have cancer associated with pregnancy, and pregnancy worsens prognosis.

Breast cancer is considered to be associated with pregnancy if it is diagnosed during pregnancy or within 1 year of delivery (3). Approximately 1 in

3000 to 10,000 women will receive a diagnosis of a malignant breast tumor that is associated with a pregnancy (4–6). In 32 series of women with breast cancer, 0.2% to 3.8% of patients had a pregnancy-associated tumor (7). So, taken in terms of all women with the disease, most of whom are post-menopausal, breast cancer in pregnancy seems to be rare. However, for pre-menopausal women, it is striking that 1 in 3 to 4 breast cancers is associated with pregnancy, according to the definition cited above (8, 9). In addition, given the several-year occult growth period of breast tumors, it is likely that many more cancers were present during and influenced by a preceding pregnancy, perhaps years before diagnosis. Association with pregnancy is a risk factor because 1) most studies confirm that the normal physiologic breast changes of pregnancy may mask a developing malignant mass and significantly delay diagnosis (10), 2) the elevated hormone levels seen in pregnancy may stimulate breast cancer growth, and 3) consideration of the developing fetus will affect the treatment options available to the mother.

Physiology and Anatomy

The breast is composed of two distinct cell populations: epithelial cells and mesenchymal cells. The epithelial cells line the ducts, and the mesenchymal cells make up the stroma. Beginning early in the course of pregnancy and continuing throughout gestation, the epithelial cells undergo rapid and profuse proliferation, altering the ratio of epithelial cells to mesenchymal cells and resulting in the dense, nodular, and engorged breasts characteristic of pregnancy (11). The lymphatics and blood vessels also increase significantly in size and number during pregnancy. Figure 11-2, A to C, shows the dramatic differences between the breasts of pregnant and nonpregnant women and a cancerous breast.

Breast hypertrophy is related to the significant increase in pregnancy-related hormones, including estradiol, estrone, estriol, progesterone, cortisol, insulin, and prolactin. Each of these hormones is involved in the increase in breast tissue and the maturation of the ducts and lobules required for lactation. Progesterone levels are increased more than 1000 times relative to nonpregnant levels, estrogen levels are increased more than 100 times, corticosteroid levels are increased 2 to 3 times, and insulin and prolactin levels are significantly elevated (12).

Steroid hormones, such as estrogen and progesterone, act through intracellular transcription factors called *steroid receptors*. Receptors for estrogen and progesterone are usually abundant in breast cancers. However, compared with breast cancers that are not associated with pregnancy, pregnancy-associated tumors have low or absent estrogen-receptor levels, a poor prognostic sign (13).

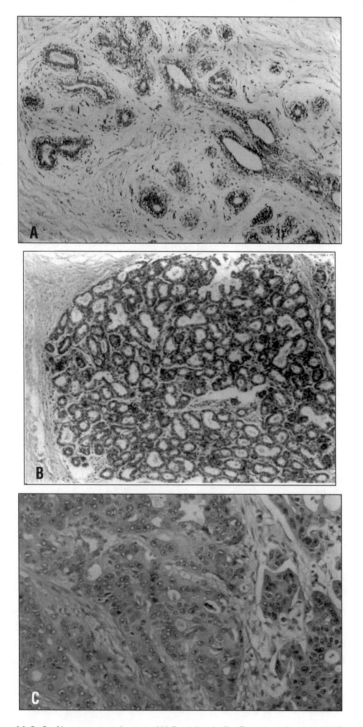

Figure 11-2 A, Nonpregnant breast; H&E stained. **B,** Pregnant breast; H&E stained. **C,** Cancerous breast; H&E stained.

The reason why low estrogen-receptor levels are characteristic of pregnancy-associated tumors is unclear. Estradiol and progesterone have been reported to downregulate estrogen receptors in the breast (14), and it is tempting to speculate that the very high circulating levels of these hormones cause the scarcity of receptors usually seen in pregnancy-associated tumors.

Why do low estrogen-receptor levels mean a worse prognosis? This question, which addresses an important area in tumor biology, has not been fully answered. It is assumed that receptors are indicative of a well-differentiated tumor, one that—like normal breast cells—depends on estrogens and progesterone to stimulate epithelial cell growth. In contrast, the tumor with few receptors or mutated receptors (15) has escaped the need for hormonal stimulation and presumably has acquired a mutation (as in a tumor suppressor gene or one leading to constitutive growth factor expression) that drives growth independent of hormones. Hormone independence characterizes breast cancers that are poorly differentiated and more anaplastic than the more common, hormone-dependent cancers. Unfortunately, they also seem to characterize tumors found during or shortly after pregnancy.

Does this mean that the hormones of pregnancy are not involved in tumor progression during pregnancy? It is hypothesized that many hormone-independent tumors were originally stimulated by hormones and expressed steroid receptors in levels adequate to promote this response (16). Therefore, although most investigators believe that hormones do not *cause* breast cancer, it is likely that the high hormone levels seen in pregnancy do drive the growth of some tumors and may be a factor in the rapid progression characteristic of certain breast cancers in pregnancy. On the other hand, the deleterious effects of pregnancy hormones on breast cancer growth have been legitimately debated because, as discussed below, the termination of pregnancy after a diagnosis of breast cancer does not seem to improve outcome in many patients.

Diagnosis

Epithelial cell hypertrophy and resultant breast enlargement make it difficult to diagnose breast cancer during pregnancy. A dominant mass is less likely to be palpable during pregnancy, and mammography—the most important diagnostic test used in the workup of a breast mass—is unreliable. Consequently, diagnosis is delayed 9 to 15 months from the time of symptom onset in pregnancy. The average tumor size at diagnosis is 3.5 cm in pregnant women and less than 2 cm in nonpregnant women. The most common symptoms experienced by women with breast cancer during pregnancy are a new dominant mass and nipple discharge.

In general, patients with a dominant mass or abnormal nipple discharge during pregnancy should have the same diagnostic workup as their nonpregnant counterparts. Many pregnant women have nipple discharge during pregnancy, but the discharge is usually clear or slightly milky and arises from multiple ducts. For the purposes of this discussion, abnormal nipple discharge is considered to be present if only one duct is involved or if the discharge is bloody or purulent. If this type of discharge is present or if a dominant mass is palpable, workup should be undertaken without delay.

In pregnancy, mammography is acceptable with regard to fetal radiation exposure. However, it is likely to be nondiagnostic because of the density of the pregnant breast, and it cannot be relied on to rule out cancer. In a study of eight pregnant women with confirmed breast cancer who had mammography, six of the eight mammograms showed negative results (17). Ultrasonography can be used to distinguish fluid-filled cysts from solid masses. If cysts are present, the fluid should be aspirated and sent for cytologic evaluation if it is bloody. Many practitioners believe that if the fluid is clear, cytologic evaluation is unnecessary. However, the mass should be monitored to ensure that fluid does not re-accumulate. Fine-needle aspiration of a solid mass is less accurate in pregnancy because of the normal hyperplastic epithelial changes associated with pregnancy, and the results of this procedure must be interpreted by an experienced pathologist. Not infrequently, fine-needle aspiration of breast masses during pregnancy is nondiagnostic and the masses may be falsely labeled malignant (18). Therefore, if a solid mass is found, surgical excision is standard and can usually be done under local anesthesia, although general anesthesia is not contraindicated in pregnancy (12). Excisional biopsy may be complicated by infections, hematomas, and milk fistulas. Therefore, prophylactic antibiotics should be given, and patients should consider discontinuation of breastfeeding if biopsy is done in the postpartum period (19).

Staging

Once carcinoma of the breast is diagnosed, staging must be done to rule out metastatic disease. This is important because a surgical cure is unlikely if metastatic disease is present. In addition to taking a complete history and doing a detailed physical examination, the physician should order laboratory tests. These tests should include a CBC and a biochemical analysis with liver function tests. Radiologic tests are also indicated, and most are within the acceptable range with respect to fetal radiation exposure (this exposure should total no more than 5 cGy [mrads] over the duration of the pregnancy). Fortunately, most screening tests result in far lower exposures. For example, chest radiography, which is indicated in the staging workup of all patients, results in an exposure of approximately 0.008 cGy when abdominal shielding is used. Nuclear magnetic resonance is currently accepted as safe in pregnancy and may be preferable to CT, but CT is not generally contraindicated in pregnancy. For clinical stage I and II disease, bone scanning is not indicated unless the patient has symptoms or serum chemistry results suggestive of bone involvement. Caution must be used in the interpretation of serum alkaline phosphatase because alkaline phosphatase from the placenta increases normal values during pregnancy. However, for clinical stage III disease, a modified bone scan done using maternal hydration, as reported by Baker and co-workers (20), will reduce fetal radiation exposure to a very acceptable 76 milirems (mrem) resulting from the isotope 99m-Tc. Unless the patient has CNS symptoms, brain scans are rarely done.

Treatment

The general approach to the treatment of breast cancer is the same in pregnant and nonpregnant patients. However, for disease that is clinically nonmetastatic according to the staging evaluation, modified radical mastectomy is standard for pregnancy-associated breast cancer. Unfortunately, lumpectomy with radiation therapy, a popular option for women with early disease who are not pregnant, provides unacceptably high doses of radiation to the fetus. The fetal radiation dose is 0.2% to 2.0% of the maternal dose (21). Thus, with the dose of 5000 cGy used in standard radiation therapy, expect the fetus to receive 10 cGy in early pregnancy and 200 cGy in late pregnancy. Because these doses exceed the recommended limit for the total pregnancy (5 cGy), breast conservation with radiation therapy is not recommended in pregnancy (22, 23).

For surgery (as stated above, this will generally be modified radical mastectomy), general anesthesia is indicated. Antacids should be given to increase the gastric pH because of the increased risk for aspiration seen in pregnancy. Prolonged preoxygenation should be done before endotracheal intubation, and intraoperative fetal monitoring should be considered so that anesthesia can be adjusted to avoid fetal hypoxia. Postoperative external uterine monitoring should be done to rule out preterm labor, and postoperative tocolysis should be instituted if necessary.

For stage II or greater disease, chemotherapy is indicated. Chemotherapy with a combination of cyclophosphamide, adriamycin, and 5-fluorouracil (CAF) rather than cyclophosphamide alone is standard. Most clinicians avoid use of the folate inhibitor methotrexate during pregnancy because reported malformation rates are 17% to 25% with methotrexate and 6% with cyclophosphamide alone (24). These figures can be compared with the baseline malformation rate of 3% in the general population. In addition to malformations, fetal growth abnormalities may result from chemotherapy. In one report (25), almost 40% of infants exposed to chemotherapy in utero were growth restricted. Therefore, one should consider delaying chemotherapy for several weeks if the diagnosis is made in the middle of the third trimester or later, after 30 to 32 weeks of gestation. This would allow time for steroids to be given to assist in fetal lung maturation before an indicated preterm delivery is performed.

The role of therapeutic abortion in the management of breast cancer in pregnancy has been debated. An evolution in thinking has occurred in the past two decades. It is now believed that a therapeutic abortion has no benefit for the mother (26, 27). However, an abortion may be indicated if significant fetal effects are expected to result from therapy—that is, if the diagnosis is made in early pregnancy.

Prognosis

Stage for stage, outcomes are the same in pregnant and nonpregnant women (28, 29). However, pregnant women present with more advanced disease: Twenty-eight percent present in stage I, 30% present in stage II, and 47% present in stages III and IV (12). Lymph node metastasis is present in 65% of patients with pregnancy-associated breast cancer. The overall survival rate is 70% (30). The 5-year survival rate for patients with negative nodes in pregnancy is 82%; this is identical to the rate seen in nonpregnant patients (10).

Effects of Subsequent Pregnancies on Prognosis in Breast Cancer

The most recent literature indicates that subsequent pregnancy does not result in a poorer outcome for women who have been treated for breast cancer (31). However, it is prudent to wait 2 to 5 years after diagnosis and treatment to ensure that recurrence is not imminent (3). It is interesting to ask: What is the effect of pregnancy on the incidence of breast cancer? In a large Scandinavian study (32), the incidence of breast cancer over a woman's lifetime significantly decreased as a function of the number of pregnancies delivered. If the hormones of pregnancy stimulate breast cancer progression and development, how can this finding be explained? Definitive answers are lacking, but it can be hypothesized that the protective nature of pregnancy is associated with extensive involution of the breast in the postpartum, postlactation period. Only at this point in a woman's reproductive life does the most complete quiescence of the breast epithelium occur. Perhaps this period of involution, associated with extensive apotosis of the breast epithelium, provides long-term protection against cancer.

REFERENCES

1. **Feuer EJ, Wun LM, Boring CC, et al.** The lifetime risk of developing breast cancer. J Natl Cancer Inst. 1993;85:848-9.

2. **Albain KS, Allred DC, Clark GM.** Breast cancer outcome and predictors of outcome: are there age differentials? Monogr Natl Cancer Inst. 1994;16:35-42.

3. **Petrek JA.** Breast cancer and pregnancy. Monogr Natl Cancer Inst. 1994;16:113-21.

4. **White TT.** Carcinoma of the breast in pregnancy. Ann Surg. 1979;139:9-18.

5. **Peete CH, Honeycutt HC, Cherny WB.** Cancer of the breast in pregnancy. N C Med J. 1966;27:514-20.

6. **Anderson JM.** Mammary cancers in pregnancy. BMJ. 1979;1:1124-7.

7. **Wallack MK, Wolf JA Jr, Bedwinek J, et al.** Gestational carcinoma of the female breast. Curr Probl Cancer. 1983;7:1-58.

8. **Horsley JS 3d, Alrich EM, Wright CB.** Carcinoma of the breast in women 35 years of age or younger. Ann Surg. 1969;196:839-43.

9. **Finn WF.** Pregnancy complicated by cancer. Bull Margaret Hague Maternity Hospital. 1952;5:2-6.

10. **Petrek JA, Dukoff R, Rogatko A.** Prognosis of pregnancy-associated breast cancer. Cancer. 1991;67:869-72.

11. **Canter JW, Oliver GC, Zaloudek CJ.** Surgical diseases of the breast during pregnancy. Clin Obstet Gynecol. 1983;26:853-64.

12. **Fiorica JV.** Special problems: breast cancer and pregnancy. Obstet Gynecol Clin North Am. 1994;21:721-32.

13. **Hubay CA, Barry FM, Marr CC.** Pregnancy and breast cancer. Surg Clin North Am. 1978;58:819-31.

14. **Berkenstam A, Glaumann H, Martin M, Gustafsson JA, Norstedt G.** Hormonal regulation of estrogen receptor messenger ribonucleic acid in T47Dco and MCF-7 breast cancer cells. Mol Endocrinol. 1989;3:22-8.

15. **Leslie KK, Tasset DM, Horwitz KB.** Functional analysis of a mutant estrogen receptor isolated from T47Dco breast cancer cells. Am J Obstet Gynecol. 1992;166:1053-61.

16. **Clarke R, Brunner N, Katzenellenbogen BS, Thompson EW, Norman MJ, Koppi C, et al.** Progression of human breast cancer cells from hormone-dependent to hormone-independent growth both in vitro and in vivo. Proc Natl Acad Sci U S A. 1989;86:3649-53.

17. **Max MH, Klamer TW.** Pregnancy and breast cancer. South Med J. 1983;76:1088-90.

18. **Finley JL, Silverman JC, Lannin DR.** Fine needle aspiration of cytology of breast masses in pregnancy and lactating women. Diagn Cytopathol. 1989;5:255-9.

19. **Byrd BF Jr, Bayer DS, Robertson JC, et al.** Treatment of breast tumors associated with pregnancy and lactation. Ann Surg. 1962;155:940-7.

20. **Baker J, Ali A, Groch MW, et al.** Bone scanning in pregnant patients with breast carcinoma. Clin Nucl Med. 1987;12:519-24.

21. National Council on Radiation Protection and Measurements Report #39. Basic Radiation and Protection Criteria. Washington, DC: National Council on Radiation Protection Productions; 1971.

22. **Donegan WL.** Pregnancy and breast cancer. Obstet Gynecol. 1977;50:244-51.

23. **International Commission on Radiological Protection and International Commission on Radiation Units and Measurements.** Exposure of man to ionizing radiation arising from medical procedures. Phys Med Biol. 1957;2:107-51.

24. **Doll DC, Ringenberg S, Yarbro JW.** Management of cancer during pregnancy. Arch Intern Med. 1988;148:2058-64.

25. **Sweet DL, Kinzie J.** Consequences of radiotherapy and antineoplastic therapy for the fetus. J Reprod Med. 1976;17:241-6.

26. **Nugent P, O'Connell TX.** Breast cancer and pregnancy. Arch Surg. 1985;120:1221-4.

27. **King RM, Welch JS, Martin JL, et al.** Carcinoma of the breast associated with pregnancy. Surg Gynecol Obstet. 1985;160:228-32.

28. **Haagensen CD.** Carcinoma of the breast in pregnancy. In: Haagensen CD, ed. Diseases of the Breast, 2d ed. Philadelphia: WB Saunders; 1971:660-8.

29. **Peters MV.** The effect of pregnancy in breast cancer. In: Forrest APM, Kunkler PB, eds. Prognostic Factors in Breast Cancer. Baltimore: Williams & Wilkins; 1968:65-80.

30. **Ribiero G, Palmer M.** Breast carcinoma associated with pregnancy: a clinician's dilemma. BMJ. 1977;2:1524-7.

31. **Wallack MK, Wolf JA Jr, Bedwinek J, et al.** Gestational carcinoma of the female breast. Curr Probl Cancer. 1983;7:1-58.

32. **Albreksten G, Heuch I, Kvale G.** The short-term and long-term effect of a pregnancy on breast cancer risk: a prospective study of 802,457 parous Norwegian women. Br J Cancer. 1995;72:480.

APPENDIX: CHEMOTHERAPEUTIC AGENTS

The table on page 658 is for reference when there is a clinical indication for treatment with one of the chemotherapeutic agents listed. Decisions about their use in pregnancy should be made on the basis of a benefit-to-risk ratio, avoiding unnecessary treatment of symptoms but with consideration of the fact that fetal well-being depends on maternal well-being. We have classified these chemotherapeutic agents as follows:

Data Suggest Agent Use May Be Justified When Indicated
When data and/or experience supports the safety of the agent.

Data Suggest Agent Use May Be Justified in Some Circumstances
When less extensive or desirable data are reported but the agent is reasonable as a second-line therapy or may be used on the basis of the severity of maternal illness.

Data Suggest Agent Use Is Rarely Justified
Use agent only when alternatives supported by more experience and/or a better safety profile are not available.

Pregnancy pharmacokinetics may necessitate a significant increase in dose or frequency, and dosing recommendations may require modification according to individual circumstances.

Chemotherapeutic Agents

	Use May Be Justified When Indicated	Use May Be Justified in Some Circumstances	Use Is Rarely Justified	Comments*/ Dose Adjustments†
Adriamycin		√		Long-term cardiac effects on fetus not known
Azathioprine	√			Teratogenic in animals; no adverse effects reported in human transplant recipients
Carboplatin		√		Case reports of renal and cardiac anomalies
Chlorambucil		√		
Corticosteroids	√			
Cyclophosphamide		√		Case reports of anomalies with 1st trimester exposure; IUGR after exposure; all alkylating agents can cause premature ovarian failure
5-Fluorouracil			√	Antimetabolites are of uncertain safety in 2nd and 3rd trimester

*Chemotherapy is contraindicated during first trimester.
†No data support dose adjustments.

CHAPTER 12

Neurologic Disorders

I. Headaches
Linda Anne Barbour, MD, MSPH

II. Cerebrovascular Disease
Lucia Larson, MD

III. Epilepsy
Linda Anne Barbour, MD, MSPH, and Jeffrey Pickard, MD

IV. Bell Palsy and Nerve Entrapment Syndromes
Lucia Larson, MD, and Richard V. Lee, MD

V. Myasthenia Gravis
Lucia Larson, MD

VI. Multiple Sclerosis
Lucia Larson, MD

I. Headaches
Linda Anne Barbour

Nearly one in five women have migraine headaches and, as a result, headache is the most common neurologic disorder seen during pregnancy (1). Migraines in women are significantly influenced by hormonal changes, including those that occur in pregnancy, and treatment must be modified accordingly. Some serious headaches more common or exclusive to pregnancy must be differentiated from migraine headaches, requiring further investigation by the practitioner.

Natural History of Migraine in Pregnancy

There is no specific entity known as "migraine of pregnancy" because in the largest studies, many women with migraine have had improvement in the second and third trimesters (Table 12-1) (2–5). If migraine worsens or occurs for the first time in association with pregnancy, it tends to do so during the first trimester or in the postpartum period, when estrogen levels fluctuate or decrease (6). Sustained high estrogen levels have been suggested as a mechanism of migraine relief, and alleviation of headache may be most common with menstrual migraine. Despite medication use, pregnant women with migraines do not have higher risks for miscarriage, congenital malformations, stillbirth, or preeclampsia–eclampsia (2).

Differential Diagnosis

Headaches other than migraines must be differentiated from migraines during pregnancy. Tension headaches are much less likely than migraines to improve over the course of gestation, and some sinus headaches may worsen and be exacerbated by the "stuffy nose of pregnancy" caused by estrogen-mediated nasal mucosal edema. Headaches that occur more often or only during pregnancy and that require immediate investigation include those associated with preeclampsia–eclampsia, choriocarcinoma, stroke, cerebral venous thrombosis (CVT), subarachnoid hemorrhage (SAH), and pituitary adenoma (Box 12-1). Idiopathic intracranial hypertension (pseudotumor cerebri) is a rare disease that occurs in women (often obese women) of childbearing age. It

Table 12-1 Natural History of Migraine in Pregnancy

	Bousser et al. (2)	Granella et al. (3)	Chen and Leviton (4)
Pregnancies with migraine	147	943	484
New migraine during pregnancy	16/147 (11%)	12/943 (1.3%)	
Previous migraine	131	571	484
Previous migraine improved	102/131 (78%)	384/571 (67%)	382/484 (79%)
Previous migraine unchanged or worse	29/131 (22%)	187/384 (33%)	102/484 (21%)

is thought by most to occur more often in pregnancy, and it may worsen during pregnancy (7, 8). Women with this condition often present with headache, blurred vision, diplopia, tinnitus, and nausea. On examination, they may show papilledema, abducens nerve palsy, and visual-field deficits.

Cerebral venous thrombosis is more common during the first 4 weeks after delivery, and headache is an almost universal symptom of CVT (9). This thrombosis is often related to cesarean section, dehydration, hypercoagulable states, infection, or hyperviscosity and can be missed by computed tomography (CT) (9, 10). Severe headache of sudden onset and extended duration may result from SAH or unruptured aneurysm. Hemorrhage from an aneurysm is often into the subarachnoid space; therefore, focal neurologic deficits may be absent, as in hypertensive encephalopathy. Premonitory headaches may occur in as many as 50% of patients (11).

The evaluation of headache during pregnancy or the postpartum period requires a thorough history and neurologic and opthalmoscopic examinations (12). If the results of these examinations are normal and the headache is chronic, no further evaluation is needed. However, especially after the first trimester, women who present with new-onset or worsened headache, progressive intractable or atypical headache, increased frequency or severity of headache, new focal headache (especially with aura), or new-onset neurologic symptoms or signs should undergo CT with or without contrast, magnetic

---

Box 12-1 Causes of Headache in Pregnancy

Common causes
  Migraine
  Tension
Causes specific to pregnancy
  Preeclampsia/eclampsia
  Choriocarcinoma
Vascular causes
  Aneurysm
  Arteriovenous malformation
  Cerebral venous thrombosis
Craniospatial causes
  Pituitary adenoma
  Pseudotumor cerebri
Other causes
  Sinusitis
  Meningitis

resonance imaging (MRI), or magnetic resonance angiography (MRA). With abdominal shielding, these procedures produce only minimal radiation to the fetus, and it is important to make the proper diagnosis without delay (1). Standard CT of the head exposes the uterus to less than 1 mrad of radiation, and MRI induces an electric field that increases core temperature by less than 1°F. Contrast angiography and MRA are also safe when indicated. Computed tomography is the study of choice for head trauma and possible nontraumatic, subarachnoid, subdural, or intraparenchymal hemorrhage. However, MRI is better for nontraumatic or nonhemorrhagic craniospatial conditions. One should use MRA to evaluate suspected vascular pathologic lesions. Lumbar puncture should be done if there is concern about infection, pseudotumor, or subarachnoid bleeding not detected on CT.

Treatment

In the treatment of migraine, it is imperative to attempt to identify and remove triggers of migraine, including sleep deprivation, stressors, and dietary changes. If the headache does not respond to rest, reassurance, ice packs, and fluids, pharmacologic treatment is indicated (1). Acetaminophen, caffeine, metaclopramide, prochlorperazine, cyproheptadine, intranasal lidocaine, narcotics (such as propoxyphene, hydromorphine, morphine, meperidine, methadone, oxycodone, butorphanol, and codeine), corticosteroids (preferably prednisone), and very brief courses (<48 hours) of nonsteroidal anti-inflammatory drugs (NSAIDs) can be used safely during pregnancy in attempts to terminate an acute migraine (see the Drug Table for Migraines at the end of this chapter). Cyclobenzaprine can be useful in tension headaches. Long-term use of NSAIDs or aspirin in analgesic doses can cause narrowing or premature closure of the PDA at term, hemostatic abnormalities in the newborn, oligohydramnios, and renal insufficiency and can inhibit labor. Vasoactive agents, such as ergotamines or sumitriptan, should be avoided altogether because of concern about uteroplacental vasoconstriction and insufficiency. Benzodiazepines or barbiturates may be used very sparingly in the second and early third trimesters; they have been associated with congenital anomalies in the first trimester and can result in respiratory depression and sedation in the newborn near term (13). Long-term use of narcotics, including intranasal butorphanol, can result in narcotic-withdrawal headaches.

Preventive treatment is justified only for the patient with increasing frequency and severity of headache who requires regular use of narcotics or for the patient who has weekly, severe headaches that are incapacitating and unresponsive to other symptomatic therapy (see the Drug Table for Migraines). Beta-adrenergic blockers, such as propanalol or atenolol, may be considered for prophylaxis, although extended use of these agents may be associated with intrauterine growth restriction (IUGR). Antidepressants, such as amitriptyline or nortriptyline, may be considered after the first trimester and may be particularly useful in severe tension or mixed vascular-tension headaches. In the collaborative perinatal project (13), no increase in congenital malformations was seen with the use of amitriptyline in the first trimester. Calcium-channel blockers, such as verapamil, are probably third-line prophylactic agents, given the minimal data on these agents in pregnancy. Methysergide is contraindicated in pregnancy because of its oxytocic action.

Headaches during pregnancy are usually migraine or tension-type headaches, but headaches produced by some disorders, such as sinusitus, stroke, CVT, preeclampsia–eclampsia, SAH, and aneurysmal or arteriovenous malformation (AVM) bleeding, may occur more often during pregnancy or the postpartum period and must be differentiated from the former. Because most women with migraine will have alleviation in the second and third trimesters, new-onset, severe, focal, unremitting headache, especially if associated with neurologic signs and symptoms, requires investigation. Computed tomography and MRI seem to be relatively safe in pregnancy, and the study that provides the most information on the concern at hand is the study of choice. Although vasoconstrictive medications should be avoided, other medications exist that should be used in pregnant women whose headaches repeatedly interfere with functional status.

REFERENCES

1. **Silberstein SD.** Migraine and pregnancy. Neurol Clin. 1997;15:209-31.

2. **Bousser MG, Ratinahirana H, Darbois X.** Migraine and pregnancy: a prospective study in 703 women after delivery [Abstract]. Neurology. 1990;40:437.

3. **Granella F, Sances G, Zanferrari C, Costa A, Martignoni E, Manzoni GC.** Migraine without aura and reproductive life events: a clinical epidemiologic study in 1300 women. Headache. 1993;33:385-89.

4. **Chen TC, Leviton A.** Headache recurrence in pregnant women with migraine. Headache. 1994;34:107-10.

5. **Stein GS.** Headaches in the first postpartum week and their relationship to migraine. Headache. 1981;21:201-5.

6. **Welch KMA.** Migraine and pregnancy. In: Neurological Complications of Pregnancy. New York: Raven Press; 1994:77-81.

7. **Peterson CM, Kelly JV.** Pseudotumor cerebri in pregnancy: case reports and review of the literature. Obst Gynecol Surv. 1985;40:323-9.

8. **Katz VL, Peterson R, Cefalo RC.** Pseudotumor cerebri and pregnancy. Am J Perinatol. 1989;6:442-5.

9. **Donaldson JO, Lee NS.** Arterial and venous stroke associated with pregnancy. Neurol Clin. 1994;12:583-99.

10. **Lanska DJ, Kryscio RJ.** Peripartum stroke and intracranial venous thrombosis in the national hospital discharge survey. Obstet Gynecol. 1997;89:413-8.

11. **Dias MS.** Neurovascular emergencies in pregnancy. Clin Obstet Gynecol. 1994;37: 337-54.

12. **Albert JR, Morrison JC.** Neurologic diseases in pregnancy. Obstet Gynecol Clin North Am. 1992;19:765-81.

13. **Briggs GG, Freeman RK, Yaffe SJ.** Drugs in pregnancy and lactation. Baltimore: Williams & Wilkins; 1998.

II. Cerebrovascular Disease
Lucia Larson

Cerebrovascular disorders (such as ischemic stroke, intracranial hemorrhage, and hypertensive encephalopathy) contribute to as many as 12% of all maternal deaths; reported maternal mortality rates associated with these disorders are as high as 30% to 40%. Although eclampsia may be present in some of these cases, a misdiagnosis of eclampsia is made in significant numbers of patients (1). An awareness of these disorders and a high index of suspicion for them are needed to prevent delay of appropriate treatment of pregnant women with cerebrovascular disease.

Subarachnoid Hemorrhage

Subarachnoid hemorrhage occurs in 1 to 5 of 10,000 pregnancies. Aneurysm and AVM are common causes of SAH, but preeclampsia and eclampsia may precipitate SAH in otherwise normal women. Cocaine use, disseminated intravascular coagulation, anticoagulant use, ectopic endometriosis, Moyamoya disease, subacute bacterial endocarditis, and choriocarcinoma may also cause and contribute to SAH.

The presentation of SAH is similar in pregnant and nonpregnant patients: Sudden onset of severe headache, often followed by nausea, vomiting, meningismus, and altered consciousness. Patients may use worrisome headache descriptions, such as "This is the worst headache of my life," "I feel as if someone hit my head with a bat," or "It feels like an explosion in my head." Associated vasospasm or intracerebral hemorrhage may be responsible for focal neurologic signs and symptoms. Seizures may develop. Hypertension may precede the event or may be secondary to increased intracranial pressure. Because 14% of patients with SAH develop albuminuria (1), this constellation of findings may erroneously suggest a diagnosis of eclampsia. However, 10% to 20% of SAHs occur in the setting of preeclampsia (2).

It is important not to delay the radiographic evaluation of this life-threatening event just because a patient is pregnant. Noncontrast head CT with abdominal shielding can be done safely, and if this shows no evidence of blood, lumbar puncture is needed to rule out erythrocytes or xanthochromia in the cerebrospinal fluid. Evaluation of the cerebral vasculature may be done by cerebral angiography or MRI–MRA once the diagnosis of SAH is confirmed.

Intracranial Aneurysm and Arteriovenous Malformation

In the general population, the most common cause of SAH is intracerebral aneurysm. This is true in the gravid population as well, but relatively more hemorrhages secondary to AVM are seen in pregnant patients than in non-pregnant patients. In one study of 154 patients who had intracranial hemorrhage during pregnancy (3), 75% of the hemorrhages were caused by an aneurysm and 25% were caused by an AVM; in the general population, the ratio of aneurysms to AVMs is 7:1. Pregnant women with an AVM tend to be younger (15 to 25 years of age) than pregnant women with aneurysms (25 to 35 years of age) (4). Half of all patients who present with a ruptured aneurysm during pregnancy have had previous pregnancies without difficulty (4), whereas patients with an AVM are more likely to be primiparous.

The risk for rupture of intracerebral aneurysm during pregnancy increases with each trimester and decreases in the postpartum period. Few aneurysms initially rupture during labor and delivery, although rebleeding may occur at this time. In contrast, the risk for rupture of AVMs peaks in the second trimester and during labor. The reason for bleeding of these lesions in pregnancy is thought to be related to the hemodynamic stresses on the vessel walls associated with the increased blood flow seen during pregnancy. Estrogen effects on vessel walls may also play a role. Transient increases in aneurysmal size during pregnancy have been noted by MRI (5). In the general population, the risk for hemorrhage from an AVM is greater during the reproductive years than at other times (6) (Table 12-2).

Bleeding of intracerebral aneurysms and AVMs is associated with high morbidity and mortality rates. The maternal mortality rate has been reported to be as high as 35%, and the fetal mortality rate is as high as 18% (2, 3). Because fetal well being depends on maternal well being, decisions about maternal treatment should be based on neurosurgical and not obstetric grounds without delay due to fetal concerns. Repair of both aneurysms and AVMs has been done successfully in pregnancy, and thromboprophylaxis may be required. Once repairs have been made, the risk for rebleeding is eliminated, and patients who have had repair are not at increased risk during the rest of the pregnancy or during labor and delivery.

Patients with aneurysms or AVMs that have not been surgically repaired are at increased risk for rebleeding. Once bleeding of an AVM has occurred in a pregnancy, the risk for rebleeding is 27% to 50% (3). There has been partic-

Table 12-2 Characteristics of Pregnant Patients with Aneurysm and Arteriovenous Malformation

Pregnant Patient with	Average Gravity	Average age at Presentation (years)	Peak Incidence of Bleeding
Aneurysm	Multiparous	25–35	Bleeding increases with each trimester and decreases post-partum
Arteriovenous malformation	Primiparous	15–25	Second trimester and postpartum

ular concern about the possibility that the Valsalva maneuver, with pushing, and the hemodynamic changes associated with labor and delivery may precipitate bleeding. Some authors recommend that these women undergo cesarean section. However, studies have shown no difference in maternal and fetal mortality rates with vaginal and surgical delivery if the hemodynamic stresses of labor are minimized by providing adequate pain control with an early epidural and if pushing is averted by a vacuum or forceps delivery (1–3). Oxytocic agents and amniotomy have been used safely in these patients (2).

Neurosurgical Treatment

Intracranial hemorrhage is life-threatening to both mother and fetus, and the benefits of many of the treatments for this event far outweigh their risks to the pregnancy. Corticosteroids are effective and safe in the management of increased intracranial pressure. Hyperventilation is also frequently used. However, allowing the Pco_2 to decrease below 25 torr or the pH to exceed 7.6 risks fetal compromise because the umbilical vessels may constrict and there is a shift of the oxyhemoglobin dissociation curve. This results in an increased affinity of maternal hemoglobin for oxygen and decreased transfer of oxygen to fetal blood. Mannitol can be problematic because it crosses the placenta and may cause fetal dehydration. Significant maternal dehydration may jeopardize placental perfusion. All calcium-channel blockers prevent vasospasm and should be used if indicated. Similarly, the clinician should not hesitate to use anticonvulsants if they are needed. During neurosurgical procedures, induced hypotension and hypothermia are often used. The effects of hypothermia on the fetus are not well delineated, but hypothermia has been used without apparent significant effects. Any hemodynamically altering treatment, such as induced hypotension, should be done in conjunction with fetal monitoring. Aminocaproic acid is often used in the treatment of AVMs that have bled. We have few data on the use of this agent in pregnancy, but there is concern that it may cause a thrombotic event. Given the serious nature of intracranial bleeding and the risks this bleeding presents to both mother and fetus, most of the usual treatment given to nonpregnant patients should be used in pregnant patients. The added measure of close fetal monitoring should also be instituted.

Ischemic Cerebrovascular Disease

Ischemic stroke is uncommon in young women but it is 7 to 13 times more common in pregnant women than in nonpregnant women (7, 8). It can occur at any time during pregnancy or the puerperium. Cesarean section and hypertension have both been noted to be predictors of peripartum stroke. The potential causes of stroke in this group of patients are many but should be aggressively investigated. Embolic events related to valvular disease, septal defects, and mural thrombi (including those associated with peripartum cardiomyopathy) are the most common causes. In pregnant patients, it is important to strongly consider the possibility that preeclampsia–eclampsia is causing neurologic symptoms, but a broad differential diagnosis must be entertained. Thrombotic strokes related to the antiphospholipid antibody syndrome and other thrombophilias have been reported. Less common pregnancy-related causes of stroke include amniotic fluid embolism and choriocarcinoma. Cardiac disorders, such as atrial septal defect, patent foramen ovale, and atrial fibrillation, should be considered in addition to vasculitic diseases, substance abuse, atherosclerosis, and other causes of stroke usually considered in nonpregnant patients. Careful evaluation should include CT with abdominal shielding, MRI–MRA, or angiography and echocardiography and is safe in pregnancy. If anticoagulation is indicated, heparin may be given during pregnancy. Warfarin is teratogenic and may cause fetal cerebrovascular bleeding (see Chapter 8).

Cerebral Venous Thrombosis

Cerebral venous thrombosis has been estimated to occur in 1 in 2500 to 1 in 10,000 deliveries. It is more common in undeveloped countries. In one report from Maduri, India, the incidence was as high as 1 in 250 pregnancies (9). The associated mortality rate may be as high as 30%, but the prognosis varies, ranging from death to complete recovery. Cerebral venous thrombosis may occur at any time in pregnancy but classically occurs in the first 3 weeks after an uncomplicated pregnancy and delivery. One study (10) found that of 67 patients with pregnancy-associated CVT, 61 developed this condition postpartum. Conditions other than pregnancy that are associated with CVT include hyperviscosity (as in dehydration, polycythemia, or sickle-cell anemia), sepsis, intracranial infection (meningitis, otitis media, or paranasal sinus infection), cancer, oral contraceptive use, and the thrombophilias (especially the prothrombin gene mutation).

Patients present with symptoms resulting from increased intracranial pressure caused by thrombosis of the sagittal sinus or draining veins. Initial worsening headache may progress to seizures and focal neurologic deficits. A mild fever and elevated leukocyte count may cause the condition to be confused with meningitis. Although CT of the head may be helpful when a delta sign is present, MRI–MRV is the test of choice.

Treatment often consists of prompt anticoagulation with intravenous standard heparin, but because of the possibility of associated hemorrhage the decision to use this treatment should be made only after careful review of central nervous system (CNS) imaging. Anticoagulation should continue throughout pregnancy and the postpartum period in a manner similar to that suggested for pregnant women with thromboembolic disease, and an evaluation for underlying hypercoagulable states should be done as described in Chapter 8.

The frequency of recurrent CVT is greatest in the year after the initial event, and there have been reports of recurrence in subsequent pregnancies. Future pregnancies carry an increased risk for a recurrent event, but the exact risk is not known. Therapeutic or prophylactic heparin may be advisable in future pregnancies. The heparin dose would depend on the severity of the individual circumstances and the presence or absence of an underlying hypercoagulable state. These patients should avoid estrogen-containing oral contraceptives because these agents increase risk for recurrent stroke.

REFERENCES

1. **Witlin AG, Friedman SA, Egerman RS, Frangieh AY, Sibai B.** Cerebrovascular disorders complicating pregnancy—beyond eclampsia. Am J Obstet Gynecol. 1997;176: 1139-48.
2. **Wilterdink JF, Feldmann E.** Cerebral hemorrhage. In: Neurologic Complications of Pregnancy. New York: Raven Press; 1994.
3. **Dias MS, Sekhar LN.** Intracranial hemorrhage from aneurysms and arteriovenous malformations during pregnancy and the puerperium. Neurosurgery. 1990;27:855-66.
4. **Wiebers DO.** Subarachnoid hemorrhage in pregnancy. Semin Neurol. 1988;8:226-9.

5. **Ortiz O, Voelker J, Eneorji F.** Transient enlargement of an intracranial aneurysm during pregnancy: case report. Surg Neurol. 1997;47:527-31.

6. **Karlsson B, Lindqvist C, Johansson A, Steiner L.** Annual risk for the first hemorrhage from untreated cerebral arteriovenous malformation. Minim Invasive Neurosurg. 1997;40:40-6.

7. **Lanska DJ, Kryscio RJ.** Peripartum stroke and intracranial venous thrombosis in the national hospital discharge survey. Obstet Gynecol. 1997;89:413-8.

8. **Barnett HJM.** Stroke in women. Can J Cardiol. 1990;6(Suppl B):11B-7B.

9. **Simolke GA, Cox SM, Cunningham FG.** Cerebrovascular accidents complicating pregnancy and the puerperium. Obstet Gynecol. 1991;78:37-42.

10. **Cantu C, Barinagarrementeria F.** Cerebral venous thrombosis associated with pregnancy and puerperium: review of 67 cases. Stroke. 1993;24:1880-4.

III. Epilepsy
Linda Anne Barbour and Jeffrey Pickard

Epilepsy is the most common neurologic complication of pregnancy. It has a prevalence of approximately 1% of the population, and 1 in 200 newborns is born to a mother with epilepsy. Seizures during pregnancy may complicate gestation for both mother and fetus, and medications used to treat epilepsy may complicate the pregnancy. Conversely, pregnancy may have an effect on both the seizure disorder and the medications used to treat it.

Effect of Pregnancy on Epilepsy

There is disagreement over the exact numbers, but approximately 50% of women with epilepsy have little or no change in the frequency of their seizures during pregnancy. Of the other 50%, roughly equal numbers have increased and decreased seizure frequency (1–5). Responses to pregnancy vary so much that it is impossible to reliably predict what will happen to seizure frequency during pregnancy on the basis of age, seizure type, drug regimen, or seizure frequency in a previous gestation (2). Whatever its effect on overall seizure frequency, pregnancy does not seem to affect the likelihood of status epilepticus.

Many factors may contribute to altered seizure frequency (Box 12-2). Despite this, less than 25% of women experience a worsening of seizures during pregnancy. Estrogen seems to be somewhat epileptogenic, and progesterone seems to have the opposite effect (2). Various metabolic changes that occur throughout gestation may play a role in the effect of pregnancy on seizures.

Box 12-2 Possible Causes of Altered Seizure Frequency in Pregnancy

---

Hormonal factors
  Estrogen levels
  Progesterone levels
Metabolic factors
Maternal factors
  Sleep deprivation
  Stress and anxiety
  Noncompliance with medication
  Alcohol and drug abuse
Antiepileptic drug factors
  Decreased absorption
  Increased volume of distribution
  Increased clearance
  Decreased albumin concentration

Increased body weight, fluid retention, sodium retention, the mild hyperventilation that results in a compensated respiratory alkalosis, and hypomagnesemia have all been suggested as factors that affect seizure frequency. However, few data show that any of these factors are important (2). Sleep deprivation and noncompliance with antiepileptic drug (AED) regimens probably have an adverse effect with respect to seizures during pregnancy, as do stress and anxiety.

The altered pharmacokinetics of AEDs during pregnancy results in lower serum total levels, although levels of unbound drug may not be significantly affected (2). The decrease in total serum levels may be due to an increased volume of distribution, impaired absorption, accelerated metabolism, and clearance. Compliance with AED regimens is often a problem during pregnancy because of the nausea and vomiting of pregnancy or because women or their physicians fear the effects of AEDs on the fetus and discontinue their use. Most AEDs are highly protein bound. As levels of some serum proteins increase, especially during the first trimester, free levels of AEDs may decrease. Conversely, albumin levels decline during pregnancy, resulting in a decrease in the total levels of AEDs but little change in unbound levels. One study (6) prospectively followed 51 women with epilepsy throughout pregnancy, measuring the total levels, free levels, and metabolites of the AEDs that the women were taking. The total concentrations of all AEDs declined as pregnancy progressed, reaching the lowest levels at term and increasing again postpartum. Free levels declined slightly as well, but the decline was significant only for phenobarbital; free levels of valproic acid actually increased. The period of greatest decline in phenytoin and phenobarbital levels occurred during the first trimester. This indicates that changes in plasma volume alone are not responsible for the decreases.

Effect of Epilepsy on Pregnancy Outcome

Although isolated seizures of short duration are generally tolerated by the fetus, epilepsy may complicate gestation and increase perinatal morbidity and mortality rates. Some studies have shown a slight increase in preeclampsia, bleeding, placental abruption, and premature labor in women with epilepsy (1, 2, 7) but others have not (3). Labor and delivery are usually unaffected in women with epilepsy, although grand mal seizures during labor may cause fetal asphyxia and bradycardia as well as reduced variability and late decelerations in fetal heart tracings; this indicates the need for urgent delivery (7). Women receiving AEDs may have slightly prolonged labor and increased bleeding at delivery because AEDs can diminish the force of uterine contractions and lower serum levels of vitamin K–dependent clotting factors (7).

Inheritance

The genetics of epilepsy is not entirely clear. The empirical risk for epilepsy is 4% to 10% for close relatives of patients with generalized epilepsy (8). This risk is too low to be monogenic and suggests polygenic transmission. Some relatives of patients with epilepsy are clinically healthy and seizure free despite abnormal electroencephalograms; this indicates that external factors may contribute to the development of seizures. Genetic factors determine the clinical variety of seizures, whereas environmental factors, such as sleep deprivation and stress, may influence the extent and severity of the clinical expression of epilepsy (8). This implies that the modification of environmental factors may be an important therapy, especially during pregnancy.

Antiepileptic Drugs

Untreated epilepsy carries an unacceptable risk for uncontrolled seizures resulting in maternal or fetal trauma, status epilepticus, miscarriage, fetal hypoxia, and lactic acidosis. Studies on the risk of AEDs have been confounded by genetic susceptibility, including both maternal and paternal factors; nutritional factors; type or severity of epilepsy; environmental factors; whether a dysmorphologist examined the newborn; and use of polypharmacy or varying doses of the AEDs. Possible mechanisms of teratogenicity in women with epilepsy who receive AEDs include 1) free radical intermediates of AEDs that cause abnormal morphogenesis, 2) enzymatic deficiencies that are genetically inherited and cause accumulation of toxic metabolites, and 3) AED-induced folate deficiency.

Mechanisms of Teratogenicity

Genetic influences clearly contribute to the malformation rate because women with epilepsy who do not receive AEDs have nearly a twofold increase in the rate of malformations (2, 9, 10). Malformations may, in part, be associated with the maternal epilepsy syndrome, and drug treatment and a "liability" gene may predispose AED-exposed fetuses to an adverse outcome (10). Reactive intermediates of AEDs, such as free radicals, are embryotoxic and are metabolized or conjugated by free radical–scavenging enzymes. Low levels of these enzymes are associated with birth defects. Unstable intermediates can be metabolized to nonreactive hydrodiols by epoxide hydrolase. This enzyme is inherited in a classic Mendelian fashion. Thus, one fourth of persons are homozygous for the recessive allele and exhibit low enzymatic activity. Fetuses with low levels of epoxide hydrolase may be at particular risk for the congenital malformations (11). Although enzymatic activity can by assayed in maternal and paternal lymphocytes and fetal amniocytes, the assay is not commercially available and its predictive power has not been adequately tested. Other possible mechanisms for free radical formation include AED overinduction of serum copper–zinc superoxide dismutase and depletion of glutathione (a scavenger of hydrogen peroxide). This leads to overproduction of hydroxyl radicals, which are reactive and can bind to nucleic acids and proteins; disrupt the synthesis of DNA, RNA, and other proteins; and ultimately disturb transcription, translation, cell division, and migration (12). Excessive exposure to free radicals through pathways that may be genetically determined increases the risk for spontaneous abortion, perinatal death, IUGR, and malformations. Some minor malformations are more strongly associated with parental phenotype than with AEDs, and 25% of AED-exposed infants who develop spina bifida have a family history of neural tube defects (9, 10).

Folic acid deficiency is another postulated mechanism of teratogenicity: All of the established AEDs, including phenytoin, phenobarbital, valproic acid, and carbamazepine, decrease folic acid levels. Folate deficiency in women without epilepsy is associated with neural tube defects and ventricular septal defects. Phenytoin, carbamazepine, and phenobarbital cause folate malabsorption, and valproic acid interferes with folate metabolism. In a collaborative, randomized, double-blind, controlled trial in healthy women (13), perinatal vitamin supplementation with 0.4 mg of folic acid before conception significantly decreased the risk for neural tube defects. The Medical Research Council (14), in a randomized, controlled trial, showed that supplementation with 4 mg of folic acid before conception in women who had previously given birth to an infant with a neural tube defect reduced the subsequent risk for another infant with a neural tube defect by 70%. To be efficacious, folate must be present between days 1 and 28 of conception, when the posterior neuropore closes. However, a missed menstrual cycle is not noticed until at least 15 days after conception, so folic acid supplementation must be given before conception. The U.S. Public Heath Service and the Centers for Disease Control and Prevention recommend that all women of childbearing age receive 0.4 mg of folic acid daily and that women with a previously affected child receive 4 mg of folic acid daily (15). Some investigators recommend the use of 4 mg of folate daily before conception for women receiving AEDs (3, 4). However, no data indicate that this supplementation will decrease the risk for neural tube defects in women using AEDs. There is no consensus on the dose of folic acid for women receiving AEDs because high levels of folic acid may increase AED metabolism and mask vitamin B_{12} deficiency (1, 9). Given the efficacy of the 4 mg dose in women with previously affected infants and given the abnormalities in vitamin metabolism known to occur with AEDs, it seems reasonable to use the higher dose in women with treated epilepsy and to monitor drug levels before conception and through the first 10 weeks of gestation in women receiving this dose.

All of the established AEDs have teratogenic effects, but the absolute risk for major malformations is 3% to 9% (a twofold to threefold increase) with monotherapy (9, 10, 16, 17). Women whose epilepsy requires treatment with a single agent can be reassured that they have at least a 90% chance of a favorable outcome. Although first recognized with phenytoin, the fetal anticonvulsant syndrome—characterized by orofacial clefting, cardiovascular and neural tube defects, gastric and urinary defects, and digital malformations—can occur with any of the established AEDs. Valproic acid and carbamazepine have been most strongly associated with neural tube defects (usually spina bifida and not anencephaly), with risks of 1% to 4% and 0.5% to 1%, respectively (1, 10, 17). Phenytoin and phenobarbital have been more strongly associated with cardiac and orofacial clefting, although these defects can occur less often with other AEDs (Table 12-3). The phenotypic expression of these defects is critically dependent on timing of drug exposure, and all occur within the first trimester, usually before a women enters prenatal care (Table 12-4). Because all of these established AEDs have been found to be more or less favorable with regard to malformations, depending on the study population and dosage used, the AED that most effectively treats epilepsy at the lowest dose is the preferred AED for a particular patient (1, 2, 4, 18).

Table 12-3 Anomalies Reported with Antiepileptic Drugs

	Phenytoin	Phenobarbital	Valproic Acid	Carbamazepine
Cardiac defects	+	+	+	+/–
Neural tube defects	+/–	+/–	+	+
Gastric and urinary defects	+	+/–	+	+/–
Orofacial clefting	+	+	+	+/–
Dysmorphic syndrome	+	+	+	+

Table 12-4 Timing of Certain Malformations

Malformation	Interval from Conception
Meningomyelocele	28 days
Cleft lip	5 weeks
Cleft palate	10 weeks
Ventrical septal defect	6 weeks

Women receiving polytherapy seem to have a higher risk for malformations in a nonlinear manner (17); one study (19) found that the risk for major malformations with four AEDs was 25%. Potentially deleterious interactions involving accelerated formation of arene oxide metabolites as well as intensified folic acid deficiency may partly explain this risk. All established AEDs have also been associated with a dysmorphic syndrome, and minor malformations that typically involve the face and digits include hypertelorism, frontal bossing, malar hypoplasia, epicanthal folds, micrognathia, broad nasal bridge, upturned nasal tip, low-set ears, and distal digital and nailbed hypoplasia. These malformations are often outgrown in the first year of life. Minor morphologic abnormalities occur in up to 15% of children born to women without epilepsy and in 30% of infants in women with epilepsy (10). Some of these have been associated with untreated epilepsy, and others (epicanthal folds, hypertelorism, and nailbed hypoplasia) seem to be more specific to women using AEDs (9, 20).

Neurodevelopmental Sequelae

Neurodevelopmental outcome and the risks of AEDs are controversial. Adverse neurodevelopmental outcome, as assessed by reduced head circumference or lower IQ, has been associated with smaller parental head circumference, lower maternal and paternal IQ, maternal seizures, presence of multiple congenital anomalies in the offspring, and environmental factors. Phenobarbital, phenytoin, and valproic acid have all been associated with neurodevelopmental delay (21–23), although all studies have been confounded by other determinants of IQ. Whether carbamazepine is problematic is unclear because one of the studies addressing this issue (24) used carbamazepine in epileptic and nonepileptic persons and compared these persons primarily with epileptic patients receiving phenytoin. Although the risk for major malformations is limited to first-trimester exposure, sustained use of AEDs later in pregnancy may cause embryogenic neurologic disorders, such as impaired cellular migration, myelin formation, or impaired metabolic processes (21).

Other Adverse Outcomes

All of the established AEDs except valproic acid induce the cytochrome p450 system. This induction significantly reduces the estradiol and progesterone in oral contraceptives, promotes metabolism of active vitamin D to inactive metabolites, and accelerates both maternal and fetal metabolism of vitamin K–dependent clotting factors. The AEDs may also interfere with the intestinal absorption of calcium. All of the established AEDs except valproic acid can cause decreases in fetal vitamin K–dependent clotting factors, which have been measured as PIVKA (products induced in vitamin K's absence); the precursors of thrombin; and factors VII, IX, and X. It has been shown that giving vitamin K to the mother normalizes the increased levels of PIVKA in the fetus and may prevent the hemorrhagic disease of the newborn seen (albeit rarely) within 48 hours of birth in infants born to mothers receiving phenobarbital, phenytoin, and carbamazepine (25–27). Most experts recommend that mothers receiving these AEDs receive 10 to 20 mg of vitamin K daily at 34 to 36 weeks gestation (1, 2, 4, 28) and receive supplementation with vitamin D at the doses found in prenatal vitamins.

Specific Antiepileptic Drugs

Phenytoin
Used to treat tonic-clonic seizures as well as partial seizures at dosages of 300 to 600 mg/d, phenytoin is 90% protein bound. Therefore, if drug levels are being monitored, it is free levels that should be checked (1 to 2 mg/L). Phenytoin induces fetal metabolism of vitamin K and may act as a competitive inhibitor of placental transport of vitamin K. By inducing the cytochrome p450 system, it increases the metabolism of other agents, including oral contraceptives. The amount of phenytoin ingested by a breastfeeding infant is probably less than 5% of the maternal dose, so phenytoin is considered compatible with nursing (29).

Phenobarbital

Primidone is metabolized to phenobarbital, which is used to treat generalized tonic-clonic seizures and (less frequently) partial seizures at doses of 60 to 240 mg. Phenobarbital is 50% protein bound, but free drug levels are not readily available and optimal drug levels vary significantly from person to person. Phenobarbital is a potent inducer of the cytochrome p450 system and has been associated with neonatal coagulopathy that results (rarely) in hemorrhagic disease in the newborn within 48 hours of birth (4). Because of phenobarbital's sedation, most patients must dose at night or divide the daytime dose to tolerate sedative side effects. Phenobarbital may produce a neonatal barbiturate withdrawal syndrome, which typically presents more than 7 days after birth because of phenobarbital's very long half-life in the neonate. Phenobarbital is excreted into breast milk and (because of reduced neonatal metabolism) serum levels can accumulate, leading to sedation and withdrawal symptoms when breastfeeding is discontinued. It is considered problematic and if nursing is elected, careful observation for sedation and drug monitoring in the neonate is recommended (29).

Carbamazepine

Previously thought to be the AED of choice, carbamazepine has been shown to cause dysmorphic features similar to those caused by phenytoin, including digital hypoplasia. Carbamazepine is also associated with a 0.5% to 1% risk for spina bifida, and it induces hepatic microsomal oxidative systems and produces similar epoxides. It is primarily used to treat partial epilepsy, especially complex partial epilepsy with or without generalization, at 600 to 2000 mg/d in two to four divided doses. Carbamazepine is approximately 70% protein bound. Free drug levels are not widely available. Approximately 25% of maternal drug levels are found in breastmilk, and carbamazepine is considered compatible with nursing (29).

Valproic Acid

Although not found to be teratogenic in early animal models, valproic acid and its sodium salt divalproex increase the risk for spina bifida 10-fold to 17-fold, to an absolute risk of 1% to 4% (1, 10, 17). Valproic acid is used primarily for primary juvenile generalized epilepsy, including tonic-clonic and absence seizures. Doses of 500 to 3000 mg are typically used, and the drug is 90% protein bound but free drug levels are rarely available. Data support dose-dependent teratogenicity, and high peak serum levels may be particularly injurious. Therefore, it is recommended that the minimum amount of valporic acid be administered in three to four doses per day. In one study (30), six of six cases of spina bifida were seen in mothers with an average daily dose of 1640 mg. In 83 valproic acid–exposed patients who had normal outcomes, the average dose was 950 mg. Neonatal excitability and neurodevelopment at 6 years may also be related to serum levels of valproic acid at birth (21). Animal models suggest that the same amount of total drug is more toxic if high peak levels form than if smaller doses are given (9). Because 25% of mothers receiving valproic acid who give birth to infants with spina bifida have family members with neural tube defects, women with a family history of neural tube defects should be given valproic acid only with extreme caution and only when it is clearly the AED of choice. Valproic acid inhibits hepatic microsomal enzymes, so it has not been associated with oral contraceptive failure or vitamin K–dependent clotting abnormalities in newborns. Approximately 15% of maternal levels are found in breastmilk; thus, valproic acid is considered compatible with nursing (29).

Ethosuxamide
Ethosuxamide is used to treat absence seizures. There is much less experience with the use of this drug during pregnancy, but minimal data suggest that it causes a constellation of problems similar to those caused by other AEDs. Ethosuxamide is minimally protein bound, induces hepatic microsomal enzymes, and can result (rarely) in a hemorrhagic syndrome in the newborn. Levels in breastmilk are similar to maternal levels, and ethosuxamide has been reported to cause poor suckling and hyperexcitability in the newborn. Therefore, ethosuxamide is considered problematic with breastfeeding (29).

Clonazepam
No guidelines are available for the drug monitoring of clonazepam, which is infrequently used to treat absence epilepsy and myoclonic seizures at dosages of 2 to 6 mg/d. Experience with clonazepam in pregnancy is limited. The drug has been associated with congenital heart disease and is sedating, potentially resulting in respiratory depression in the newborn. Clonazepam is excreted into breastmilk and is therefore considered problematic.

New Antiepileptic Drugs
Most of the new AEDs (e.g., felbamate, gabapentin, lamotrigine) have lower protein binding and do not induce the cytochrome p450 system. Therefore, the pregnancy-related increases in hepatic metabolism will not affect concentrations of these AEDs and these drugs are less likely to affect vitamin K metabolism and levels of sex steroids in oral contraceptives. The lower concentrations of arene oxide metabolites may improve pregnancy outcome, but human data are insufficient to allow risk to be determined. Lamotrigine does not seem to have an antifolate effect, but the effects of the other agents are unknown. Animal studies show no teratogenicity of these AEDs, with the exception of vigabatrin, which has been associated with orofacial abnormali-

ties. However, animal studies may be poor predictors of human teratogenicity. A prospective registry for lamotrigine has been established by Glaxo-Well-come, but the new AEDs are often used with other AEDs. Of 60 women who used lamotrigine in the first trimester, two liveborn infants and two pregnancy terminations complicated with neural tube defects occurred in women who also received other AEDs (31). Before 1993, women of childbearing age were excluded from investigational drug trials, and information on teratogenicity has depended on a voluntary reporting system. It is estimated that only 10% of medication-related adverse effects are reported (10). Physicians and other health care providers should report any pregnant women receiving AEDs to the Epilepsy Drug Registry (telephone, 888-233-2334) so that women of child-bearing age will have adequate information on the risks of these agents.

Monitoring Drug Levels

The practice of monitoring drug levels is controversial, and no agreement exists among experts. Although the American College of Obstetrics and Gynecology (28) recommends that trough drug levels be checked frequently, others believe that the lack of availability of free drug levels, the fact that most women with epilepsy do not have increased seizures during pregnancy, and concern about dose-related toxicity argue against frequent drug monitoring except for clinical indications (21, 32). Two studies (32, 33) found no clear-cut relation between seizure control and plasma concentrations of AEDs during pregnancy. Free drug levels correlate better than total levels with seizure control, but not all laboratories have the ability to measure free drug levels, and such measurement may be costly. Reasons to monitor drug levels include the need to ascertain compliance, assess the possibility of toxicity, and evaluate women whose seizures are inadequately controlled or who have a clear seizure threshold at a particular drug level. Given the problems with drug monitoring and the fact that the best therapeutic strategy for minimizing adverse effects is to use the lowest dose of an AED that prevents seizures, individual monitoring for special circumstances seems reasonable.

Antenatal Testing

Women receiving AEDs should be offered antenatal testing, especially if diagnosis of a major malformation would influence their desire to maintain the pregnancy or would affect the delivery plan. Transvaginal ultrasonography at 11 to 13 weeks of gestation may be able to visualize a neural tube defect early. Maternal serum alpha-fetoprotein (MSAFP) testing is usually offered at about 16 weeks, and a formal anatomy scan and four-chamber view of the heart and cardiac outflow tract are done at 18 to 20 weeks. Fetal echocardiography can be repeated at 20 to 22 weeks if the four-chamber view is suboptimal or suspicious (4). Expertly targeted ultrasonography visualizing the CNS and neural tube can identify up to 95% of neural tube defects. The combination of normal MSAFP and normal targeted ultrasonography results in a risk for an open neural tube defect of less than 1%. Therefore, amniocentesis to measure fetal alpha-fetoprotein is usually reserved for cases with suspicious anatomy, increased MSAFP, or suboptimal anatomic views. Ultrasonography to measure serial growth is indicated for the usual troubling clinical variables, including inappropriate fundal height. Nonstress tests are usually reserved for women with poorly controlled seizures or evidence of IUGR (3, 4).

Labor and Delivery and Postpartum Concerns

Approximately 1% to 2% of women with epilepsy have seizures during labor and delivery. If oral medications cannot be taken, intravenous phenytoin 10 to 15 mg/kg at a rate of less than 50 mg/min should be administered with cardiac monitoring. Alternatively, if the woman has been receiving phenobarbital, an intramuscular dose of 60 to 90 mg can be given. Treatment of status epilepticus is unchanged in pregnancy, and the clinician should remember to place the woman on her left side with displacement of the uterus off the inferior vena cava to improve fetal circulation. Eclampsia should be ruled out because the treatment of choice for eclamptic seizures is magnesium sulfate. Levels of AEDs should be checked within 48 hours postpartum and again at 1 and 2 weeks, especially if dosages were increased during pregnancy, because toxicity can occur rapidly. Vitamin K administration is the standard of care for all neonates. Neonates should be monitored closely for drug withdrawal or respiratory depression, especially if exposed to phenobarbital or clonazepam. All established AEDs except for phenobarbital, clonazepam, and ethosuximide are considered compatible with breastfeeding; close monitoring of the infant is required if nursing is to be attempted with any of these three agents. Mothers should be advised against bathing infants alone and should perform feeding and changing on the floor with padded mattresses and cushions.

Postpartum contraception is critical, and if oral contraceptives are taken by women receiving phenytoin, phenobarbital, and carbamazepine, 50-µg estrogen pills should be used (34–37). Failures are less common with this dose, although they have been reported. If breakthrough bleeding is noted or women desire very high effectiveness, a spermicidal gel or foam or other barrier method should be added. Depomedroxyprogesterone has not been associated with contraceptive failures (35), although some recommend increasing the frequency of the dose to every 2 months. However, more than 30 accidental pregnancies have been reported with levornorgestrol implants in women using AEDs, so these implants should not be recommended.

Box 12-3 summarizes the recommendations at three stages for pregnant women with epilepsy: before conception, during pregnancy, and at delivery and postpartum.

Box 12-3 Recommendations for Pregnant Women with Epilepsy

Before conception
Determine whether AED regimen is needed
Use monotherapy, if possible at lowest dose
Discuss risks of poorly controlled seizures and risks of AED regimen
Provide folate at 1–4 mg per day
Determine needed for contraception while optimizing epilepsy management

During pregnancy
Emphasize AED therapy goal to prevent generalized seizures
Emphasize avoidance of sleep deprivation, alcohol, tobacco, and drugs, and discuss strategies to reduce stress
Use monotherapy, if possible at lowest dose
Divide dosing of valproic acid to tid–qid
Continue folate throughout first trimester
Individualize monitoring of AED levels (use free level for monitoring phenytoin)
Do transvaginal ultrasonography at 11–13 weeks to visualize neural tube
Maternal serum alpha-fetoprotein (MSAFP) at 15–20 weeks
Targeted fetal anatomy ultrasound at 18–20 weeks with four-chamber view of heart
Fetal echocardiogram at 20–22 weeks if four-chamber view suboptimal or suspicious
Amniocenteses before 20 weeks for abnormal MSAFP or inadequate fetal ultrasound
Fetal surveillance for poorly controlled seizures or fetal growth restriction
Give mother vitamin K 10–20 mg daily at 34–35 weeks

At delivery and postpartum
Give IV phenytoin or phenobarbital if oral AEDs cannot be taken
Give infant vitamin K 1 mg
Monitor maternal AED levels at 48 hours and 1–2 weeks postpartum
Examine infant for anomalies or withdrawal symptoms and report to Epilepsy Registry
Monitor breast-fed infants for AED effects or withdrawal symptoms
Advise mothers against bathing infant alone or feeding or changing infant on elevated surfaces
Determine need for appropriate contraception

REFERENCES

1. **Delgado-Escueta AV, Janz D.** Consensus guidelines: Preconception counseling, management, and care of the pregnant woman with epilepsy. Neurology. 1992;42(Suppl 5):149-60.

2. **Yerby MS, Devinsky O.** Epilepsy and pregnancy. In: Devinsky O, Feldmann E, Hainline B. Neurological Complications of Pregnancy. New York: Raven Press; 1994.

3. **Eller DP, Patterson A, Webb GW.** Maternal and fetal implications of anticonvulsive therapy during pregnancy. Obstet Gynecol Clin North Am. 1997;24:523-34.

4. **Malone FD, D'Alton ME.** Drugs in pregnancy: anticonvulsants. Semin Perinatol. 1997;21:114-23.

5. **Devinsky O, Yerby MS.** Women with epilepsy: reproduction and effects of pregnancy on epilepsy. Neurol Clin. 1994;12:479-95.

6. **Yerby MS, Friel PN, McCormick K.** Antiepileptic drug disposition during pregnancy. Neurology. 1992;42(Suppl 5):12-6.

7. **Hiilesmaa VK.** Pregnancy and birth in women with epilepsy. Neurology. 1992; 42(Suppl 5):8-11.

8. **Janz D, Beck-Mannagetta G, Sander T.** Do idiopathic generalized epilepsies share a common susceptibility gene? Neurology. 1992;42(Suppl 5):48-55.

9. **Lindhout D, Omtzigt JGC.** Teratogenic effects of antiepileptic drugs: implications for the management of epilepsy in women of childbearing age. Epilepsia. 1994;35(Suppl 4):19-28.

10. **Morrell MJ.** The new antiepileptic drugs and women: efficacy, reproductive health, pregnancy, and fetal outcome. Epilepsia. 1996;37(Suppl 6):34-44.

11. **Buehler BA, Delimont D, van Waes M, Finnel R.** Prenatal prediction of the risk of the fetal hydantoin syndrome. N Engl J Med. 1990;332:1567-72.

12. **Liu CS, Wu HM, Kao SH, Wei YH.** Phenytoin-mediated oxidative stress in serum of female epileptics: a possible pathogenesis in the fetal hydantoin syndrome. Hum Exp Toxicol. 1997;16:177-81.

13. **Czeizel AE, Dudas I.** Prevention of the first occurrence of neural-tube defects by periconceptional vitamin supplementation. N Engl J Med. 1992;327:1832-5.

14. **Medical Research Council Vitamin Study Research Group.** Prevention of neural tube defects: results of the Medical Research Council Vitamin Study. Lancet. 1991;338:131-7.

15. **Centers for Disease Control and Prevention.** Recommendations for the use of folic acid to reduce the number of cases of spina bifida and other neural tube defects. MMWR Morb Mortal Wkly Rep. 1992;41(RR-14):1-7.

16. **Jick SS, Terris BZ.** Anticonvulsants and congenital malformations. Pharmacotherapy. 1997;17:561-4.

17. **Samren EB, can Duijn CM, Hiilesmaa VK, Klepel H, Bardy AH, Mannagetta GB, et al.** Maternal use of antiepileptic drugs and the risk of major congenital malformation: a joint European prospective study of human teratogenesis associated with maternal epilepsy. Epilepsia. 1997;38:981-90.

18. **Waters CH, Belia Y, Gott PS, Shen P, De Giorgio CM.** Outcomes of pregnancy associated with antiepileptic drugs. Arch Neurol. 1994;51:250-3.

19. **Nakane Y, Okuma T, Takahashi R.** Multi-institutional study on the teratogenicity and fetal toxicity of antiepileptic drugs: report of a collaborative study group in Japan. Epilepsia. 1980;21:663-80.

20. **Nulman I, Scolnik D, Chitayat D, Farkas LD, Koren G.** Findings in children exposed in utero to phenytoin and carbamazepine monotherapy: independent effects of epilepsy and medications. Am J Med Genet. 1997;68:18-24.

21. **Koch S, Jager-Roman E, Losche G, Nau H, Rating D, Heige H.** Antiepileptic drug treatment in pregnancy: drug side effects in the neonate and neurological outcome. Acta Pediatr. 1996;85:739-46.

22. **Reinisch JM, Sanders SA, Mortensen EL, Psych C, Rubin DB.** In utero exposure to phenobarbital and intelligence deficits in adult men. JAMA. 1995;274:1518-25.

23. **van der Pol MC, Hadders-Algra M, Huisjes HJ, Touwen BCL.** Antiepileptic medication in pregnancy: late effects on the children's central nervous system development. Am J Obstet Gynecol. 1991;164:121-8.

24. **Scolnik D, Nulman I, Rovet J, Gladstone D, Czuchta D, Gardner HA, et al.** Neurodevelopment of children exposed in utero to phenytoin and carbamazepine monotherapy. JAMA. 1994;271:767-70.

25. **Thorp JA, Gaston L, Caspers DR, Pal ML.** Current concepts and controversies in the use of vitamin K. Drugs. 1995;49:376-87.

26. **Cornelissen M, Steegers-Theunissen R, Kolle L, Eskes T, Vogels-Mentink G, Motohara K, et al.** Increased incidence of neonatal vitamin K deficiency resulting from maternal anticonvulsant therapy. Am J Obstet Gynecol. 1993;168:923-8.

27. **Cornelissen M, Steegers-Theunissen R, Kollee L, Eskes T, Motohara K, Monnens L.** Supplementation of vitamin K in pregnant women receiving anticonvulsant therapy prevents neonatal vitamin K deficiency. Am J Obstet Gynecol. 1993;168:884-8.

28. **American College of Obstetricians and Gynecologists.** Seizure disorders in pregnancy. ACOG Technical Bulletin. 1996;231.

29. **Committee on Drugs.** The transfer of drugs and other chemicals into human milk. Pediatrics. 1994;93:137-50.

30. **Omtzigt JCC, Los EJ, Grobbee DE.** The risk of spina bifida perta after first trimester valproate exposure in a prenatal cohort. Neurology. 1992;42(Suppl 5):119-25.

31. **Mackay FJ, Wilton LV, Pearce GL, Freemantle SN, Mann RD.** Safety of long-term lamotrigine in epilepsy. Epilepsia. 1997;38:881-6.

32. **Lander CM, Eadie MJ.** Plasma antiepileptic drug concentration during pregnancy. Epilepsia. 1991;32:257-66.

33. **Tomson T, Lindbon U, Ekqvist B, Sundqvist A.** Epilepsy and pregnancy: a prospective study of seizure control in relation to free and total plasma concentrations of carbamazepine and phenytoin. Epilepsia. 1994;35:122-30.

34. **Shuster EA.** Epilepsy in women. Mayo Clin Proc. 1996;71:991-9.

35. **Krauss GI, Brandt J, Campbell M, Plate C, Summerfield M.** Antiepileptic medication and oral contraceptive interactions: a national survey of neurologists and obstetricians. Neurology. 1996;46:1534-9.

36. **Corson SL.** Contraception for women with health problems. Int J Fertil. 1996;41:77-84.

37. **Jones KP, Wild RA.** Contraception for patients with psychiatric or medical disorders. Am J Obstet Gynecol. 1994;170:1575-80.

IV. Bell Palsy and Nerve Entrapment Syndromes
Lucia Larson and Richard V. Lee

Nerve entrapments and compressive injuries are common during pregnancy and parturition (Box 12-4). Although obstetric nerve palsies are common, clinicians must remember that toxic and metabolic neuropathies are not alleviated by pregnancy and that the nutritional demands of pregnancy may exacerbate pre-existing neuropathies (1–3). Persons with type 1 insulin-dependent diabetes and diabetic neuropathy may have worsening symptoms during pregnancy and may be more susceptible to entrapment or compressive injury. Pregnancy increases peripheral nerve susceptibility to local anesthetics by potentiating inhibition of impulse conduction (4), and this may contribute to the frequency of neuropathic symptoms and syndromes among pregnant women.

Five nerve entrapment syndromes occur often enough during gestation, usually in the latter half of pregnancy, to warrant special attention: Bell palsy, brachial plexus (thoracic outlet syndrome), carpal tunnel syndrome, abdominal wall stretching and hypochondral pain, and meralgia paresthetica (compression of lateral femoral cutaneous nerve). Nerve compression injuries occurring during labor and delivery include peroneal nerve compression and lumbosacral plexus injury.

Nerve Entrapment Syndromes Beginning During Pregnancy

Bell Palsy

Bell palsy is a disturbance of cranial nerve VII (facial nerve) that leaves patients with unilateral facial weakness. At times, loss of taste on the anterior

---

Box 12-4 Common Nerve Entrapment and Compression Syndromes of Pregnancy and Parturition

Nerve entrapments beginning during pregnancy
  Bell palsy
  Brachial plexus (thoracic outlet syndrome)
  Carpal tunnel syndrome
  Abdominal wall stretching and hypochondral pain
  Meralgia paresthetica (compression of lateral femoral cutaneous nerve)
Nerve compression injuries occurring during labor and delivery
  Peroneal nerve compression
  Lumbosacral plexus injury

two thirds of the tongue and hyperacusis develop. Sir Charles Bell first noted the association of pregnancy with seventh-nerve palsy in 1830, but it was Hilsinger and colleagues (5) who quantified this risk in 1975, finding that Bell palsy is 3.3 times more likely to occur during pregnancy and the puerperium. Incidence estimates vary, but Bell palsy probably occurs in approximately 1 in 2600 pregnancies (6).

The facial nerve lesion is thought to occur near the stylomastoid foramen or within the bony canal. In nonpregnant patients, Bell palsy has been associated with numerous disease processes, including Lyme disease, herpetic infection, otitis media, trauma, tumors, sarcoidosis, diabetes, and leukemia. The reason why Bell palsy's incidence is increased in pregnancy is not known, but it has been postulated that the increase may be due to viral infection (especially herpes simplex virus infection), hypertension, fluid retention, an immune process, pathologic changes involving the vasovasorum, or a combination of these factors (7–10). Some authors have suggested an increased incidence in primigravidas because of the increased prevalence of preeclampsia, but the association between primigravid status and Bell palsy is unclear.

The course, evaluation, and treatment of Bell palsy are the same in pregnant and nonpregnant women. Two thirds of patients recover within 2 weeks, and most recover within 6 months. Persons more likely to have incomplete recovery are older, have more severe initial paralysis, or have hyperacusis or diminished taste. Steroids have been reported to improve the rate of recovery if given early in the disease course, but this is controversial. There is no reason to withhold steroid treatment during pregnancy or breastfeeding. Eye patching and methylcellulose drops may be required to prevent corneal injury.

Most pregnancy-related cases of Bell palsy occur in the third trimester or postpartum, and cases may be associated with preeclampsia in multiparous patients. Recurrence in more than one subsequent pregnancy has also been noted. There seem to be no increased risks during pregnancy in women with pre-existing idiopathic facial nerve palsy (11, 12). Bilateral facial palsies have been reported, but this raises concern about other, underlying systemic diseases. Regional anesthetics may be given safely because studies have not shown an association (13), although case reports describing the development of Bell palsy after epidural blood patch have been published (14, 15). This has not been proven to represent a true association.

Pregnant women with Bell palsy are especially distressed and concerned that they have had a stroke or that the fetus is in danger. Any time taken to provide reassurance and patient education is time well spent.

Brachial Plexopathy (Thoracic Outlet Syndrome)

The brachial plexus and subclavian artery may be compressed by 1) the increased pressure of brassiere straps resulting from increased weight of the breasts, 2) additional supraclavicular adipose tissue, and 3) postural changes of pregnancy (such as sagging and stooped shoulders or exaggerated lumbar lordosis). Shoulder and neck aches, paresthesias (especially in the ulnar nerve distribution), and vascular symptoms of the hand, including cyanosis and blanching, may occur in up to 5% of pregnant women. A patient may induce the symptoms by working with the arm elevated or working at a keyboard machine. Attempts to produce symptoms by postural manipulation, such as the Adson maneuver, may give inconsistent results unless the examiner has the patient in her usual clothes and posture. Attention to head, shoulder, and arm position and removal of constricting straps can be helpful, simple management techniques. Patients who have the thoracic outlet syndrome before pregnancy may have severely increased symptoms during pregnancy but improve after delivery and cessation of lactation.

Carpal Tunnel Syndrome

The carpal tunnel syndrome has been reported in 5% to 10% of pregnant women (16). One retrospective study of 1000 consecutive postpartum patients found that 25% had had symptoms of carpal tunnel compression during their pregnancy (17). Most women have bilateral symptoms, but symptoms in the dominant hand are usually more severe. The bothersome paresthesias and diminished fine-motor capacity of the hand are often nocturnal or morning-awakening symptoms that are often alleviated by proper wrist and hand splints (18). The edema of pregnancy seems to play a pathogenetic role, but diuretic therapy is not indicated. Resolution after delivery is slow and not always complete. Tobin (19) reported that 15% of patients did not obtain full postpartum recovery. Recurrence in subsequent pregnancies is expected, and surgical carpal tunnel release may be indicated for the woman with refractory symptoms, especially if she is considering another pregnancy. Consideration of surgical management should be left until postpartum resolution, if any, has stabilized. Diabetes and hypothyroidism should be considered as possible underlying causes.

Patients with upper-extremity neuropathies can have overlapping and confusing symptoms and physical findings. Having the patient mark the location of her symptoms on a diagram of the hand is a useful technique that has obviated nerve conduction studies in male and nonpregnant female patients. Nerve conduction studies may be necessary, however, to distinguish between syndromes caused by thoracic outlet and carpal tunnel compression and those caused by metabolic neuropathies.

Abdominal Wall Nerve Entrapment

As the uterus rises above the umbilicus, the abdominal wall is stretched, and the greatest tension is placed on the attachment of the fascial and muscular layers to the costal margin. The spinal nerves supplying sensory innervation to the upper abdomen traverse and penetrate the abdominal wall and can be compressed or stretched by the shearing forces between the different fascial and muscular layers produced by the stretching of the abdominal wall. The result is a characteristic syndrome of annoying dysethesia of the upper abdomen. The pain worsens during the last 6 weeks of pregnancy, interferes with sleep, and is unrelieved by postural changes. Patients may be subjected to sonography for renal, liver, and gallbladder disease or suspected uterine injury. The clinical clue is the presence of hypesthesia or anesthesia and superficial dysesthesia along with a history of parethesias in the distribution of the perforating abdominal branches of the thoracic spinal nerves. Occasionally, nerve blocks are needed to provide transient relief. Delivery initiates steady recovery.

Meralgia Paresthetica

Dysesthesia and hypesthesia or anesthesia of the anterior lateral thigh is a common but usually minor problem during pregnancy. Use of the lateral decubitus position aggravates the condition by compressing the anterior branch of the lateral femoral cutaneous nerve as it penetrates the tensor fascia lata. The discomfort of the paresthesias and dysesthesia of meralgia paresthetica may interfere with the postural management recommended for patients with edema, varicosities, and preeclampsia. Avoidance of prolonged compression of the lateral thigh by constricting circumferential garments is helpful. Even moderately tight slacks can exacerbate the syndrome if the patient is seated for a long time.

Nerve Compression
Syndromes Related to Labor and Delivery

Compressive peripheral nerve injuries are most likely to occur during labor and delivery. Peroneal nerve injury caused by malpositioning of the patient in the lithotomy position may not be apparent until 24 to 48 hours postpartum. Occasionally, the foot drop produced by compression of the peroneal nerve against the fibular head will require a short leg brace for a few weeks. Most often, the patient will have local tenderness and paresthesias or hypesthesia of the dorsum of the foot and anterolateral leg. Careful attention to padding on the knee stirrups and freeing of the parturient woman's legs from the knee stirrups can prevent the problem. Patients with cephalopelvic disproportion or those who require a difficult midforceps delivery may sustain injury to the anterior divisions of the L4 or L5 portions of the lumbrosacral trunk (20). The patient may have buttock or leg pain that intensifies with uterine contractions and may develop paresthesias, gastrocnemius, or anterior tibialis weakness postpartum. Spontaneous recovery from these "pinched nerve injuries" is the rule.

REFERENCES

1. **Massey EW, Cefalo RC.** Neuropathies of pregnancy. Obstet Gynecol. 1979;34:489-92.
2. **Massey EW.** Mononeuropathies in pregnancy. Semin Neurol. 1988;8:193-6.
3. **Fox MW, Harms RW, Davis DH.** Selected neurologic complications of pregnancy. Mayo Clin Proc. 1990;65:1595-618.
4. **Butterworth JF, Walker FO, Lysak SZ.** Pregnancy increases median nerve susceptibility to lidocaine. Anesthesiology. 1990;72:962-5.
5. **Hilsinger R, Adour K, Doty H.** Idiopathic facial paralysis, pregnancy and the menstrual cycle. Ann Otol Rhinol Laryngol. 1975;84:433-42.
6. **Walling AD.** Bell's palsy in pregnancy and the puerperium. J Fam Pract. 1993;36:559-63.
7. **Danielides V, Skevas A, Van Cauwenberge P, Vinck B, Tsanades G, Plachouras N.** Facial nerve palsy during pregnancy. Acta Otorhinolaryngol Belg. 1996;50:131-5.
8. **Morgan M, Nathwani D.** Facial palsy and infection: the unfolding story. Clin Infect Dis. 1992;14:263-71.
9. **Gboloade B.** Recurrent lower motor neurone facial paralysis in four successive pregnancies. J Laryngol Otol. 1994;108:587-8.
10. **Deshpande AD.** Recurrent Bell's palsy in pregnancy. J Laryngol Otol. 1990;104:713-4.
11. **Falco NA, Eriksson E.** Idiopathic facial palsy in pregnancy and the puerperium. Surg Gynecol Obstet. 1989;169:337-40.
12. **McGregor JA, Guberman A, Amer J, Goodlin R.** Idiopathic facial nerve paralysis (Bell's Palsy) in late pregnancy and the early puerperium. Obstet Gynecol. 1987;69:435-8.
13. **Dorsey DL, Camann W.** Obstetric anesthesia in patients with idiopathic facial paralysis (Bell's Palsy): a 10-year survey. Anesth Analg. 1993;77:81-1.
14. **Perez M, Olmos M, Garrido FJ.** Facial nerve paralysis after epidural blood patch. Reg Anesth. 1993;18:196-8.
15. **Lowe DM, McCullough AM.** 7th nerve palsy after extradural blood patch. Br J Anaesth. 1990;65:721-2.
16. **Massey EW.** Carpal tunnel syndrome in pregnancy. Obstet Gynecol Surv. 1978;33:145-8.
17. **Voitk AJ, Mueller JC, Farlinger DE, et al.** Carpal tunnel syndrome in pregnancy. Can Med Assoc J. 1983;128:277-9.
18. **Katz JN, Larson MG, Sabra A, et al.** The carpal tunnel syndrome: diagnostic utility of the history and physical examination findings. Ann Intern Med. 1990;112:321-7.
19. **Tobin SM.** Carpal tunnel syndrome in pregnancy. Am J Obstet Gynecol. 1967;97:493-8.
20. **Whittaker WG.** Injuries to the sacral plexus in obstetrics. Can Med Assoc J. 1958;79:622-6.

V. Myasthenia Gravis
Lucia Larson

Myasthenia gravis (MG) is an uncommon disease with an incidence of 40 cases per million (1, 2). Its prevalence in pregnancy has been reported to be 1 in 20,000 (3). The peak onset of MG is during the reproductive years in women but during the 60s and 70s in men. It is an autoimmune disease associated with antibodies directed against the nicotinic acetylcholine receptors at the neuromuscular junction, which are thought to block acetylcholine. Detectable levels of these antibodies are found in as many as 90% of patients with MG. Approximately 10% to 15% of patients with MG have an associated thymoma and, conversely, 30% of patients with thymoma have MG. Myasthenia gravis is often associated with other autoimmune diseases, such as Hashimoto thyroiditis or systemic lupus erythematosus.

Patients with MG present with symptoms of muscle weakness and fatigability. Usual symptoms include ptosis, diplopia, dysphagia, and facial and limb weakness, especially after repetitive motions. The diagnosis of MG is often strongly suggested by history and physical examination. However, the edrophonium (Tensilon) test, assays for serum acetylcholine receptor antibodies, and electromyography may also be useful in making the diagnosis. All of these studies may be done safely in pregnancy. Associated thymic pathology can be ruled out by MRI.

Effect of Pregnancy on Myasthenia Gravis

Because MG is uncommon, it is not surprising that no prospective studies have evaluated the effect of pregnancy on the course of MG. From the limited data available, various authors have come to various conclusions about this effect (4–9). What can be said is that MG is as unpredictable in pregnancy and the puerperium as it is outside of pregnancy. Some women have significant exacerbations, and others have entirely uneventful pregnancies and postpartum courses. When exacerbations occur, they may present during any trimester or during the puerperium. Exacerbations may be precipitated by identifiable factors, such as systemic illness or changes in medications, or may occur without clear precipitants. In keeping with the unpredictability of the disease, the course of MG in a previous pregnancy does not predict the course of MG in a subsequent pregnancy.

Treatment of Myasthenia Gravis in Pregnancy

In general, patients with MG should be treated in the same way whether they are pregnant or not (10). The anticholinesterases are important medications for these patients, and their use should be continued during pregnancy. Because of the physiologic changes associated with pregnancy, doses and the frequency of administration may need to be increased. If required, neostigmine and pyridostigmine may be given intramuscularly or intravenously. Overmedication with anticholinesterases can cause increased weakness and other symptoms of a cholinergic crisis, such as pallor, sweating, nausea, vomiting, hypersalivation, abdominal pain, and meiosis. Corticosteroid treatment is also important in the management of myasthenia but, when instituted for an exacerbation, it may cause temporary worsening before improvement is noted. Monitoring for hyperglycemia during pregnancy when corticosteroids are used is advised. Stress steroid doses are required at delivery if steroids have been used for more than 3 weeks during the year before delivery. Plasmapheresis is useful in the treatment of myasthenic crisis and has been used successfully in pregnancy. Thymectomy is associated with improvement or remission of MG in 85% of patients, but sometimes only months or years after surgery. It can be done during the second trimester but ideally should be done before conception or delayed until after delivery.

Effect of Myasthenia Gravis on Pregnancy

Myasthenia gravis neither affects fertility nor significantly increases the risk for miscarriage or congenital malformations. Slight increases in preterm labor have been reported (4, 5). Intrauterine fetal MG from transplacental passage of IgG antibodies is rare and is manifested by decreased fetal movement, which may be associated with joint contractures (arthrogryposis). Polyhydramnios, presumably related to impaired swallowing, has been reported, as has pulmonary hypoplasia related to decreased chest expansion. A woman with two previous pregnancies complicated by neonatal deaths associated with myasthenia was treated in subsequent pregnancies with plasmapheresis and prednisone. As her antibody titers changed, fetal breathing movements were noted to appear and disappear (6).

Special Management Issues
in Pregnancy, Labor, and Delivery

During pregnancy, it is important to monitor for changes in disease status by evaluating maternal muscle strength and measuring vital capacity. Changes in medication doses related to the physiologic changes of pregnancy are likely to be required even if the activity of MG is unchanged. Conditions that frequently exacerbate MG, including hyperthyroidism, hypothyroidism, and occult infection, should be meticulously sought. Asymptomatic bacteriuria must be aggressively screened for and treated. Similarly, prompt treatment of respiratory infections should be instituted. Adequate rest is advised. Attention should be paid to the numerous medications that have been noted to exacerbate muscle weakness in patients with MG (Box 12-5), particularly magnesium sulfate and beta-adrenergic agents such as terbutaline.

Because the uterus consists of smooth muscle, which is unaffected by MG, labor in women with MG proceeds normally. During the second stage of labor, however, voluntary striated muscles may tire and a forceps or vacuum delivery may be required. Cesarean section should be done for obstetric indications only. It is important to continue intravenous or intramuscular anticholinesterase therapy if patients are not receiving oral medications or if gastric absorption is likely to be impaired. Consultation with an experienced anesthetist is desirable. Epidural anesthesia may be given, but the metabolism of the ester-type anesthetics may be impaired in women treated with anticholinesterases. Although general anesthesia may be given, ether, halothane, and the nondepolarizing muscle relaxants (such as curare) should be avoided.

Box 12-5 Drugs Associated with Worsening Muscle Weakness in Myasthenia Gravis

---

Penicillamine

Corticosteroids

Anticonvulsants (phenytoin, trimethadione)

Antibiotics (aminoglycosides, ampicillin, erythromycin, polymixin, ciprofloxacin, clindamycin)

Narcotics

Barbiturates

Inhalation anesthetics (ether, halothane, trichlorethylene)

Neuromuscular blocking agents (curare, pancuronium, succinylcholine)

Beta-adrenergic agent (terbutaline, ritodrine)

Magnesium sulfate

Anticholinergic drugs

Beta-blockers (including eye drops)

Calcium-channel blockers (verapamil)

Iodinated contrast agents

Psychotropics (chlorpromazine, phenelzine)

Lithium

Antiarrythmics (procainamide, quinidine, lidocaine)

Effect of Maternal Myasthenia Gravis on the Neonate

Maternal IgG antibodies to acetylcholine receptors cross the placenta, and approximately 10% to 20% of neonates born to women with MG develop neonatal myasthenia from this passive transfer of antibodies. Severity varies, but the infant usually has generalized muscle weakness, difficulty in feeding, and feeble cry. Respiratory distress may develop, necessitating ventilatory support. Infants usually become symptomatic within the first 24 hours of life and often recover completely by 6 weeks. A few infants may not become symptomatic for 3 to 4 days; this may be related to the transplacental transfer of anticholinesterase medications used to treat the mother. Infants with neonatal myasthenia are not at increased risk for MG later in life.

Of note, the development of neonatal MG cannot be predicted by using antibody titers or maternal disease status. Case reports exist of asymptomatic women who delivered several affected babies and only later were diagnosed with MG (7). The reason for this is uncertain but may be related to developmental differences in acetylcholine receptors or differences in the antibodies themselves (3). There is also evidence to suggest that the neonates produce their own autoantibodies (8).

Breastfeeding

The breastmilk of women with MG contains antibodies to acetylcholine receptors. The importance of the potential transfer of these antibodies to the neonate through breastfeeding is in question because much larger quantities of these antibodies reach the infant through transplacental transfer. There are reports of women with MG who have breastfed with no apparent effect (2). It may be reasonable to allow breastfeeding, with close observation, of infants who do not have neonatal myasthenia. However, the breastfeeding of affected neonates, who are already more likely to have feeding difficulties, should be approached with greater caution.

Summary

Myasthenia gravis is unpredictable in pregnancy, and women with MG who are considering pregnancy should be aware of this. These women may not have exacerbations during pregnancy or the postpartum period, but they should be prepared for the possibility. They may require assistance in the care of their newborn. In addition, 15% to 20% of newborns are affected by neonatal MG, which usually resolves by 6 weeks after birth. The medications used to treat MG should be continued during pregnancy, and dosage adjustments may be required. Medications that exacerbate MG, such as magnesium sulfate and terbutaline, should be avoided.

REFERENCES

1. **Mitchell FJ, Bebbington M.** Myasthenia gravis in pregnancy. Obstet Gynecol. 1992; 80:178-81.
2. **Kurtzke JF.** Epidemiology of myasthenia gravis. Adv Neurol. 1978;19:545-66.
3. **Giacoia GP, Azubuike K.** Autoimmune diseases in pregnancy: their effect on the fetus and newborn. Obstet Gynecol Surv. 1991;46:723-32.
4. **Fennell DF, Ringel SP.** Myasthenia gravis and pregnancy. Obstet Gynecol Surv. 1987;41:414-21.
5. **Plauche WC.** Myasthenia gravis in mothers and their newborns. Clin Obstet Gynecol. 1991;34:82-99.
6. **Carr SR, Gilchrist JM, Abuelo DN, Clark D.** Treatment of antenatal myasthenia gravis. Obstet Gynecol. 1991;78(3 pt 2):485-9.
7. **Barnes PRJ, Kanabar DJ, Brueton L, Newsomdavis J, Huson SM, Mann NP, Hilton-Jones D.** Recurrent congenital arthrogryposis leading to a diagnosis of myasthenia gravis in an initially asymptomatic mother. Neuromuscul Disord. 1995;5:59-65.
8. **Pilkington C, Lefvert AK, Rook GAW.** Neonatal myasthenia gravis and the role of agalactosyl IgG. Autoimmunity. 1995;21:131-5.
9. **Gilchrist J.** Muscle disease in the pregnant women. In: Neurologic Complications in Pregnancy. New York: Raven Press; 1994:193-208.
10. **Wittbrodt ET.** Drugs and myasthenia gravis. Arch Intern Med. 1997;157:399-408.

VI. Multiple Sclerosis
Lucia Larson

Multiple sclerosis (MS) is an acquired demyelinating disease that affects approximately 250,000 persons in the United States. It affects twice as many women as men and tends to present during the reproductive years. It is characterized by exacerbations and remissions of neurologic symptoms related to multiple lesions in the brain and spinal cord white matter. Common presenting symptoms include visual blurring secondary to optic neuritis, diplopia, ataxia and sensory symptoms, and weakness of the limbs. Courses vary from patient to patient, but MS often presents with a relapsing–remitting pattern and becomes a secondarily progressive disease with time. Approximately one third of patients will have a progressive course from onset. Poor prognostic signs include older age at onset, significant paresis or tremor, poor response to corticosteroid treatment, and male sex. Unfortunately, many patients and their families experience significant psychosocial and economic difficulties related to the physical problems brought on by the disease.

The cause of MS is unknown but may be related to an immune response to an infectious agent in a genetically susceptible person. Pathologic specimens show plaques in the white matter of the brain and spinal cord; these plaques begin as focal areas of demyelination that are followed by reactive gliosis. They develop at different times and are scattered throughout the CNS. Evidence of genetic susceptibility is supported by studies of twins and adopted children. The offspring of patients with MS have a 30- to 50-fold increased risk for MS (1). That environmental factors play a role is suggested by the observation that the incidence of MS increases with northern latitude.

Diagnosis

The diagnosis of MS requires evidence of two lesions occurring in different parts of the CNS at different times. Findings supporting the diagnosis include oligoclonal bands in the cerebrospinal fluid and prolonged visual, auditory, and somatosensory evoked responses. Studies to elicit these findings may be done safely in pregnancy. Magnetic resonance imaging is helpful diagnostically in evaluating clinically silent lesions and in quantitating the burden of disease over time. It has been done safely in pregnancy, although gadolinium is usually omitted because little information is available on the use of gadolinium in pregnancy (2).

Effect of Pregnancy on the Course of Multiple Sclerosis

Patients with MS in the early 20th century were counseled against pregnancy because of the impression that pregnancy adversely affected the course of MS. Since that time, many studies have attempted to determine the effect of pregnancy on MS. Multiple sclerosis is difficult to study because its course is unpredictable and variable both within an individual patient and from patient to patient. Quantitating disease activity is not easy. For instance, measurement of the number of relapses in relapsing–remitting disease may evaluate short-term disease activity but does not necessarily relate to the rate of sustained disability or account for patients with chronic progressive disease. Many of the studies done on MS in pregnancy have been retrospective and subject to recall bias and other limitations. Most prospective studies have small numbers of patients and limited follow-up. Further, earlier studies did not use clear diagnostic criteria and many did not distinguish between relapsing–remitting and chronic progressive disease. The severity of MS may influence reproductive decisions: Women with less severe MS may be more likely than those with severe MS to choose pregnancy.

Despite these limitations, several conclusions may be drawn. First, no evidence suggests that pregnancy alters the risk for long-term disability (3–7). Second, there seems to be a decreased rate of relapse during pregnancy. Third, approximately 20% to 40% of patients have relapse in the first 6 months postpartum (3–6, 8–10); this represents a statistically significant increase compared with the rate of relapse in nonpregnant periods (5). Information on the severity of relapse during pregnancy and the postpartum period is limited, but some investigations suggest that attacks may be more severe in the postpartum period. In one study (11), 27 of 91 patients (30%) were unable to care for their newborns. We have an important report of two patients who became pregnant during a serial MRI study in which disease activity was found to decrease during pregnancy and active lesions reappeared postpartum (12). The tendency toward improvement during pregnancy and exacerbation postpartum is mirrored in other immune-mediated diseases, such as rheumatoid arthritis and Graves disease. It is thought that the immune changes of pregnancy that allow tolerance of paternal antigens may be responsible for the effects of pregnancy on these diseases.

Effect of Multiple Sclerosis on Pregnancy

As a group, women with MS have not been found to have an increase in obstetric complications. Their rates of miscarriage, congenital malformation, preeclampsia, prematurity, and infant death do not differ from those of the general population. Obstetric issues that are common in the general population may be treated in the usual manner in patients with MS. In particular, magnesium sulfate and the sympathomimetics still used for tocolysis in some centers, such as terbutaline, may be used (9).

Special Management Concerns in Pregnancy

In general, women with mild MS should enjoy pregnancies without complications, but several issues should be addressed in women with more severe disease and greater disability. A woman with a neurogenic bladder may have worsening symptoms because of the mechanical effects of the gravid uterus and the hormonally induced changes of the urinary tract. These patients must be carefully evaluated for bacteriuria and may require frequent urinary catheterization or antibiotic prophylaxis. Constipation may worsen. Less-mobile patients may develop skin breakdown. It may be reasonable to consider giving prophylactic heparin to significantly immobile patients, whose risk for thromboembolic disease is further increased in pregnancy. In addition, patients with a marginal ability to ambulate or make transfers before pregnancy may be challenged even further as they face the progressive physical changes of pregnancy. Fatigability is a factor in any woman's pregnancy but may be more prominent in women with MS.

Treatment of Multiple Sclerosis in Pregnancy

The medications used in the treatment of MS may prevent relapse, prevent progression of disease, or treat symptoms. Corticosteroids are important in the treatment of MS relapse and can be used safely in pregnancy. A pregnant woman receiving a significant steroid dose during pregnancy should be monitored for hyperglycemia. In addition, stress-dose steroids should be given during labor and delivery to women who received steroids for 3 or more weeks in the year before delivery. Interferon has proven useful in the management of MS, but there is less experience with its use in pregnancy and it has been found to have abortifacient activity in monkeys at high doses. Glatiramer acetate is used as an alternative to interferon-beta in the treatment of MS, but no data are available on its use in pregnancy. Other agents that have been used to treat relapsing and progressive MS include azathioprine, intravenous immune globulin, methotrexate, cyclophosphamide, and cyclosporine. The information available on their use in pregnancy and lactation is summarized in the Drug Table for Seizures and Multiple Sclerosis at the end of this chapter (2, 13), which also lists the drugs used to treat neurogenic bladder and muscle spasm. Decisions about the use of these drugs in pregnancy should involve a careful weighing of the potential benefits and risks.

Parturition and Postpartum

In general, labor and delivery may proceed normally in patients with MS, although a woman with more disabling disease may be unable to adequately push. Early intervention with forceps may be required in some cases. Cesarean section should be done only for obstetric indications. Some patients may develop increased spasticity in labor secondary to visceral stimuli from the bladder, bowel, and uterine contractions. There has been concern that regional anesthesia may cause an exacerbation of MS, possibly through a direct neurotoxic effect of the agents used. However, current studies have found no increased rate of relapse in patients who have received epidural anesthesia (8, 14). In a study by Bader and associates (14), the women who had postpartum relapse had received higher concentrations of bupivacaine. This led the authors to recommend that lower concentrations of anesthetics be used. Multiple sclerosis is not an absolute contraindication to regional anesthesia, and the benefits of this anesthesia need not be denied to patients with MS. After delivery, a patient with MS may need help caring for her newborn. The rate of relapse of MS is particularly increased in the first 3 months postpartum but remains elevated for 6 months. No study has correlated such variables as physical and emotional stress or sleep deprivation with the incidence of relapse, but rest is certainly recommended. One study treated women with intravenous immunoglobulin for the first 3 months postpartum in an attempt to decrease postpartum exacerbations. Of the nine patients treated, none had relapse within 6 months but three had relapse at 8 and 10 months postpartum (15). Further research is needed to examine possible treatments to prevent postpartum relapse. Breastfeeding is not contraindicated and should be encouraged and supported if desired (8, 16). The American Academy of Pediatrics considers prednisone compatible with breastfeeding, but many other commonly used immunosuppressive agents are not recommended in breastfeeding mothers.

Summary

Most women with multiple sclerosis do well during pregnancy and have the same risk for obstetric complications as women in the general population. Labor and delivery may be expected to proceed normally, and regional anesthesia may be given. Women with MS may be reassured that no evidence suggests that pregnancy increases the overall rate of progression to long-term disability. Patients should know that while the rate of relapse during pregnancy is decreased, 20% to 40% of women will have relapse in the first 6 months postpartum and this may interfere with the ability to care for the newborn. Breastfeeding need not be discouraged on the basis of MS alone, although it may not be advisable with certain medications. It should be noted that the children of women with MS have a 3% risk for contracting MS in their lifetime. Pregnancy is not contraindicated in women with MS, but a woman should be encouraged to consider her personal circumstances before beginning a pregnancy. Considerations may include baseline disability and the resources available to the woman and her family if her disease should progress.

REFERENCES

1. **Rudick RA, Cohen JA, Weinstock-Guttman B, Kinkel RP, Ransohoff RM.** Management of multiple sclerosis. N Engl J Med. 1997;337:1604-11.

2. The Reprotox System. Reproductive Toxicology Center, Micromedex Computerized Clinical Information Center; 1998.

3. **Damek D, Shuster E.** Pregnancy and multiple sclerosis. Mayo Clin Proc. 1997;72:977-89.

4. **Weinreb JH.** Demyelinating and neoplastic diseases in pregnancy. Neurol Clin. 1994; 12:509-26.

5. **Cook SD, Toiano R, Bansil S, Dowling PC.** Multiple sclerosis and pregnancy. In: Neurologic Complications in Pregnancy. New York: Raven Press; 1994:83-95.

6. **Worthington J, Jones R, Crawford M, Forti A.** Pregnancy and multiple sclerosis—a 3 year prospective study. J Neurol. 1994;241:228-33.

7. **Sadovnick AD, Eisen K, Hashimoto SA, Farquhar R, Yee IM, Hooge L, et al.** Pregnancy and multiple sclerosis: a prospective study. Arch Neurol. 1994;51:1120-4.

8. **Confavreux C, Hutchinson M, Hours MM, Cortinovis-Tourniaire P, Moreau T.** Pregnancy in multiple sclerosis group: rate of pregnancy-related relapse in multiple sclerosis. N Engl J Med. 1998;339:285-91.

9. **Davis R, Maslow A.** Multiple sclerosis in pregnancy: a review. Obstet Gynecol Surv. 1992;47:290-6.

10. **Birk K, Rudick R.** Pregnancy and multiple sclerosis. Arch Neurol. 1986;43:719-26.

11. **Poser S, Poser W.** Multiple sclerosis and gestation. Neurology. 1983;33:1422-7.

12. **van Walderveen MAA, Tas MW, Barkhof F, Polman CH, Frequin STFM, Hommes OR, Valk J.** Magnetic resonance evaluation of disease activity during pregnancy in multiple sclerosis. Neurology. 1994;44:327-9.

13. **Briggs G, Freeman R, Yaffe S.** Drugs in Pregnancy and Lactation. Baltimore: Williams & Wilkins; 1998.

14. **Bader AM, Hunt CO, Datta S.** Anesthesia for the obstetric patient with multiple sclerosis. J Clin Anesth. 1988;1:21-21.

15. **Achiron A, Rotstien Z, Noy S, Mashiach S, Dulitzky M, Achiron R.** Intravenous immunoglobulin treatment in the prevention of childbirth-associated acute exacerbations in multiple sclerosis: a pilot study. J Neurol. 1996;243:25-8.

16. **Nelson L, Franklin GM, Jones MC.** Risk of multiple sclerosis exacerbation during pregnancy and breast-feeding. The Multiple Sclerosis Study Group. JAMA. 1988;259:3441-3.

APPENDIX: DRUGS FOR MIGRAINE AND SEIZURES/MULTIPLE SCLEROSIS

The drug tables on pages 699 and 700 are for reference when there is a clinical indication for treatment with one of the medications listed. Decisions about medication use in pregnancy should be made on the basis of a benefit-to-risk ratio, avoiding unnecessary treatment of symptoms but with consideration of the fact that fetal well-being depends on maternal well-being. Because the U.S. Food and Drug Administration is working on a new classification system for the use of medications in pregnancy, we have classified medications as follows:

Data Suggest Drug Use May Be Justified When Indicated
When data and/or experience supports the safety of the drug.

Data Suggest Drug Use May Be Justified in Some Circumstances
When less extensive or desirable data are reported but the drug is reasonable as a second-line therapy or may be used on the basis of the severity of maternal illness.

Data Suggest Drug Use Is Rarely Justified
Use drug only when alternatives supported by more experience and/or a better safety profile are not available.

Pregnancy pharmacokinetics may necessitate a significant increase in dose or dosing frequency, and dosing recommendations may require modification according to individual circumstances.

Drugs for Migraine

	Use May Be Justified When Indicated	Use May Be Justified in Some Circumstances	Use Is Rarely Justified	Comments/Dose Adjustment
Treatment				
Analgesics (narcotic)	√			All can cause neonatal withdrawal syndrome if used near delivery
Meperidine				
Oxycodone				
Codeine				
Morphine				
Analgesics (simple)	√			
Acetaminophen, caffeine				
Analgesics (simple)	√			
Aspirin, NSAIDs				
Antiemetics	√			Preferred agent
Metoclopramide				
Prochlorperazine, trimethobenzamide, promethazine		√		
Barbiturates		√		
Butalbital				
Corticosteroids				
Prednisone	√			Preferred agent
Dexamethasone		√		Fetal adrenal suppression
Prophylaxis				
Amitriptyline	√			Preferred prophylactic agent
Atenolol		√		
Cyproheptadine	√			
Vasoactive agents		√		Adverse effect on placental blood flow
Ergotamine				
Dihydroergotamine				
Methysergide				
Sumatriptan				
Veramapil, diltiazem				
Vitamin B_6		√		Preferred prophylactic agent

Drugs for Seizures and Multiple Sclerosis

	Use May Be Justified When Indicated	Use May Be Justified in Some Circumstances	Use Is Rarely Justified	Comments/Dose Adjustment
Drugs for Seizures				
Antiepileptic agents (i) Phenytoin Phenobarbital Carbamazepine	√			See Section III; all AEDs probably are teratogenic and associated with neonatal coagulopathy, but their use is preferable to uncontrolled seizures
Antiepileptic agents (ii) Valproic acid		√		Early first-trimester use is associated with 10- to 17-fold increase in neural tube defects
Newer antiepileptic agents Lamotrigine Gabapentin Felbamate		√		Limited data available
Drugs for Multiple Sclerosis				
Cyclobenzaprine		√		Preferred muscle relaxant
ACTH and corticosteroids	√			Human studies show no increase in anomalies
Beta-interferon		√		Abortifacient in monkeys; no human data
Baclofen			√	Ossification abnormalities; neural tube defects in animals
Hyoscyamine		√		

CHAPTER 13

Infectious Disease

I. Introduction
Richard V. Lee

Pregnancy does not protect a woman from the microbes of the world. In fact, the biological and behavioral effects of gestation may enhance a woman's risk for infection by microbes and by toxin-producing multicellular organisms (Box 13-1).

Because of their adverse effects on pregnancy outcome, certain food-related infections and intoxications, upper and lower respiratory tract infec-

---

Box 13-1 Gestational Effects That Influence the Clinical Manifestation of Infections

---

Altered cell-mediated immune function
Diminished gastrointestinal motility
    Delayed gastric emptying
    Esophageal relaxation
    Slow passage through colon
    Decreased peristalsis of biliary tract; dilation of gallbladder
Increased vascularity of the skin
    Increased blood flow
    Telangiectasia
    Increased surface temperature
Intrapartum and postpartum soiling of perineum

---

tions, urinary tract infections, sexually transmitted infectious diseases, and infections that can cause transplacental or intrauterine infection are of particular concern during gestation (Table 13-1 and Figure 13-1). Preterm, premature rupture of membranes, premature labor and delivery, intrauterine infection with fetal demise or persisting neonatal infection, and infection of the neonate acquired during delivery are major continuing problems caused by maternal infection with a variety of microbes (Table 13-2).

After reviewing antimicrobial drug use and immunizations during pregnancy, this chapter discusses genitourinary tract infections, sexually transmitted diseases and HIV, and upper respiratory and pulmonary infections; a review of unusual infections closes the chapter.

Antimicrobial Drugs

Anti-infective agents are, after vitamins, the drugs most commonly prescribed for pregnant women. Gestational effects alter patterns of infection and the pharmacokinetics of antimicrobial drugs. Increases in maternal plasma volume, total body water, and the glomerular filtration rate result in an increased volume of distribution and an increased rate of clearance of almost all antimicrobial drugs. Serum concentrations of antibiotics tend to be lower in pregnant than in nonpregnant women, and adjustments in dosing intervals and dosage quantities, guided by appropriate serum levels, are necessary (1–6). Infections that traverse the placenta to infect the fetus require

Table 13-1 Effects of Some Common Maternal Infectious Diseases on Pregnancy

	Preterm, Premature Rupture of Membranes	Premature Labor and Delivery	Transplacental Infection	Neonatal Infection
Sexually transmitted diseases	Chlamydia gonococcus, bacterial vaginosis, Trichomonas vaginalis	Chlamydia gonococcus, bacterial vaginosis, Trichomonas vaginalis	Syphilis	Herpes simplex, group B streptococci
Food-borne infections		Listeria monocytogenes, Campylobacter sp., Shigella sp., Salmonella sp.	Listeria monocytogenes; Toxoplasma gondii; Salmonella sp.	Listeria monocytogenes, Campylobacter sp., Shigella sp., Salmonella sp., hepatitis B, enteroviruses, Taenia solium (tapeworm in mother, cysticercosis in child)
Urinary tract infections	Upper and lower UTI with E. coli	Pyelonephritis (various organisms)		
Pneumonia		Multi-lobe pneumonia (various organisms)		
Vector-borne infections		Malaria	Malaria (Plasmodium falciparum), Trypanosoma cruzi (Chagas disease)	
Air-borne infections		Active untreated tuberculosis	Parvovirus B19, rubella, varicella	Active untreated tuberculosis

treatment with antibiotics that can produce therapeutic levels in both the maternal and the fetoplacental compartments. Although all antibiotics cross the placenta to some extent, only a few are transported efficiently enough to be efficacious or toxic in the fetus (3).

Studies of new antimicrobial drugs in pregnant women are limited, and this further complicates management decisions in the gravid woman with a serious infectious disease (1). The philosophy of this book is to use the most efficacious drug or drugs available—regardless of theoretical or possible but unproved adverse effects on the fetus and pregnancy outcome—in cases of life-threatening maternal or fetal infection. There is nothing to be gained and everything to be lost by withholding necessary but toxic antibiotics from pregnant women with multidrug-resistant tuberculosis, Plasmodium falciparum malaria, or staphylococcal infection. Similarly, unthinkingly prescribed antibiotic treatment of self-limited viral infections is both futile and dangerous. Very few contemporary antibiotics are absolutely contraindicated in pregnancy. The Drug Table for Infectious Diseases at the end of this chap-

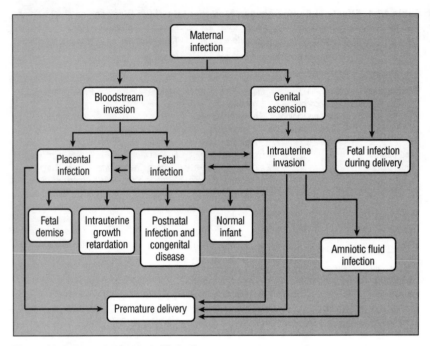

Figure 13-1 Dangers of maternal infection.

ter lists the classes of antimicrobial drugs that are most often thought to be associated with fetotoxicity (1–6).

Anxiety and inertia also surround the use of antimicrobial agents by lactating mothers. Maternal anti-infective drugs are secreted into breastmilk in small amounts and pose no particular threat to nursing infants. The concentrations of common antimicrobial drugs in breastmilk in relation to those in maternal serum are shown in Table 13-3. Even when they occur in breastmilk in concentrations similar to maternal plasma concentrations, antibiotics that are necessary for effective maternal therapy but potentially risky for the infant should be used. For example, the infants of breastfeeding mothers who are receiving isoniazid (INH) for active tuberculosis should receive supplemental vitamin B_6 while continuing to receive breastmilk.

Immunizing Pregnant Women

One of the truly illustrious accomplishments of 20th century medicine was the development of effective vaccines for immunoprophylaxis. One of the saddest failures of 20th century medicine was the incomplete and erratic delivery of vaccines to populations at risk (7). In the United States a substantial mi-

Table 13-2 Pathogens with Particular Risks for Maternal, Fetal, and Neonatal Problems

Organism	Maternal Problems	Fetal Problems	Neonatal Problems
Bacteria			
Listeria mono-cytogenes	Bacteremia, sepsis, amnionitis	Intrauterine infection, granulomatosis infantisepticum, IUFD, stillbirth	Sepsis, meningitis
Group B streptococci	Chronic GU carriage, UTI, sepsis		Early-onset sepsis and pneumonia, meningitis
Treponema pallidum	Syphilis	Intrauterine infection, IUFD, stillbirth	Congenital syphilis
Viruses			
HIV	AIDS	Vertical transmission to fetus and neonate	Vertical transmission to fetus and neonate
Hepatitis B	Chronic infection, fulminant hepatitis	Vertical transmission to fetus and neonate	Vertical transmission to fetus and neonate
Hepatitis E	Fulminant hepatitis, maternal death		
Parvovirus B19	Arthralgias, rash, minor symptoms, fever; can be asymptomatic	Hydrops fetalis	Anemia
Rubella	Rash, arthralgias, minor symptoms, fever	Congenital rubella syndrome	Congenital rubella syndrome
Herpes simplex	Primary infection HSVI: gingivolabial HSVII: genital and pharyngeal Incandescent active infection		Disseminated herpes simplex
Parasites			
Toxoplasma gondii	Often asymptomatic	Intrauterine fetal infection, abortion, IUFD, congenital sequelae	
Plasmodium falciparum	Malaria	Intrauterine fetal infection	
Trypanosoma cruzi	Chagas disease	Intrauterine fetal infection with congenital sequelae	
Taenia solium	Pig tapeworm		Cysticercosis

nority of young women are not rubella immune, and around the world measles remains a major cause of death.

Anxiety about the adverse effects of vaccines on the fetus has led to confusion and overcaution about the use of vaccines during pregnancy. An experienced, educated maternal immune system is still the first line of defense against devastating maternal, fetal, and neonatal infections. Ideally, women entering their reproductive careers should be fully immunized against common infections. Unfortunately, antagonism to immunization remains a serious obstacle to control of preventable infectious disease in the industrialized and developed world. The terrible cost of preventable deaths resulting from neonatal tetanus (8), childhood diphtheria, and measles is ignored or denied.

Immunization is very specific. Immunization against measles will not protect the recipient against tetanus. Patients must understand that the human immune system is, by nature, a wonderfully specific recognition system and that multiple immunizations are required to protect against multiple diseases. Many adults are reluctant to be vaccinated because of misconceptions about the need for multiple vaccines. Common but invalid excuses for avoiding vaccination include being pregnant or living in a household with a pregnant woman, breastfeeding or caring for an infant, currently being ill, currently using antimicrobial therapy, recently having been exposed to an infectious disease, having a family or personal history of local reactions to vaccine, and having a family or personal history of atopic allergies or food intolerance.

Protective immunity can be gained by 1) exposing a patient's immune system to the key antigens of a pathogen so that protective antibodies or lymphocytes are produced (active immunization) or 2) providing antibodies preformed in humans or animals (passive immunization). Because incubation of an infection can take less time than the development of active immunity,

Table 13-3 Antibiotic Excretion in Breastmilk in Relation to Maternal Serum Concentration

<10%	10%–50%	>50%
Penicillin	Erythromycin	Metronidazole
Amoxicillin	Clindamycin	Ciprofloxacin
Imipenem	Azithromycin	Ofloxacin
Cefazolin	Doxycycline	Isoniazid
Cephalexin	Rifampin	Ethambutol
Cefotaxime	Nitrofurantoin	
Aztreonam		
Sulfamethoxazole		
Trimethoprim		
Amantadine		

Data from Briggs GG, Freeman RK, Yaffe SJ. Drugs in Pregnancy and Lactation, 5th ed. Baltimore: Williams & Wilkins; 1998; and Duff P. Antibiotic selection in obstetric patients. Infect Dis Clin North Am. 1997;11:1-12.

passive immunization may be desirable when a patient will be immediately immersed in an epidemic situation. Pooled human gamma globulin has become increasingly scarce, limiting the availability of passive immunization against pathogens for which specific active immunization is available. Moreover, the production of human immune globulins for a variety of pathogens has made passive immunization more specific and has reduced the risk for complicating serum sickness and anaphylaxis from animal-derived antiserums.

Passive Immunization

Most animal antiserums—for example, those for black widow spider bites, botulism, diphtheria, and snake bites—come from horses. Scorpion-venom antiserum is raised in goats. Human immunoglobulin has been prepared for hepatitis A, hepatitis B, rabies, Rh antigen, varicella, and tetanus (Table 13-4).

Table 13-4 Passive Immunization Using Human Immunoglobulin

Disease	Preparations	Use
Hepatitis A	Pooled immune gamma globulin 0.02–0.06 mL/kg IM for 3 months of protection 0.02 mL/kg IM up to 2 weeks after exposure Start hepatitis A virus vaccine at a different site	Active immunization with hepatitis A virus vaccine is preferred for travelers because pooled immunoglobin is increasingly scarce
Hepatitis B	HBIG 0.06 mL/kg as soon as possible after exposure Hepatitis B virus vaccine series started simultaneously If no vaccine, repeat HBIG in 3–4 weeks	For parental or mucosal exposure or for neonates of mothers who are chronic carriers of hepatitis B
Rabies	Rabies IgG 20 U/kg: half infiltrated locally, half IM Begin rabies virus vaccine series	Must be given within hours of suspected bite for best effect
Tetanus	Tetanus IgG Wound prophylaxis: 250–500 U IM Tetanus therapy: 3000–6000 U IM Begin tetanus toxoid series or give booster at different site	For unimmunized patients with wounds at risk for tetanus
Varicella	Varicella zoster IgG 1 vial/10 kg IM for a maximum of 5 vials	Give to exposed susceptible pregnant women to modify course of natural infection; best given within 5 days of exposure For neonates of mothers with active varicella for 5 days before or 2 days after delivery

Anaphylactic reactions and serum sickness are almost exclusively complications of the use of animal antiserum. A history of treatment with horse serum or of reactions to antiserum injections is important, but the clinician should be prepared for an adverse reaction regardless of history or the results of skin testing for immediate hypersensitivity.

Active Immunization

A variety of vaccines to induce humoral and cellular immunity are available, and more are being prepared for general use (9–14). These vaccines range from toxoids of bacterial toxins to attenuated live viruses and live bacteria. If a patient does not have allergic hypersensitivity to a vaccine's constituents, only live viral and live bacterial vaccines are contraindicated in pregnancy (see the Drug Table for Immunizations at the end of this chapter).

The inadvertent administration of rubella and yellow fever vaccines to pregnant women has been followed by evidence of transplacental fetal infection with vaccine virus but no evidence of fetal injury or persisting infection (13, 15). Inadvertent live-virus vaccination is not, therefore, an indication for pregnancy termination. In keeping with standard practice, vaccines are best given after the end of the first trimester. However, if an epidemic or pandemic (such as an influenza pandemic) is a potential concern, pregnant women at risk should be vaccinated immediately, even in the first trimester.

Viral Exanthems

Measles

Where childhood immunization programs are consistently and widely applied, measles during pregnancy is rare. Before the widespread use of measles vaccine, most persons had measles before puberty and the incidence of measles during pregnancy was estimated to be about 4 to 6 cases per 100,000 pregnancies. Currently, about one third of cases of measles are in persons of reproductive age, and the attack rate in pregnant women is much higher than it used to be (>700 cases per 100,000 pregnancies) (16). Maternal pneumonia, premature labor and spontaneous abortion, and low birthweight are the most common recorded complications of gestational measles (17). Maternal infection 2 to 3 weeks before delivery results in congenital infection in about one third of newborns. The effect of congenital infection on the newborn is inversely proportional to gestational age, with a 56% mortality rate in premature infants and a 20% mortality rate in full-term infants. The morbidity and mortality rate associated with measles in areas where measles is common are greatly influenced by the nutritional and comorbid status of the patient. Pregnancy loss, primary measles pneumonia, and maternal death are more common in malnourished populations with heavy infectious disease burdens. In a well-fed, basically healthy population, pregnancy only marginally enhances the severity of infection.

Mumps

Mumps is less contagious than measles, varicella, and rubella. Before widespread vaccine use, about one fourth of 10-year-old children were susceptible to mumps, and the incidence of mumps during gestation was about 80 to 100 cases per 100,000 pregnancies (18). The incidence of mumps in women of reproductive age has declined with vaccine use. Both vaccine virus and wild virus cross the placenta, but no specific pattern of teratogenesis or developmental abnormality has emerged. The severity of maternal illness is not magnified by pregnancy, but mumps mastitis can be particularly unpleasant when it develops during gestation or lactation.

Rubella

The rubella virus was the first virus shown to have teratogenic and fetotoxic effects (19). German or soft measles (as opposed to rubeola or hard measles) in unvaccinated populations is an endemic infection of school-age children: About half of children 9 to 11 years of age have serologic evidence of infection. In unvaccinated populations, 80% to 85% of women of childbearing age have antibody to the rubella virus. Vaccination programs have changed rubella from a childhood to an adulthood infection (20). By 1992–93, 46% to 65% of reported cases were in persons older than 20 years of age. It is estimated that in the United States 10 million women of reproductive age are susceptible to rubella.

Pregnancy does not magnify the severity of maternal illness, and as many as 25% of infections are subclinical. The clinical expression of rubella (fever, maculopapular rash, lymphadenopathy, and arthralgias) is mimicked by the clinical expression of parvovirus B19 infection. One fourth of mothers of children with congenital rubella infection had no complaint of illness during pregnancy, and only 45% reported an illness with a skin rash during pregnancy (21). The practice of obtaining rubella antibody studies as an essential component of early antenatal care has focused clinical surveillance on rubella-susceptible patients. However, it is important to note that reinfection, despite existing immunity, can occur, especially in epidemic settings with intense exposure (21–24). Moreover, maternal antibody does not provide complete protection against transplacental infection of the fetus. Congenital infection and the congenital rubella syndrome were present in a small but not insignificant number of the infants of rubella-reinfected mothers. Maternal immunity, nevertheless, is preferable to nonimmunity. Occasional maternal reinfection is not a reason to discard rubella vaccination and antenatal screening for rubella antibody.

It is useful to recognize congenital rubella infection and the congenital rubella syndrome as distinct clinical entities. Congenital rubella infection can occur at any time after implantation and the creation of a maternal–fetal placental blood supply in the endometrium. The congenital rubella syndrome is the result of fetal damage by wild-virus congenital infection in the first half of gestation. After weeks 20 to 24 of gestation, congenital infection is common but teratogenesis and developmental abnormalities are rare. Rubella vaccination inadvertently given during pregnancy has resulted in congenital infection with attenuated vaccine virus without the complications of the congenital rubella syndrome (25).

Reinfection with rubella during pregnancy is a diagnostic and management dilemma. With polymerase chain reaction technology, specimens of fetal blood and amniotic fluid can be examined for evidence of fetal rubella infection, but a positive result does not accurately predict congenital rubella infection injury and fetotoxicity. The choice of pregnancy termination in this setting remains with the mother and the family.

Wild rubella virus continues to circulate in the United States. Pregnant women who are exposed to rubella are usually exposed to children or adults with acquired rubella. However, babies with congenital infections shed virus for as long as 4 months and are an important reservoir. Of particular concern is the survey finding that almost two thirds of obstetric office practices do not require documentation of rubella immunity for office staff, nurses, or physicians (26). The same survey found that about one fifth of respondents did not have documentation of rubella immunity. Because internists and family physicians may think of rubella as a childhood problem, they may consider the immunization of adults to be a low priority. Nothing could be further from the truth.

Chickenpox

Varicella-zoster virus (VZV), a DNA herpes virus, is the pathogen that causes chickenpox and reactivation shingles, or herpes zoster. Like measles, varicella is highly communicable, but the clinical attack rate is lower and asymptomatic or very mild infection is common. Although chickenpox is a childhood disease, the number of susceptible persons of childbearing age is increasing, and chickenpox during pregnancy has become more common (27, 28). The advent of live attenuated varicella virus vaccine is likely to further alter the demographic characteristics of the population with chickenpox. Changing epidemiology and the frequency of serologic evidence of immunity with no history of clinical disease makes screening for varicella antibody a useful preconception or prenatal test.

Chickenpox or primary VZV infection, not herpes zoster, poses risks to the pregnant patient. There is controversy over whether age or gestation is responsible for the fact that the incidence of varicella pneumonia complicating gestational chickenpox is approximately 20% (29, 30). It should be noted that the 25% to 40% mortality rate from varicella pneumonia during pregnancy far exceeds the mortality rate of varicella pneumonia in nonpregnant patients.

The timing of maternal viremia has implications for the fetus (Figure 13-2). Early in pregnancy, there is a small but definite risk for fetal infection that produces fetopathy (31). Late in pregnancy, transplacental passage of virus to the fetus can result in congenital chickenpox or chickenpox in the neonate. If fetal infection is acquired before maternal antibody responses have begun, there is a risk that the neonate will develop lesions 5 to 10 days postpartum and will have an aggressive, sometimes fatal course.

For all of these reasons, it is prudent to determine the mother's immune status and to use varicella-zoster immune globulin (VZIG) for susceptible mothers exposed to persons with varicella infection (29). It is best to give

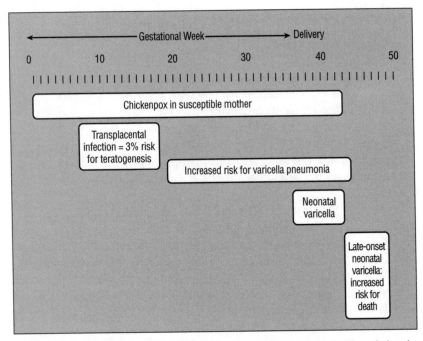

Figure 13-2 Varicella infection during pregnancy according to time of maternal viremia. Incubation period from viremia to lesions ranges from 10 to 20 days.

VZIG within 96 hours of exposure. Although VZIG will not always prevent fetal or maternal infection, it will attenuate the severity of the clinical course. The recommended dose is 125 U/10 kg of body weight. Varicella pneumonia should be treated with intravenous acyclovir 10 mg/kg every 8 hours for a minimum of 7 days (32).

Parvovirus B19 Infection

The parvoviruses, which are small DNA viruses, are common pathogens of a variety of animals. Only parvovirus B19 causes human disease (33, 34). It binds to the P antigen on bone marrow cells (erythroblasts and megakaryocytes), endothelial cells, and synovial and placental cells. Persons without the P-system blood group antigen are resistant to parvovirus B19 infection. The organism produces three characteristic clinical syndromes (35). The most common is the childhood disease erythema infectiosum (fifth disease) with fever and erythematous rash (especially the "slapped cheeks" appearance). In adults, the usual clinical syndrome is arthralgias, dependent edema, and low-grade fever, occasionally progressing to frank arthritis involving the hands, wrists, feet, and knees. However, about 20% of adult infections are asymptomatic. In susceptible pregnant women, parvovirus B19 can traverse the placenta to cause intrauterine fetal infection without causing clinical illness in the mother. The third clinical disease relates to the virus's predilection for erythroid precursors in bone marrow. The characteristic hematologic picture is transient anemia with some hemolysis but without reticulocytosis. Occasionally, pancytopenia occurs. Persons with active bone marrow erythropoiesis, like sickle-cell disease, hereditary spherocytosis, thalassemia, or some hematologic cancers, are at particular risk for protracted aplastic anemia. The fetus is at particular risk after it begins to produce erythrocytes (36). Fetal erythrocytes have a half-life of 50 to 75 days, and fetal erythrocyte production is commensurately intense. Parvovirus marrow suppression can cause severe fetal anemia and the development of heart failure and nonimmune hydrops fetalis.

Parvovirus B19 circulates among school-age children and causes outbreaks, usually in late winter and spring. The infection is highly contagious and is spread by secretions in the air, on fingers, and on fomites. Viremia occurs about 7 days after inoculation and lasts for up to 4 days. Clinical symptoms begin about 7 to 10 days after the viremia. By the time the child develops the classic erythema infectiosum rash, the susceptible exposed gravida will already have acquired the virus. Lasting immunity mediated by IgG develops after infection. IgM can persist for up to a year.

About half of the population at puberty and 60% of adults have serologic evidence of previous infection. The attack rate among exposed susceptible persons is related to the intensity of exposure (37, 38). Household exposures result in infection in 50% to 60% of cases. Nurses, teachers, and cafeteria workers in schools have a 20% to 30% infection rate.

A substantial minority of pregnant women are susceptible. If exposure occurs, the results of serologic tests for IgG and IgM antibody against parvovirus B19 determine clinical management (Figure 13-3). A patient with IgG only is immune and does not need further follow-up. A patient with no antibody is susceptible and must be cautioned about exposure and monitored

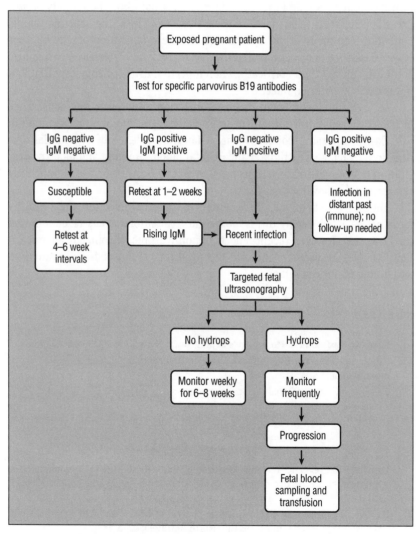

Figure 13-3 Management of parvovirus B19.

with regular testing if exposure cannot be avoided. Patients with both IgG and IgM antibodies should be retested (quantitative titers should be obtained) at 1 to 2 weeks. Increasing IgM titers suggest very recent infection and the need for fetal monitoring. A patient with IgM alone has had an acute infection and requires fetal monitoring.

Infection early in gestation may cause spontaneous abortion. Fetal infection after the first trimester is usually self-limited and without fetotoxic or teratogenic effect. However, if fetal infection progresses, effects on the fetus can develop rapidly, so frequent ultrasonographic evaluation for signs of myocardial dysfunction and hydrops fetalis is essential (39). The rapidity of progression suggests that viral myocarditis, not just the anemia alone, contributes to the hydrops. Spontaneous in utero resolution of fetal hydrops is well described and suggests that the severity of fetal congestive heart failure is multifactorial (40). Fetal death, when it occurs, usually happens within 3 to 6 weeks after maternal infection.

Serologically documented maternal infection followed by the appearance of fetal hydrops requires frequent, even daily, ultrasonographic examination (33, 34). Progressing congestive heart failure, evidence of myocardial dysfunction, or fetal arrhythmia mandate fetal blood sampling and fetal transfusion. In fetuses with such serious problems, fetal transfusion has significantly reduced fetal mortality rates (41).

A mother with serologically documented maternal infection and a healthy fetus on repeated weekly ultrasonographic evaluations needs to be followed for 12 weeks. However, recent reports of nonhydropic, chronically anemic infants of infected mothers indicate the need for careful pediatric evaluation and follow-up for the infant.

REFERENCES

1. **Koren G, Pastuszak A, Ito S.** Drugs in pregnancy. N Engl J Med. 1998;338:1128-37.

2. **Briggs GG, Freeman RK, Yaffe SJ.** Drugs in Pregnancy and Lactation, 5th ed. Baltimore: Williams & Wilkins; 1998.

3. **Edwards MS.** Antibacterial therapy in pregnancy and neonates. Clin Perinatol. 1997; 24:251-66.

4. **Duff P.** Antibiotic selection in obstetric patients. Infect Dis Clin North Am. 1997;11:1-12.

5. The choice of antibacterial drugs. Med Lett. 1998;40:33-42.

6. **Loebstein R.** Pregnancy outcome following gestational exposure to fluoroquinolones: a multicenter prospective controlled study. Antimicrob Agents Chemother. 1998;42:1336-9.

7. **Hayden GF, Henderson RH.** Worldwide control of disease through immunization: progress and prospects. Infect Dis Clin North Am. 1990;4:245-58.

8. **Centers for Disease Control and Prevention.** Neonatal tetanus—Montana 1998. MMWR Morb Mortal Wkly Rep. 1998;47:928-30.

9. Guide for Adult Immunizations, 3d ed. Philadelphia: American Coll Physicians; 1994.

10. **Ruben FL.** Now and future influenza vaccines. Infect Dis Clin North Am. 1990;4:1-10.

11. **Edwards KM.** Diphtheria, tetanus, and pertussis immunization in adults. Infect Dis Clin North Am. 1990;4:85-103.

12. **LaForce FM.** Poliomyelitis vaccines: success and controversy. Infect Dis Clin North Am. 1990;4:75-83.

13. **Wharton M, Cochi SL, Williams WL.** Measles, mumps, and rubella vaccines. Infect Dis Clin North Am. 1990;4:47-73.

14. **Hadler SC.** Vaccines to prevent hepatitis B and hepatitis A. Infect Dis Clin North Am. 1990;4:29-46.

15. **Tsai TF, Paul R, Lynberg MC, Letson GW.** Congenital yellow fever virus infection after immunization in pregnancy. J Infect Dis. 1993;168:1520-3.

16. MMWR Morb Mortal Wkly Rep. 1994;43:391.

17. **Almar RL, Englund JA, Hammill H.** Complications of measles in pregnancy. Curr Infect Dis. 1992;14:217-26.

18. **Gershon AA.** Chickenpox, measles, and mumps. In: Remington JS, Klein JO, eds. Infectious Diseases in the Fetus and the Newborn Infant. Philadelphia: WB Saunders; 1990:395-445.

19. **Sever JL, White LR.** Intrauterine viral infections. Annu Rev Med. 1968;19:471-86.

20. **Schluter WW, Reef SE, Redd SC, Dykewicz CA.** Changing epidemiology of congenital rubella syndrome in the United States. J Infect Dis. 1998;178:636-41.

21. **Morgan-Capner P, Miller E, Vurdien JE, et al.** Outcome of pregnancy after maternal reinfection with rubella. Commun Dis Rep. 1991;1:1257-9.

22. **Best JM.** Rubella reinfection. Virology. 1993;2:35-40.

23. **Horstmann DM, Liebhaber H, LeBouvier G, et al.** Rubella reinfection of vaccinated and naturally immune persons exposed to an epidemic. N Engl J Med. 1970;283:771-6.

24. **Robinson J, Lemay M, Vandry WL.** Congenital rubella after anticipated maternal immunity: two cases and a review of the literature. Pediatr Infect Dis. 1994;13:812-5.

25. **Sheppard S, Smithells RW, Peckham CS, et al.** National congenital rubella surveillance, 1971-1975. Health Trends. 1997;9:38-41.

26. **Schoenhoff DD, Lane TW, Hansen CJ.** Primary prevention and rubella immunity: overlooked issues in the outpatient obstetric setting. Infect Control Hosp Epidemiol. 1997;18:633-6.

27. **Miller E, Vurdien J, Farrington P.** Shift in age in chickenpox. Lancet. 1993;341:308-9.

28. **Choo PW, Donahue JG, Manson JE, Platt R.** The epidemiology of varicella and its complications. J Infect Dis. 1995;172:706-12.

29. **Brunell PA.** Varicella in pregnancy, the fetus and the newborn: problems in management. J Infect Dis. 1992;166(Suppl. 1):542-7.

30. **Lawal O, Nathan AT, Hartwell R, Dodd P.** Varicella pneumonia complicating pregnancy. J Obstet Gynaecol. 1997;17:166-7.

31. **Pastuszak A, Schick-Boschetto B, Zuber C, et al.** Pregnancy outcome following first trimester exposure to fluoxetine (Prozac). JAMA. 1993;269:2246-8.

32. **Smego RA, Asperilla MO.** Use of acyclovir for varicella pneumonia during pregnancy. Obstet Gynecol. 1991;78:1112-6.

33. **Levy R, Weissman A, Blomberg G, Hagay ZJ.** Infection by parvovirus B19 during pregnancy: a review. Obstet Gynecol Surv. 1997;52:254-9.

34. **Rodis JF.** Parvovirus infection in pregnancy. Curr Obstet Med. 1995;3:159-81.

35. **Garcia-Tapia AM, delAlama CF, Giron JA, Mira J, et al.** Spectrum of parvovirus B19 infection: analysis of an outbreak of 43 cases in Cadiz, Spain. J Infect Dis. 1995;21: 1424-30.

36. **Gratacos E, Torres P, Vidal J, Antolin E, et al.** The incidence of human parvovirus B19 infection during pregnancy and its impact on perinatal outcome. J Infect Dis. 1995;171:1360-3.

37. **Public Health Laboratory Service Working Party on Fifth Disease.** Prospective study of human parvovirus infection in pregnancy. BMJ. 1990;300:1166-8.

38. **Centers for Disease Control.** Risks associated with human parvovirus B19 infection. MMWR Morb Mortal Wkly Rep. 1989;38:81-4.

39. **Lowden E, Weinstein L.** Unexpected second trimester pregnancy loss due to maternal parvovirus B19 infection. South Med J. 1997;90:702-4.

40. **Kelly T, Mathers A.** Early presentation and spontaneous resolution of hydrops fetalis, secondary to parvovirus B19 infection. J Obstet Gynaecol. 1998;18:190-1.

41. **Farley CK, Smoloniec JS, Carl O, Miller E.** Observational study of effect of intrauterine transfusions on outcome of fetal hydrops after parvovirus B19 infection. Lancet. 1995;346:1335-7.

II. Genitourinary Tract Infections, Sexually Transmitted Diseases, and HIV

Richard V. Lee, Carol A. Stamm, James A. McGregor, Janice I. French, Ronald Gibbs, and Ellen D. Mason

Urinary Tract Infections

Urinary tract infections (UTIs) are one of the most common infectious complications of pregnancy (1–3). Sexual intercourse—the usual prerequisite for gestation—is associated with an increased risk for UTIs. Many sexually transmitted pathogens (*Ureaplasma, Gardnerella, Chlamydia,* and *Trichomonas* species, and group B streptococci) may colonize the vulva and urethra and foster the ascent of urinary tract pathogens to the bladder. Gestational changes in ureteral mechanisms produce hydroureter, hydropelvis, and alterations in urinary flow, bladder capacity, and bladder emptying, so that pregnant women have, in essence, a single open urinary collecting system. Bacteria colonizing any portion of the urinary tract can readily and rapidly spread throughout. Pregnancy and delivery are therefore a time of heightened risk for serious upper UTI, and pyelonephritis is a risk factor for premature, preterm labor (4). Bacteriuria, whether symptomatic or asymptomatic, is an important clinical event (1–3) that predisposes pregnant women to pyelonephritis.

The evaluation of every pregnant patient with acute recurrent UTI should include an assessment of urinary tract anatomy and renal function to exclude the possibility of underlying urinary tract abnormalities unrelated to pregnancy (1–3, 5, 6). This is particularly important in patients who have repetitive symptomatic UTIs or persistent asymptomatic bacteriuria despite repeated treatment.

In patients without pre-existing renal disease, urinary tract abnormalities, vaginal pathogens, or bacteriuria, pregnancy does not predispose to bacteriuria (2). Only 1% to 2% of healthy women who have sterile urine early in pregnancy will develop a symptomatic UTI (1–3). Of women with bacteriuria (including that with genital pathogens), 20% to 40% will develop an acute UTI at some point during gestation if they remain untreated. Antibiotic treatment reduces the incidence of symptomatic UTI by 80% to 90% (1, 2, 7, 8) so treatment of asymptomatic bacteria is required.

The organisms that cause UTIs during pregnancy are no different from the pathogens that cause it in nonpregnant patients. Therefore, the choice of antibiotics for pregnant patients is limited only by the need to avoid 1) antibiotics that are contraindicated during gestation and 2) antibiotics to which the infecting organism is resistant. Because pregnancy causes functional and anatomic abnormalities of the urinary tract and because the lower genital and urinary tracts are considered a single anatomic unit in pregnant women, short-course antibiotic regimens are inadequate. Antibiotic treatment for less than 5 to 7 days, even for lower UTIs, is inappropriate.

Failure to eradicate bacteriuria forces the clinician to consider and, usually, to prescribe continuing suppressive treatment, with its risk for antimicrobial resistance and adverse drug reactions. Unfortunately, no studies have compared continuous suppressive therapy with episodic intense antimicrobial treatment for acute pyelonephritis.

Despite anxiety about aminoglycosides, the management of acute pyelonephritis in a pregnant patient requires prompt, aggressive antibiotic therapy. Until the antimicrobial sensitivities of the pathogen are known, parenteral therapy should include an aminoglycoside in combination with a beta-lactam antibiotic, such as ampicillin or cephalosporin. The vast majority of patients respond within 72 hours. Therapy with the best oral agent, according to culture and sensitivity testing, should be continued to complete a 2-week course. Some experts recommend suppressive therapy be continued until delivery for all pregnant patients with a single episode of pyelonephritis.

Genital Tract Infections:
Chorioamnionitis and Sexually Transmitted Diseases

Sexually transmitted infectious diseases (STDs) and sex-associated microbial conditions, including bacterial vaginosis (BV) and cervicitis, are the most common, and potentially the most morbid, complications of pregnancy. Common STDs and BV are often unrecognized during pregnancy and should be routinely screened for and treated at the initial antenatal examination. All treated pregnant women should be given tests of cure. All partners should be screened and, if infection is diagnosed, should be treated appropriately according to updated guidelines from the Centers for Disease Control and Prevention (CDC).

Common STDs and BV can adversely affect pregnancy outcomes for both mother and baby. Common complications of clinical and subclinical reproductive tract infections include preterm birth, premature rupture of membranes (PROM), fetal and newborn infections, and maternal infections during pregnancy and the postpartum period. Of these complications, preterm birth is the most prevalent and potentially the most costly.

Fully 11% of births in the United States are preterm (9). Chronic sequelae of many children who survive preterm birth include respiratory insufficiency, cerebral palsy, mental retardation, blindness, deafness, and need for supportive services. The direct and indirect costs of prematurity can be immense and include liability for failure to prevent preterm birth due to reproductive tract infection.

Primary fetal infections, including syphilis, herpes simplex virus infection, and cytomegalovirus infection, are less common but cause intrauterine death, preterm birth, and congenital infections. Inexpensive, easy-to-use diagnostic tests and safe, effective treatments are available for most common STDs. Guidelines from the CDC (10) should be followed. All treated pregnant women should be offered tests of cure approximately 1 month after treatment. Women at risk for reinfection or relapse should be rescreened at approximately 28 weeks of gestation or later. Partners and sexual contacts should be identified and treated, if necessary, in accordance with CDC guidelines and also offered tests of cure. Prevention of STD during pregnancy is paramount because STDs acquired during pregnancy are the most dangerous to the developing fetus. (The combination of Screening, Treatment, and Prevention may be remembered as the acronym STP.)

The CDC guidelines recommend screening all pregnant women for syphilis, hepatitis B, and HIV infection. Women deemed "at risk" should be routinely screened for BV, gonorrhea, and chlamydia.

Table 13-5 lists common sexually transmitted and sex-associated infections in pregnancy. These are discussed in detail below.

Table 13-5 Common Sexually Transmitted and Sex-Associated Infections in Pregnancy

Condition	Comments	Diagnosis	Treatment
Bacterial vaginosis	Associated with prematurity, PROM, postpartum febrile morbidity	Amsel criteria on wet mount	Metronidazole 250 mg tid for 7 days
Chlamydia trachomatis	Associated with prematurity, PROM, postpartum endometritis	EIA; PCR or LCR preferred	Erythromycin base 500 mg qid for 7 days or amoxicillin 500 mg tid for 7 days or azithromycin 1 g PO in a single dose
Trichomoniasis	Associated with prematurity and PROM	Identification of motile trichomonads on wet mount	Metronidazole 2 g PO in a single dose
Gonorrhea	Associated with prematurity, PROM, endometritis	Culture	Cefixime 400 mg PO in a single dose or ceftriaxone 125 mg IM single dose or azithromycin 1 g PO in a single dose
Syphilis	Associated with congenital syphilis, preterm labor, stillbirths	Dark-field microscopy or serologic test VDRL or RPR plus confirmatory FTA-ABS	Long-acting penicillin G; dose dependent on duration of disease
Primary syphilis			Benzathine penicillin G 2.4 million units IM in a single dose
Secondary syphilis			Benzathine penicillin G 2.4 million units IM in a single dose
Latent syphilis of unknown duration			Benzathine penicillin G 2.4 million units IM in a single dose at 1-week intervals for penicillin G total of three doses
Tertiary syphilis			Aqueous crystalline penicillin G 18–24 million units a day; given as 3–4 million units IV every 4 h for 10–14 days
HBV	Associated with neonatal infection, cirrhosis, hepatocellular carcinoma	HBsAg	HBIG and vaccination for newborn (interferons for nonpregnant patients only)
HCV	Associated with neonatal infection rarely, with a risk of cirrhosis, hepatocellular carcinoma	HCV antibody test with RIBA II confirmatory test	Not yet developed

Adapted from Centers for Disease Control and Prevention. 1998 guidelines for treatment of sexually transmitted diseases. MMWR Morb Mortal Wkly Rep. 1998;47(RR-1):8-75.

Bacterial Vaginosis

Bacterial vaginosis is the most common cause of vaginal discharge. It is best considered a massive microbial alteration of cervicovaginal microecology. It is marked by a characteristic "set" of microflora, including *Gardnerella vaginalis*, anaerobes, and mycoplasmas with a concomitant decrease in hydrogen peroxide–producing lactobacilli. Approximately half of women with BV, however, are asymptomatic. Bacterial vaginosis is best considered a sex-associated microbial alteration; treatment of partners is not beneficial. Black women are at increased risk for BV and for preterm birth of microbial cause.

Clinical diagnosis is based on Amsel's criteria (11). Three of Amsel's criteria are required for diagnosis: "milky" homogenous discharge, amine (fishy) odor, and identification of more than 20 "clue" cells on wet preparation on microscopy. Alternatively, a diagnosis may be made by Speigel's or Nugent's criteria in Gram stain, a positive result on a probe test for *G. vaginalis* (Affirm III, B-D), or a combination of pH greater than 4.5 and a positive amine test (Fem Card, Cooper Surgical).

More than 20 studies show that BV in pregnant women is associated with a risk for preterm birth that is 1.5 to 7 times greater than baseline risk (12, 13). Other studies show that the presence of BV at the initial antepartum visit is a marker for second-trimester birth and miscarriage (14, 15). Bacterial vaginosis in pregnancy is associated with increased risk for PROM, postpartum endometritis, and post–cesarean section infection (16). In each of these settings, BV-associated micro-organisms are the most common microbes isolated.

Production of proteases (including mucinase and sialidase) and phospholipase A_2 and C by vaginosis-associated microbes may help microbes enter the uterus. Microbes and host inflammatory molecules can influence the release of prostaglandin and directly weaken amniotic membranes in vitro (17–19).

Multiple intervention studies show a reduction in preterm birth after the treatment of BV during pregnancy (20–22). Antibiotic treatment to prevent preterm labor may be analogous to antimicrobial treatment of periodontal and peptic ulcer disease (23). One placebo-controlled intervention trial of metronidazole 500 mg twice daily for 7 days and enteric-coated erythromycin 300 mg twice daily for 7 days in patients with a history of preterm delivery or low maternal weight decreased the risk for preterm birth by approximately one third in patients with asymptomatic BV (20). Morales and co-workers were able to reduce the incidence of preterm birth and PROM by more than 60% by giving metronidazole alone to women with BV and previous preterm birth (21). A study of 1200 pregnant women in an urban population in Denver, Colorado (14), showed that routine screening and treatment of BV reduced the occurrence of preterm birth and PROM by approximately 50%. In this study, combinations of infections (such as BV and *Trichomonas vaginalis* infection or chlamydia) resulted in a preterm birth rate greater than 30%; specific treatment reduced this rate by 50%. The CDC (10) recommends that women at risk for prematurity be screened and treated for BV and that all symptomatic women with BV be similarly screened and treated.

The presence of BV may increase susceptibility to HIV infection (24). Detection and treatment of asymptomatic BV may soon be mandated to reduce risk for HIV transmission. Reproductive tract infections and chorioamnionitis are known to increase risk for vertical transmission of HIV, and it is now hypothesized that screening and treatment of BV in pregnancy can reduce risk for perinatal HIV infection.

The recommended regimen for pregnant women with BV who are at high risk for preterm delivery is metronidazole 250 mg orally three times daily for 7 days. Metronidazole decreases bacterial virulence factor production. Alternative regimens include oral metronidazole 2 g in a single dose or oral clindamycin 300 mg twice daily for 7 days (10). For pregnant women with symptomatic BV, these regimens are all acceptable. Metronidazole gel 0.75% given in a 5-g dose intravaginally twice daily for 5 days has also been approved (10). Other topical treatments are not currently recommended during pregnancy. Tests of cure should be done, and retreatment with an alternative regimen should be given if BV recurs.

Trichomoniasis

Trichomoniasis is caused by *Trichomonas vaginalis*, a flagellated protozoan. It is very common during pregnancy. Symptomatic patients with trichomoniasis present with a yellow or green malodorous vaginal discharge. The symptoms are most marked in women; many men are asymptomatic (10). Approximately 5% of female infants of infected mothers show evidence of trichomoniasis, which usually resolves as maternal estrogen influence diminishes.

Identification of affected pregnant patients is important because of the association of trichomoniasis with PROM and preterm delivery. A 40% increased risk for premature delivery of a low-birthweight infant was seen in the Vaginal Infections and Prematurity study (25) in pregnant women with trichomoniasis. Compared with no infection, *T. vaginalis* infection has been associated with a twofold increased risk for PROM and low-birthweight infants (26). Phospholipase A_2 and other proteolytic enzymes produced by *T. vaginalis* may be partly responsible for the association of *T. vaginalis* with preterm labor (27, 28). It has been shown that *T. vaginalis* reduces amniochorionic tensile strength in vitro (28).

The preferred treatment is oral metronidazole 2 g in a single dose. Ninety percent to 95% of patients are cured with one treatment. Some patients may be infected with *T. vaginalis* strains that seem resistant to metronidazole, but most of these patients respond to higher metronidazole doses (10). If patients are allergic to metronidazole, desensitization is recommended because metronidazole is the preferred therapy. Sexual partners require treatment. As with all STDs, patients should avoid sexual intercourse until both partners have received appropriate medication and are cured. It is appropriate to treat pregnant patients, and metronidazole can be safely given in pregnancy for this use.

Chlamydia

Chlamydia trachomatis infection is the most common bacterial STD during pregnancy. Mucopurulent cervicitis and urethral infection are most often asymptomatic. Screening for chlamydia in pregnancy is recommended (10). The prevalence of chlamydia in pregnant women is approximately 5% and does not reflect socioeconomic status, race, or ethnicity (10).

Infection with *C. trachomatis* is associated with preterm birth, PROM, and postpartum endometritis in the mother. Chorioamnionitis has been described with chlamydia. In addition, chlamydia causes pelvic inflammatory disease, increased risk for ectopic pregnancy, infertility, and chronic pelvic pain. A recent prospective study in the Kaiser managed care population (29) showed that screening of asymptomatic young women leads to treatment and decreases risk for pelvic inflammatory disease.

Diagnosis is optimized by the use of nucleic acid–based testing, preferably with PCR or LCR. During pregnancy, the mother should be sampled from the cervix. Half of affected newborns are identified at birth, and one in six may have conjunctivitis or pneumonitis (10). Silver nitrate or antibiotic solution prevents neonatal gonococcal ophthalmia but not chlamydial disease (10). The strongest evidence of an association of maternal chlamydia with preterm birth comes from a prospective study at Johns Hopkins. This study involved 801 women at 22 to 30 weeks of gestation who were cultured for a variety of genital pathogens (30). Colonization with *C. trachomatis* was significantly related to preterm delivery (odds ratio, 1.6; 90% CI, 1.01 to 2.05) and to intrauterine growth restriction (IUGR) (odds ratio, 2.4; 90% CI, 1.32 to 4.18).

Significant reductions in low-birthweight infants occurred when antenatal treatment for *C. trachomatis* was given in one retrospective study (31). Another retrospective study (32) showed a reduction in the incidence of preterm birth among women who were treated for evidence of chlamydial disease. For women who had chlamydia and received erythromycin rather than placebo in the Vaginal Infections and Prematurity study (33), the incidence of PROM was reduced.

Gonococcal Infection

Although its incidence is declining, new infection with *Neisseria gonorrhoeae* occurs in 600,000 persons in the United States each year (10). Gonorrhea is often asymptomatic in pregnancy but may be associated with endometritis postpartum.

In pregnancy, gonorrhea is associated with an increased perinatal mortality rate (34), a higher rate of premature labor and birth (34–36), and PROM (34, 37). A case of gonococcal chorioamnionitis associated with perinatal sepsis has been described (38). All pregnant women should be routinely screened for gonorrhea, and affected pregnant women and their partners should be treated to reduce risk for prematurity (39), ophthalmia neonatorum, and postpartum infection.

Other sequelae of gonococcal infection include infertility from tubal injury, increased risk for ectopic pregnancy, and chronic pelvic pain. All women at high risk for STDs should be screened for gonococcal infection.

Often, patients with gonorrhea also have chlamydia, so it is reasonable to cover both infections. There have been increasing reports of infection with quinolone-resistant *N. gonorrhoeae*, so culture and sensitivity testing for this organism should be done in cases of treatment failures (10). Recommended regimens include oral cefixime 400 mg in a single dose, ceftriaxone 125 mg intramuscularly in a single dose, and oral azithromycin 1 g in a single dose (10).

Genital Herpes Simplex Virus Infection

Genital herpes simplex virus (HSV) infection occurs in one fifth of the population (40). Forty-five million persons in the United States have had this infected diagnosed (10), and many more affected persons do not know that they are infected.

The risk that a previously unaffected pregnant woman will acquire HSV-1 or HSV-2 infection is approximately 2%, as determined by Western blot assays for antibodies to HSV-1 and HSV-2 (41). The risk for acquisition of HSV is roughly 30% in all trimesters (41). Overall, the estimated risk for transmission to the neonate from a pregnant women who has a primary HSV infection during pregnancy is less than 3% (41). The risk for neonatal infection due to past maternal HSV infection is much less, approximately 1 in 2000 to 20,000 births. Each year, 1500 to 2200 babies in the United States develop neonatal herpes (42). Sequelae include death, mental retardation, and cerebral palsy.

Perinatal HSV transmission may be caused by hematogenous spread of uterine infection but is most commonly ascribed to direct contact with infectious secretions around the time of birth. Most cases of neonatal transmission involve an asymptomatic or subclinical genital HSV infection (43, 44). Use of fetal scalp electrodes seems to increase neonatal risk for HSV infection and should be avoided in the presence of HSV (45). The risk for perinatal infection is greatest if the mother acquired primary genital HSV just before labor (41).

Both genital HSV acquisition in pregnancy and asymptomatic HSV shedding have been linked to preterm delivery (46). Additional complications in association with HSV acquisition in pregnancy include IUGR and spontaneous abortion. Possible explanations may be related to chorioamnionitis and uteroplacental insufficiency (47).

Diagnosis of genital herpes depends primarily on the recognition of typical fluid-filled blisters on an erythematous base ("dew drops on a rose petal") or, more commonly, atypical lesions (painful papules and ulcers). Viral culture is appropriate to confirm the diagnosis.

Routine viral cultures during pregnancy for persons with HSV are not recommended because they do not identify mothers or neonates at risk (48). It may be useful to 1) culture women with recent outbreaks to ensure that the infection is completely resolved before labor ensues and 2) consider acyclovir treatment to reduce viral shedding (47) and increase the likelihood of vaginal delivery. Serologic diagnosis done using glycoprotein antibody or Western blot analysis may be an effective way to confirm the clinical diagnosis or make a serologic diagnosis. Development of protective antibodies to HSV typically takes 4 to 6 weeks (41).

Primary or secondary genital herpes during pregnancy is generally treated with acyclovir because this agent seems to be safe in pregnancy and in neonates. Acyclovir does not seem to be teratogenic. Any patient with disseminated disease in pregnancy requires acyclovir treatment for disseminated disease. Intravenous acyclovir 5 mg/kg every 8 hours is recommended for disseminated HSV disease, encephalitis, pneumonitis, or hepatitis (10). Patients with active HSV lesions or prodromal symptoms should have cesarean section, if possible, before membrane rupture. Some evidence suggests that cesarean section should occur within 4 to 6 hours for maximum benefit (49). The patient should be counseled that abdominal delivery will not completely prevent neonatal infection, although it will decrease risk for it.

The management of patients who have PROM at less than 32 weeks of gestation can be individualized. Conservative management, intravenous acyclovir, and intramuscular betamethasone to hasten fetal lung maturation are reasonable (49). For patients who have PROM at or after 34 weeks of gestation, immediate cesarean section or cesarean section with documented fetal lung maturity and maternal acyclovir administration is recommended (48).

Syphilis

Syphilis is increasingly uncommon in North America, but approximately 30 cases of congenital syphilis still occur each year. Most of these cases are due to failure to screen and treat. Syphilis is caused by the spirochete *Treponema pallidum*. An initial painless chancre, which is highly contagious, is often not noticed by the patient. In the secondary stage, many patients present with fever, lymphadenopathy, and a very contagious macular rash over the palms and soles. Tertiary-stage disease may include neurologic, cardiac, or ophthalmic symptoms, and gummas may be present.

Transplacental passage of spirochetes may occur during each trimester (50). Fetal and neonatal complications in an untreated pregnant patient include preterm labor, stillbirth, IUGR, abnormal skeletal and tooth development, hepatosplenomegaly, and dermatitis (10).

Diagnosis is dependent on screening and rescreening of high-risk patients or on a high index of suspicion. Dark-field microscopy with identification of spirochetes is the definitive diagnostic method. Serologic tests include the nontreponemal Venereal Disease Research Laboratory (VDRL) test and the rapid plasma reagin test. If the diagnosis is made with one of these tests, a confirmatory fluorescent treponemal antibody absorption test (FTA-ABS) is required because false-positive results can occur with diseases such as systemic lupus erythematosus.

Most patients will have nonreactive nontreponemal tests after treatment. However, some patients have persistent titers and are considered to be serofast (10). Reactive treponemal tests remain reactive in most patients after treatment (10). It is important not to use treponemal test antibody titers to gauge the effectiveness of treatment: The titers show poor correlation with disease activity (10). Patients with AIDS may fail to seroconvert.

Patients with neurosyphilis usually have abnormal cerebrospinal fluid (CSF). Usually, the cell or protein count is abnormal or the CSF VDRL test is reactive (10). The CSF leukocyte count is often greater than 5 cells/mm^3 at the time of diagnosis and is a sensitive indicator of therapeutic (10). The CSF FTA-ABS is less specific than the CSF VDRL (10).

The treatment of choice is long-acting parenteral penicillin G, the efficacy of which is supported by four decades of evidence (10). Pregnant patients and patients with neurosyphilis who have penicillin allergy should undergo desensitization with parenteral penicillin G.

Follow-up titers at 6 and 12 months are recommended. Persistent signs or symptoms or a persistent fourfold increase in the nontreponemal test titer indicates patients with treatment failure or reinfection (10). It is prudent to evaluate these patients for HIV infection and to offer retreatment (10). Retreatment should consist of three weekly intramuscular injections of benzathine penicillin G 2.4 million U. Treatment of sexual partners is mandatory; many states require the reporting of persons with syphilis, and this reporting can help identify persons who require treatment.

The Jarish-Herxheimer reaction may be a concern in the treatment of patients with syphilis, particularly pregnant patients. There seems to be no successful way to avoid this reaction (51), which is thought to be caused by massive treponemal death. The affected person often presents with chills, fever, headache, tachycardia, and even hypotension approximately 8 to 12 hours after the start of treatment (52). Supportive care for the pregnant patient is appropriate and often sufficient.

A retrospective study (53) involving 71 pregnancies among Australian aborigines offers the best modern glimpse into the impact of syphilis. Twenty-eight percent of women in this study were positive for maternal syphilis, and the perinatal mortality rate was 48 per 1000 live births (relative risk for stillbirth, 4). The odds ratio for a preterm delivery with maternal syphilis was 21.5.

Low-birthweight infants were found in association with syphilis in multivariate regression analysis in a South African black population (35).

Hepatitis B and Hepatitis C

Infectious hepatitis is common in pregnant women. The hepatitis B virus (HBV) is a widespread and preventable cause of hepatitis in pregnancy. It can cause the unfortunate sequelae of cirrhosis and hepatocellular carcinoma. Hepatitis B occurs in 0.1% to 0.2 % of all pregnant women in the United States (54); 0.5% to 1.5% of pregnant women are chronic carriers of HBV (54) and many are asymptomatic. The mechanism for acquisition of hepatitis B for most women is heterosexual intercourse, but blood transfusion was previously a common cause (55). Needle sharing is another common method of acquisition (55). All pregnant patients at high risk for hepatitis should be screened initially and again in the third trimester.

Most patients with hepatitis B have asymptomatic or subclinical infection. Those who are symptomatic may present with nausea, vomiting, abdominal pain, or jaundice. The aspartate aminotransferase and alanine aminotransferase levels are particularly elevated. Detection of hepatitis B surface antigen (HBsAg) indicates the presence of HBV in the body; blood and other body secretions are infectious. If the patient also has hepatitis B e antigen (HBeAg), infectivity is markedly increased.

In early pregnancy, HBV can be transmitted through the placenta (55). However, most vertical transmission occurs around parturition with exposure to blood or infected genital tract secretions. It is unknown whether avoidance of fetal membrane rupture, fetal scalp sampling, or fetal scalp electrode placement can reduce risk for vertical HBV transmission. What is clear is that perinatal transmission occurs in 90% of HBeAg-positive mothers and in up to 20% of HBeAg-negative mothers.

Perinatally infected children can, unfortunately, have an accelerated HBV disease course: persistent hepatitis, cirrhosis, and early progression to hepatocellular carcinoma. Significantly, giving IgG specific to hepatitis B to the neonate promptly after birth and initiating the series of three injections of HBV vaccine can reduce vertical transmission of HBV by 70% to 90% (55). In addition, the efficacy of the vaccine does not differ in full-term and preterm babies (56). Breastfeeding seems reasonable if the neonate has received the immunoglobulin and has started the vaccine series (54). Unfortunately, only 89% of neonates at risk for vertical transmission of HBV actually receive the vaccine and immunoglobulin after birth, and only 50% receive the required series of three immunizations (57). It is now recommended that HBV vaccination begin in the newborn period.

Family members and sexual contacts of index cases should be screened for anti-HBsAg and HBsAg and vaccinated if serosusceptible. It is assumed that regular use of barrier contraceptives can prevent sexual transmission of HBV. Fulminant cases of HBV infection have occurred in pregnancy: These cases require intensive care and, occasionally, liver transplantation. The likelihood of symptomatic and chronic disease is increased with supra-infection with hepatitis delta virus (HDV) (55), a defective RNA virus that only infects in the presence of ongoing HBV infection. One should assay for HDV if a patient's condition worsens or if chronic active hepatitis is evident clinically but HBeAg serologic test results are negative (58). Perinatal transmission of HDV has been reported (54).

Interferon is the only therapy approved by the Food and Drug Administration (FDA) for HBV infection, but pregnant patients are excluded from interferon treatment because of theoretical concerns about possible augmentation of fetal–maternal immune interactions.

The hepatitis C virus (HCV) causes approximately 90% of cases of posttransfusion hepatitis (59, 60). Transmission of HCV primarily occurs through direct injection of blood products or through use of infected needles; it occurs through contact with infectious body secretions much less often. Vertical and sexual transmission of HCV is uncommon, approximately 0% to 5% (59). Universal screening in pregnancy is not recommended because most patients with hepatitis C have an easily identifiable risk factor for the disease, such as intravenous drug use or previous blood transfusion, and selective screening of high-risk patients seems very reasonable (52). The current antibody test may produce a false-positive result, so a confirmatory recombinant immunoblot assay is recommended unless the patient has obvious risk factors for the disease (55).

After infection, the patient with hepatitis C often has a mild subclinical illness that may last 6 to 9 weeks. Often, antibodies are not detectable until 3 to 5 months afterward. Patients who have acquired HCV through blood transfusion are the most likely to develop chronic infection, which may lead to continuing liver damage and cirrhosis.

Current evidence suggests that vertical transmission is unlikely but that maternal co-infection with HIV and certain HCV genotypes may increase risk for vertical transmission (61). In one study (54), patients without detectable HCV RNA in their blood did not transmit HCV to their neonates. Alanine aminotransferase levels do not seem to predict risk for vertical transmission (62). The risk for transmission through breastfeeding has been inadequately researched. No HCV immunoglobulin or vaccine is yet available to prevent the spread of HCV disease.

Genital Tract Infections:
Group B Streptococci in Pregnancy and Newborn

Group B streptococci (GBS) are commonly found in the lower genital tracts of females, but they are an important cause of both maternal and neonatal infection (63–66). Over the past 10 years, interest in these organisms has increased, and national guidelines for the prevention of GBS infection have been developed (65, 66).

Epidemiology

Group B streptococci are present in the rectovaginal cultures of approximately 20% of pregnant women when cultures are obtained by using optimal techniques. Before the institution of wide-scale preventive programs, approximately 1.5 per 1000 live-born infants developed early-onset neonatal sepsis. Thus, it may be calculated that the attack rate of early-onset neonatal sepsis due to GBS is about 1% among infants born to culture-positive mothers.

Recognized risk factors for GBS neonatal sepsis include prematurity, intrapartum fever, duration of rupture of membranes greater than 18 hours, a previous infant with invasive GBS disease, and GBS bacteriuria in the current pregnancy (63, 65).

Approximately 80% of cases of neonatal sepsis due to GBS are early onset (within the first week of life); the remaining 20% are late onset (65). Manifestations of neonatal GBS sepsis include bacteremia, meningitis, or both. Although prematurity is a major risk factor, approximately 80% of all cases of early-onset neonatal GBS sepsis occur in term infants (because these infants make up the vast majority of births). Approximately 9% of cases occur in infants born at 30 to 36 weeks of gestation, and 12% occur in infants born at less than 34 weeks.

Diagnosis

The gold standard for the diagnosis of GBS is culture. The optimal technique for detecting GBS carriage includes rectovaginal culturing and use of selective media (65). Selective media are commercially available and usually contain a nutrient broth plus antibiotics to suppress other genital flora. Numerous rapid diagnostic techniques are available, but these are all insensitive for the detection of carriage (67).

Treatment

Treatment of the symptomatic neonate has suboptimal results (64). This is particularly true in preterm infants, in whom—even with modern antibiotic and supportive therapy—the mortality rate is 16% to 28%. Among term infants with invasive GBS disease, the mortality rate is much lower (<5%). Because most cases of early-onset GBS infection are established in utero, many infants who subsequently develop signs and symptoms of early-onset neonatal sepsis are already bacteremic at birth (63).

Prevention

Given the limited efficacy of the practice of waiting for symptoms before beginning neonatal antibiotic therapy, the emphasis in the past decade has been on prevention. Overall preventive strategies include antenatal detection and treatment of maternal GBS carriers; intrapartum prophylaxis of women; antibiotic prophylaxis for neonates at risk; and maternal vaccination (68–70). Because of the limitations of the antenatal and neonatal approaches and because we lack an effective vaccine, the current approach uses intrapartum antibiotic prophylaxis. After nearly 10 years of debate, national consensus was attained in 1996 when the CDC and the American College of Obstetricians and Gynecologists (ACOG) issued national guidelines (65, 66). These guidelines offer two approaches. One is based on screening for maternal carriage at 35 to 37 weeks of gestation and then giving prophylaxis to all carriers at term and to all persons with risk factors before term. The alternative approach is to give prophylaxis to all women with risk factors. Algorithms for these approaches are shown in Figures 13-4 and 13-5.

HIV and AIDS

The number of women infected by HIV has increased steadily in all countries since the onset of the global epidemic. Most affected women are of reproductive age. Practitioners who care for women in this age group are responsible for routinely screening for, counseling on, and testing for HIV infection. Recently, with the advent of complex combination antiretroviral therapies and advances in the technology used to follow and treat HIV disease and its complications, a debate has developed over whether HIV-infected persons can be adequately cared for by primary care practitioners, including general internists (71). The debate continues to rage, but it is very clear that generalists of all types who work in the field of women's health will continue to play a critical role in preventing and diagnosing HIV infection and in initially evaluating HIV-infected women. They are also likely to be on the front line in counseling women in reproductive decision making. In addition, primary care providers are often part of the multidisciplinary team that manages the HIV-positive woman during pregnancy.

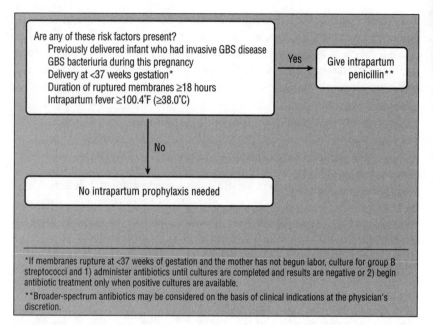

Are any of these risk factors present?
Previously delivered infant who had invasive GBS disease
GBS bacteriuria during this pregnancy
Delivery at <37 weeks gestation*
Duration of ruptured membranes ≥18 hours
Intrapartum fever ≥100.4°F (≥38.0°C)

Yes → Give intrapartum penicillin**

No ↓

No intrapartum prophylaxis needed

*If membranes rupture at <37 weeks of gestation and the mother has not begun labor, culture for group B streptococci and 1) administer antibiotics until cultures are completed and results are negative or 2) begin antibiotic treatment only when positive cultures are available.
**Broader-spectrum antibiotics may be considered on the basis of clinical indications at the physician's discretion.

Figure 13-4 Algorithm for prevention of early-onset group B streptococcal (GBS) disease in neonates, using risk factors. (Data from Centers for Disease Control and Prevention. Prevention of perinatal group B streptococcal disease: a public health perspective. MMWR Morb Mortal Wkly Rep. 1996;45(RR-7):1–24.)

Epidemiology

As of December 1997, the World Health Organization estimated that 30.6 million infected adults and children worldwide were living with HIV infection. Since the middle of 1995, 70,000 women have been diagnosed with AIDS and several hundred thousand are seropositive for HIV (72). The mortality rate from HIV-related disease in women has continued to increase, and HIV infection is now the third leading cause of death in U.S. women 25 to 44 years of age (73). Particularly high mortality rates have been seen in black and Hispanic women.

Data on HIV seroprevalence among pregnant women in the United States are derived from anonymous testing of neonatal blood spots for HIV antibodies. Aggregate data, which are collected and analyzed through the CDC, indicate an overall seroprevalence rate of 1.5 per 1000 childbearing women in the United States (74, 75). Although the highest seroprevalence rates in U.S. women are seen in the Northeast, Florida, California, and Texas, the proportion of cases reported in the Midwest and South is increasing, indicating the spread of the epidemic into previously less-affected areas.

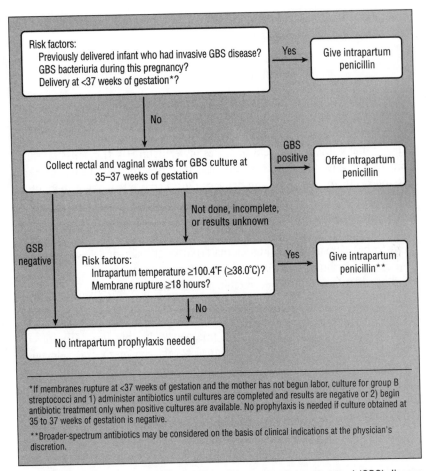

Risk factors:
   Previously delivered infant who had invasive GBS disease?   **Yes** → Give intrapartum penicillin
   GBS bacteriuria during this pregnancy?
   Delivery at <37 weeks of gestation*?

↓ **No**

Collect rectal and vaginal swabs for GBS culture at 35–37 weeks of gestation   **GBS positive** → Offer intrapartum penicillin

Not done, incomplete, or results unknown ↓

GSB negative

Risk factors:
   Intrapartum temperature ≥100.4°F (≥38.0°C)?   **Yes** → Give intrapartum penicillin**
   Membrane rupture ≥18 hours?

↓ **No**

No intrapartum prophylaxis needed

*If membranes rupture at <37 weeks of gestation and the mother has not begun labor, culture for group B streptococci and 1) administer antibiotics until cultures are completed and results are negative or 2) begin antibiotic treatment only when positive cultures are available. No prophylaxis is needed if culture obtained at 35 to 37 weeks of gestation is negative.

**Broader-spectrum antibiotics may be considered on the basis of clinical indications at the physician's discretion.

Figure 13-5 Algorithm for prevention of early-onset group B streptococcal (GBS) disease in neonates, using screening at 35 to 37 weeks of gestation. (Data from Centers for Disease Control and Prevention. Prevention of perinatal group B streptococcal disease: a public health perspective. MMWR Morb Mortal Wkly Rep. 1996;45(RR-7):1–24.)

Effect of Human Immunodeficiency Virus Infection on Pregnancy

In developing countries, HIV-infected pregnant women who are evaluated prospectively have increased rates of low birthweight, preterm labor, and infectious disease (76). In the United States, increased rates of hematologic abnormalities, infections (such as postpartum endometritis and STDs), and stillbirth have been noted (77). As it is in many medical conditions that occur during pregnancy, maternal status is highly correlated with perinatal outcome. The effects on a developing fetus of opportunistic infections and the medications used to treat them are still largely unknown and continue to be an area of investigation and concern.

Vertical Transmission

Given the grave prognosis of pediatric HIV infection, extensive investigations into the mechanisms underlying perinatal HIV transmission and into ways in which such transmission can be reduced have been ongoing. Earlier studies indicate that without intervention, rates of perinatal HIV transmission range from 25% to 35% (78, 79). It is estimated that 70% to 90% of cases of transmission occur during labor and delivery (80). Factors that seem to facilitate HIV transmission during pregnancy include a history of STDs during pregnancy, prolonged rupture of membranes (>4 hours), and invasive obstetric procedures such as amniocentesis (Box 13-2) (81, 82). Transmission rates seem to be increased with higher maternal viral loads and lower maternal CD4 counts, although perinatal transmission has been documented even in cases in which no virus was detectable in maternal plasma (83).

In 1994, a landmark multicenter study by AIDS Clinical Trials Group 076 showed that perinatal transmission of HIV was significantly decreased by the administration of zidovudine during pregnancy. In this trial, HIV-infected pregnant women were randomly assigned to placebo or to oral zidovudine therapy at 14 weeks of gestation. The treatment group took zidovudine 200 mg five times daily throughout pregnancy and received intravenous zidovudine infusions during labor and delivery. Neonates born to women in the treatment group received oral zidovudine syrup for 2 weeks after birth (84). Of infants

---

Box 13-2 Risk Factors for Mother-to-Child Transmission of Human Immunodeficiency Virus

Viral load
Advanced disease (p24 antigenemia, lower CD4 count)
Duration of rupture of membranes >4 hours
History of sexually transmitted disease
Invasive obstetric procedures
Chorioamnionitis
Illicit drug use and smoking (placental disruption)
Prematurity and very low birthweight
HIV-1 in cervicovaginal secretions
Vaginal delivery
Breastfeeding

born to mothers in the placebo group, 25.5% were HIV-infected; the rate of mother–infant transmission in the zidovudine-treated group was 8.3%. The results of this trial gave rise to a general recommendation that zidovudine be offered to all pregnant HIV-infected women after 14 weeks of gestation. Widespread dissemination and implementation of the protocol in the United States has shown impressive decreases in the rates of HIV infection in infants born to HIV-infected women. A CDC study showed perinatal HIV infection rates of 21% before the 1994 Public Health Service guidelines were issued and 11% in 1995 (85).

Studies published more recently have documented 1) further decreases of 3% to 5% in vertical transmission rates and 2) declines in the number of new cases of perinatally acquired HIV infection when this standard of care is implemented. A recent national survey (86) found that the number of children diagnosed with AIDS in the first year of life decreased from 8.4 per 100,000 in 1992 to 5.1 per 100,000 in 1996. The reason why rates of infection are decreasing so quickly is unclear. The use of multidrug therapy in some infected patients may be part of the explanation. Increased precautions to prevent exposure of the fetus or neonate to maternal secretions during labor, delivery, and the postpartum period may also be helping.

Effect of Pregnancy on Human Immunodeficiency Virus Infection

Although pregnancy is associated with increased rates of morbidity and mortality from some viral infections, available data do not indicate that pregnancy accelerates the course of HIV disease (87). Retrospective studies of frozen serum specimens from the early 1980s show that the natural history of HIV infection includes a long period of viral replication with clinical quiescence after primary infection (88). In general, persons who are less immunocompetent have more opportunistic infections and cancers. In the United States, anemia, pneumonia (bacterial, tubercular, viral, and parasitic), symptomatic STDs, esophageal candidiasis, and the wasting syndrome are all common in HIV-infected pregnant women (89–91). The incidence of these complications of pregnancy correlates with high maternal viral loads and low CD4 counts.

Management of HIV in Pregnancy

Initial Evaluation
Patients newly found to be positive for HIV during pregnancy should be carefully evaluated. A complete medical history should be taken, with an emphasis on symptoms that suggest advanced disease. Specific questions should be asked about fever, rash, diarrhea, night sweats, weight loss, cough, and fatigue. Any history of previous STDs, recurrent vaginal candidiasis, or abnormal Papanicolaou (Pap) smears should be carefully documented.

The physical examination should document any signs of lymphadenopathy, oral thrush or vaginal candidiasis, visceromegaly, pneumonia, or dermatologic abnormalities. Standard obstetric assessment of fetal gestational age and morphology should be done. In addition to the usual prenatal laboratory tests, assays for lymphocyte profile (CD4 count, CD4 percentage, and ratio of CD4 to CD8 cells), HIV-1 RNA viral load, cytomegalovirus, and *Toxoplasma* IgG titers; hepatitis B and C serologic tests; and a purified protein derivative (PPD) test with anergy battery should be ordered (Box 13-3). A high incidence of abnormal Pap smears is seen in HIV-positive women, so careful assessment for cervical dysplasia, including repeated Pap smears and colposcopy, is warranted (92). If antiretroviral therapy or opportunistic prophylaxis is begun, the patient should be carefully monitored for toxicities and adverse effects associated with the medication being given. An important example pertaining to pregnancy is the potential effect of protease inhibitors on carbohydrate metabolism and lipid levels. These inhibitors are associated with the develop-

---

Box 13-3 Laboratory Evaluation and Testing for Human Immuno-deficiency Virus

---

At initial evaluation, test for or measure:
HIV viral load (RNA copies)
Lymphocyte profile (CD4 count, CD4%, CD4:CD8 ratio)
Cytomegalovirus
Toxoplasma IgG titers
Hepatitis B and C serology
Purified protein derivative with anergy panel
CBC
Electrolytes, BUN, creatinine
Liver transaminase
Amylase
Cholesterol and tryglycerides (if patient on protease inhibitor)
Early 1-hour glucola diabetes screen (if patient on protease inhibitor)
At follow-up evaluation (at least once each trimester), test for or measure:
HIV viral load
CBC
Electrolytes, BUN, creatinine
Liver transaminase
Amylase
Cholesterol and tryglycerides (if patient on protease inhibitor)
Repeat 1-hour glucola diabetes screen (especially if patient on protease inhibitor)

ment of carbohydrate intolerance and hyperlipidemia in many patients. Given the diabetogenic nature of pregnancy, repeated glucose challenges and serial lipid profiles may be necessary in women taking these medications.

Pharmacotherapy

The use of antiretroviral medication during pregnancy has two critical objectives. Treatment of the HIV-infected woman should include chemoprophylaxis to reduce risk for vertical transmission of HIV-1 to the fetus. Equally important, therapies of known benefit for maternal disease should not be withheld during pregnancy unless their potential adverse effect on the fetus is thought to outweigh the benefit to the mother. Combination antiretroviral therapy, usually consisting of two nucleoside analogue reverse transcriptase inhibitors and a protease inhibitor, is the currently recommended standard for HIV-1–infected adults who are not pregnant. Federal guidelines state that pregnancy should not preclude the use of optimal therapeutic regimens (93). Additional medications may be required to treat or prevent opportunistic infections.

Information on the safety and efficacy of all antiretroviral agents, including zidovudine, is limited. The available data on antiretroviral treatment in pregnancy are presented in a comprehensive review by Minkoff and Augenbraun (94). These authors emphasize that antiretroviral therapy should be started in pregnancy and outside of pregnancy for the same clinical indications (low CD4 counts and viral loads >20,000). If possible, therapy should be started after the first trimester (95). Similarly, appropriate prophylaxis against opportunistic infections, such as *Pneumocystis carinii* and *Mycobacterium avium-intracellulare* infections, should be started during pregnancy according to the same guidelines that apply to nonpregnant adults, given the grave nature of these infections.

Efforts are ongoing to gather prospective data on pregnancy outcomes in women who use antiretroviral agents during pregnancy. A collaborative prospective registry has been started by several pharmaceutical companies, and its findings should be available in the near future.

Pregnant women with HIV infection need a lengthy discussion about the medication regimens available to them, and this discussion should include full disclosure of the risks, benefits, and unknown effects of the medications in pregnancy. Those who opt for zidovudine monotherapy should be made aware of the theoretical concern that monotherapy may select for resistant viral strains and lessen the efficacy of zidovudine later in life.

Counseling and Testing

It is projected that, by the year 2000, 10 million women and children will be HIV infected (96). A major strategy to combat the spread of HIV among women and particularly among children is *prevention:* prenatal HIV counseling and testing. Universal prenatal counseling accomplishes two important objectives. First, it provides an opportunity for clinicians to 1) educate all prenatal patients about the major modes of HIV transmission and 2) initiate practical discussions about risk reduction with uninfected women. Second, it allows HIV infection to be diagnosed in all HIV-infected pregnant women while there is still time to initiate pharmacologic interventions that may prevent vertical transmission.

However busy a clinician may be, it is mandatory that he or she use a rapid but comprehensive module for counseling antenatal patients before and after testing for HIV infection. In pretest counseling, the clinician must give the rationale for HIV testing in pregnancy, review modes of HIV transmission (distinguishing between HIV infection and AIDS), and discuss options for maternal treatment and fetal prophylaxis in the event of a positive test result. The patient should be assured of the confidentiality of the counseling and test results. Post-test counseling may include advice to retest if the patient had a possible exposure less than 3 months before the test or has a negative or indeterminate test result. All positive test results should include referral to appropriate medical and social services (97).

Information given to patients during pre- or post-test counseling may be specified by state law or guidelines (98–100). The CDC, ACOG, and most state health departments provide guidelines to assist clinicians in counseling (101, 102). Most states require that informed consent be given before routine antenatal HIV testing is done. Nonconsensual testing of newborns may occur in the near future according to provisions of the Ryan White Care Act, passed by the U.S. Congress in 1996. This act (which would, in effect, be the same as nonconsensual testing of pregnant women) requires each state to 1) reduce rates of pediatric AIDS cases by 50% compared with data from 1993 or 2) have knowledge of the HIV serostatus of 95% of pregnant women who obtained prenatal care before 34 weeks of gestation (103).

Reproductive Decision Making and Contraception

For HIV-positive women, the usual contraceptive options may involve risks not faced by HIV-negative women. Debate continues as to whether estrogen-containing contraceptives have an immune-enhancing or immune-suppressing effect. No convincing evidence for or against is compelling enough to remove these agents from the list of birth control options for HIV-positive women. Intrauterine devices are considered inappropriate for HIV-positive women because of the increased risk for infection during insertion and the higher rates of pelvic inflammatory disease that are associated with these devices (104). Barrier methods of contraception are highly effective in preventing pregnancy and STDs when used consistently. Nonoxynol 9, which is a common component of contraceptive foam and latex condoms, has been reported to cause vaginal inflammation in some women (105). It is thought that local vaginal inflammation may enhance transmission of HIV and other sexually transmitted infectious organisms. Female condoms were approved by the FDA in 1993. They do not seem to be effective in preventing pregnancy. Their primary use is in the prevention of sexual transmission of HIV and other infectious organisms; this may be an important issue in the protection of male sexual partners.

REFERENCES

1. **Norden CW, Kass EH.** Bacteriuria of pregnancy: a critical appraisal. Annu Rev Med. 1968;19:437-8.

2. **Andriole VT, Patterson TE.** Epidemiology, natural history, and management of urinary tract infections in pregnancy. Med Clin North Am. 1991;75:359-73.

3. **Patterson TF, Andriole VT.** Detection, significance, and therapy of bacteriuria in pregnancy. Infect Dis Clin North Am. 1997;11:593-608.

4. **Brumfitt W, Davies BI, Rosser E.** Urethral catheter as a cause of urinary tract infection in pregnancy and puerperium. Lancet. 1961;2:1059-61.

5. **Gilstrap LC, Cunningham FG, Whalley PJ.** Acute pyelonephritis in pregnancy: an anterospective study. Obstet Gynecol. 1981;57:409-14.

6. **Gilstrap LC, Leveno KJ, Cunningham FG.** Renal infection and pregnancy outcome. Am J Obstet Gynecol. 1981;141:709-14.

7. **Harris RE.** The significance of eradication of bacteriuria during pregnancy. Obstet Gynecol. 1979;53:71-4.

8. **Gratacos E, Torres PJ, Vila J, Alonso PL, et al.** Screening and treatment of asymptomatic bacteriuria in pregnancy prevent pyelonephritis. J Infect Dis. 1994;169:1390-2.

9. **Goldenberg RL, Rouse DJ.** Prevention of premature birth. N Engl J Med. 1998;339:313-20.

10. **Centers for Disease Control and Prevention.** 1998 guidelines for treatment of sexually transmitted diseases. MMWR Morb Mortal Wkly Rep. 1998;47(RR-1):8-75.

11. **Amsel R, Totten PA, Spiegel CA, et al.** Nonspecific vaginitis: diagnostic criteria and microbial and epidemiologic associations. Am J Med. 1983;74:14-22.

12. **McGregor JA, French JI.** Evidence-based prevention of preterm birth and rupture of membranes: infection and inflammation. J Soc Obstet Gynaecol Can. 1997;19:835-52.

13. **Hillier SL, Nugent RP, Eschenbach DA, et al.** Association between bacterial vaginosis and preterm delivery of a low-birth-weight infant. N Engl J Med. 1995;333:1737-42.

14. **McGregor JA, French JI, Parker R, et al.** Prevention of premature birth by screening and treatment for common genital tract infections: results of a prospective controlled evaluation. Am J Obstet Gynecol. 1995;173:157-67.

15. **Hay PE, Lamont RF, Taylor-Robinson D, et al.** Abnormal bacterial colonization of the genital tract and subsequent preterm delivery and late miscarriage. BMJ. 1994;308:295-8.

16. **Gravett MG, Nelson HP, DeRouen T, Critchow C, Eschenbach DA, Holmes KK.** Independent associations of bacterial vaginosis and *Chlamydia trachomatis* infection with adverse pregnancy outcome. JAMA. 1986;256:1899-903.

17. **McGregor JA, French JI, Lawellin D, et al.** Bacterial protease-induced reduction of chorioamniotic membrane strength and elasticity. Obstet Gynecol. 1987;69:167-74.

18. **Sbarra AJ, Thomas GB, Cetrulo CL, et al.** Effect of bacterial growth on the bursting pressure of fetal membranes in vitro. Obstet Gynecol. 1987;70:107-10.

19. **Schoonmarker JN, Lawellin DW, Lunt B, et al.** Bacteria and inflammatory cells reduce chorioamniotic membrane integrity and tensile strength. Obstet Gynecol. 1989; 74:590-6.

20. **Hauth JC, Goldenberg RL, Andrews WW, DuBard MB, Copper RL.** Reduced incidence of preterm delivery with metronidazole and erythromycin in women with bacterial vaginosis. N Engl J Med. 1995;333:1732-6.

21. **Morales WJ, Schorr S, Albritton J.** Effect of metronidazole in patients with preterm birth in preceding pregnancy and bacterial vaginosis: a placebo-controlled, double-blind study. Am J Obstet Gynecol. 1994;171:345-7.

22. **McGregor JA, French JI.** Chlamydia trachomatis infection during pregnancy. Am J Obstet Gynecol. 1991;164:1782-9.

23. **Offenbacher S, Katz V, Fertik G, et al.** Periodontal infection as a possible risk for preterm low birthweight. J Periodontal. 1996;67(Suppl. 10):1103-13.

24. **Sewankambo N, Grag RH, Wavier MJ, et al.** HIV-I infection associated with abnormal vaginal feva morphology and bacterial vaginosis. Lancet. 1997;350:546-50.

25. **Cotch MF, for the Vaginal Infections and Prematurity Study Group.** Carriage of Trichomonas vaginalis is associated with adverse pregnancy outcome [Abstract]. Presented at the 30th Annual Meeting of the Interscience Conference on Antimicrobial Agents and Chemotherapy, October 21-24, 1990, Atlanta, Georgia.

26. **Grice AC.** Vaginal infection causing spontaneous rupture of the membranes and premature delivery. Aust N Z J Obstet Gynecol. 1974;14:156-8.

27. **Alderete JF, Newton E, Dennis C, et al.** Antibody in sera of patients infected with Trichomonas vaginalis is to trichomonad proteinases. Genitour Med. 1991;67:331-4.

28. **Draper D, Jones W, Heine RP, et al.** Trichomonas vaginalis weakens human amnio-chorion in an in vitro model of premature membrane rupture. Infect Dis Obstet Gynecol. 1995;2:267-74.

29. **Scholes D, Stergachis A, Heidrich FE, Andrilla H, Holmes KK, Stamm WE.** Prevention of pelvic inflammatory disease by screening for cervical chlamydial infection. N Engl J Med. 1996;334:1362-6.

30. Association of Chlamydia trachomatis and Mycoplasma hominis with intrauterine growth retardation and preterm delivery. The Johns Hopkins Study of Cervicitis and Adverse Pregnancy Outcome. Am J Epidemiol. 1989;129:1247-57.

31. **Ryan GM Jr, Adbella TN, McNeeley SG, et al.** Chlamydia trachomatis infection in pregnancy and effect of treatment on outcome. Am J Obstet Gynecol. 1990;162:34-9.

32. **Cohen I, Veille J-C, Calkins BM.** Improved pregnancy outcome following successful treatment of chlamydial infection. JAMA. 1990;263:3160-3.

33. **Martin DH, and the VIP Study Group.** Erythromycin treatment of Chlamydia trachomatis infection during pregnancy [Abstract]. Presented at the 30th Annual Interscience Conference on Antimicrobial Agents and Chemotherapy. October 21-24, 1990, Atlanta, Georgia.

34. **Amstey MS, Stedman KT.** Asymptomatic gonorrhea and pregnancy. J Am Vener Dis Assoc. 1976;3:14-6.

35. **Donders GG, Desmyter J, DeWet DH, Van Assche FA.** The association of gonorrhea and syphilis with premature birth and low birthweight. Genitour Med. 1993;69:98-101.

36. **Elliott B, Brunham RC, Laga M, Piot P, Ndinya-Achola JO, Maitha G, et al.** Maternal gonococcal infection as a preventable risk factor for low birth weight. J Infect Dis. 1990;161:531-6.

37. **Ekwo EE, Gosselink CA, Woolson R, Moawad A.** Risks for premature rupture of amniotic membranes. Int J Epidemiol. 1993;22:495-503.

38. **Smith LG Jr, Summers PR, Miles RW, Biswas MK, Pernoll ML.** Gonococcal chorioamnionitis associated with sepsis: a case report. Am J Obstet Gynecol. 1989;160: 573-4.

39. **Charles AG, Cohen S, Kass MB, et al.** Asymptomatic gonorrhea in prenatal patients. Am J Obstet Gynecol. 1981;57:479-82.

40. **Prober CG, Arvin AM.** Genital herpes and the pregnant woman. In: Remington JS, Swartz M, eds. Current Clinical Topics in Infectious Diseases, v. 10. Boston: Blackwell Scientific Publications; 1989:1-26.

41. **Brown ZA, Selke S, Zeh J, Kopelman J, Maslow A, Ashley RL, et al.** The acquisition of herpes simplex virus during pregnancy. N Engl J Med. 1997;337:509-15.

42. **Stone KM, Brooks CA, Guinan ME, Alexander ER.** National surveillance for neonatal herpes simplex virus infection. Sex Transm Dis. 1989;16:152-6.

43. **Prober CG, Corey L, Brown ZA, Hensleigh PA, Frenkel LM, Bryson Y, et al.** The management of pregnancies complicated by genital infections with herpes simplex virus. Clin Infect Dis. 1992;15:1031-8.

44. **Stagnos S, Whitley RJ.** Herpes virus infections of pregnancy. Part II: Herpes simplex virus and varicella-zoster virus infections. N Engl J Med. 1985;313:1327-30.

45. **Brown ZA, Benedetti J, Ashley R, et al.** Neonatal herpes simplex virus infection in relation to asymptomatic maternal infection at the time of labor. N Engl J Med. 1991; 324:1247-52.

46. **Brown ZA, Benedetti J, Selke S, Ashley R, Watts H, Corey L.** Asymptomatic maternal shedding of herpes simplex virus at the onset of labor: relationship to preterm labor. Obstet Gynecol. 1996;87:483-8.

47. **Brown ZA, Vontver LA, Benedetti J, Critchlow CW, Sells CJ, Berry S, Corey L.** Effects on infants of a first episode of genital herpes during pregnancy. N Engl J Med. 1987;317:1246-51.

48. **Prober CG, Hensleigh PA, Boucher FD, Yasukawa LL, Au DS, Arvin AM.** Use of viral cultures at delivery to identify neonates exposed to herpes simplex virus. N Engl J Med. 1988;318:887-91.

49. **Nahimas AJ, Josey WE, Naib ZM, Freeman MG, Fernandez RJ, Wheeler JH.** Perinatal risk associated with maternal genital herpes simplex virus infection. Am J Obstet Gynecol. 1971;110:825-37.

50. **Harter C, Bernirschke K.** Fetal syphilis in the first trimester. Am J Obstet Gynecol. 1976;124:705-11.

51. **Brown ST.** Adverse reactions in syphilis therapy. J Amer Vener Dis Assoc. 1976;3:172-6.

52. **Gelfand JA, Elin RJ, Berry FW, Frank MM.** Endotoxemia associated with the Jarisch-Herxheimer reaction. N Engl J Med. 1976;295:211-3.

53. **How JH, Bowditch JD.** Syphilis in pregnancy: experience from a rural aboriginal community. Aust N Z J Obstet Gynaecol. 1994;34:383-9.

54. **Dinsmoor MJ.** Hepatitis in the obstetric patient. Infect Dis Clin North Am. 1997; 11:77-91.

55. **Centers for Disease Control and Prevention.** Prevention of perinatal hepatitis B through enhanced case management. MMWR Morb Mortal Wkly Rep. 1996;45:584.

56. **Lee WM.** Hepatitis B infection. N Engl J Med. 1997;337:1733-45.

57. **Belloni C, Chirico G, et al.** Immunogenicity of hepatitis B vaccine in term and preterm infants. Acta Paediatr. 1998;87:336-8.

58. **Smedile A, Farci P, et al.** Influence of delta infection on severity of hepatitis B. Lancet. 1982;2:945-7.

59. **Dienstag JL.** Sexual and perinatal transmission of hepatitis C. Hepatology. 1997;26: 66S-70S.

60. **Bohnman VR, Stettler R, et al.** Seroprevalence and risk factors for hepatitis C virus antibody in pregnant women. Obstet Gynecol. 1992;80:609.

61. **Zuccoth GV, Jribero M, et al.** Effect of hepatitis C genotype on mother-to-infant transmission of virus. J Pediatr. 1995;127:278.

62. **Resti M, Azan C, et al.** Mother-to-infant transmission of hepatitis C virus. Acta Paediatr. 1995;84:251.

63. **Boyer KM, Gotoff SP.** Prevention of early-onset neonatal GBS infection. N Engl J Med. 1986;314:1665-9.

64. **Weisman LE, Stoll BJ, Cruess DF.** Early-onset group B streptococcal sepsis: a current assessment. J Pediatr. 1992;121:428-33.

65. **Centers for Disease Control and Prevention.** Prevention of perinatal group B streptococcal disease: a public health perspective. MMWR Morb Mortal Wkly Rep. 1996; 45(RR-7):1-24.

66. **ACOG Committee OB Practice.** Committee Opinion Number 173. Prevention of early-onset group B streptococcal disease in newborns. June 1996.

67. **Yancey MK, Armer T, Clark P, Duff P.** Assessment of rapid identification tests for genital carriage of group B streptococci. Obstet Gynecol. 1992;80:1038-47.

68. **Coleman RT, Sherer DM, Maniscalco WM.** Prevention of neonatal group B streptococcal infections: advances in maternal vaccine development. Obstet Gynecol. 1992; 80:301-9.

69. **Gibbs RS, McDuffie RS Jr, McNabb F, Fryer GE, Miyoshi T, Merenstein G.** Neonatal group B streptococcal sepsis during 2 years of a universal screening program. Obstet Gynecol. 1994;84:496-500.

70. **Rouse DJ, Goldenberg RL, Cliver SP, Cutter GR, Mennemeyer ST, Fargason CA Jr.** Strategies for the prevention of early-onset neonatal group B streptococcal sepsis: a decision analysis. Obstet Gynecol. 1994;83:483-94.

71. **Soloway B.** Primary care and specialty care in the age of HAART. AIDS Clinical Care. 1997;9:37-9.

72. **Centers for Disease Control and Prevention.** First 500,000 AIDS cases—United States, 1995. MMWR Morb Mortal Wkly Rep. 1995;44(RR-7):1-15.

73. **National Center for Health Statistics.** Annual summary of birth, marriages, divorces and deaths: United States, 1994. Monthly Vital Statistics Report, v. 43. Hyattsville, MD: Department of Health and Human Services, Public Health Service; 1994.

74. **Gwinn M, Pappaioanou M, George JR, et al.** Prevalence of HIV infection in childbearing women in the United States: surveillance using newborn blood samples. JAMA. 1991;265:1204.

75. **Karon JM, Rosenberg PS, McQuillan G, et al.** Prevalence of HIV infection in the United States—1984 to 1992. JAMA. 1996;276:126.

76. **Leroy V, Msellati P, Lepage P, et al.** Four years of natural history of HIV-1 infection in African women. J Acquir Immune Defic Syndr Hum Retrovirol. 1995;9:415.

77. **Tenerman M, Epahntua NC, Jackoniah N, et al.** Maternal human immunodeficiency virus-1 infection and pregnancy outcome. Obstet Gynecol. 1994;83:495-501.

78. **Cowan MJ, Walker C, Culver K, et al.** Maternally transmitted HIV infection in children. AIDS. 1988;2:437-41.

79. **European Collaborative Study.** Mother to child transmission of HIV infection. Lancet. 1988;2:1039-42.

80. **Centers for Disease Control and Prevention.** US Public Health Service recommendations for human immunodeficiency virus counseling and voluntary testing for pregnant women. MMWR Morb Mortal Wkly Rep. 1995;44(RR-7):1-15.

81. **Landesman SH, Kalish LA, Burns DN, et al.** Obstetrical factors and the transmission of human immunodeficiency virus type 1 from mother to child. N Engl J Med. 1996;334:1617-23.

82. **Mandelbrot L, Marguax MJ, Bongain A, et al.** Obstetric factors and mother to child transmission of human immunodeficiency virus type 1. The French Perinatal Cohort. Am J Obstet Gynecol. 1996;175(pt 1):661.

83. **Sperling RS, Shapiro DE, Coombs RW.** Maternal viral load, zidovudine treatment and the risk of transmission of human immunodeficiency virus type 1 from mother to child. N Engl J Med. 1996;335:1621-9.

84. **Conner EM, Sperling RS, Gilbert R, et al.** Reduction of maternal infant transmission of human immunodeficiency virus type 1 with zidovudine treatment. N Engl J Med. 1994;331:1173-89.

85. **National Institute of Allergy and Infectious Diseases.** News. Bethesda, MD: National Institutes of Health; 1996.

86. Pediatric AIDS surveillance. MMWR Morb Mortal Wkly Rep. 1997;46:1086.

87. **Berreb A, Kobuch WE, Puel J, et al.** Influence of pregnancy on human immunodeficiency virus infection. Am J Obstet Gynecol. 1990;160:910-20.

88. **Mellors JW, Rinaldo CR Jr, Gupta P, et al.** Prognosis in HIV-1 infection predicted by the quantity of virus in plasma. Science. 1994;272:1915-21.

89. **Alger L, Farley JJ, Robinson BA, et al.** Interactions of human immunodeficiency virus infection and pregnancy. Obstet Gynecol. 1993;82:878-796.

90. **Hirshtick RE, Glassroth J, Jordan MC, et al.** Bacterial pneumonia in persons infected with the human immunodeficiency virus. N Engl J Med. 1995;333:845-51.

91. **Minkoff HL, Henderson C, Nendez H, et al.** Pregnancy outcomes among mothers infected with the human immunodeficiency virus and uninfected control subjects. Am J Obstet Gynecol. 1991;163:1201-6.

92. **DelPriore G, Maag T.** The value of cervical cytology in HIV infected women. Gynecol Oncol. 1995;56:495-398.

93. Public Health Service Task Force recommendations for the use of antiretroviral drugs in pregnant women infected with HIV-1 transmission in the United States. MMWR Morb Mortal Wkly Rep. 1998;47(RR-2).

94. **Minkoff H, Augenbraun M.** Antiretroviral therapy for pregnant women. Am J Obstet Gynecol. 1997;176:478-89.

95. Human immunodeficiency virus infection during pregnancy. ACOG Bulletin No 232; 1997.

96. **Chin J.** Current and future dimensions of the HIV/AIDS pandemic in women and children. Lancet. 1991;336:221-4.

97. **Rips J.** Establishing a successful HIV counseling and testing service: a blueprint for preventing pediatric HIV infections and translating research into clinical practice. Obstet Clin North Am. 1997;4:873-97.

98. Fla Stat Ann 384.31 ("The prevailing professional standard of care in the state requires each health care provider to counsel the woman to be tested for human immunodeficiency virus (HIV)").

99. NJ Stat Ann 26: 5-C-16 (West 1997).

100. NY Comp Codes R & Regs Tit 10 63 (1997).

101. **Centers for Disease Control and Prevention.** Recommendations for human immunodeficiency virus counseling and voluntary testing for pregnant women. MMWR Morb Mortal Wkly Rep. 1995;44:1-15.

102. **American College of Obstetricians and Gynecologists.** Human immunodeficiency virus infections in pregnancy. ACOG Educational Bulletin 232; 1997:1-7.

103. USCA 300ff-34 (1996).

104. **Kelley P.** Fertility, menstruation and birth control in HIV. Treatment Issues. 1992;6:10-4.

105. **Bird A.** The use of spermicide containing nonoxynol 9 in the prevention of HIV infection. AIDS. 1991;5:791-6.

III. Upper Respiratory Infections, Pneumonia, and Tuberculosis
Richard V. Lee and Linda Anne Barbour

Respiratory Viruses

The many serotypes of respiratory viruses and the antigenic lability of these viruses contribute to cycles of epidemic upper respiratory infection (URI) (1–4).

We have no reliable or available vaccines for respiratory viruses, with the exception of the influenza virus. Complete isolation is impossible, and URIs in pregnant women are common. Preventive care principally consists of common sense, and good public health information enhances common sense. The major route of transmission of respiratory viruses is skin-to-skin contact (5).

About half of all episodes of pneumonia in pregnant women are preceded by an acute URI (6). Although URIs are usually mild infections, they must be regarded as predecessors of potentially serious complications of pregnancy and the puerperium (7). All gravid women have an enhanced risk for bacterial sinusitis and eustachian tube dysfunction during or after viral URIs. Normal pregnancy can increase severity of symptoms and susceptibility to the complications of viral respiratory infections (8).

The Common Cold

The management of colds during pregnancy is supportive and directed at excluding treatable nonviral infections, such as *Mycoplasma pneumoniae* infection and group A beta-hemolytic streptococcal infection. Throat culture for group A streptococci and serologic tests for *Mycoplasma* species are helpful if fever, persistent cough, and pharyngeal exudates complicate a cold.

Antihistamines, decongestants, and nasal sprays should be avoided. Antihistamines thicken secretions and predispose to diminished clearance of secretions from the nose and sinuses (9, 10). A variety of fetal anomalies have been attributed to antihistamines, and neonatal withdrawal has been attributed to regular maternal use of antihistamines (11). Of all of the decongestants, only pseudoephedrine and oxymetalazone (Afrin) has shown no association with adverse fetal effects. Systemic vasoconstrictors should be avoided during pregnancy, especially in women with labile or elevated blood pressure.

Lower Respiratory Infections

Bronchitis and pneumonia are uncommon in nonsmoking, young, healthy women. Smoking tobacco and illicit substances like crack cocaine, amphetamines, and marijuana produce acute and chronic tracheobronchial irritation and inflammation, interfere with mucociliary clearance, and foster bronchial colonization with mixed aerobic-anaerobic flora (including *Haemophilus influenzae* and *Branhamella* and *Moraxella* species). Smoking is the principal risk factor for lower respiratory tract infection in otherwise healthy young women. Teenage females are the largest group of new tobacco smokers and, although the prevalence of cigarette smoking in general has stabilized or decreased, many women enter their reproductive years with subtle established bronchial disease due to smoking.

Pregnancy enhances the risk for lower respiratory infections because of gastroesophageal reflux and attendant aspiration. Alterations in cell-mediated immunity and pulmonary vascular circulation may permit the establishment and extension of bronchopulmonary colonization into parenchymal infection once normal host clearance mechanisms have been compromised. Pregnancy is a special risk for primary viral pneumonia with influenza and varicella infections.

Heavy alcohol consumption is a well-known risk factor for pneumonia, especially pneumococcal infection. Injection of narcotics can produce a talc or particulate granulomatous pneumonia. Altered consciousness during pregnancy, such as intoxication with alcohol or heroin, magnifies risk for aspiration.

The reported incidence of pneumonia ranges from 1.0 to 2.5 episodes per 1000 pregnancies. Prevalence is increased during periods of epidemic respiratory infection, such as influenza. Occupational exposures to respiratory infections are seen among teachers, medical and nursing personnel, and persons working in jobs that involve intense public contact.

No respiratory pathogens are unique to pregnancy. Community-acquired and nosocomial pathogens infect pregnant women and nonpregnant patients in similar patterns. What is special about pregnancy is the frequent occurrence of aspiration and the predisposition to more aggressive clinical illness with organisms that are usually contained or eliminated by cell-mediated immunity.

Recurrent themes in the care of pregnant patients with respiratory infections are the suitability of chest radiography and the selection of antibiotics. Pregnancy should never be a reason to avoid diagnostic chest radiography. Shielding of the abdomen provides some protection for the fetus against the very small amounts of radiation needed for standard anterior, posterior, and lateral chest radiographs. Antibiotics should be chosen according to the susceptibility of the organism. Close monitoring of maternal Po_2 to ensure adequate fetal oxygenation is important.

Aspiration Pneumonia

Aspiration of gastric contents is common in pregnant women and can precipitate bronchospasm. New-onset asthma or an increased frequency of episodic wheezing in patients with established asthma should suggest gastroesophageal reflux. Postural maneuvers and antacids for reflux dyspepsia often suffice; H_2-receptor blockers can be used if needed. Motility-enhancing agents, such as metoclopramide and cisapride, may be necessary for intransigent gastroesophageal reflux. Aspiration pneumonia is discussed in Chapter 7.

Bronchitis

Bronchitis during pregnancy warrants antibiotic treatment if a patient is febrile and has increases in sputum amount and purulence. Antibiotics should be aimed at the usual flora found in chronic bronchitis: *Streptococcus* species, *Haemophilus influenzae*, and a variety of oropharyngeal organisms.

Viral Pneumonia

Invasion of the lung parenchyma is unusual for respiratory viruses, except for VZV, adenoviruses, enteroviruses, and influenza viruses.

Gestation-induced alterations in cell-mediated immunity may diminish the pregnant patient's ability to contain viral pathogens once they have entered the lung parenchyma. The physiologic and immunologic circumstances of pregnancy seem to combine to predispose pregnant women to a greater risk for and a more severe course of viral pneumonia, especially late in pregnancy, when physiologic and anatomic alterations are at their greatest. In contrast, pregnancy does not alter the risk for or course of bacterial pneumonia for which phagocytic cells and antibodies are the principal host defenses.

The course of primary viral pneumonia during pregnancy can be dramatic and may be associated with acute lung injury or the acute respiratory distress syndrome. Isolation or immunization are the only effective prophylactic measures.

After the pneumonic process has started, little can be done except to provide ventilatory support, prevent or treat superimposed bacterial infection, and monitor fetal status to rescue the fetus in time if the mother's death should become imminent. Premature surgical delivery has not been shown to benefit maternal morbidity or mortality.

Influenza

Immunity to influenza follows naturally occurring infection and experimental challenge with live virus (12–16). Secretory IgA and circulating IgM and IgG are produced, and immunity to reinfection and illness with homologous virus persist for decades. Diminished cell-mediated immunity is likely to be associated with aggressive influenza virus infection.

The most severe illness is caused by novel strains of virus for which the population and the individual host have little or no cross-reactive immunity. The most seriously affected persons, regardless of the prevalent viral strain causing infection, are pregnant patients and patients with preexisting lung and heart disease that cause congestive heart failure or pulmonary congestion (12–18). There are two categories of complications. The first and most common category is bacterial superinfections: sinusitis, otitis, and pneumonia. An unusual superinfection complication, the toxic shock syndrome, was reported in 1987 (19, 20). The second category of complications follows dissemination of the virus and infection of tissues other than the respiratory epithelium: primary influenza pneumonia (21, 22), myositis, myocarditis, encephalitis, and transplacental fetal infection.

The spectrum of influenza ranges from inapparent infection to fulminant viral pneumonia (12–17). Though a large portion of the population has at least partial immunity, about 20% of infections are inapparent and another 30% of persons have only coryza without fever. Febrile influenza occurs in about 50% of infected persons, and about 5% of these patients have lower respiratory tract involvement.

The effect of influenza on pregnant women has been most dramatic during major pandemics. In 1918, the mortality rate for all pregnant women was

27%; among women contracting influenza in the last month of gestation, the mortality rate was in excess of 60% (23, 24). Nonpregnant patients with influenza complicated by pneumonia had a 30% mortality rate; more than 50% of pregnant patients with pneumonia died. During the 1957–58 Asian flu epidemic in New York City, half of the young women who died of influenza were pregnant (25). Throughout the United States, a sharp increase in the maternal mortality rate was associated with the 1957–58 influenza outbreak, but this increase was not as marked as the increase seen in the 1918 pandemic (26). Women in the last few weeks of gestation were at greatest risk. As a general rule, excess maternal morbidity and mortality occur during the early months of epidemic influenza, in association with the appearance of new antigenic variants (27, 28). Over the past 30 years, there has been a reduction in mortality from influenza during pregnancy (27). The decline in maternal mortality rates associated with influenza may be related to the absence of completely novel pandemic strains of influenza since the last great pandemic of "Hong Kong flu" in 1968–70 as well as to improved respiratory care and immunization practices.

An increase in stillbirths, prematurity, and congenital anomalies associated with severe maternal influenza has been reported during every major influenza epidemic of the 20th century (29–42). No consistent pattern of congenital anomalies or fetal injury is discernible; this suggests that the fetal effects of influenza virus, if any, are multifactorial (43).

Transplacental fetal infections have been documented. McGregor and colleagues (44) reported a woman who had acute A/Bangkok (H3N2) influenza with uterine tenderness suggesting chorioamnionitis; the virus was isolated from nasal washings and from amniotic fluid. The healthy infant delivered 3 weeks after maternal recovery had no virus isolated from the placenta, amniotic fluid, or nasal washings. Cord blood contained IgM and IgA antibodies against the infecting virus. Fetal influenza infection with recovery does occur, but fetal infection has not been found in most reports describing disseminated maternal influenza virus infection (45, 46). In some fatal maternal cases, influenza virus has been recovered from both maternal and fetal tissue (47, 48).

Supportive care—rest, fluids, humidity, acetaminophen, and frequent reassurance—is the only solace for pregnant patients with influenza. Antibiotics are indicated only for secondary bacterial infection. Patients should be monitored for changes in chest examination, dyspnea, and changes in secretions that might indicate superimposed bacterial infection or aggressive viral disease. Pneumonia warrants admission and closer observation.

Amantadine and rimantadine block replication of influenza A virus but not influenza B virus. They have been used prophylactically and to treat infected high-risk patients (13). Unfortunately, these agents are embryotoxic and teratogenic in rodents and cannot be recommended for general use in pregnancy. During epidemics, however, some high-risk pregnant patients with valvular heart disease and chronic lung disease should be offered amantadine or rimantadine prophylaxis if they are susceptible. In this circumstance, the benefits probably outweigh the risks. Newer agents for influenza have not been evaluated in pregnant women.

A better solution is to immunize high-risk patients with multivalent influenza vaccine before conception or, if necessary, during pregnancy (49–54). The only real contraindication to influenza immunization is allergy to eggs, which are used for propagating the virus (53). New split-antigen vaccines have been proven even safer (52). Women have been immunized safely during gestation and have rapidly produced high titers of transplacentally transmitted protective influenza-specific antibody (51). Whether all pregnant women should receive influenza vaccine is debatable. However, when an antigenic shift in influenza virus occurs and an increase in influenza in the general population can be expected, vaccination of pregnant women makes good sense (55).

Bacterial Pneumonias

Bacterial pulmonary infection ranges in extent from patchy, discrete infiltrates (bronchopneumonia) to the dense lobar infiltrates of classic pneumococcal pneumonia to the diffuse "white out" of aggressive viral pneumonia and the adult respiratory distress syndrome. The infecting pathogen and the underlying pulmonary status of the patient determine the pattern of the pulmonary lesions (56).

For community-acquired pneumonia other than the pregnancy-related events that predispose to respiratory tract infections or contribute to the severity of pneumonic infection, pregnant patients can be managed like nonpregnant patients (56–59). Empiric antibiotic choices are not substantially restricted by pregnancy. Careful attention to fetal status is the only difference. Decisions to intubate and to institute ventilatory support may be influenced by deterioration of fetal status, especially when maternal hypoxia or hypercapnea or acidosis supervene (60).

Tuberculosis

Tuberculosis is a serious health problem in women of childbearing age. The number of cases in the United States increased 41% between 1985 and 1992, and a similar increase was seen among children (61). The rapid increase in numbers of HIV-infected women as well as a marked increase in the rate of tuberculosis in foreign-born persons has translated into an increasing number of pregnant women with tuberculosis. New York City reported an incidence of 94.8 cases of tuberculosis per 100,000 deliveries in 1991–92; in 1985–90 it was 12.4 cases per 100,000 deliveries. Six of the 16 cases reported were extrapulmonary, 11 of the women tested were HIV-positive, and only 40% of the patients had positive results on skin tests for tuberculosis (62). A more intensive screening strategy to diagnose tuberculosis is mandated to prevent an increasing number of cases of neonatal and infant tuberculosis, which is often fatal (63).

Effect of Pregnancy on Tuberculosis

The effect of tuberculosis on pregnancy was controversial in the pre-antibiotic era. Many believed that pregnancy and the postpartum period posed unacceptable risks for progression and that pregnancy termination was appropriate. However, a 1953 report that described 250 pregnant tuberculous women suggested that pregnancy does not seem to exacerbate tuberculosis, although a slightly increased risk for progression may be seen postpartum (64). However, since the antibiotic era, the largest series suggest that with adequate treatment pregnant women with tuberculosis have a prognosis similar to that of nonpregnant women (65). The combination of the anatomic extent of disease, susceptibility, and the immune status of the patient seems to be a stronger predictor of outcome than pregnancy alone.

The clinical presentation of tuberculosis may be somewhat altered in pregnancy because there seems to be a higher incidence of asymptomatic cases. In one series (66), one half to two thirds of pregnant women were asymptomatic and unaware of their disease. Symptoms may be nonspecific in nature, mimicking the physiologic changes of pregnancy. Cough or shortness of breath (74%), weight loss (41%), fever (30%), and malaise and fatigue (30%) were the most common clinical manifestations. Because of the lack of specificity and severity of symptoms, only 10 of 26 mothers who gave birth to neonates with congenital tuberculosis had tuberculosis diagnosed before their infants did (67). A series in Rhode Island (68) found that pregnant women with pulmonary tuberculosis were more likely than nonpregnant women with culture-positive tuberculosis in the same age group to be found by routine screening and to be asymptomatic. In addition, pregnant women were more likely to have unilateral, noncavitary, smear-negative disease. Extrapulmonary tuberculosis does not seem to be more common among pregnant women but is more common in HIV-positive persons.

Effect of Tuberculosis on Pregnancy

Maternal tuberculosis does not cause congenital malformations but may increase risk for prematurity, fetal and perinatal loss, and low-birthweight infants, especially with late diagnosis, inadequate treatment, and advanced pulmonary lesions (69). With early diagnosis and adequate treatment, pregnancy outcome should be favorable.

Congenital tuberculosis, which is defined as vertical transmission to the infant in utero or during labor and delivery, is rare but may be increasing in the HIV-infected population. Such transmission can occur through fetal ingestion of infected amniotic fluid, fetal aspiration of infected amniotic fluid, or hematogenous infection via the umbilical vein in mothers who have tuberculosis involving the placenta or genital tract tuberculosis. The revised criteria for diagnosis of congenital tuberculosis mandate that tuberculous lesions in the neonate be culture proven and that at least one of the following criteria be present: 1) a lesion in the first week of life, 2) primary hepatic complex or caseating hepatic granuloma, 3) tuberculous infection of the placenta or genital tract, and 4) exclusion of the possibility of postnatal transmission. The largest report of neonatal tuberculosis over a 1-year period was reported in South Africa, where the incidence of maternal tuberculosis is 413 cases per 100,000 deliveries (70). Of 77 neonates investigated for perinatal tuberculosis, 11 were culture positive and 6 of the 11 met the criteria for congenital tuberculosis. Six of the 11 mothers were seropositive for HIV, and 1 neonate and 2 mothers died within 3 months after delivery. Seven of the 11 mothers had evidence of current or past tuberculosis or close contact with tuberculosis, and genital tuberculosis was detected in only 1 mother (probably because of this condition's subclinical nature).

Infection to the newborn is most often postnatal and due to airborne inoculation secondary to exposure to the infected mother, an infected family member, or another infected caregiver. Symptoms and signs in the neonate do not usually present until several weeks after birth and are often confused with hyaline membrane disease, pulmonary air leak disease, and bronchopulmonary dysplasia in a preterm infant. The purified protein derivative (PPD) test result is usually negative, and the infant often presents with fever, irritability, lethargy, poor feeding, respiratory symptoms, failure to thrive, lymphadenopathy, splenomegaly, biliary obstruction, or central nervous system (CNS) and middle-ear involvement. Death ensues within weeks to months without treatment, and a literature review of 26 infants with perinatally acquired tuberculosis (67) reported a mortality rate of 46%; 9 of the infants who died were untreated and had the diagnosis established postmortem. Preterm infants may be immunologically immature and are often managed with ventilation. Their hyperoxic lungs are ideal for the rapid proliferation of tuberculosis.

Tuberculosis in Women with Human Immunodeficiency Virus Infection

In the United States, 46% of persons in a tuberculosis clinic were found to be HIV-positive; HIV positivity increases the risk for tuberculosis 500-fold (71).

The risk for developing active disease increases by 8% annually in patients with positive PPD test results. Figure 13-6 presents an algorithm for evaluating asymptomatic women with a positive PPD test result. Progression to active and sometimes fulminant tuberculosis can occur within days (72). Extrapulmonary tuberculosis is more prevalent in the HIV-infected population at approximately 50%. This condition increases the risk for congenital tuberculosis and is more difficult to diagnose (62). Anergy is high but does not seem to be higher in pregnancy, according to the Women and Infants Transmission Study (73). The risk for active tuberculosis did not seem to differ in pregnant and nonpregnant HIV-infected women in a case–control study (74). The risk to the infant seems to be higher (62, 70), mandating a thorough investigation (including chest radiography and sputum sampling) to detect tuberculosis in HIV-infected women who are negative on PPD testing but have a known exposure to or symptoms compatible with tuberculosis. Prophylaxis should be continued for 12 months in HIV-positive patients, and treatment for active disease should be continued until the sputum culture is negative for at least 6 months.

Screening

The substantial number of pregnant women with asymptomatic or minimally symptomatic disease supports the idea that pregnant women with tuberculosis will not be identified unless they are screened. Given the increasing incidence of tuberculosis in children, women of childbearing age should be targeted for appropriate screening, prevention, and treatment. Although many authorities recommend screening for all pregnant women, the CDC recommends that, at the very least, all pregnant women who are members of high-risk groups receive a PPD test (75) (Table 13-6). Prenatal clinics with a high proportion of medically underserved low-income patients, foreign-born persons, immunosuppressed persons, or persons with substance abuse or malnutrition should strongly consider a universal screening policy. For many high-risk women, prenatal or peripartum care is their only contact with the health care system. For all pregnant women, the history taken at the first prenatal visit should include questions about a previously positive tuberculin skin-test result, previous treatment for tuberculosis, and current symptoms compatible with tuberculosis. Questions about exposure or an increased likelihood of developing disease once infected should also be asked.

The results of the PPD test, which is an intradermal injection of 0.1 mL of 5 tuberculin unit-strength PPD, do not seem to be affected by pregnancy (76). Women with HIV infection should receive two controls to determine anergy (77). The Advisory Committee for the Elimination of Tuberculosis and the American Thoracic Society (78) recommend that a pregnant woman with a varying PPD test reaction (5, 10, or 15 mm) be considered for preventive ther-

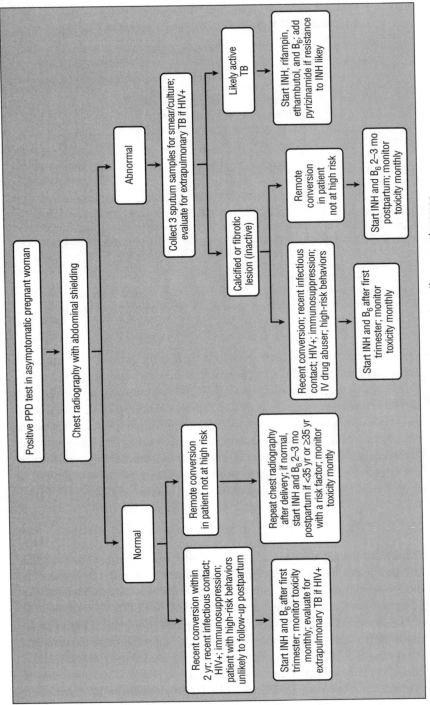

Figure 13-6 Algorithm for positive purified protein derivative (PPD) test in asymptomatic pregnant woman.

Table 13-6   Centers for Disease Control and Prevention Criteria for Determining Need for Preventive Therapy for Persons with Positive Tuberulin Reactions

	Age Group	
Category	<35 Years	≥35 Years
With risk factor*	Treat if PPD test result is ≥10 mm (or ≥5 mm and patient recently had contact with an infected person, is HIV infected, or has radiographic evidence of previous tuberculosis	Same as for <35 years
No risk factor (high-incidence group)†	Treat if PPD test result is ≥10 mm	Do not treat
No risk factor (low-incidence group)	Treat if PPD test result is ≥15 mm ‡	Do not treat

* Risk factors include HIV infection or suspended HIV infection, recent contact with a person with a newly diagnosed infection, skin test conversion within 2 years, abnormal chest radiographs showing fibrotic lesions, intravenous drug abuse, medical conditions (including diabetes mellitus) conditions requiring immunosuppressive therapy, leukemia, Hodgkin disease, end-stage renal disease, and undernutrition.
† High-incidence groups include foreign-born persons, medically undeserved low-income populations, and residents of long-term care facilities.
‡ Lower or higher cut-points may be used to define positive reactions, depending on the relative presence of *Mycobacterium tuberculosis* infection and nonspecific cross-reactivity in the population.

apy according to age and high-risk category, as is the case with nonpregnant persons (Table 13-7). Similarly, patients who have received bacille Calmette-Guérin (BCG) vaccine should be considered for treatment because tuberculin reactivity caused by BCG wanes with the passage of time. A 10-mm reaction is unlikely to persist 10 years after vaccination in the absence of tuberculosis (79). Chest radiography with abdominal shielding should be done after the first trimester but before delivery in PPD-positive women, both to determine the extent of maternal infection and to obviate temporary separation of the mother from the infant for radiography just after delivery (77).

Prophylaxis

Prophylaxis has usually been delayed until after delivery unless the patient is HIV positive or has had a PPD skin-test conversion within 1 to 2 years, although this is controversial (80). Isoniazid seems to be safe to the fetus, but concerns about hepatotoxicity in the mother led the CDC to recommend that perinatal use of INH prophylaxis be avoided except in women at high risk for tuberculosis. These concerns are based on case reports and case–control data suggesting that INH hepatotoxicity may be increased during pregnancy and during the 6 months after delivery, particularly in Hispanic and black women (81, 82). Unfortunately, adherence to INH therapy seems to be low if treatment is initiated 3 to 6 months postpartum. This may be because patients

Table 13-7   American Thoracic Society Dosage Recommendations for Initial Treatment of Tuberculosis

Drug	Dosage (mg/kg)	
	Daily	**Twice Weekly**
Isoniazid	5 (maximum, 30 mg)	15 (maximum, 900 mg)
Rifampin	10 (maximum, 600 mg)	10 (maximum, 600 mg)
Ethambutol	15–25	50
Pyrazinamide	15–30 (maximum, 2 g)	50–70 (maximum, 4 g)

perceive the therapy to be unimportant because a treatment delay is allowed and because care is transferred from one segment of the health care system to another (83). Prophylaxis with 300 mg of INH and 50 mg of pyridoxine (vitamin B_6) should be initiated in patients who have a recent PPD skin-test conversion, are immunodeficient, or at high risk for developing active disease. Monthly liver function tests are recommended so that INH treatment can be stopped if aminotransferase levels increase fivefold.

Treatment of Active Tuberculosis

The CDC recommends that the treatment of active tuberculosis include a regimen of at least three drugs, because of multidrug resistance (84). The preferred initial treatment is INH, rifampin, and ethambutol with 50 mg of pyridoxine (see Figure 13-6) for 9 months or for at least 3 months after a negative sputum culture. When the drug sensitivity of the bacteria is known, use of one of the drugs may be discontinued after 1 to 2 months. Some international tuberculosis organizations also recommend pyrizinamide. If resistance to INH or rifampin is suspected, pyrizinamide should be considered as part of an initial four-drug regimen. Management reports to the CDC from state and large-city tuberculosis control programs have shown that approximately 25% of patients failed to complete therapy within 12 months. Therefore, directly observed therapy may be given after the first 2 months of treatment under the supervision of a health care worker on a twice weekly basis (77). All cases of active tuberculosis should be reported to a public health department or the CDC so that household contacts can be thoroughly investigated.

Isoniazid reaches levels in the fetal circulation that are similar to those in the maternal circulation, but no increase in malformations has been reported in animal and human data as long as pyridoxine is also given. The actions of rifampin to inhibit DNA-dependent RNA polymerase created initial concerns, but the likelihood of teratogenic risk seems to be low (4.4% of 204 pregnancies) (85). Rifampin induces cytochrome P-450 microsomal hepatic enzymes, often renders low-dose oral contraceptives ineffective, and may decrease vitamin K levels in mother and infant. Vitamin K 10 to 20 mg/d for at least 3 weeks beginning at 32 to 34 weeks of gestation is recommended. Ethambutol use in pregnancy has generated concerns about optic neuritis, but in 320 infants exposed during the first trimester the incidence of malformations was not increased (2.2%). No cases of optic neuritis in the fetus were found (85). No adequate animal or human epidemiologic studies of pyrizinamide in pregnancy have been done, but no adverse effects have been reported. Streptomycin-induced ototoxicity in the fetus is possible, and in a review of 206 exposed infants (85) 17% had significant eighth-nerve damage. If streptomycin is necessary, levels must be carefully monitored to avoid high peak concentrations. We have inadequate data on the use of second-line antituberculous agents, including ethionamide, kanamycin, capreomycin, paraaminosalicylic acid, and cycloserine, during pregnancy. Therefore, these agents should be reserved for mothers whose strains have multidrug resistance to first-line agents.

Hepatotoxicity caused by antituberculosis drugs may be more common in pregnancy than in nonpregnant women. If *above normal* is defined as 50% greater than the upper limit of normal, 22% of pregnant patients have at least one abnormal hepatic aminotransferase level (17). Liver function tests should be done monthly during pregnancy; of 64 patients with an SGOT elevated fivefold, only 17 were symptomatic.

All of the agents, including streptomycin, are compatible with breastfeeding; streptomycin is very poorly absorbed from oral administration (86). The percentage of drug that an infant receives in breastmilk is no more than 20% for INH, less than 1% for rifampin, and less than 11% for streptomycin, kanamycin, cycloserine, and ethambutol.

Infants rarely need to be separated from their mothers unless the mother is contagious (according to a positive sputum smear result) (77). Once an infant is receiving appropriate chemotherapy or the mother is judged to be noncontagious, separation should continue only if the mother is ill enough to require hospitalization, if she is expected to be noncompliant with treatment, or if she is thought to be infected with a multidrug-resistant strain. Use of INH should be continued in an infant who has been exposed to active tuberculosis until the mother is culture negative for at least 3 months. At that time, the infant should have a skin test. If the result is positive, the infant should be extensively evaluated for tuberculosis.

Summary

Health care providers involved in the care of pregnant women are in a position to favorably affect 1) the increasing incidence of tuberculosis in women of childbearing age and 2) the high mortality rate associated with undiagnosed, perinatally acquired tuberculosis. Many women at high risk for tuberculosis enter the health care system only for prenatal care and for labor and delivery. Broader tuberculosis screening and evaluation for active disease during pregnancy is warranted given the minimally symptomatic nature of the disease in pregnancy and the gravity of the tuberculosis epidemic in young women and their infants.

REFERENCES

1. **Lee RV.** Viral respiratory diseases: an overview. In: Gleicher NB, ed. Principles of Medical Therapy in Pregnancy, 3d ed. Norwalk, CT: Appleton & Lange; 1998:777-9.

2. **Lee RV.** Important clinical syndromes caused by respiratory viruses. In: Gleicher NB, ed. Principles of Medical Therapy in Pregnancy, 3d ed. Norwalk, CT: Appleton & Lange; 1998:779-82.

3. **Lee RV.** Common endemic respiratory viruses. In: Gleicher NB, ed. Principles of Medical Therapy in Pregnancy, 3d ed. Norwalk, CT: Appleton & Lange; 1998:782-5.

4. **Lee RV.** Epidemic and pandemic respiratory virus: influenza. In: Gleicher NB, ed. Principles of Medical Therapy in Pregnancy, 3d ed. Norwalk, CT: Appleton & Lange; 1998:787-91.

5. **Gwaltney JM Jr.** The common cold. In: Mendell GL, Bennett JE, Dolin R, eds. Principles and Practice of Infectious Diseases, 4th ed. New York: Churchill Livingstone; 1995:561-6.

6. **Hopwood HG.** Pneumonia in pregnancy. Obstet Gynecol. 1965;25:875.

7. **Leontic EA.** Respiratory disease in pregnancy. Med Clin North Am. 1977;61:111.

8. **Lee RV, DiMaggio LA, Lippes HA.** The aches and pains of pregnancy: common complaints of pregnant and postpartum women. In: Lee RV, ed. Current Obstetric Medicine, v. 2. St. Louis, MO: Mosby–Year Book; 1993:221-4.

9. **Gaffey MJ, Gwaltney JM, Sastre A, et al.** Intranasally and orally administered antihistamine treatment of experimental rhinovirus colds. Am Rev Respir Dis. 1987;136:556.

10. **Gaffey MJ, Kaiser DL, Hayden FG.** Ineffectiveness of oral terfenadine in natural colds: evidence against histamine as a mediator of common cold symptoms. Pediatr Infect Dis J. 1988;7:223.

11. **Lee RV, Garner PR, Coustan DR, Cotton D, W.M. B.** Current Obstetric Medicine, v. 1. Chicago: Mosby–Year Book; 1995.

12. **Glezen WP, Cough RB.** Influenza viruses. In: Evans AS, ed. Viral Infections of Humans, 3d ed. New York: Plenum; 1989:419.

13. **LaForce M, Nichol KL, Cox NJ.** Influenza: virology, epidemiology, disease, and prevention. Am J Prev Med. 1994;10:31.

14. **Gross PA.** Preparing for the next influenza pandemic: a reemerging infection. Ann Intern Med. 1996;124:682.

15. **Hers JF, Mulder J.** Broad aspects of the pathology and pathogenesis of human influenza. Am Rev Respir Dis. 1961;83:84.

16. **Noble GR.** Epidemiological and clinical aspects of influenza. In: Beare AS, ed. Basic and Applied Influenza Research. Boca Raton, FL: CRC Pr; 1982:11.

17. **Sweet C, Smith H.** Pathogenicity of influenza virus. Microbiol Rev. 1980;44:303.

18. **Naficy K.** Human influenza infection with proved viremia: report of a case. N Engl J Med. 1963;269:964.

19. **Sperber SJ, Francis JB.** Toxic shock syndrome during an influenza outbreak. JAMA. 1987;257:1086.

20. **MacDonald KL, Osterholm MT, Hedberg CW, et al.** Toxic shock syndrome: a newly recognized complication of influenza and influenza-like illness. JAMA. 1987;257:1053.

21. **Petersdorf RG, Fusco JJ, Harter DH, Albrink WS.** Pulmonary infections complicating Asian influenza. Arch Intern Med. 1959;103:106.

22. **Newton-John HF, Yung AP, Bennett N, Forbes JA.** Influenza virus pneumonitis: a report of ten cases. Med J Aust. 1971; 2:1160.

23. **Frost WH.** The epidemiology of influenza. JAMA. 1919;73:313.

24. **Harris JW.** Influenza occurring in pregnant women. JAMA. 1919;72:978.

25. **Greenberg M, Jacobziner H, Pakter J, et al.** Maternal mortality in the epidemic of Asian influenza, New York City, 1957. Am J Obstet Gynecol. 1957;76:897.

26. **Martin CM, Junin CM, Gottlieb LS, et al.** Asian influenza A in Boston, 1957–1958. Arch Intern Med. 1959;103:515.

27. **Mullooly JP, Barker WH, Nolan TF.** Risk of acute respiratory disease among pregnant women during influenza A epidemics. Public Health Rep. 1986;101:205.

28. **Griffiths PD, Ronalds CJ, Heath RB.** A prospective study of influenza infections during pregnancy. J Epidemiol Community Health. 1980;34:124.

29. **Wynne Griffith G, Adelstein AM, Lambert PM, Weatherall JAC.** Influenza and infant mortality. BMJ. 1972;2:553.

30. **Stanwell-Smith R, Parker AM, Chakravarty P, et al.** Possible association of influenza A with fetal loss: investigation of a cluster of spontaneous abortions and stillbirths. Commun Dis Rep. 1994;4:28.

31. **Widelock D, Csizmas L, Klein S.** Influenza, pregnancy, and fetal outcome. Public Health. 1963;78:1.

32. **Campbell WAB.** Influenza in early pregnancy. Effects of the fetus. Lancet. 1959;1:173.

33. **Coffey VP, Jessop WJE.** Maternal influenza and congenital deformities: a progressive study. Lancet. 1959;2:935.

34. **Wilson MG, Heins HL, Imagawa DT, et al.** Teratogenic effects of Asian influenza. JAMA. 1959;171:638.

35. **Doll R, Hill AB, Jakula J.** Asian influenza in pregnancy and congenital defects. Br J Prev Soc Med. 1960;14:167.

36. **Leck I.** Incidence of malformations following influenza epidemics. Br J Prev Soc Med. 1963;17:70.

37. **Coffey VP, Jessop WJ.** Maternal influenza and congenital deformities: a follow-up study. Lancet. 1963;1:748.

38. **Wilson MG, Stein AM.** Teratogenic effects of Asian influenza. JAMA. 1969;219:336.

39. **Hakosalo J, Saxen L.** Influenza epidemic and congenital defects. Lancet. 1971;2:1346.

40. **MacKenzie JS, Houghton M.** Influenza infections during pregnancy: association with congenital malformations and with subsequent neoplasma in children, and potential hazards of live virus vaccines. Bacteriol Rev. 1974;38:356.

41. **Hardy JG, Azarowicz EN, Mannini A, et al.** The effect of Asian influenza on the outcome of pregnancy. Am J Public Health. 1961;51:1182.

42. **Conover PT, Roessmann U.** Malformation complex in an infant with intrauterine influenza viral infection. Arch Pathol Lab Med. 1990;114:535.

43. **Walker WM, McKee AM.** 633 women with Asian flu antibodies. No congenital malformations. Obstet Gynecol. 1959;13:394.

44. **McGregor JA, Burns JC, Levin MJ, et al.** Transplacental passage of influenza A/Bangkok (H3N2) mimicking amniotic fluid infection syndrome. Am J Obstet Gynecol. 1984;149:856.

45. **Monif GRG, Sowards DL, Eitzman DV.** Serologic and immunologic evaluation of neonates following maternal influenza infection during the second and third trimesters of gestation. Am J Obstet Gynecol. 1972;114:239.

46. **Ramphal R, Donnelly WH, Small PA Jr.** Fatal influenzal pneumonia in pregnancy: failure to demonstrate transplacental transmission of influenza virus. Am J Obstet Gynecol. 1980;138:347.

47. **Yawn DH, Pyeatte JC, Joseph JM, et al.** Transplacental transfer of influenza virus. JAMA. 1971;216:1022.

48. **Ruben FL, Thompson DS.** Cord blood lymphocyte in vitro responses to influenza A antigens after an epidemic of influenza A/Port Chalmers/73 (H3N2). Am J Obstet Gynecol. 1981;141:443.

49. **Brokstad KA, Cox RJ, Olofsson J, et al.** Parenteral influenza vaccination induces a rapid systemic and local immune response. J Infect Dis. 1995;171:198.

50. **Puck JM, Glezen WP, Frank AL, et al.** Immunoprophylaxis: protection of infants from infection with influenza A virus by transplacentally acquired antibody. J Infect Dis. 1980;142:844.

51. **Englund JA, Mbawnike IN, Hammill H, et al.** Maternal immunization with influenza or tetanus toxoid vaccine for passive antibody protection in young infants. J Infect Dis. 1993;168:647.

52. **Ruben FL.** Now and future influenza vaccines. Infect Dis Clin North Am. 1990;4:1-10.

53. Prevention and control of influenza: recommendations of the Advisory Committee of Immunization Practices (ACIP). MMWR Morb Mortal Wkly Rep. 1995;44:1.

54. **Patriarca PA, Strikas RA.** Influenza vaccine for healthy adults? [Editorial] N Engl J Med. 1995;333:933.

55. **Philit F, Cordier JF.** Therapeutic approaches of clinicians to influenza pandemic. Eur J Epidemiol. 1994;10:491.

56. **Berkowitz K, LaSala A.** Risk factors associated with the increasing prevalence of pneumonia during pregnancy. Am J Obstet Gynecol. 1990;163:981.

57. **Bartlett JG, Mundy LM.** Community acquired pneumonia. N Engl J Med. 1995;333:1618-24.

58. **Rickey SD, Roberts SW, Ramkin KD.** Pneumonia complicating pregnancy. Obstet Gynecol. 1994;84:525.

59. **Riley L.** Pneumonia and tuberculosis in pregnancy. Infect Dis Clin North Am. 1997;11:119-33.

60. **Madinger NE, Greenspoon JS, Gray EH.** Pneumonia during pregnancy: has modern technology improved maternal and fetal outcome? Am J Obstet Gynecol. 1989;161:657.

61. **Cantwell MF, Shehab ZM, Costello AM, Sands L, Green WF, Ewing EP, et al.** Brief report: congenital tuberculosis. N Engl J Med. 1994;330:1051-4.

62. **Margono F, Mroueh J, Garely A, White D, Duerr A, Minkoff HL.** Resurgence of active tuberculosis among pregnant women. Obstet Gynecol. 1994;83:911-4.

63. **Barbour LA.** Tuberculosis. Current Obstetric Medicine. Mosby–Year Book; 1996:19-33.

64. **Hedvall E.** Pregnancy and tuberculosis. Acta Med Scand. 1953;147(Suppl 2/86):1-101.

65. **Schaefer G, Zervoudakis IA, Tucks FF.** Pregnancy and pulmonary tuberculosis. Obstet Gynecol. 1975;46:706-15.

66. **Wilson EA, Thelin TJ, Dilts PV.** Tuberculosis complicated by pregnancy. Am J Obstet Gynecol. 1973;115:526-9.

67. **Hageman J, Shulman S, Schreiber M.** Congenital tuberculosis: critical reappraisal of clinical findings and diagnostic procedures. Pediatrics. 1980;66:980-4.

68. **Carter EJ, Mates S.** Tuberculosis during pregnancy: the Rhode Island experience, 1987-1991. Chest. 1994;106:1466-70.

69. **Jana N, Vasishta K, Jindal SK, Khunnu B, Ghosh K.** Perinatal outcome in pregnancies complicated by pulmonary tuberculosis. Int J Gynecol Obstet. 1994;44:119-24.

70. **Adhikari M, Pillay T, Pillay DG.** Tuberculosis in the newborn: an emerging disease. Pediatr Infect Dis J. 1997;16:1108-12.

71. **Saade GR.** Human immunodeficiency virus (HIV)-related pulmonary complications in pregnancy. Semin Perinatol. 1997;21:336-50.

72. **Daley CL, Small PM, Schecter GF.** An outbreak of tuberculosis with accelerated progression among persons infected with the human immunodeficiency virus. N Engl J Med. 1992;326:231-5.

73. **Mofenson LM, Rodriguez EM, Hershow R, Fox HE, Landesman S, Tuomala R, et al.** *Mycobacterium tuberculosis* infection in pregnant and nonpregnant women infected with HIV in the Women and Infants Transmission Study. Arch Intern Med. 1995;155:1066-72.

74. **Espinal MA, Reingold AL, Lavandera M.** Effect of pregnancy on the risk of developing active tuberculosis. J Infect Dis. 1996;173:488-91.

75. **Centers for Disease Control.** Screening for tuberculosis and tuberculous infection in high risk populations and the use of preventive therapy for tuberculosis infection in the United States. MMWR Morb Mortal Wkly Rep. 1990;39(Suppl):1-12.

76. **Present PA, Comstock GW.** Tuberculin sensitivity in pregnancy. Am Rev Respir Dis. 1975;112:413-6.

77. **Anderson GD.** Tuberculosis in pregnancy. Semin Perinatol. 1997;21:328-35.

78. **American Thoracic Society.** Treatment of tuberculous infection in adults and children. Am J Respir Crit Care Med. 1994;149:1359-74.

79. **Vallejo JG, Starke JR.** Tuberculosis and pregnancy. Clin Chest Med. 1992;13:693-707.

80. **Centers for Disease Control.** The use of preventive therapy for tuberculosis infection in the United States. Recommendations of the Advisory Council for Elimination of Tuberculosis (ACET). MMWR Morb Mortal Wkly Rep. 1993;39:9-12.

81. **Moulding TS, Redeker AG, Kanal GC.** Twenty isoniazid-associated deaths in one state. Am Rev Respir Dis. 1989;140:700-5.

82. **Franks AL, Blinkin NJ, Snider DE.** Isoniazid hepatitis among pregnant and postpartum Hispanic patients. Public Health Rep. 1989;104:151-5.

83. **Starke JR.** Tuberculosis. An old disease but a new threat to the mother, fetus and neonate. Clin Perinatol. 1997;24:107-27.

84. **Centers for Disease Control.** Initial therapy for tuberculosis in the era of multi-drug resistance. Recommendations of the Advisory Council for the Elimination of Tuberculosis (ACET). MMWR Morb Mortal Wkly Rep. 1993;42:1-8.

85. **Brost BC, Newman RB.** The maternal and fetal effects of tuberculosis therapy. Obstet Gynecol Clin North Am. 1997;24:659-73.

86. **Snider DE, Powell KE.** Should women taking antituberculosis drugs breastfeed? Arch Intern Med. 1984;144:589-90.

IV. Unusual Infections
Richard V. Lee

Food-Borne and Gastrointestinal Infections

Food can be a vehicle for the transmission of microbes or the toxic products of microbial metabolism. The prevalence of foodborne illness is difficult to state with precision because many episodes occur in individual persons or in small outbreaks that are not investigated or reported (1). It is estimated that there are millions of cases of foodborne illness and thousands of deaths related to this illness each year in the United States, where infections caused by foodborne organisms are second in prevalence to respiratory infections.

Diminished gastrointestinal motility results in delayed gastric and colonic emptying, which prolongs contact between infectious pathogens and the gastrointestinal mucosa. The increased vascularity of mucosal surfaces and increased cardiac output contribute to rapid incorporation and dissemination of toxins and pathogens. Liberal antacid therapy for gastroesophageal reflux neutralizes an important host defense against ingested microbes. Decreased peristaltic action of the gallbladder can facilitate ascending colonization and infection of the biliary duct system by bile tolerant organisms, such as *Salmonella* species.

Except for listeriosis, infections by tissue-invasive parasites, and enteric fever caused by *Salmonella* species, infections caused by foodborne organisms lead to acute syndromes characterized by altered gastrointestinal motility: nausea, vomiting, and diarrhea. Maternal dehydration and electrolyte imbalance are important consequences and require careful oral or parenteral fluid and electrolyte resuscitation and maintenance. Diarrhea is a protective and restorative response, and antispasmodics may prolong the carriage of some intestinal pathogens so they are not recommended.

Infectious Diarrhea

Campylobacter species are now the most common culture-proven cause of dysenteric diarrhea in North America. *Campylobacter* species infections are a recognized cause of transplacental infection, with septic abortion and still-birth, in both animals and humans (2, 3). Neonatal infection can occur when delivery proceeds during active maternal gastrointestinal infection with soiling of the perineum by *Campylobacter*-contaminated feces (4). Gastroenteritis caused by *Campylobacter jejuni* may be an antecedent to the Guillain-Barré syndrome (5). Pregnancy does not seem to affect risk for postinfection complications. Treatment consists of azithromycin or erythromycin. Experience is insufficient to allow the statement that treatment of the mother reduces risk for transplacental infection. However, because of the postinfection risks, treatment during pregnancy is recommended.

Shigella dysenteriae and *Escherichia coli* 0157:H7 are toxin-producing organisms that cause dysentery and serious acute systemic complications, including the hemolytic-uremic syndrome and disseminated intravascular coagulopathy (1, 6, 7). In some survivors, postinfection arthropathy can develop. Both *S. dysenteriae* and *E. coli* 0157:H7 are virulent, highly infectious organisms: Ingestion of as few as 200 viable cells can initiate infection (7).

Trimethoprim–sulfamethoxazole is the usual antibiotic recommended, but the prevalence of resistant strains is increasing. Infection with less-virulent species is usually self-limited, and rehydration is the only important therapy. However, the severity of complications from Shiga toxin–producing organisms requires prompt and vigorous supportive treatment.

Certain *Salmonella* (8) and *Vibrio* (9) species are common causes of systemic infection with substantial morbidity and mortality rates. Fortunately, transplacental infection and fetotoxicity are rare, perhaps because older patients with serious comorbid conditions, such as alcohol-related liver disease, are the most susceptible and the most common victims.

Enteric Fever

Enteric fever (8) is caused by several invasive *Salmonella* species: *S. typhi*, *S. paratyphi A* and *B*, *S. typhimurium*, and *S. choleraesuis*. Ascending infection through the biliary tree and invasion of mesenteric lymphatics are important in the pathogenesis of enteric fever and in establishment of the chronic carrier state. Pregnancy, because of changes in gallbladder function and an increased incidence of gallstones and gallbladder sludge, is a risk factor for chronic carriage of enteric fever *Salmonella* organisms. Travel to areas where *Salmonella* infection is endemic—southern Asia, portions of Central and South America, and Africa—is a risk factor that is often neglected in medical history taking of pregnant women.

Enteric fever poses a particular problem for the care of pregnant patients because, worldwide, multiple antibiotic resistance among *Salmonella* organisms has become common.

Vibrio Septicemic Disease

Vibrio vulnificus is a vicious tissue toxin producer that is probably the most common cause of serious illness from *Vibrio* species in the United States (9). Mild gastroenteritis among otherwise healthy eaters of raw shellfish is common. Raw oysters are the most common source of the infection, but crabs, crayfish, and shrimp have also been implicated.

Treatment is directed at the bacteremia and the local wound infection. The choice of antibiotics is limited: semisynthetic tetracyclines, quinolones, and cephalosporins. A pregnant patient with septicemic *V. vulnificus* infection deserves uninhibited antibiotic treatment and intense topical therapy of the metastatic cutaneous infection.

Listeria monocytogenes

The foodborne, gram-positive bacillus *Listeria monocytogenes* poses particular risks for pregnant women and their newborns (10, 11). Pregnant women are prone to bacteremic infection with proliferation of the organism in the placenta and in the fetus after transplacental infection of the fetus (12, 13). Premature labor is common with maternal listeriosis, and 22% of perinatal *Listeria* species infections result in intrauterine or neonatal death. Intrauterine infection can cause spontaneous abortion, IUFD and neonatal death from the disseminated listerial infection, and granulomatosis infantisepticum, characterized by microabscesses and granulomas, especially in the liver and spleen (12, 13). More commonly, neonatal *Listeria* infection after transplacental transmission presents as an early-onset sepsis syndrome. Neonatal infection acquired during delivery through a colonized birth canal is most often a late postpartum meningitis.

Pregnant women account for almost two thirds of cases of *L. monocytogenes* infection in persons 10 to 40 years of age. Twenty-seven percent of all cases occur in pregnant women (13). The vast majority of cases, excluding cases of perinatal infection, occur in patients receiving corticosteroids, transplant rejection therapy, chemotherapy, or retroviral therapy for AIDS. In nonpregnant patients, the organism has tropism for brain tissue and most often produces meningitis and meningoencephalitis (13). *Listeria monocytogenes* is the fifth most common pathogen causing meningitis, after *H. influenzae*, *S. pneumoniae*, *N. meningitides*, and group G streptococci. Meningitis caused by *L. monocytogenes* has the highest mortality rate of all types of meningitis. For unknown reasons (perhaps because of greater affinity of the organism for the placenta), listerial CNS infection is rare in pregnancy.

Listeria monocytogenes has been found in most foods: raw vegetables, unpasteurized dairy products, poultry, meat, and fish. The potential for exposure is high among pregnant women. The relative benignity of the often nondescript acute febrile illness in gravid women is particularly ominous because the correct diagnosis is so easily missed, even when the fetus is compromised. Early diagnosis and antibiotic treatment of the mother can result in the birth of a healthy infant, but the clinician must be alert to the possibility of listerial infection. Persistent fever can occur when the infected fetoplacental unit acts as a focus of continuing infection, even in the face of antibiotic treatment. Rarely, in these circumstances, delivery of the fetus and placenta are necessary to cure the mother.

For any febrile illness during pregnancy, the clinician should inquire about diet and the existence of other cases of febrile gastroenteritis or unexplained flu-like illnesses. Febrile gastroenteritis in a pregnant patient warrants blood and stool cultures for *L. monocytogenes* and other bacteria, such as *Salmonella*, *Shigella*, and *Campylobacter* species.

Listeria organisms are susceptible to penicillin and amoxicillin. Amoxicillin is the preferred penicillin. Trimethoprim–sulfamethoxazole is an effective second choice. However, only the penicillins are likely to produce intrauterine and fetal levels high enough to be relatively effective in treating or protecting the fetus from infection.

Foodborne Parasites (Protozoa)

Entamoeba histolytica is not known to cause intrauterine and fetal infection. However, evidence suggests that invasive amebiasis during pregnancy may adversely affect the fetus and successful completion of the pregnancy (14). Amebic dysentery and colitis, especially when accompanied by subserosal infection or localized bowel perforation, may produce pelvic peritoneal scarring and adhesions that may adversely affect fertility or predispose to ectopic pregnancy.

Neonates are at risk for acquiring the organisms by ingesting cysts on maternal skin or in contaminated food. Amebic infections in children younger than 6 months of age are not common; this suggests that some protective factors, possibly passively transferred maternal antibodies or secretory antibodies in breastmilk, are present (15).

Optimal management during pregnancy includes early diagnosis and treatment. If the risk for reinfection can be minimized, luminal amebiasis in pregnant patients can be treated with paromomycin. Paromomycin is a poorly absorbed aminoglycoside antibiotic that is active against luminal amebae and against the gut flora that are necessary for persistence of *E. histolytica*; its dosage is 500 mg three times daily for 7 to 10 days. Other luminally active drugs, diiodohydroxyquin and diloxanide furoate, have been used successfully during pregnancy, but neither is recommended as a first-choice agent for amebiasis in pregnant patients.

The pregnant patient with amebic dysentery, fever, and constitutional symptoms should receive at least two drugs: one active against trophozoites in the lumen and superficial mucosa and one active against the trophozoites that invade the deeper layers of the colon and (possibly) other viscera. The luminal agent can be paromomycin, diloxanide furoate, or diiodohydroxyquin. Metronidazole or another nitroimidazole should be the tissue-active or extraluminal drug. Chloroquine phosphate 1 g/d for 2 days and then 0.5 g/d for 2 to 3 weeks can be used instead of metronidazole.

Giardiasis

Giardia lamblia, also called *Giardia duodenalis* or *Giardia intestinalis*, is the *Giardia* species that infects humans (16, 17). Infection of the proximal small intestine by *G. lamblia* produces illness that ranges from an absence of symptoms to severe diarrhea with malabsorption and weight loss. The cysts may be spread in water, in food, and by direct contact. The risk for infection is directly proportional to the duration of exposure and the number of cysts ingested (18).

In the United States, *G. lamblia* is the most commonly detected intestinal parasite; it is seen in 3% to 9% of stool specimens sent for parasitologic examination (19). Infection of pregnant women with *G. lamblia* is therefore not uncommon. However, serious clinical illness among pregnant women with *G. lamblia* infection has heretofore been diagnosed only rarely. In the United States, acquisition of *G. lamblia* during travel or trekking is less common than transmission of these organisms within the household. For the obstetric clinician, this means that giardiasis should be ruled out in the evaluation of diarrheal syndromes in mothers of young children. Moreover, if the diagnosis is documented, the mother should be advised to inform her child's pediatrician.

Giardiasis has not been shown to be injurious to pregnancy beyond having an adverse nutritional and constitutional effect on the mother (20). A heavy parasite burden may compete for essential micronutrients, such as vitamin A, folic acid, and vitamin B_{12}, and may interfere with digestion and absorption of disaccharides, essential fatty acids, fat-soluble vitamins, and amino acids. Continuing severe acute disease with weight loss, malabsorption, ketosis, and fluid and electrolyte imbalance necessitates vigorous supportive therapy and antiparasitic chemotherapy during pregnancy.

Subacute or chronic disease may plague the pregnant patient with recurrent bouts of vague gastrointestinal distress and lassitude that may be attributed to morning sickness or may be considered psychosomatic. Recurrent nausea and vomiting with weight loss and ketosis may be mistakenly attributed to hyperemesis gravidarum. Chronic infection may prevent adequate weight gain, amplifying iron and folic acid needs and enhancing the appearance of anemia.

Metronidazole or another nitroimidazole is the treatment of choice (16, 18, 21). Metronidazole has been used widely and safely during pregnancy (16, 20). A single dose of oral metronidazole 2 g eradicated symptomatic giardiasis in a small, uncontrolled trial of Laotian and Cambodian refugees in two refugee camps in Thailand (22).

Clinical reports since the early 1960s indicate that paromomycin is effective against both *E. histolytica* and *G. lamblia* as well as against tapeworms and a wide array of anaerobic and aerobic bacteria. Paromomycin is poorly absorbed. Early studies showed no antibacterial activity in the plasma of patients receiving 2 g/d for as long as 50 days. Paromomycin should be the first drug selected to treat the pregnant patient with giardiasis.

Cryptosporidiosis

Cryptosporidium are highly infectious and are a common cause of diarrhea worldwide (23, 24). Clinical illness is most prominent in debilitated and immunocompromised patients, but infection occurs in normal persons during waterborne outbreaks and in young children residing in areas with poor sanitation and water supplies. Infection among family members and health care workers caring for clinically ill patients is common.

Pregnancy by itself has not yet been identified as an immunologic risk factor for progressive or severe cryptosporidiosis. No excess morbidity among pregnant women has been reported from studies of large waterborne outbreaks of cryptosporidiosis.

The presence of a woman with cryptosporidiosis in the labor and delivery suite or in the antepartum or postpartum inpatient units requires the use of procedures to protect staff, patients, and newborns.

Cyclosporidiosis

Cyclospora causing diarrhea in adventure travelers have alerted the medical community to another "new" enteric pathogen (25). Widespread outbreaks of cyclosporidiosis from contaminated raspberries in 1997 brought cyclospora to public attention. The clinical course of cyclosporal diarrheal disease in normal hosts can be much longer than that seen with cryptosporidial or isosporal infection. Like *Isospora* organisms, *Cyclospora* organisms respond to trimethoprim–sulfamethoxazole. Treatment of pregnant patients with supplemental folic acid may become desirable if the patient has a prolonged illness.

Toxoplasmosis

Epidemiology

Toxoplasma gondii is a global zoonotic parasite of felines. All cat species may be infected, and the domestic cat is the greatest source of human infection.

The importance of toxoplasmosis to obstetricians resides in the ability of *T. gondii* to produce parasitemia and transplacental intrauterine infection while causing clinically vague or silent infection in the mother (26, 27). The incidence of congenital toxoplasmosis is approximately 1 in 1000 live births in the United States (27).

Clinical Course

Infection with *T. gondii* is common; clinical disease is uncommon (26–28). The manifestations of *T. gondii* infection are determined by the size of the inoculum, by the immune status of the host, and possibly by differences in virulence among strains of *Toxoplasma* (28, 29). The most severe acute disease occurs in immunocompromised or immunoimmature hosts, such as patients with AIDS, patients with cancer, transplant recipients, and fetuses.

Primary infection is almost always accompanied by parasitemia. The most common clinical illness is febrile lymphadenopathy, which may be accompanied by atypical lymphocytosis, splenomegaly, and skin rash. The adenopathy may be localized or generalized and, characteristically, the posterior cervical chain is involved. The lymph nodes are not usually tender and do not suppurate. As the acute illness subsides over several weeks or months, host responses confine the parasite to tissue cysts.

Transplacental infection is possible only when the mother has circulating tachyzoites. The risk for intrauterine fetal infection is greatest in nonimmune mothers with primary infection, which may last for several months without treatment (30), and occasionally in chronically infected immune-incompetent mothers with reactivation.

Evidence suggests that some chronically infected mothers have foci of *Toxoplasma* in the uterus. Whether this can result in congenital infection of the fetus or in abortion is not clear. No conclusive evidence from animal or human studies shows that *Toxoplasma* organisms can cause abortion in chronically infected immunocompetent women.

Reactivation of latent infection requires serious disruption of immune function. Pregnancy by itself is not known to reactivate latent *Toxoplasma* infection. Chronically infected pregnant women with AIDS have an increased risk for transmitting *T. gondii* to the fetus. As of 1994, all infants of HIV-infected mothers reported to have congenital toxoplasmosis have also had HIV infection (27).

The French Toxoplasmosis Research Group (31–36) has followed pregnant women who acquired toxoplasmosis before and during pregnancy. Women infected before conception had no evidence of abortion, stillbirth, or congenital infection caused by *Toxoplasma* species. Of the offspring of 542 women who acquired toxoplasmosis during pregnancy, 61% had evidence of congenital infection (32). Six percent had perinatal death, 5% had severe clinical disease,

9% had mild clinical disease, and 41% had subclinical disease. Abortion, stillbirth, or severe congenital infection occurred almost exclusively when women acquired primary infection early in pregnancy.

As with other intrauterine infections, the risk of *Toxoplasma* infection for the fetus and the severity of the disease produced are related to the time during pregnancy at which maternal and transplacental infection occur. The differences in severity of clinical disease depend on the immune capacity of the fetus at the time when fetal parasitemia occurs. If the mother is infected early in pregnancy, transmission to the fetus is uncommon. However, survivors of intrauterine infection acquired early in pregnancy have the most severe residual effects of congenital infection: cerebral calcifications, hydrocephaly or microcephaly, abnormal CSF, chorioretinitis, seizures, fever, hepatosplenomegaly, and jaundice. Fetal infection is most common when maternal infection is acquired in the last trimester, but the illness in the child is more likely to be subclinical (32). Two thirds of congenitally infected infants have no symptoms, and the infection is recognized only by use of serologic tests (27, 32). About 10% of congenitally infected newborns with toxoplasmosis have signs and symptoms of complications of their transplacentally acquired disease. The most common finding in the overtly infected neonate is chorioretinitis. The manifestations of toxoplasmosis in the newborn can mimic infection by almost any pathogen producing intrauterine disease, especially syphilis, cytomegalovirus infection, and rubella.

Diagnostic Tests

The obstetrician must determine whether the infection is recent and acute (and therefore a hazard for the fetus) or old and quiescent. Various new diagnostic techniques have been developed that supplement standard serologic tests and have a special place in obstetric practice (26–28).

Isolation of the organism from blood or body fluids by animal inoculation establishes acute infection. *Toxoplasma* DNA has been detected with PCR amplification in serum, amniotic fluid, and tissue during acute toxoplasmosis. The PCR assays have emerged as the best method for confirming toxoplasmosis.

Serologic tests for specific antibodies have been the standard diagnostic method. Various serologic tests have been developed, but only a few are clinically available and all require recognition of vagaries and variations in sensitivity and reliability (26–28). Anti-*Toxoplasma* IgG may persist in titers of 1:16 to 1:256 for the lifetime of an infected person. Levels of IgM usually begin to decline several months after resolution of the acute infection. A single measurement of anti-*Toxoplasma* IgG does not confirm the diagnosis (37). The absence of IgM *Toxoplasma* antibody probably excludes the diagnosis of acute toxoplasmosis in an immunologically healthy patient. An increasing IgM fluorescent antibody titer or a titer of 1:512 or more seems to correlate well with recent onset of infection. Rheumatoid factors and antinuclear antibodies may cause false-positive indirect immunofluorescence test results for IgM.

Physicians can give practical advice that helps pregnant patients avoid toxoplasmosis: to cook meats thoroughly; to avoid handling raw meat; to avoid touching mucous membranes or eyes if handling raw meat; to keep utensils and cooking areas scrupulously clean, especially after processing raw meat; to use gloves when gardening or cleaning; and to avoid travel to areas where toxoplasmosis is endemic.

Management

The clinician has three questions to answer for each pregnant patient: Is the patient susceptible and not infected? Does the patient have a chronic latent infection? Does the patient have a recent, active infection that may be hazardous to the fetus? The initial screening tests for pregnant women should include tests for IgG and IgM. Negative test results identify a noninfected but susceptible woman who needs 1) instruction about prevention and follow-up and 2) serial screening to identify seroconversion. Diagnosis begins with serologic tests for IgG and IgM. The IFA tests are widely used for screening, and a positive result requires repeated examination with both IFA and enzyme-linked immunosorbent assay (ELISA). The absence of IgM with stable titers of IgG indicates chronic infection preceding conception with little or no risk for intrauterine infection. Anti-*Toxoplasma* IgM can persist for more than a year after acute infection, so when IgM is present further testing with ELISA-IgA and ELISA-IgE on two samples 2 weeks apart can help exclude acute infection.

When recent or active infection is documented, the patient and her physicians have three options. First, if infection occurs early in pregnancy and obstetric and ethical circumstances permit, the patient may elect to terminate the pregnancy. Second, careful evaluation of the fetus, including amniocentesis and chordocentesis and use of PCR techniques, can be done (38, 39). If the fetus is thriving and no evidence of infection is found, therapy can be withheld. If fetal infection is shown, therapy or termination is indicated (26, 33–35, 39). The third option is to treat presumptively with or without attempts to document fetal infection. Current technology allows for a reasonably safe assessment of the fetus for active infection and for sequential sonographic evaluation of the fetus at risk. Antibiotic options for toxoplasmosis have expanded so that inaction or blind maternal therapy are no longer satisfactory alternatives (36).

The antibiotic spiramycin has been widely used in Europe and has reduced risk for fetal infection by as much as 60% (27). Spiramycin reaches high concentrations in the placenta and has not been proven to be teratogenic in humans. The standard dosage of spiramycin is 3 g/d. The treatment can be given in an interrupted course (3 weeks of therapy alternating with 2 weeks of no therapy) and can be given continuously until delivery. Some centers have added pyrimethamine and a sulfonamide or trimethoprim–sulfamethoxazole and folinic acid supplements when fetal infection has been proven. Clindamycin and azithromycin are also effective in combination with pyrimethamine.

Epidemiology and Prevention

The prevalence of antibodies to *Toxoplasma* species in pregnant women ranges from 85% in Paris to 12.5% in Oslo. In New York, London, and Finland, 22% to 32% of pregnant women have positive results on serologic tests for *Toxoplasma* organisms (22, 40). In the United States, the prevalence of toxoplasmosis ranges from 20% to 70%, depending on the area of the country and style of living (especially with respect to the keeping of pets). The frequency of positive serologic test results increases with age, regardless of sex. In one national survey (40), 38% of women of childbearing age had antibodies to *Toxoplasma* species. Practitioners can expect that 50% to 60% of their female patients who reach childbearing status may be susceptible to primary *Toxoplasma* infection. Serologic examination to identify subclinical infection in women of reproductive age in an exposed group is of value (41).

Preconception toxoplasmosis testing and counseling are useful components of routine health care for childbearing women. A nonpregnant woman found to have antibody to *Toxoplasma* can be reassured that intrauterine fetal infection is rare and is unlikely to occur if she does conceive. A woman found to be susceptible should be advised to avoid cats, cat litter, and uncooked meat and should be urged to have repeated serologic tests done during pregnancy if she is at risk (42). All physicians have an obligation to alert women to the risks of toxoplasmosis (just as they have an obligation to alert them to the risks of rubella) and to pursue the epidemiologic detection of cases. The purpose of preconception and prenatal screening of susceptible women is to reduce risk for acute maternal infection with the attendant risk for congenital infection and to identify the acutely infected mother early enough to allow a choice of acceptable management options.

In the United States, the losses and costs resulting from caring for persons with congenital toxoplasmosis have been estimated to be as high as 8.8 billion dollars per year (using a prevalence of 1 case in 1000 live births) (22). These figures were derived by calculating the medical costs for newborn care and disabilities (mental retardation, visual loss, and hearing loss), costs for special education and residential care, and loss of income. Projections from countries other than the United States have shown that routine perinatal screening and antenatal testing of susceptible mothers is cost effective (27).

Infections with Foodborne Intestinal Nematodes

Infection by foodborne intestinal nematodes is rare in pregnant women (43). Enterobiasis and trichinosis are discussed below.

Enterobiasis
The major clinical manifestation of pinworm infection is itching: pruritus ani and pruritus vulvae. Migrant female worms may ascend the vagina to the pelvic peritoneum, producing vaginitis and (rarely) acute granulomatous pelvic inflammatory disease. Pregnancy may increase symptoms of vaginitis and pruritus vulvae but does not exacerbate pinworm infestation.

Trichinosis
Intrauterine trichinosis in humans has been reported, as has intrauterine trichinosis in experimental animals (44). Rare instances of abortion, premature labor, and stillbirth have been recorded. No evidence suggests that pregnancy exacerbates the acute disease or the chronic stage of larval cyst carriage.

Treatment includes supportive care and, when severe illness occurs, corticosteroids. There is no reason to withhold albendazole during pregnancy complicated by trichinosis with CNS involvement, myocarditis, or evidence of placental or transplacental infection.

Infection with Cestodes (Tapeworms, Cysticercosis, and Hydatid Cysts)

Infection with Adult Tapeworms
Human tapeworm infection follows ingestion of raw or undercooked meat that contains the larvae of *Taenia saginata* (the beef tapeworm), *Taenia solium* (the pork tapeworm), or *Diphyllobothrium latum* (the fish tapeworm) (45–47). Treatment can be niclosamide, paromomycin, or albendazole. However, unless the tapeworm causes serious medical or psychological problems, it is probably safest to withhold specific treatment until after delivery. The pregnant woman with *D. latum* infection should receive vitamin B_{12}, folic acid, and other vitamins and minerals. The tapeworm has high concentrations of folic acid and vitamin B_{12}, and competition for these essential nutrients may produce megaloblastic anemia.

Infection with Larval Tapeworms
Ingestion of *T. solium* eggs can be followed by the development of larvae that invade and encyst in muscles, heart, eyes, and brain. Uteroplacental cysticerci are very rare. Symptoms of a mass lesion or seizures may follow cerebral invasion with cysticerci, which can be fatal. Treatment with praziquantel can kill the cysticerci, but patients should be hospitalized because reactive edema is common. Careful monitoring with magnetic resonance imaging and doses of systemic corticosteroids are usually required.

Hydatid Cysts

Humans may serve as an abnormal intermediate host for the larvae of the carnivore tapeworm, *Taenia echinococcus*. In humans, the larvae form large cysts (hydatid cysts), most often in the liver. Echinocccal cysts of the pelvic organs may rupture during pregnancy or labor with the risk for anaphylaxis and peritoneal dissemination of daughter cysts. Pelvic cysts may impair fertility and impede labor and delivery (48). During pregnancy, albendazole may kill the cysticerci and daughter cysts but should be used only for anatomically precarious lesions.

Environmental Infections and Intoxications

A recent report describing hospitalizations during pregnancy in the United States in 1991 and 1992 found that infections, parasitic diseases, injuries, and poisonings accounted for 0.4 hospitalizations per 100 deliveries, or about 1 hospitalization for every 250 deliveries (49).

Table 13-8 lists infections acquired by direct contact with soil, water, and animals and their effects on pregnancy.

Infections from Pet Bites

Pasteurella multocida, which is gram positive, is part of the normal oral flora of dogs and cats. In the United States, cellulitis and rapidly ascending lymphangitis with bacteremia are the most common bite-related infections. In utero infection and fetal demise are rare complications (50, 51). Treatment is with penicillin or ampicillin; cephalosporins and macrolide antibiotics are alternatives.

Establishing the diagnosis of cat-scratch fever (bartonellosis) and treating the infected mother is a principal clinical dilemma. Delay of therapy is appropriate when serologic tests document the presence of bartonellosis. However, painful lymphadenopathy should be treated with a cephalosporin and an aminoglycoside.

Rabies

Rabies is a worldwide threat that circulates among wild and domestic carnivores and omnivores (52). In North America and western Europe, wild canines (foxes and coyotes), raccoons, skunks, and bats are the principal species that pose a risk for rabies.

Postexposure management of high-risk bite wounds requires meticulous wound cleaning, human rabies immune globulin, and a rabies vaccine series. Pregnancy is not a contraindication to any of these treatments, and they are given in the same dosage and sequence used for nonpregnant patients (53).

Table 13-8 Risk to Pregnancy from Infections Acquired by Direct Contact with Soil, Water, and Animals

Disease	Organism	Source(s)	Risk to Pregnancy	Treatment
Rabies	Rhabdovirus	Bite: canine, skunk, raccoon, bat; aerosol: bat	Invariably fatal	Supportive
Cellulitis, lymphangitis	*Pasteurella multocida*	Bite: cat, dog	Bacteremia, sepsis, placental infection, abortion	Penicillin
Cat-scratch fever	*Bartonella henslae*	Cats	Maternal lymphadenopathy, CNS involvement	Doxycycline, azithromycin, rifampin
Q fever	*Coxiella burnetii*	Aerosol: sheep, cattle, dogs, humans	Placental infection, transplacental infection, maternal hepatitis, pneumonia, endocarditis	Doxycycline, rifampin, azithromycin
Psittacosis	*Chlamydia psittaci*	Aerosol: sheep, cattle, birds	Placental infection	Azithromycin, erythromycin
Brucellosis	*Brucella* species	Aerosol, contact, ingestion: sheep, cattle	Placental infection: abortion, stillbirth	Doxycycline, rifampin, aminoglycoside
Hemorrhagic fever	Arenavirus	Rodents: aerosol, direct contact with urine, feces	Renal failure, hemorrhage	Supportive
Pulmonary syndromes	Hantavirus	Rodents: aerosol, direct contact with urine, feces	Progressive pneumonia, respiratory failure	Supportive
Leptospirosis				
With jaundice	*Leptospira icterohaemorrhagiae*	Rodents: aerosol, direct contact with urine, feces	Jaundice, hemorrhagic syndrome, renal disease	Penicillin, ampicillin
Anicteric	*Leptospira interrogans*	Rodents, dogs, livestock: direct contact with urine, feces; aerosols, contaminated water	Aseptic meningitis	Penicillin, ampicillin
Hookworm	*Ancylostoma,* Nectar, *Strongyloides*	Contaminated soil with infective larvae	Heavy infection: malnutrition, anemia, hypoproteinemia	Nutrition, antihelminthic drugs, ivermectin
Schistosomiasis	*Schistosoma mansoni, S. haematobium, S. japonicum, S. mekongi*	Contact with water containing snails, intermediate hosts	Acute infection with fever, eosinophilia, neurologic symptoms	Praziquantel
Pneumocystosis	*Pneumocystis carinii*	Aerosol, contact with human carriers, ?other animal reservoirs	Progressive pneumonia	Trimethoprim sulfamethoxazole

Q Fever

Q fever, caused by the obligate intracellular rickettsia *Coxiella burnetii*, is a worldwide zoonosis well known to be a placental and transplacental pathogen in domestic animals (54). Infection in humans is usually self-limited, often asymptomatic, and rarely diagnosed. Q fever is prevalent among sheep, cattle, and poultry farmers, and infection during pregnancy is a serious risk to the fetus (54, 55).

The risk for placental infection seems to be greatest with acute infection. However, chronic low-grade infection may recrudesce during gestation with rickettsemia and placental inoculation (56). Most acute and chronic infections produce mild illness only and are frequently missed, making Q fever an unrecognized cause of prematurity, stillbirth, and abortion.

The preferred treatment is doxycycline. Active infection during pregnancy can be treated with rifampin and erythromycin or azithromycin, but clinical studies and reports on this treatment are scarce. Greater attention to Q fever as a cause of maternal illness and pregnancy loss is needed.

Other Infections of Livestock Transmissible to Humans

Brucella species are small gram-negative rods that cause undulant fever in humans and cause septic abortion and mastitis, with contamination of milk, in livestock (goats, sheep, cattle, and camels) (57, 58). Humans acquire infection through direct contact with infected tissue or by drinking unpasteurized milk. The infection can be indolent with episodes of fever, splenomegaly, and debilitation. Bacteremia and high fever are signs of increased risk for transplacental infection. The diagnosis is confirmed by serologic tests and cultures. The usual antibiotics are doxycycline and rifampin. For pregnant patients, trimethoprim–sulfamethoxazole combined with rifampin or gentamicin is preferred.

Chlamydia psittaci is a common pathogen in birds and domestic animals. The most common source of human *C. psittaci* infection (usually pneumonia) is psittacine birds, but psittacosis is a cause of placental infection and abortion in livestock. Pregnant women who assist with lambing, especially with stillbirths, have subsequently sustained abortion (59). *Chlamydia psittaci* infection can be diagnosed by serologic tests and cultures if it is suspected. During pregnancy, azithromycin or erythromycin is the antibiotic of choice.

Infections from Contact with Rodents

Rodents are a recognized reservoir for numerous human infections (60). Rodent pathogens transmitted by arthropod vectors are discussed in the section on vector-borne infections. Direct contact with excreta or with trapped or dead rodents is a source of hemorrhagic fevers (from *Arenavirus* species infection), pulmonary syndromes (from hantavirus infections), and leptospirosis.

Like all spirochetes, those that cause leptospirosis can produce transplacental infection of the fetus, resulting in abortion, stillbirth, and congenital neonatal infection (61, 62). Bacteremic disease with jaundice and bleeding is most dangerous for mother and fetus. Anicteric leptospirosis is rarely associated with transplacental infection. Icteric leptospirosis may be confused with severe preeclampsia. Early diagnosis by blood and urine culture and prompt treatment with penicillin are essential. Antibiotic treatment late in the disease course may not affect the outcome of the illness.

Pneumocystis carinii

The management of *Pneumocystis carinii* infection in pregnancy is reviewed in Section II.

Strongyloides stercoralis

Strongyloides stercoralis (63) is a tiny hookworm with a life cycle similar to that of its larger cousins. However, larval development can occur within the host's gastrointestinal tract, so autoinfection and hyperinfection are possible. Gastrointestinal hypomotility and immune compromise often predispose to the sometimes fatal hyperinfection syndrome.

Eosinophilia, urticaria, fever, malabsorption, and anemia are prominent features. Infection with *Strongyloides stercoralis* should always be treated. Thiabendazole or ivermectin can be used.

Pregnancy, because of altered gastrointestinal motility, predisposes to autoinfection. Ivermectin, not thiabendazole, is probably the best choice for treatment. A single dose of ivermectin 200 µg/kg is as effective as thiabendazole 25 mg/kg given twice or three times daily.

Venoms and Toxins from Food Poisonings, Stings, and Bites

The alterations in gait, skin surface, and gastrointestinal motility caused by pregnancy may enhance a woman's risk for both food poisoning and envenomation. In general, the largest numbers of toxin-mediated episodes result from the ingestion of food spoiled by microbial action or by the accumulation of toxins produced during growth or preparation of the food. Syndromes mediated by toxins produced by organisms multiplying in the gastrointestinal tract, such as cholera or enterotoxigenic *E. coli* infection, are discussed elsewhere in this section. Envenomation from arthropod, coelenterate, reptile, or animal bites usually evokes anxiety about exotic toxins and concerns about secondary infection.

Systemic Toxic Syndromes from Food

Serious and sometimes fatal illness follows the consumption of toxic plants and fungi and food containing the toxins produced by bacteria, dinoflagellates, and phytoplankton (Tables 13-9 and 13-10). Death is most common with the paralytic neurotoxins of botulism and shellfish poisoning and the hepatotoxins of *Amanita* mushrooms.

Ingestion of preformed toxins produces three principal syndromes: gastrointestinal distress, systemic visceral dysfunction and failure, and combined gastrointestinal and systemic symptoms. The quantity and variety of poisonous plants, fungi, arthropods, coelenterates, mollusks, and fish are enormous. The reader is referred to standard toxicology, emergency medicine, and wilderness medicine texts for greater detail and specificity (64, 65). Clinicians must keep these surprisingly frequent and important poisoning events in mind when confronted by a perplexing patient. Travel and dietary histories may need to be obtained.

Risks to pregnancy are related to 1) dehydration and electrolyte imbalance resulting from gastrointestinal dysfunction and 2) injuries produced in the organs targeted by systemic toxins. Delayed gastric emptying fosters increased absorption of preformed toxins. Liberal use of antacids or acid-reducing medication (taken to counter reflux esophagitis) may worsen the severity of the pregnant patient's intoxication. The volume-expanded state of gestation

Table 13-9 Poisoning from Bacterial Toxins

Organism	Usual Source	Incubation	Clinical Features
Staphylococcus aureus	Cream desserts, poultry, meat, salads, vegetables, fruits (melons)	2–6 h	Cramps (upper and lower abdominal pain), vomiting, and diarrhea, sometimes simultaneously; usually resolves after 12–24 h
Bacillus cereus			
Staphylococcal-type toxin	Rice, vegetables, meat	2–6 h	Vomiting, upper abdominal cramps, diarrhea
E. coli-type toxin	Rice, vegetables, meat	6–12 h	Diarrhea, lower abdominal cramps, vomiting
Clostridium species (usually *C. perfringens*)	Meat, poultry: especially smoked foods, cooked and cooled dishes	6–12 h	Diarrhea, lower abdominal cramps
Clostridium botulinum	Home canned/ preserved foodstuffs, commercial foodstuffs packed or prepared with anaerobic foci	Hours to days	Diplopia, dysphonia, blurred vision, dysarthria, ataxia, symmetric flaccid paralysis, respiratory muscle weakness

Table 13-10 Seafood Intoxications

Name	Toxic Substance	Origin	Food Source	Symptoms Onset	Clinical Syndromes	Risk to Fetus and Neonate
Ciguatera poisoning	Ciguatoxins: heat, cold, acid stable	Toxins produced by dinoflagellate *Gambierdiscus toxicus*, accumulates in herbivorous fish without metabolic degradation, increasing content in carnivorous fish	Tropical coral reef fish: barracuda, grouper, red snapper	1–6 h	Abdominal cramps, pain, diarrhea, vomiting, paresthesia, hot-cold sensory reversal, myalgia, weakness, tachycardia, labile blood pressure; alcohol may exacerbate symptoms; may persist up to 6–8 wk	Ciguatoxins are found in breast milk
Scombroid fish poisoning	Histamine: heat, cold, acid stable	Bacterial putrefaction of dark or red-fleshed fish produces large amounts of histamine; imparts a metallic or peppery taste	Tuna, mackerel, bonito, mahi-mahi, bluefish, skipjack, yellowtail	Minutes to hours, usually less than 60 min	Severe headache, itching, flushing, urticaria, wheezing, vomiting, nausea, vertigo, light-headedness, abdominal cramps, diarrhea; usually resolves in 8–12 h without treatment	Transient fetal distress
Paralytic shellfish poisoning	Saxitoxin and other dinoflagellate toxins: water soluble, heat and acid stable	Species of dinoflagellates (*Protogonylaux, Ptychodiscus,* and *Gymnodinum*) produce saxitoxin and other neurotoxins during a "bloom"; the organism and toxins are ingested and concentrated in filter feed bivalves	Bivalve shellfish: clams, oysters, mussels, scallops	Usually within minutes, up to 3 h	Paresthesia, vomiting, diarrhea, dysphonia, dysphagia, ataxia, progressing to respiratory failure and death; survival for 12 h usually a good prognosis	Transient fetal distress, absent movement
Amnesic shellfish poisoning	Domoic acid: heat stable, water soluble	Produced by phytoplankton, *Nitzschia* species, during a bloom; the organism and toxin are ingested by filter feed bivalves and some crabs	Bivalve shellfish: mussels, clams, crab	Minutes, up to 24–30 h	Vomiting, diarrhea, headache, seizures, coma, paralysis, arrhythmia, permanent loss of short-term memory	Not known
Tetrodotoxin fish poisoning	Tetrodotoxins: acid stable, water soluble	Toxin produced by commensal bacteria/fish accumulate in skin and liver; only small amounts in muscle	Pufferfish, globefish (fugu)	Minutes, up to 4 h	Paresthesia: perioral initially, then generalized progressing to dysphonia and dysphagia, ataxia, hypotension, weakness, respiratory paralysis, and death; occasional DIC; survival past 24 h is good prognostic sign	Fetal paralysis

requires vigorous restoration of fluid and electrolyte losses resulting from diarrhea and emesis. Maternal acidosis and hypotension are serious threats to fetal well-being. Unfortunately, we have little information on the fetal effects of many toxins and venoms. Monitoring of fetal status is an integral component of caring for the acutely intoxicated woman.

Arthropod Stings and Bites

Hymenoptera Stings

Stings by hymenopteran insects are common. The annual incidence is as high as 10% in adults, and incidence peaks in late summer and early autumn. A history of systemic reaction is seen in as many as 4% of adults, and 40% to 60% of these patients can be expected to have repeated systemic reactions.

Bees, wasps, hornets, yellow jackets, and fire ants are stingers. Yellow jackets are particularly pernicious and are the most common offending creature. Local inflammation at the site of the sting occurs with all hymenopteran stings, but the inoculum and the potency of the venom vary, producing lesions that range from minor erythema to large, painful, indurated erythematous lesions with local bruising. Topical ice and corticosteroid creams may suffice. Oral antihistamines and nonsteroidal anti-inflammatory agents are welcome for relief of localized pain, pruritus, and induration.

Multiple stings (hornets and yellow jackets, unlike honeybees, can sting more than once) can produce systemic intoxication. Nausea, vomiting, diarrhea, hypotension, syncope, muscle cramps, and seizures usually resolve within 48 hours. However, occasional deaths occur, especially in small children and petite adults. Urticaria, wheezing, and cough may persist for days. Systemically envenomed patients should be admitted for observation, intravenous fluids, and parenteral antihistamines or corticosteroids if needed.

Rapid-onset anaphylactic shock can occur with any hymenopteran sting in a sensitized patient. Management of anaphylaxis during pregnancy requires prompt and repetitive administration of epinephrine (66). Pregnant patients known to be allergic to hymenopteran stings should carry and use epinephrine kits and should be reassured that prompt self-administration of epinephrine is the proper and safe response to a sting. They should seek medical attention immediately, and treatment with intravenous fluids, antihistamines, and corticosteroids should be started if necessary. Continuous fetal monitoring should be implemented.

Venom immunotherapy is almost 100% effective in reducing anaphylactic reactions in patients with established hypersensitivity. There is minimal risk (5%) for inducing a systemic allergic response that requires epinephrine at the onset of immunotherapy. Pregnancy is not a contraindication for starting or continuing venom immunotherapy, but patients receiving immunotherapy must continue to carry and, if necessary, use their epinephrine kits.

Serum sickness, with headache, lymphadenopathy, arthralgias, urticaria, and low-grade fever, is a late systemic reaction that begins 10 to 14 days after the sting. Antihistamines and nonsteroidal anti-inflammatory agents give symptomatic relief. Corticosteroids may be necessary for severe cases. Venom immunotherapy reduces the risks and severity of the serum sickness syndrome.

Antivenin prepared in animals (and therefore carrying risk for serum sickness and anaphylaxis) is available from the Antivenin Production Laboratory at Arizona State University. It should be used to supplement supportive care for patients with grade 3 or 4 envenomation.

Spider Bites

Spiders are venomous arachnids, and almost all species have venom-producing glands. Although most spiders are poisonous, very few cause harm to human beings: Only *Lactrodectus* and *Loxosceles* species regularly cause serious human illness (67, 68).

The black widow spider, *Lactrodectus mactans*, is the perpetrator of all reported cases of spider bite poisoning in pregnancy. Its venom is neurotoxic and causes generalized muscle cramps with pain and weakness, abdominal cramps progressing to rigidity, and trismus (69). Sympathetic disarray can produce flushing, salivation, and hypotension. Pregnant patients may feel as if they are in labor, although premature labor has not occurred in reported cases (70). The pregnant woman having a severe reaction to a black widow spider bite should be hospitalized and should have uterine and fetal monitoring (70). Antivenin can be used if respiratory arrest, hypertension, or seizures occur. Some experts recommend the use of antivenin because the maternal mortality rate has been as high as 5% among reported cases of spider bite poisoning in pregnancy. Considering the worldwide distribution of black widow spiders and the paucity of reported cases of spider bite poisoning in pregnant women, it seems reasonable to conclude that *Lactrodectus* venom does not interfere with gestation and that pregnancy does not enhance the toxicity of *Lactrodectus* venom.

Marine Envenomation

Cardiac arrest in pregnant patients who are stung by marine organisms and are slow to leave the water has resulted in deaths (71). Rinsing the area of the sting with seawater and applying ice packs may reduce continued firing of residual nematocysts. Vinegar inactivates nematocyst venom and should be poured liberally on the affected area.

Pregnant patients usually wear bathing suits that cover their torsos, and they are particularly susceptible to sea bather's eruption. The free-swimming microscopic larvae of several coelenterates ("sea lice") contain nematocysts and become trapped between the bathing suit fabric and the skin. Within an hour or two, the patient develops a bathing suit–distribution rash of pruritic, stinging, erythematous wheals that can persist for up to 2 weeks. Extensive contact occasionally produces systemic symptoms or anaphylaxis. Topical therapy is usually all that is needed.

Snake Bites

Snake bites during pregnancy are rare; only 62 cases are described in the literature (70, 72). The venomous snakes native to North America are pit vipers (*Crotalidae* species) and coral snakes (*Elapidae* species), and serious envenomation during pregnancy is rare. Around the world, bites by cobras, kraits, mambas, vipers, and sea snakes have caused maternal death and abortion.

Vector-Transmitted Infections

One feature of the "emerging infections" crisis of the 1990s is a reawakened respect for and interest in infections caused by organisms transmitted by arthropod vectors (73). The control of yellow fever, a triumph of medicine and public health a century ago, has allowed the emergence of complacency about mosquitoes, ticks, and other biting bugs. Lyme disease and dengue are now prominent emerging diseases that may pose risks to pregnancies. Recently identified tick-borne species, *Rickettsia* and *Ehrlichia* species, pose additional threats to the pregnant woman and her fetus (74, 75).

Tick-Borne Infections

Either tick phobia has intensified over the last quarter of the 20th century or infections caused by organisms transmitted by ticks have become more prevalent and better known.

Lyme Disease

All spirochetes that infect humans can cause transplacental infection. The treponeme of syphilis is the most virulent spirochete, and the example of intrauterine fetal infection and congenital syphilis has influenced professional and public concern about *Borrelia burgdorferi*, the cause of Lyme disease (76).

Inoculation of *B. burgdorferi* by an ixodid tick is followed by regional infection and systemic dissemination, which set in motion a chronic infection with a sequence of clinical manifestations not unlike the course of syphilis. Early infection is characterized by skin lesions, lymphadenopathy, and spirochetemia. Late infection is signaled by diminution of spirochetes and immunologically mediated inflammatory lesions of the skin, CNS, joints, and vasculature. The risk for transplacental infection is greatest during the more intense spirochetemia of early infection (76, 77). Most but not all patients develop the distinctive skin lesions, erythema chronicum migrans (ECM). As many as 20% to 40% of infected patients do not have a diagnostic clinical presentation and, because the ixodid tick is tiny, many do not recall a tick bite. Fever, fatigue, and arthralgias are common but are not diagnostic during early infection. Serologic testing using ELISA for screening and Western blot or PCR for confirmation is important in diagnosis, especially in patients without characteristic skin lesions.

Despite considerable anxiety, transplacental fetal infection by *B. burgdorferi* is rare. Several documented congenital and placental infections have been reported, but careful seroepidemiologic studies in high-prevalence areas have found very low rates of congenital infection and congenital anomalies (78–80). The risk for silent maternal Lyme disease with transplacental infection of the fetus is minimal. No evidence indicates a benefit of routine serologic screening during pregnancy.

On the other hand, when a pregnant woman develops Lyme disease, antibiotic treatment is indicated. It is in untreated mothers with active borreliosis that placental and fetal infection have developed. Only one case of congenital infection in an infant born to a mother inadequately treated with oral penicillin for ECM has been reported. Treatment of Lyme disease early in pregnancy should consist of amoxicillin or ampicillin 2 to 4 g/d for 3 weeks. Erythromycin and azithromycin are suitable alternatives.

The pregnant patient who has a tick (or has had one) but no clinical or serologic evidence of *Borrelia* infection poses a clinical quandary. Identification of the tick is immensely useful in decisions about antibiotic prophylaxis, but absence of the tick makes this identification impossible. Most patients, terrified by the tick, cannot clearly document whether it was attached or whether it had taken a blood meal. Because the risk for transplacental infection with active disease is small, watchful waiting is clinically appropriate for the tick-burdened patient. Because patient distress and the risk for presumptive legal action are great, ACOG recommends prophylaxis with oral amoxicillin for 3 weeks.

The new Lyme disease vaccine is appropriate for women who live in high-risk areas. The series of three injections should be given before conception. No data are available on use of the vaccine during pregnancy.

Ehrlichiosis and Babesiosis

Ehrlichiosis and babesiosis have rarely been reported in pregnancy. The appearance of thrombocytopenia, elevated liver enzyme levels, and abnormal CNS findings can easily be labeled as severe preeclampsia. When a high fever is present, clinicians may suspect chorioamnionitis superimposed on the HELLP syndrome (*h*emolysis, *e*levated *l*iver enzyme concentrations, and *l*ow *p*latelet count). A history of tick bite and a careful examination of the peripheral blood smear, looking for schistocytes and for morulae, may help in the differential diagnosis.

Mosquito-Borne Infections

Dengue

Vertical transmission of dengue virus, both intrauterine and intrapartum, has occurred (81, 82). In three Southeast Asian cases of maternal dengue close to term, one infant developed profound transient thrombocytopenia, one infant died with respiratory distress and uncontrollable intracerebral bleeding, and one infant had anti-dengue IgM at birth but no clinical disease.

Because the incidence and the range of dengue viruses and their mosquito vectors are increasing, the chances of a pregnancy complicated by dengue are also increasing. Treatment is supportive, and no vaccine is available.

Malaria

Malaria (83) is caused by four *Plasmodium* species that are transmitted from human to human by the bites of female anopheline mosquitoes. It is characterized by relapsing fever, rigors, splenomegaly, and anemia and continues to be a worldwide health problem. It is endemic in many parts of tropical and subtropical Africa, Asia, and Central and South America, where environmental features (including temperature, humidity, bodies of water, and agriculture) support breeding of mosquito vectors and frequent contact between mosquitoes and humans.

The clinical attack causes fever, chills, and splenomegaly, and malaria in the mother can cause profound anemia; predispose to serious incurrent illness; cause intrauterine infection and placental insufficiency; and contribute to IUGR, prematurity, low birthweight, abortion, and stillbirth (84–88).

Congenital malaria may occur in the absence of clinical evidence of maternal malaria (14–16). Parasites are found in the placenta in most patients who have *P. falciparum* malaria during pregnancy (89, 90). In one study from a malaria-endemic region in West Africa (87), 40% of mothers had demonstrable parasitemia but 16% had parasites only in the placenta and not in the maternal or cord blood. The incidence of congenital malaria is about 0.3% in the infants of immune mothers residing in malarious areas, but it is 1% to 4% in the children of nonimmune mothers living in the same regions. *Plasmodium falciparum* is the most common cause of congenital malaria, and this reflects the organism's position as the most common cause of serious maternal infection and placental sequestration of infected erythrocytes.

In the neonate, congenital malaria is often evident 48 to 72 hours after birth. Parasitemia, fever, hepatosplenomegaly, jaundice, anemia, seizures, and (occasionally) pulmonary edema may occur. There may be a prolonged latent phase and clinical signs may not develop until several weeks after delivery, even though parasites are present in the placenta and cord blood. Spontaneous clearance of *P. falciparum* in congenitally infected infants may be common. Indeed, a series of recent studies from Malawi in southeast Africa suggests that once separated from the placenta, both mother and infant can spontaneously clear parasites from the peripheral blood (88, 89).

Several factors seem to explain the common finding of placental parasitization and the relative rarity of fetal or neonatal infection (86). Maternal antibody coating the merozoites may favor rapid clearance by the fetal reticuloendothelial system. Soluble malaria antigens crossing to the fetus may elicit protective IgM and cellular fetal immune responses. *Plasmodium falciparum* does not thrive in erythrocytes containing fetal hemoglobin. The nondeformable, sticky, parasitized erythrocyte may be unable to migrate through the placental circulation into the fetal circulation.

As a general rule, clinicians working in areas where malaria is endemic can expect a high proportion of pregnant women to have malaria (84). Nonimmune mothers can be expected to have severe clinical attacks, intense parasitemia, and dense parasitization of the placenta with risk for intrauterine infection and fetal death. Young primiparous women will have more severe clinical attacks and more intense placental infection than will older, multiparous women, who are more likely to have subclinical infection. Congenital infection is unusual. Women who receive prophylaxis against malaria throughout pregnancy have larger placentas, larger babies, and less anemia than untreated women (91, 92).

Management

Clinical attacks of malaria during pregnancy should be treated promptly (93, 94). Maternal *P. falciparum* infection should always be considered a lifethreatening problem.

The recommended treatment for malaria (except for drug-resistant *P. falciparum* infection) during pregnancy is chloroquine phosphate, 1 g initially, 0.5 g after 6 hours, and then 0.5 g once daily for 2 days (95, 96). Because all species that produce human malaria, except *P. falciparum*, have a prolonged exoerythrocytic phase, primaquine phosphate 26.3 mg/d orally for 14 days should be given to prevent relapse of malaria caused by *P. vivax*, *P. malariae*, and *P. ovale*. However, primaquine should be used with caution, preferably after delivery and after testing for G6PD deficiency.

Pregnant patients with drug-resistant *P. falciparum* infection should receive a regimen appropriate for the sensitivities of the strain present in the region where the patient was infected (Box 13-4) (96–99). Chloroquineresistant *P. falciparum* is now found in Southeast Asia, Africa, the northern

---

Box 13-4 Oral Chemotherapy for Multidrug-Resistant *Plasmodium falciparum* Malaria in Pregnancy

---

Africa and America

Mefloquine 1.0 g or 25 mg/kg as initial dose

  plus

Quinine PO4 600 mg PO q8h for 3–7 days

  or

Artesunate 10 mg/kg over 3 days

  or

Combination therapy may include clindamycin, sulfadoxine-pyrimethamine (Fansidar), arizthromycin

Asia

Mefloquine 25 mg/kg as single dose

  plus

Artesunate 10 mg/kg over 3 days

  or

Quinine PO4 600 mg PO q8h for 3–7 days

  or

Combination therapy including doxycycline and clindamycin

---

areas of the Amazon Basin, and some Pacific islands. Fansidar, a combination of sulfadoxine and pyrimethamine, has been used for years as an alternative for the treatment and prophylaxis of chloroquine-resistant *P. falciparum* malaria. Among Cambodian and Burmese refugees in Southeast Asia, however, strains of *P. falciparum* resistant to mefloquine, sulfadoxine, and pyrimethamine have emerged. Indeed, some cases of *P. falciparum* malaria in Southeast Asia have failed to respond to quinine and tetracycline. In these areas, treatment of *P. falciparum* malaria is a major clinical problem. Mefloquine has been used to treat multidrug-resistant *P. falciparum* malaria during pregnancy with good results and safety (93, 100, 101). Considering the desperate circumstances of a pregnant patient unfortunate enough to have acquired multidrug-resistant *P. falciparum* malaria, it is probably wisest to treat the patient in the United States with quinine or quinidine and mefloquine (Box 13-5). Liberal folic acid supplementation and meticulous attention to maternal blood sugar, blood pressure, and electrocardiograms are essential (102, 103).

Many clinical reports document the safety of older antimalarial drugs given during pregnancy for appropriate medical indications (93, 94). However, all antimalarial agents may have adverse effects on the fetus. Chloro-

---

Box 13-5 Parenteral Chemotherapy for Severe Multidrug-Resistant
Plasmodium falciparum **Malaria in Pregnancy**

Quinine IM or IV 20 mg/kg initially, then 10 mg/kg q8h for 3–7 days; monitor EKG and blood pressure

or

Quinidine IV 10 mg/kg over 2 h; 0.02 mg/kg/min thereafter for 3–7 days; monitor EKG and blood pressure

plus

Artemether (in oil; not available in USA) IM 4 mg/kg initially, then 2 mg/kg q8h

or

Mefloquine PO 25 mg/kg as single dose or divided into 2 doses 4 hrs apart

---

quine can cause retinal and cochleovestibular damage in both mother and fetus. Quinine is ototoxic and minimally oxytocic and can produce profound maternal hypoglycemia. Mefloquine can cause neurologic symptoms—even seizures, although these are rare. Primaquine causes methemoglobinemia and hemolysis in susceptible persons. Other recommended drugs, such as sulfonamides, sulfones, tetracycline, pyrimethamine, and trimethoprim, are not without potential dangers.

Chemoprophylaxis

The best prophylaxis is to avoid travel to malarious areas. Conscientious chemoprophylaxis during and after travel to such areas is mandatory if traveling cannot be postponed until after delivery. Any person traveling or residing in a malarious area should not be allowed to overlook the need to take precautions (use of insect repellent and mosquito netting) against mosquitoes. The standard chemoprophylactic regimen for sensitive *Plasmodium* species is 500 mg of chloroquine phosphate orally once a week. This regimen should be started 1 week before departure to an endemic area and should be continued for 8 weeks after departure from the area. Chloroquine alone suppresses the erythrocytic phase of infection but does not affect the liver or tissue phases. Thus, chloroquine treatment must be continued for 2 months after the patient leaves a malarious area.

Pregnancy is a contraindication to travel or residence in areas known to have drug-resistant *P. falciparum*. However, if such travel is unavoidable, it is probably best for the patient to take mefloquine 250 mg/wk. Pregnant patients residing in holoendemic areas should probably receive prophylaxis, especially if they are expatriate women without immunity. The benefit of avoiding chloroquine-resistant *P. falciparum* malaria far outweighs the problems associated with effective chemotherapy (104).

Infections Transmitted by Other Arthropod Vectors

African Trypanosomiasis

Abortions and stillbirths are reported in pregnancies complicated by infections with African trypanosomes (105, 106). The placenta can be heavily parasitized, and this can contribute to IUGR and prematurity. Maternal survival, completion of pregnancy, and delivery of a congenitally infected infant are more likely with *Trypanosoma brucei gambiense* infection. Congenital infection in the neonate presents as fever, anemia, and meningoencephalitis; lymphadenopathy is absent, and parasites may be difficult to detect in the blood. Even if trypanosomes are not found in the cord blood, they may be found in the child's CSF.

In residents of endemic areas, diagnosis may not be difficult. Clinicians must consider trypanosomiasis in the differential diagnosis of unexplained fever and lymphadenopathy in any patient who has traveled (however briefly) in an area where this infection is endemic. Examination of thick and thin blood smears of material aspirated from lymph nodes and bone marrow is standard. Serologic tests are available, but trypanosomiasis is often diagnosed by examination of the CSF. Lumbar puncture is an essential guide to therapy in the patient with documented infection.

American Trypanosomiasis

From the southwestern United States to Argentina, more than 20 million people are infected by *Trypanosoma cruzi* (107–111). This infection, also known as Chagas disease, is acquired in three ways: 1) from hematophagous reduviid insects that deposit *T. cruzi*–containing feces while biting; 2) from blood transfusion (109); and 3) through transplacental transfer of trypanomastigotes from an infected mother (110, 111). The prevalence of *T. cruzi* infection among pregnant women residing in areas where *T. cruzi* is endemic ranges from 2% to 51% in cities and from 23% to 81% in rural areas. The disease may be present in nonendemic areas because of migration. In Buenos Aires, where it is not endemic, 6% to 8% of women giving birth at public hospitals have reactive serologic tests for *T. cruzi*, and about 3% to 4% of these women bear congenitally infected infants (108).

Transplacental passage may occur at any stage of the disease. In most cases, the mother has been asymptomatic. In a Brazilian study (110), 49% of 71 chronically infected women had parasitemia on at least one occasion and 11% had positive results on xenodiagnostic tests at least three times during pregnancy. *Trypanosoma cruzi* can produce chronic placentitis with focal necrosis. Amastigotes may be found in placental macrophages.

Congenital infection is well known (108). More than 200 cases have been reported in the literature. The true incidence of congenital infection and the adverse effects of this infection on pregnancy are not known because of inadequate surveillance and reporting. In endemic areas, the estimated incidence of congenital disease in newborns weighing less than 2 kg is about 2%. It is assumed that Chagas disease contributes to IUGR, but the prevalence of serious nutritional and socioeconomic distress in the infected population makes the association difficult to document.

Clinical findings in the neonate are related to the time during pregnancy at which transplacental parasitemia occurred (111). The earlier in gestation the fetus is infected, the more likely the fetus is to have evidence of infection at birth. Hepatosplenomegaly, anemia, jaundice, meningoencephalitis, and gastrointestinal symptoms (including impaired esophageal motility) are the principal problems. Parasites may not be present in the blood or CSF, and xenodiagnosis may be required. Serologic and PCR assays using direct agglutination, indirect hemagglutination, and indirect IgM immunofluorescence may be helpful (112, 113). The prognosis is poor, even with treatment. Twenty-seven of 60 patients with documented congenital infection died, most before reaching the age of 4 months (108). It is not known whether the asymptomatic, congenitally infected infant will develop late manifestations. Transmission of the trypanosomes through breastmilk has been shown in animals. The role of this route of infection in human disease is not clear.

Nifurtimox is useful and safe for both pregnant women and congenitally infected infants. Allopurinol, benznidazole, ketoconazole, and itraconazole are options (114). A new agent, D0870 (a *bis*-triazole derivative), has produced parasitologic cures in animal studies and offers hope for more effective therapy in the future (115).

Because of the risk for congenital infection, prematurity, miscarriage, and progression to serious chronic disease, pregnant women with parasitemia and acute disease should be treated. Whether a pregnant patient with asymptomatic chronic or latent infection should be treated is not clear. The role of amniocentesis and examination of amniotic fluid for parasites in the diagnosis and management of the pregnant patient with Chagas disease has not been unexplored.

Leishmaniasis

The immunologic aberrations induced by pregnancy may predispose to disseminated leishmaniasis in immune women. Diminution in the clearance and containment of mastigotes by the reticuloendothelial system permits intrusion of the parasite into the placental and fetal circulation. Although rarely reported, intrauterine infection does occur. Visceral leishmaniasis acquired during pregnancy should be treated despite the risks of treatment. Pregnant women, especially if they are nonimmune and do not live in endemic areas, may have faster and more aggressive progression of newly acquired infection with risk for intrauterine infection of the fetus.

Pregnancy is unusual in women with established, untreated visceral leishmaniasis. Pregnant patients with untreated visceral leishmaniasis are often so ill that they cannot meet the nutritional, physiologic, and emotional demands of pregnancy. Nutritional repair of inanition and vitamin deficiencies is essential. Despite the risks, the best course is to initiate or maintain chemotherapy (this may take as long as 4 to 6 weeks) and to terminate the pregnancy if the patient's clinical condition warrants this step.

The "New World" *Leishmania* species cause more persistent and aggressive mucocutaneous disease and usually require chemotherapy with pentavalent antimony (116). Amphotericin B and ketoconazole can be used if antimonial agents are not effective. Pregnant women with new-world cutaneous leishmaniasis should be carefully observed, and treatment should be withheld during pregnancy unless there is progression of the infection with the appearance of new, distant metastasis or progressive destruction of nasopharyngeal structures. The pregnant patient with progressive mucocutaneous leishmaniasis should receive antimony. Other drugs can be tried if response is inadequate but, in this case, termination of the pregnancy to restore full immune competence and permit aggressive antimonial chemotherapy should be considered.

Fungal Infections

Increased vascularity of the skin and the tendency toward edema resulting from diminished plasma oncotic pressure and the mechanical effects of the gravid uterus predispose pregnant patients to vulvar irritation, almost always with the presence of various yeasts (*Monilia* and *Torulopsis* species). A host of topical antifungal preparations are available: Nystatin and the various imidazoles (miconazole, ketoconazole, clotrimazole, and butaconazole) have been used in all trimesters with no consistent pattern of adverse effects (see Drug Table for Unusual Infectious Diseases).

Systemic antifungal therapy may be necessary for immunodeficient women, especially those with AIDS. Amphotericin B is the only drug for which sufficient clinical experience has accumulated; no fetotoxic or teratogenic effects have been seen with this agent. Pregnancy does not affect the incidence or severity of the toxicities from amphotericin B in the mother.

The newer triazoles (ketoconazole, fluconazole, and itraconazole) have been used as systemic antifungal agents in only a few pregnant patients (117). Ketoconazole is known to inhibit gonadal and adrenal steroid synthesis. All of the triazoles (as well as griseofulvin and flucytosine) have embryotoxic and teratogenic effects in large doses in experimental animals. Until more experience has accumulated, none of these drugs should be used systemically for fungal infections during pregnancy.

Onychomycosis is a cosmetic issue, and the use of even very low doses of systemic imidazole and triazole drugs during pregnancy is not condoned. Systemic antifungal drugs should be used only for life-threatening maternal infections.

REFERENCES

1. **Tauxe RV.** Emerging foodborne diseases: an evolving public health challenge. Emerg Infect Dis. 1997;3:425-34.

2. **Eden AN.** Perinatal mortality caused by *Vibrio* fetus: review and analysis. J Pediatr. 1966;68:297-301.

3. **Gribble MJ, Salit IE, Isaac-Renton J, et al.** *Campylobacter* infection in pregnancy. Am J Obstet Gynecol. 1981;140:423-5.

4. **Vesokari T, Huttman L, Malci R.** Perinatal *Campylobacter* fetus *Jejuni* enteritis. Acta Paediatr Scand. 1981;70:261-3.

5. **Cornick NA, Gorbach SL.** *Campylobacter.* Infect Dis Clin North Am. 1988;2:643-54.

6. **Schlager TA, Guerrant RL.** Seven possible mechanisms for *Escherichia coli* diarrhea. Infect Dis Clin North Am. 1988;2:607-24.

7. **DuPont HL.** *Shigella.* Infect Dis Clin North Am. 1988;2:599-605.

8. **Goldberg MB, Rubin RH.** The spectrum of *Salmonella* infection. Infect Dis Clin North Am. 1988;2:571-98.

9. **Holmberg SD.** *Vibrio* and *Aeromonas.* Infect Dis Clin North Am. 1988;2:655-76.

10. **Seuchat A.** Listeriosis and pregnancy: food for thought. Obstet Gynecol Surv. 1997; 53:721-2.

11. **Schlech WF.** *Listeria* gastroenteritis: old syndrome, new pathogen. N Engl J Med. 1997;336:130-2.

12. **Dalton CB, Austin CC, Sobel J, et al.** An outbreak of gastroenteritis and fever due to *Listeria monocytogenes* in milk. N Engl J Med. 1997;336:100-5.

13. **Lorber B.** Listeriosis. Clin Infect Dis. 1997;24:1-11.

14. **Czeizel D, Hancsok M, Palkovich I, et al.** Possible relation between fetal death and *E. histolytica* infection of the mother. Am J Obstet Gynecol. 1966;96:264.

15. **Gillon FD, Reiner DS, Wang C.** Human milk kills parasitic intestinal protozoa. Science. 1983;221:1290.

16. **Hill DR.** Giardiasis: issues in diagnosis and management. Infect Dis Clin North Am. 1993;7:503-25.

17. **Roberts-Thomson IC.** Genetic studies of human and murine giardiasis. Clin Infect Dis. 1993;16(Suppl):98-104.

18. **Ortega YR, Adam RD.** *Giardia*: overview and update. Clin Infect Dis. 1997;25:545-50.

20. **Kreutner NK, Del Bene VE, Amstey MS.** Giardiasis in pregnancy. Am J Obstet Gynecol. 1981;140:895.

21. **Jokipii L, Jokipii AMM.** Giardiasis and balantidiasis. In: Braude AI, ed. Medical Microbiology and Infectious Diseases. Philadelphia: WB Saunders; 1981:1075.

22. **Roberts T, Murrell KD, Marks S.** Economic losses caused by foodborne parasitic diseases. Parasitol Today. 1994;10:419-23.

23. **Clark DP, Sears CL.** The pathogenesis of cryptosporidiosis. Parasitol Today. 1996;12: 221-5.

24. **Dupont HL, Chappell CL, Sterling CR, Okhuysen PC, Rose JB, Jakubowski W.** The infectivity of *Cryptosporidium parvum* in health volunteers. N Engl J Med. 1995;332: 885-859.

25. **Soave R.** *Cyclospora:* an overview. Clin Infect Dis. 1996;23:429-37.

26. **Alger LS.** Toxoplasmosis and parvovirus B19. Infect Dis Clin North Am. 1997;11:55-75.

27. **Wong S, Remington JS.** Toxoplasmosis in pregnancy. Clin Infect Dis. 1994;18:853-61.

28. **McCabe R, Chiruvgi V.** Issues in toxoplasmosis. Infect Dis Clin North Am. 1993;7:587-604.

29. **Howe DK, Sibley LD.** *Toxoplasma gondii* comprises three clonal lineages: correlation of parasite genotype with human disease. J Infect Dis. 1995;172:1561-6.

30. **Vogel N, Kirisits M, Michael E, Bach H, et al.** Congenital toxoplasmosis transmitted from an immunologically competent mother infected before conception. Clin Infect Dis. 1996;23:1055-60.

31. **Desmonts G, Couvreur J.** Congenital toxoplasmosis: a prospective study of 378 pregnancies. N Engl J Med. 1974;290:1110.

32. **Desmonts G, Couvreur J.** Congenital toxoplasmosis: a prospective study of the offspring of 542 women who acquired toxoplasmosis during pregnancy: pathophysiology of congenital disease. In: Thalhammer O, Baumgarden K, Pollak A, eds. Perinatal Medicine. Stuttgart: Georg Thieme; 1979:51.

33. **Daffos F, F. F, Capella-Pavlovsky M, et al.** Prenatal management of 746 pregnancies at risk for congenital toxoplasmosis. N Engl J Med. 1988;318:271.

34. **Desmonts G, Forestier F, Thulliez PH, et al.** Prenatal diagnosis of congenital toxoplasmosis. Lancet. 1985;1:500.

35. **Couvreur J, Desmonts G, Thulliez PH.** Prophylaxis of congenital toxoplasmosis: effects of spiramycin on placental infection. J Antimicrob Chemother. 1988;22:193.

36. **Hahlfeld P, Daffos F, Thulliez P, et al.** Fetal toxoplasmosis: outcome of pregnancy and infant follow up after in utero treatment. J Pediatr. 1989;115:765.

37. **Cotty F, Descamps P, Body G, Richard-Lenoble D.** Prenatal diagnosis of congenital toxoplasmosis: the role of *Toxoplasma* IgA antibodies in amniotic fluid. J Infect Dis. 1995;171:1384-5.

38. **Teutsch SM, Sulzer AJ, Ramsey JE, et al.** *Toxoplasma gondii* isolated from amniotic fluid. Obstet Gynecol. 1980;55:2.

39. **Hohlfeld P, Daffos F, Costa J, Thulliez P, Forestier F, Vidand M.** Prenatal diagnosis of congenital toxoplasmosis with a polymerase-chain-reaction test on amniotic fluid. N Engl J Med. 1994; 331:695-9.

40. **Sever JL.** Perinatal infections affecting the developing fetus and newborn. In: Eichenwald H, ed. The Prevention of Mental Retardation Through Control of Infectious Diseases. Washington, DC: US Gov Printing Office; 1968:37: Public Health Service Publication no. 1692.

41. **Luft BJ, Remington JS.** Acute *Toxoplasma* infection among family members of patients with acute lymphadenopathic toxoplasmosis. Arch Intern Med. 1984:144-53.

42. **Foulon W, Naessens A, Derde MD.** Evaluation of the possibilities for preventing congenital toxoplasmosis. Am J Perinatol. 1994;11:57-62.

43. **Lin LX, Weller PF.** Strongyloidiasis and other intestinal nematode infections. Infect Dis Clin North Am. 1993;7:655-82.

44. **Gould SE.** Trichinosis in Man and Animals. Springfield, IL: Charles C Thomas; 1970.

45. **Cook GC.** Taeniasis and cysticercosis. J R Soc Med. 1998;91:534-5.

46. **Botero D, Tanowitz HB, Weiss LM, Wittner M.** Taeniasis and cysticercosis. Infect Dis Clin North Am. 1993;7:683-97.

47. **Kammerer WS, Schantz PM.** Echinococcal disease. Infect Dis Clin North Am. 1993; 7:605-18.

48. **Bickers WM.** Hydatid disease of the female pelvis. Am J Obstet Gynecol. 1970;107:477.

49. **Bennett TA, Kotelchuck M, Cox CE, Tucker MJ, Nadeau DA.** Pregnancy-associated hospitalizations in the United States in 1991 and 1992: a comprehensive view of maternal morbidity. Am J Obstet Gynecol. 1998;178:346-54.

50. **Rollof J, Johansson PJ, Holst E.** Severe *Pasteurella multocida* infections in pregnant women. Scand J Infect Dis. 1992;24:453-8.

51. **Waldor M, Roberts D, Kazanjian P.** In utero infection due to *Pasteurella multocida* in the first trimester of pregnancy: case report and review. Clin Infect Dis. 1992;14:497-502.

52. **Fishbein DB.** Rabies. Infect Dis Clin North Am. 1991;5:53-72.

53. **Chutivongse S, Wilde H, Benjavongkulchai M, et al.** Post exposure rabies vaccination during pregnancy: effect on 202 women and their infants. Clin Infect Dis. 1995;20: 818-20.

54. **Raoult D, Marrie T.** Q fever. Clin Infect Dis. 1995;20:489-96.

55. **Guo HR, Gilmore R, Waag DM, Shireley L, et al.** Prevalence of *Coxiella burnetii* infections among North Dakota sheep producers. J Occup Environ Med. 1998;40:999-1006.

56. **Bental T, Fejgin M, Keysary A, Rzotkiewicz S, et al.** Chronic Q fever of pregnancy presenting in *Coxiella burnetii* placentitis: successful outcome following therapy with erythromycin and rifampin. Clin Infect Dis. 1995;21:1318-21.

57. **Figueroa DR, Rajas RL, Marcano TES.** Brucellosis in pregnancy: course and perinatal results. Ginecol Obstet Mex. 1995;63:190-5.

58. **Oscherwitz SL.** Brucellar bacteremia in pregnancy. Clin Infect Dis. 1995;21:714-5.

59. **Jorgensen DM.** Gestational psitticosis in a Montana sheep rancher. Emerg Infect Dis. 1997;3:191-4.

60. **Mills JN, Childs JE.** Ecologic studies of rodent reservoirs: their relevance for human health. Emerg Infect Dis. 1998;4:529-37.

61. **Shaked Y, Shpilberg O, Samra D, Famra Y.** Leptospirosis in pregnancy and its effect on the fetus: case report and review. Clin Infect Dis. 1993;17:241-5.

62. **Farr RW.** Leptospirosis. Clin Infect Dis. 1995;21:1-8.

63. **Liu LX, Weuer PF.** Strongyloidiasis and other intestinal nematode infections. Infect Dis Clin North Am. 1993;7:655-82.

64. **Auerbach PS.** Wilderness Medicine, 3d ed. St. Louis, MO: Mosby; 1995.

65. **Ellenhorn MJ.** Ellenhorn's Medical Toxicology, 2d ed. Baltimore: Williams & Wilkins; 1997.

66. **Schwartz HJ, Golden DB, Lockey RE.** Venom immunotherapy in the *Hymenoptera* allergic pregnant patient. J Allergy Clin Immunol. 1990;85:709-15.

67. **Boyer Hassen LV, McNally JT.** Spider bites. In: Auerbach PS, ed. Wilderness Medicine, 3d ed. St. Louis, MO: Mosby; 1995:769-86.

68. **Minton SA, Bechtel HB.** Arthropod envenomation and parasitism. In: Auerbach P, ed. Wilderness Medicine, 3d ed. St. Louis, MO: Mosby; 1995:742-68.

69. **Scalzone JM, Wells SL.** *Lactroductus mactans* (black widow spider) envenomation: an unusual cause for abdominal pain in pregnancy. Obstet Gynecol. 1994;83:830-1.

70. **Pantanowitz L, Guidozzi F.** Management of snake and spider bites in pregnancy. Obstet Gynecol Surv. 1996;51:615-20.

71. **Auerbach PS.** Marine envenomation. In: Auerbach PS, ed. Wilderness Medicine, 3d ed. St. Louis, MO: Mosby; 1995:1327-74.

72. **Dunnihoo DR, Rush BM, Wise RB, et al.** Snakebite poisoning in pregnancy. J Reprod Med. 1992;37:653-8.

73. **Telford SR, Pollack RJ, Spielman A.** Emerging vector-borne infections. Infect Dis Clin North Am. 1991;5:7-18.

74. **Centers for Disease Control and Prevention.** African tick-bite fever among international travelers—Oregon, 1998. MMWR Morb Mortal Wkly Rep. 1998;47:950-2.

75. **Azad AF, Beard CB.** Rickettsial pathogens and their arthropod vectors. Emerg Infect Dis. 1998;4:179-86.

76. **Silver HM.** Lyme disease during pregnancy. Infect Dis Clin North Am. 1997;11:93-7.

77. **Maraspin V, Cimperman J, Lotric-Furlan S, et al.** Treatment of erythema migrans in pregnancy. Clin Infect Dis. 1996;22:788-93.

78. **Nadal D, Hunziker U, Bucher H, et al.** Infants born to mothers with antibodies against *Borrelia burgdorferi* at delivery. Eur J Pediatr. 1989;148:426.

79. **Strobino B, Williams C, Abid S, et al.** Lyme disease and pregnancy outcome: a prospective study of two thousand perinatal patients. Am J Obstet Gynecol. 1993;169:367.

80. **Williams C, Strobino B, Weinstein A, et al.** Maternal Lyme disease and congenital malformations: a cord blood serosurvey in endemic and control areas. Pediatr Perinatol Epidemiol. 1995;9:320.

81. **Chye JK, Lim CT, Ng KB, Lin JMH, et al.** Vertical transmission of dengue. Clin Infect Dis. 1997;25:1374-7.

82. **Thaithumyanon P, Thisyakorn U, Deeroinawong J, Innis BL.** Dengue infection complicated by severe hemorrhage and vertical transmission in a paturient woman. Clin Infect Dis. 1994;18:248-9.

83. **Lee RV.** Protozoan infections. In: Gleicher NB, ed. Principles of Medical Therapy in Pregnancy, 3d ed. Norwalk, CT: Appleton & Lange; 1998:823-48.

84. **Menendez C.** Malaria during pregnancy: a priority area of malaria research and control. Parasitol Today. 1995;11:178-83.

85. **Steketee RW, Wirima JJ, Slutsker L, et al.** The problem of malaria and malaria control in pregnancy in sub-Saharan Africa. Am J Trop Med Hyg. 1996;55:2-7.

86. **Quinn TC, Jacobs RF, Mertz GI, et al.** Congenital malaria: a report of four cases and a review. J Pediatr. 1982;101:229.

87. **McGregor IA, Wilson ME, Billewicz WZ.** Malaria infection of the placenta in Gambia, West Africa: its incidence and relationship to stillbirth, birthweight, and placental weight. Trans R Soc Trop Med Hyg. 1983;77:232.

88. **Meuris S, Piko BB, Eerens P, et al.** Gestational malaria: assessment of its consequences on fetal growth. Am J Trop Med Hyg. 1993;48:603-9.

89. **Redd SC, Wirima JJ, Steketee RW, et al.** Transplacental transmission of *Plasmodium falciparum* in rural malaria. Am J Trop Med Hyg. 1996;55:57-60.

90. **Yamada M, Steketee R, Abramivsky C, et al.** *Plasmodium falciparum* associated placental pathology: a light and electron microscopic and immunohistologic study. Am J Trop Med Hyg. 1989;41:161.

91. **Steketee RW, Wirima JJ.** Malaria prevention in pregnancy: the effects of treatment and chemoprophylaxis on placental malaria infection, low birth weight, and fetal, infant and child survival. Am J Trop Med Hyg. 1996;55:1-100.

92. **Bouvier P, Breslow N, Doumbo O, Robert CF, et al.** Seasonality, malaria, and impact of prophylaxis in a West African village: I. Effect on anemia in pregnancy, II. Effect on birthweight. Am J Trop Med Hyg. 1997;56:378-89.

93. **Parke A.** Antimalarial drugs and pregnancy. Am J Med. 1988;85:30.

94. **White NJ.** Treatment of malaria. N Engl J Med. 1996;335:800-6.

95. **Wolfe MS, Cordero JF.** Safety of chloroquine in chemosuppression of malaria during pregnancy. BMJ. 1985;290:1466.

96. **Steketee RW, Wirima JJ, Slutsker L, et al.** Malaria treatment and prevention in pregnancy: indications for use and adverse events associated with the use of chloroquine or mefloquine. Am J Trop Med Hyg. 1996;55:50-6.

97. **Nosten F, Luxemburger C, terKuile FO, et al.** Treatment of multi-drug resistant *Plasmodium falciparum* malaria with three day artesunate-mefloquine combination. J Infect Dis. 1994;170:971-7.

98. **Hien TT, Day NPJ, Phu NH, et al.** A controlled trial of artemether or quinine in Vietnamese adults with severe *P. falciparum* malaria. N Engl J Med. 1996;335:76-83.

99. **Hoffman SL.** Artemether in severe malaria—still too many deaths (Editorial). N Engl J Med. 1996;35:124-6.

100. **Phillips-Howard PA, Steffen R, Kerr L, Vanhanwere B, et al.** Safety of mefloquine and other antimalarial agents in the first trimester of pregnancy. J Travel Med. 1998;5:121-6.

101. **Vanhanwere B, Maradit H, Kerr L.** Post-marketing surveillance of prophylactic mefloquine (Lariam) use in pregnancy. Am J Trop Med Hyg. 1998;58:17-21.

102. **Okitolonda W, Delacollette C, Malengreau M, Henquin JC.** High incidence of hypoglycemia in African patients treated with intravenous quinine for severe malaria. BMJ. 1987;295:716.

103. **White NJ, Warrell DA, Chanthavanich P, et al.** Severe hypoglycemia and hyperinsulinemia in *P. falciparum* malaria. N Engl J Med. 1983;309:61.

104. **Nosten F, terKuile PO, Maelankiri L, et al.** Mefloquine prophylaxis prevents malaria during pregnancy: a double-blind placebo-controlled study. J Infect Dis. 1994;169:595-603.

105. **Kirchoff LV.** Agents of African trypanosomiasis (sleeping sickness). In: Mandell GL, Bennett JE, Dolin R, eds. Principles and Practice of Infectious Diseases. New York: Churchill Livingstone; 1995:2450-5.

106. **Olowe SA.** A case of congenital toxoplasmosis in Lagos. Trans R Soc Trop Med Hyg. 1975;69:57.

107. **Kirchoff LV.** Chagas' disease: American trypanosomiasis. Infect Dis Clin North Am. 1993;7:487-502.

108. **Freilij H, Altech J.** Congenital Chagas' disease: diagnostic and clinical aspects. Clin Infect Dis. 1995; 21:551-5.

109. **Grant IH, Gold JWM, Wittner M, et al.** Transfusion associated acute Chagas' disease acquired in the United States. Ann Intern Med. 1989;111:849.

110. **Bittencourt AL.** Congenital Chagas' disease. Am J Dis Childhood. 1976;130:97.

111. **Russomando G, Petomassone MMC, DeGuillen I, Acosta N, et al.** Treatment of congenital Chagas disease diagnosed and followed up by the polymerase chain reaction. Am J Trop Med Hyg. 1998;59:487-91.

112. **Laraja FS, Dias E, Nobrega G, et al.** Chagas' disease: a clinical, epidemiologic, and pathologic study. Circulation. 1956;14:1035.

113. **Szarfman A, Cossio PM, Arana RM, et al.** Immunologic and immunopathologic studies in congenital Chagas' disease. Clin Immunol Immunopathol. 1975;4:489.

114. **Apt W, Aquilera X, Arribada A, Perez C, et al.** Treatment of chronic Chagas disease with itraconazole and allopurinol. Am J Trop Med Hyg. 1998;59:133-8.

115. **Urbino JA, Payares G, Molina J, et al.** Cure of short- and long-term experimental Chagas' disease using D0870. Science. 1996;273:969-71.

116. **Herwaldt BL, Stokes SL, Juranek DD.** American cutaneous leishmaniasis in US travelers. Ann Intern Med. 1993;118:779-84.

117. **King CT, Rogers PD, Cleary JD, Chapman SW.** Antifungal therapy during pregnancy. Clin Infect Dis. 1998;27:1151-60.

APPENDIX: IMMUNIZATIONS, DRUGS FOR INFECTIOUS DISEASES, AND DRUGS FOR UNUSUAL INFECTIOUS DISEASES

The drug tables on pages 793 to 795 are for reference when there is a clinical indication for one of the immunizations or medications listed. Decisions about medication use in pregnancy should be made on the basis of a benefit-to-risk ratio, avoiding unnecessary treatment of symptoms but with consideration of the fact that fetal well-being depends on maternal well-being. Because the U.S. Food and Drug Administration is working on a new classification system for the use of medications in pregnancy, we have classified medications as follows:

Data Suggest Drug Use May Be Justified When Indicated

When data and/or experience supports the safety of the drug.

Data Suggest Drug Use May Be Justified in Some Circumstances

When less extensive or desirable data are reported, but the drug is reasonable as a second-line therapy or may be used on the basis of the severity of maternal illness.

Data Suggest Drug Use Is Rarely Justified

Use drug only when alternatives supported by more experience and/or a better safety profile are not available.

Pregnancy pharmacokinetics may necessitate a significant increase in dose or dosing frequency, and dosing recommendations may require modification according to individual circumstances.

Immunizations

	Use May Be Justified When Indicated	Use May Be Justified in Some Circumstances	Use Is Rarely Justified	Comments/Dose Adjustment
Diptheria	√			Toxoid
Hepatitis A	√			
Hepatitis B	√			Also used for neonates of chronic carrier mothers
Immunoglobulin	√			
Inactivate polio	√			
Influenza	√			Indicated for all pregnant women
MMR (Measles, Mumps, Rubella)			√	Live attenuated virus may cross placenta
Meningococcal disease	√			Polysaccharides
Pneumococcal disease	√			
Rabies	√			Inactivated virus
Sabin polio vaccine (oral)			√	
TB (PPD/Tine)	√			Not altered by pregnancy
Tetanus	√			Same indications as for nonpregnant patient
Varicella			√	Live attenuated virus may cross placenta
Varicella-Zoster IgG (VZIG)	√			Give to exposed susceptible pregnant woman within 5 days of exposure; for neonates of mothers with active varicella, give 5 days before or 2 days after delivery

Drugs for Infectious Diseases

	Use May Be Justified When Indicated	Use May Be Justified in Some Circumstances	Use Is Rarely Justified	Comments/Dose Adjustments
Acyclovir	√			Indicated for systemic herpes and varicella infections
Aminoglycosides		√		May require greater dose frequency; no data to support 24-hour dosing in pregnancy; potential fetal ototoxicity
Antiretroviral agents (other than AZT)		√		See Section II; use for same clinical indications as in nonpregnant patient
Azithromycin	√			
AZT, zidovudine	√			Should be part of all prophylactic regimens for HIV+ mothers to prevent vertical transmission
Cephalosporins (1st & 2nd generation)	√			
Cephalosporins (3rd generation)		√		Protein binding may displace bilirubin in neonate
Clarithromycin			√	
Doxycycline, tetracycline			√	Staining of bone/teeth; use for serious infection; sensitive to tetracycline only (*Rickettsia, Ehrlichia*)
Erythromycin (except estolate)	√			Estolate not desirable due to hepatic toxicity
Ethambutol		√		No adverse fetal effects found
Fluoroquinolines			√	Adverse effect on cartilage and collagen development in animals
Isoniazid (INH)		√		Safe to fetus but may increase hepatic toxicity in mother
Macrodantin	√			Used for UTI prophylaxis; hemolysis with G6PD deficiency
Penicillins	√			Preferred drug
Rifampin		√		May interfere with oral contraceptives; lowers fetal and maternal VIMC levels
Sulfonamides		√		
Trimethoprim		√		Folic acid supplementation desirable
Trimethoprim sulfamethoxazole		√		Use for *Pneumocystis carinii* prophylaxis
Vancomycin	√			

Drugs for Unusual Infectious Diseases

	Use May Be Justified When Indicated	Use May Be Justified in Some Circumstances	Use Is Rarely Justified	Comments/Dose Adjustment
Antifungals (nystatin, amphotericin, topical agents)		√		Amphotericin preferred systemic antifungal; preferred mode of administration is topical
Antifungals (fluconazole, ketoconazole)			√	Use indicated for fungemia and systemic fungal infection only
Ivermectin		√		Preferred drug for strongyloides
Paromomycin	√			Tapeworms
Piperazine		√		Ascaris with a heavy worm burden
Praziquantel	√			Use for symptomatic CNS, cystircercosis, schistosomiasis
Pyrantel		√		No teratogenicity reported
Thiabendazole, mebendazole		√ 2nd & 3rd trimesters	√ 1st trimester	Trichinosis with systemic involvement or severe hookworm; use only in 2nd or 3rd trimester

CHAPTER 14

Dermatology

Richard V. Lee, MD

Skin Problems Specific to Pregnancy

Pruritis is the common clinical denominator of skin eruptions related to pregnancy (Box 14-1) (1). Of the many discomforts of pregnancy, pruritis can be the most annoying, the most discouraging, and the most difficult to treat. Antihistamines are usually not very helpful and can produce both maternal and fetal somnolence, and some may be fetotoxic or teratogenic. Topical therapy can give relief, but when the itch or the eruption is generalized, topical agents have limited value. Cool baths, good humor, and emotional support are always welcome.

Pruritus Gravidarum

Generalized itching without skin lesions, associated with the retention of bile acids and other constituents of bile, is a common problem in the second half of pregnancy (2–4). Cholestasis of pregnancy is the accepted pathophysiology, and elevated alkaline phosphatase and serum bile acid levels are biochemical markers. Pregnancy-related cholestasis and pruritus are found worldwide, but Chile, Scandinavia, and China have unusually high incidences of these conditions (3). Because progressive cholestasis of pregnancy is associated with increased risks for low birthweight, prematurity, and stillbirth, generalized gestational pruritus requires regular, frequent monitoring of both fetus and mother (2). Women with elevated bilirubin levels and increasing alkaline phosphatase levels are at risk for intrapartum and postpartum hemorrhage, which are probably due to vitamin K deficiency.

Box 14-1   Pruritic Dermatologic Conditions Related to Gestation

---

Pruritus of pregnancy (pruritus gravidarum)
Cholestasis of pregnancy (increased risks for prematurity and postpartum
   hemorrhage due to vitamin K deficiency)
Pruritic folliculitis of pregnancy
Pruritic papules of pregnancy
Pruritic urticarial papules and plaques of pregnancy (PUPPP)
Herpes gestationis

Oral cholestyramine binds bile acids in the gastrointestinal tract and can relieve itching in some patients, but it does not affect the intrahepatic process and can exacerbate the constipation that plagues many pregnancies. Ursodeoxycholic acid has alleviated symptoms of pruritis in a few patients and may be a helpful alternative (5). Phototherapy and narcotic antagonists, such as naloxone, have relieved pruritus in pregnant patients but have not been systematically or carefully studied. Delivery is followed by prompt resolution of the itch and gradual decreases in the biochemical measures of cholestasis. Cholestasis and itching tend to recur in subsequent pregnancies.

Folliculitis

A few women develop a pruritic acneiform eruption on the trunk, shoulders, arms, and neck that is not related to cholestasis (6, 7). Topical therapy with 0.5% to 1.0% hydrocortisone cream and low-potency benzoyl peroxide may give some relief.

Papular Lesions (Prurigo of Pregnancy)

Pruritic papules, without cholestasis, urticaria, and coalescence into plaques, are an occasional problem (6). Topical hydrocortisone cream usually provides relief. As in pruritus gravidarum, delivery produces rapid resolution.

Pruritic Urticarial Plaques and Papules of Pregnancy

In the United Kingdom, pruritic urticarial plaques and papules of pregnancy (PUPPP)—a characteristic, intensely pruritic rash—is known as *polymorphic eruption of pregnancy* (6, 8). It is seen in 1 of 120 to 240 pregnancies and is therefore the most common pruritic eruption that occurs during pregnancy.

Usually in the second half of pregnancy, patients with abdominal striae develop small papules on the abdomen that become urticarial, enlarge, and coalesce. Erythematous urticarial papules crop up on the arms, thighs, trunk, and buttocks and expand or coalesce to form erythematous, slightly indurated plaques. Many early lesions have blanched halos. Excoriation and small vesicles are common. Histopathologic examination of skin biopsy specimens shows a perivascular infiltrate with mononuclear cells and eosinophils. No consistent biochemical, immunologic, or hematologic abnormalities are seen. The process can resolve in a few weeks during or after pregnancy. The condition should be distinguished from erythema multiforme, drug-induced eruptions, and pityriasis rosea. Topical, medium-potency steroids can give transient relief. Other than producing extraordinary distress from itching and rash, PUPPP has no known adverse effects on fetus or mother. It is not a recurring problem, although a few patients have recurrence in subsequent pregnancies.

Herpes Gestationis

Herpes gestationis has nothing at all to do with herpesviruses. It is an autoimmune bullous dermatosis with antibody and complement binding to basement membrane. It establishes urticaria, erythema, and intense pruritus followed by vesicle and bullae formation (3, 6, 9). Fortunately, it is rare; it affects about 1 in 50,000 pregnancies.

Lesions often begin on the periumbilical skin and spread centripetally to the breasts, trunks, arms, legs, palms, and soles. Facial and scalp lesions are unusual. Erythema and then urticaria develop in expanding polymorphous lesions, which develop vesicles that progress to bullae at the margins of the erythematous, edematous plaques. If no superimposed bacterial infection is present, the lesions heal without scars. Histopathologic examination of biopsied lesions characteristically shows an infiltrate of histiocytes, lymphocytes, and eosinophils and immunofluorescent, linear deposition of C3 complement and IgG in the basement membrane.

Onset of the rash follows implantation and the appearance of an IgG that cross-reacts with placental and skin antigens, the *herpes gestationis factor*. Lesions can appear in the first 6 weeks or as late as 1 week postpartum. Most patients have HLA-DR$_w$3 and an increased incidence of other autoimmune conditions such as Graves disease. Once established, the herpes gestationis diathesis almost always causes lesions in subsequent pregnancies or with the use of hormonal contraception.

Herpes gestationis factor IgG can cross the placenta and produce lesions in the fetus and neonate. Neonatal herpes gestationis is infrequent (it is seen in 2% to 5% of pregnancies) and is less severe than the maternal lesions. The lesions resolve within 4 weeks without treatment. Histopathologic examination of the erythematous papules and vesicles shows deposition of C3 complement and IgG in the basement membrane. Maternal steroid treatment can reduce the quantity of herpes gestationis factor so that the dermal and constitutional effects of immunologically mediated inflammation in the fetus can be diminished.

The important option in the differential diagnosis of herpes gestationis is PUPPP. The early lesions and their distributions are similar in the two conditions, so when questions arise, biopsy and immunofluorescence studies are the only tests that distinguish between herpes gestationis and PUPPP.

Herpes gestationis is the only pruritic eruption of pregnancy that is best treated with systemic as well as topical steroids. Prednisone 40 mg/d usually initiates a response, and treatment can then be tapered to maintenance doses. Peripartum flares can occur and may require transient increases in the steroid dosage.

Skin Problems Complicated by Pregnancy

Melanoma

Pregnancy is marked by increases in pigmentation. Darkening of the aureolae, freckles, melanocytic nevi, the linea nigra, and the "mask of pregnancy," or melasma, are common. Gestational hyperpigmentation is the source of the incorrect idea that pregnancy fosters the malignant transformation of benign pigmented lesions.

Because of the close relation between sun exposure and malignant melanoma, women with a history of blistering sunburn and protracted sun exposure should be considered at risk for melanoma during gestation. Women with familial dysplastic nevus syndrome and a family history of multiple atypical nevi and melanoma are at risk for malignant transformation with hormonal treatments and with pregnancy (10, 11). These women should have regular dermatologic examinations and careful documentation of lesions with serial photographs. Whether patients with familial dysplastic nevi who develop malignant melanoma during pregnancy should subsequently become pregnant or use hormonal contraception is uncertain, but most clinicians advise against both options.

The general experience indicates that women who receive a diagnosis of malignant melanoma during pregnancy tend to be diagnosed at a later stage of disease than nonpregnant patients do. The clinical message is clear: Increased awareness, careful surveillance, and early diagnosis are fundamental. Management of melanoma is no different because of pregnancy, and the termination of pregnancy does not improve maternal outcome.

Hirsutism and Hair Loss

Pregnancy promotes an increase of hair in the anagen or growing phase (12). Many women notice an increase in fine, light-colored hair, especially on the face, during gestation. After delivery, the amount of anagen hair decreases and the amount of telogen or resting hair increases, and hair loss usually occurs 2 to 4 months postpartum. The fine hair growth of pregnancy disappears, and a generalized shedding of scalp hair is seen. This *telogen effluvium* can be distressing but necessitates only reassurance. Complete regrowth occurs within 6 to 18 months postpartum.

Skin Infections of Concern

A few troubling skin infections can tax the clinician who cares for pregnant women (Table 14-1). The most common of these are infections by sexually transmitted viruses and ectoparasites that affect the external genitalia and pubic skin.

Genital warts (condyloma acuminatum), caused by strains of human papillomavirus, can expand greatly during gestation. They can cause problems with local hygiene but rarely interfere with vaginal delivery (13). Derivatives of podophyllin are the classic treatment but are contraindicated in pregnancy. Careful laser surgery or topical trichloroacetic acid are acceptable alternatives. With exuberant, fleshy lesions, treatment should be staged.

Scabies and crab lice are generally benign nuisances, but for personal and consortial hygiene, treatment is desirable. Both can cause bothersome itching and may be confused with pruritus gravidarum. Neither type of organisms is a vector for other pathogens. Direct microscopic identification of mites, nits, or *Phthirus pubis* makes the diagnosis. However, the presence of scabies in the household or the presence of crab lice on the patient's consort is enough of an indication for treatment. Permethrin cream is the best agent for the treatment of scabies during pregnancy. Crotamiton and lindane may have adverse effects on the fetus if used repeatedly. The permethrin cream or lotion is applied "all over" except on the face and eyes, is left on for 8 to 18 hours, and is then washed off. A single session of therapy is usually all that is needed. Clothing and bedclothes should be washed and either ironed or boiled. Permethrin as a shampoo or lotion works well for crab lice, but its application should be repeated in 7 to 10 days, even if the consort is treated and clothing is sterilized. Crab lice not uncommonly attach to eyelash and eyebrow hair and should be sought in those locations. Physostigmine liquid applied with a cotton swab will paralyze the adult organisms. Treatment must usually be repeated in a week or so, after the residual nits hatch.

Established leprosy shifts from the tuberculoid to the lepromatous pole as gestational changes in cell-mediated immunity develop. This is usually not a

Table 14-1 Skin Infections That Are Problems During Pregnancy and Puerperium

Infection	Source	Risks to Pregnancy	Management
Viral infections			
External genital warts (condyloma acuminatum)	Sexual transmission	May proliferate and interfere with vaginal delivery	Podophyllin contraindicated during pregnancy; laser surgery; trichloroacetic acid
Molluscum contagiosum	Sexual transmission	None	Watchful waiting
Bacterial infections			
Group A streptococcal infections			
Necrotizing fasciitis Toxic shock syndrome	Postoperative wound infection	Destructive, progressive lesions; often polymicrobial	Wide debridement; beta-lactam antibiotic with synergistic aminoglycoside
Mycobacterial infections			
Leprosy (*Mycobacterium leprae* infection)	Pre-existing infection	Shift from tuberculoid to lepromatous polar form	Continue all appropriate medications except thalidomide
Yeast and fungal infections			
Moniliasis (*Monilia* and *Torulopsis* infections)	Indigenous flora	Minor irritation associated with bacterial vaginosis	
Parasite infections			
Scabies (*Sarcoptes scabiei* infection)	Close contact	Secondary infection	Soap, water, and topical permethrin, crotamiton
Crab lice (*Phthirus pubis* infection)	Sexual transmission	None	

serious problem; however, women with lepromatous leprosy may be receiving thalidomide to prevent the type S lepra reaction, erythema nodosum leprosum (ENL). If the pregnancy is planned, thalidomide treatment should be stopped before conception. If not, the patient and the clinician are confronted with an ethical dilemma. Type 2 reactions, ENL, may be exacerbated by pregnancy and by the abrupt cessation of thalidomide therapy.

Erythema Nodosum

Painful inflammatory skin nodules, usually on the extensor surfaces of the extremities, accompany numerous infections and granulomatous inflammatory conditions, including sarcoidosis, inflammatory bowel disease, and fungal infections such as coccidioidomycosis. Normal pregnancy can also trigger the onset of erythema nodosum. However, because underlying infection or inflammatory disease is potentially harmful to mother and fetus, a careful evaluation, including shielded anteroposterior and lateral chest radiography, is always necessary.

REFERENCES

1. **Furhoff AK.** Itching in pregnancy. Acta Med Scand. 1974;196:403-10.
2. **Klein NA, Riely CA.** Liver disease. Curr Obstet Med. 1991;1:99-124.
3. **Reyes H.** The spectrum of liver and gastrointestinal disease seen in cholestasis of pregnancy. Gastroenterol Clin North Am. 1992;21:95-921.
4. **Reyes H, Simon FR.** Intrahepatic cholestasis of pregnancy: an estrogen-related disease. Semin Liver Dis. 1993;13:289-301.
5. **Palma J, Reyes H, Ribalta J, et al.** Effects of ursodeoxycholic acid in patients with intrahepatic cholestasis of pregnancy. Hepatology. 1992;15:1043-6.
6. **Holmes RC, Black M.** The specific dermatoses of pregnancy. J Am Acad Dermatol. 1983;8:405-12.
7. **Zoberman E, Farmer E.** Pruritic folliculitis of pregnancy. Arch Dermatol. 1981;117:20-2.
8. **Lawley TJ, Hertz KC, Wade TR, et al.** Pruritic urticarial papules and plaques of pregnancy. JAMA. 1979;241:1696-9.
9. **Shornick JK.** Herpes gestationis. J Am Acad Dermatol. 1987;17:539-56.
10. **Slingluff CLJ, Reintgen DS, Vollmer RT, et al.** Malignant melanoma arising during pregnancy. Ann Surg. 1990;211:582-9.
11. **Wong DJ, Strassner HT.** Melanoma in pregnancy. Clin Obstet Gynecol. 1990;33:782-91.
12. **Lynfield YL.** Effect of pregnancy on the human hair cycle. J Invest Dermatol. 1960;35:323-7.
13. **Beutner KR, Reitano MV, Richwald GA, Wiley DJ, et al.** External genital warts: report of the American Medical Association Consensus Conference. Clin Infect Dis. 1998;27:796-806.

CHAPTER 15

Postpartum Disorders

Karen Rosene-Montella, MD,
Linda Anne Barbour, MD, MSPH,
and Lucia Larson, MD

The postpartum period is a time of both exhilaration and exhaustion for new mothers and their families. Sleep deprivation and rapid shifts in hormone levels make mood disturbances common, and it is frequently difficult to elicit an adequate history. Night sweats, urinary frequency, and breast engorgement are often normal during the postpartum period. The importance of carefully listening to the patient and her family during this chaotic time cannot be overemphasized.

The puerperal period (usually defined as 42 days after delivery) or the postpartum period (up to 6 months after delivery) may bring increased risk for flares of chronic medical conditions or for the onset of new conditions. Rebound of cell-mediated immunity may partly account for exacerbations in autoimmune diseases. Dramatic changes in hormonal levels, coagulation factors, volume shifts, and vascular reactivity may result in neurologic and vascular events. Numerous profound psychological and physical challenges may precipitate conditions that had been clinically silent. Some conditions thought to have obstetric causes, such as preeclampsia–eclampsia and peripartum infection, may take time to resolve or may present for the first time. Others conditions that may be identified first during pregnancy, such as the antiphospholipid antibody syndrome or gestational diabetes, may have significant implications for the health of the woman for the remainder of her life. Women with immunologic disorders, such as rheumatoid arthritis, systemic lupus erythematosus, multiple sclerosis, myasthenia gravis, thyroiditis, and Graves disease, are at risk for postpartum exacerbations. This chapter reviews normal postpartum changes and highlights the most common disorders that may arise in the postpartum period. Most of these disorders are discussed in further detail in other chapters.

Breastfeeding

It is widely accepted that breastfeeding is the preferred source of nourishment for the newborn. The American Academy of Pediatrics recommends that breastfeeding begin within 1 hour of birth and continue throughout the first year of life. Although breastfeeding certainly is natural, many new mothers find it far from easy and wonder how the human race survived when it depended solely on the breast to feed its young. Some new mothers present to their internists with problems such as sore breasts or with questions about how their medical problems or medications may affect breastfeeding. Many women have a strong wish to breastfeed but want to be certain that it is safe for their babies; others simply prefer not to nurse. Bottle feeding in the United States is quite safe. Some women need to have this reinforced because they feel that they are harming (or at least not doing their best for) the newborn if they do not breastfeed. If the internist provides good information and support to patients who have concerns about breastfeeding, the patient and her baby will be well served during this special time.

Most breastfeeding mothers, at some point, have sore nipples; this is frequently a result of improper positioning at the breast. The nipple should be centered, and as much of the aureole as possible (approximately 1 inch) should be in the baby's mouth during nursing. Rotating among different feeding positions may be helpful. A lactation consultant or books may be useful resources. Other helpful measures include taking acetaminophen or ibuprofen 30 minutes before feeding, wearing a cotton bra, air-drying the nipples after feeding, and keeping the flaps of a nursing bra open beneath a cotton top to allow air circulation. Because milk production is determined by supply and demand, supplementing feedings with formula may adversely affect the milk supply. It is better to suggest frequent, shorter nursings, which are better for sore nipples than longer, infrequent feedings. Starting on the least-sore breast may help because infants suck more vigorously early in a feeding. Cool, wet compresses after feeding may be helpful. Many over-the-counter creams and ointments should be avoided, but pure lanolin made for nursing mothers is useful and does not need to be removed before nursing. Mothers who have burning nipples may have thrush or eczema; thrush can also occur in the infant, so both mother and infant should be treated.

It is not uncommon for a woman who uses a medication for an acute or chronic medical problem to present to an internist with questions about the advisability of breastfeeding during treatment. Often, a woman may continue treatment safely while breastfeeding, but several pharmacokinetic factors influence the advisability of use of specific drugs. Almost all drugs taken by the mother enter the breastmilk, but the amount is usually less than 2% of the maternal dose (1). Because it is the free drug that enters the milk, drugs that are more protein bound are less likely to be transferred, and the greater the lipid solubility, the greater the transfer. Of note, molecular size is a less-important factor. The composition of breastmilk varies both over the course of the day and within each feeding, so variations in milk protein and lipid content lead to variations in drug delivery to the breastmilk. Once the drug is delivered to the neonate, it must be absorbed and metabolized. Infants have lower gastric acid secretion than adults do, and they also have longer gastric emptying times that may affect absorption. Premature neonates may have nonselective gastrointestinal permeability and may absorb molecules that are not usually absorbed. Enzyme metabolism and renal excretion are also lower in neonates, so drugs may accumulate, particularly in younger babies. Generally, however, if the mother has taken a given drug during pregnancy, neonatal exposure is far less than fetal exposure. Several sources (2–4) review specific drugs for use during lactation or provide general information.

The level of drug in breastmilk correlates with serum drug levels because drugs may be freely transferred between breastmilk and blood. It has been stated that the best time to take a drug is immediately after a feeding and that after a dose is taken, feedings should be withheld for at least 1 to 2 hours or even longer, depending on the feeding schedule. This may be ideal, but it may not be practical or even necessary with many medications.

It should be noted that the radionucleotides used in many radiologic studies are transferred to breastmilk. Whenever a mother undergoes an investigation that uses these agents, she is advised to prevent the exposure of her infant by 1) bottle feeding and 2) pumping and discarding breastmilk for as long as the radionuclide is excreted. The necessary length of time varies with the radionucleotide but may be in the range of 24 to 48 hours. Some mothers may wish to collect and freeze breastmilk ahead of time so that they do not need to use formula during the excretion period. These mothers appreciate a discussion about the measures they will need to take with regard to breastfeeding before the procedure.

Some mothers wonder whether a particular medical condition alone, regardless of medication use, prohibits them from breastfeeding. The vast majority of women need not be restricted. For mothers with conditions that make it impossible to maintain good nutritional status, breastfeeding may be inadvisable. Women infected with organisms (such as HIV) that may be transmitted through the breastmilk or through bloody fluids from cracked nipples should plan on bottle feeding, especially in the United States, where bottle feeding is so safe. In countries where the formula supply is less safe, breastfeeding may be preferable even in infected mothers.

Although breastfeeding is less widespread in the United States than in other countries, many U.S. women wish to nurse their babies. Even the most motivated mother who plans to feed her baby naturally may find breastfeeding surprisingly difficult. The internist can give support to such women and help those who have medical problems that require medication or radiologic testing to nurse successfully and safely.

Postpartum Fever

When an internist is asked to evaluate a patient for postpartum fever, the request may come from the patient herself or from an obstetrician. Ambulatory patients are not scheduled to see their obstetricians until the routine postpartum visit: 2 weeks after cesarean section or 6 weeks after vaginal delivery. Referrals by obstetricians may be made for ambulatory or hospitalized patients and often represent difficult diagnostic problems. The most frequent cause of postpartum fever is uterine infection, and this infection should be suspected in all cases, even when pelvic infection seems to have been excluded by the obstetrician. Causes of postpartum fever are summarized in Table 15-1. Seemingly benign conditions may worsen quickly and warrant close follow-up. In a recent review, the major causes of septic shock during pregnancy were pyelonephritis, chorioamnionitis, and postpartum endometritis. Less common causes were necrotizing fasciitis, septic abortion, and toxic shock syndrome, all of which were related to postpartum infection (5).

Postpartum Endometritis

Postpartum endometritis (PPE) occurs in 3% to 5% of patients after vaginal delivery and in 10% to 20% of patients after cesarean section, even when antibiotic prophylaxis has been used. Studies done before the use of antibiotic prophylaxis reported prevalence rates as high as 50%. Bacteremia rates range from 8% to 20%, and serious complications occur in 2% to 5% of patients with confirmed uterine infection.

Risk factors for PPE (Box 15-1) are those that increase the exposure of the upper genital tract to bacteria from the lower genital tract, reflecting the pathophysiology of PPE. Thus, infectious factors that increase the size or virulence of the inoculum will further contribute to the risk for PPE. Data from numerous excellent studies confirm that the isolation of specific microorganisms from the antepartum patient is associated with an increased risk

Table 15-1 Causes of Postpartum Fever

Site	Diagnosis
Uterus and pelvis	Endometritis
	Retained products of conception
	Wound infection
	Episiotomy infection
	Necrotizing fasciitis
	Myonecrosis
Breast	Engorgement
	Mastitis
	Abscess
Genitourinary system	Urinary tract infection
	Pyelonephritis
	Trauma to bladder, ureters, or urethra during delivery
Pulmonary system	Pneumonia
	Aspiration pneumonia
	Atelectasis
	Transfusion-related cause
Rheumatologic system	Flare of systemic lupus erythematosus
	Flare of rheumatoid arthritis
Gastrointestinal system	Cholecystitis
	Flare of inflammatory bowel disease
Hematologic system	Venous thromboembolism
	Septic pelvic thrombophlebitis
	Thrombotic thrombocytopenia purpura
	Lymphoproliferative disorders

Box 15-1 Risk Factors for Postpartum Endometritis

Maternal age ≤25 years

Ruptured membranes

Prolonged labor

Greater number of vaginal examinations

Bacterial vaginosis

Chorioamnionitis

Cesarean section

Antepartum isolation of group B streptococci, *Chlamydia*, or *Mycoplasma*

Failure to use prophylactic antibiotics

---

for postpartum infection. These microorganisms include group B streptococci, *Chlamydia trachomatis*, *Mycoplasma hominis*, and, more recently, the microorganisms associated with bacterial vaginosis (*Gardnerella vaginalis*, *Bacteroides* species, and *Peptostreptococcus* species) (6).

The criteria for diagnosis of PPE are simple: 1) body temperature 38.5°C or more in the first 24 hours postpartum or body temperature 38°C for at least 4 consecutive hours more than 24 hours postpartum and 2) lower abdominal tenderness greater than expected. The postpartum uterus should be nontender on examination after vaginal delivery, and an area apart from the incision should be equally nontender after cesarean section. A postpartum uterus palpable at or above the umbilicus, tender abdominally, or associated with abdominal distention or ileus is abnormal and requires further investigation.

The normal postpartum uterus returns to its nongravid size by 6 to 8 weeks after delivery. Small amounts of intrauterine blood or fluid are normally seen on postpartum ultrasonography, and intrauterine air is visible in 20% of healthy postpartum women (7). Imaging is required only if patients have persistent fever despite treatment or persistent or unusually severe or localized pain. Retained products of conception are seen on pelvic ultrasonography as an echogenic mass that may contain calcifications. Visualization of blood flow into the mass confirms the placental origin of the mass. Retained products of conception must be removed by dilatation and curettage because they are an ongoing nidus for infection. Identification of other causes of persistent pain or fever may require computed tomography (CT) or magnetic resonance imaging (MRI). These other causes include ovarian venous thrombosis, abscess (intrauterine, parametrial, or broad-ligament), and hematoma (uterine, bladder flap, subfacial, rectus sheath, or intraperitoneal), all of which are more common after cesarean section.

Postpartum endometritis is almost always a polymicrobial infection, and the most likely etiologic agent differs at different postpartum stages (Box 15-2). Within 24 to 48 hours postpartum, gram-positive and gram-negative aerobes prevail. At 48 hours, involvement of anaerobic bacteria is likely, and by 7 days, C. trachomatis is often found (8). Rational treatment requires an understanding of the etiologic organisms and a review of antepartum risk factors. For example, if bacterial vaginosis or streptococcal infection was present antepartum, PPE is probably the result of spread of the infectious agents into the upper genital tract; treatment would be modified accordingly. Chlamydial endometritis can be an indolent infection but is an important cause of postpartum tubal dysfunction and subsequent sterility. Therefore, it is essential that an agent active against Chlamydia be included in any regimen used to treat late PPE. Ideally, treatment should follow the careful acquisition of an endometrial sample and culture of the sample by a double- or triple-lumen technique that prevents vaginal and cervical contamination (9). Antibiotic treatment regimens for PPE are outlined in Table 15-2. Recent data confirm the validity of once-daily dosing of gentamicin in the treatment of PPE (10). Once a patient with early PPE has been afebrile for 48 hours and tenderness has resolved, antibiotic use can be discontinued. No evidence indicates that outcome is improved or risk for recurrence decreased if oral therapy is given

---

Box 15-2 Bacterial Isolates in Postpartum Endometritis

Facultative gram-positive organisms
  *Group B streptococci
  *Other streptococci—hemolytic, group D, *Streptococcus viridans*
  Enterococci
  Staphylococcus aureus
Facultative gram-negative organisms
  Gardnerella vaginalis
  Escherichia coli
  Enterobacter species
  Klebsiella species
  Proteus mirabilis
  Haemophilus influenzae, Citrobacter species, *Pseudomonas* species
Anaerobic gram-positive organisms
  Peptostreptococci
  Peptococcus species
  Peptococcus asaccharolyticus
  Clostridium perfringens
Anaerobic gram-negative organisms
  Bacteroides bivius
  Bacteroides fragilis
Other organisms
  Other *Bacteroides* species
  Fusobacterium species
  Ureaplasma urealyticum
  Mycoplasma hominis
  Chlamydia trachomatis

*Most frequent isolate.

---

upon discontinuation of intravenous therapy, so oral therapy is not recommended. Late infection requires a 14-day course of an agent active against *Chlamydia*, such as doxycycline. Use of a shorter course of azithromycin for late PPE is being studied.

Wound, Soft Tissue, and Episiotomy Infection

Wound infections complicate 2% to 8% of cesarean sections. Factors associated with an increased risk for wound infection include preoperative fever, amniotic fluid infection, prolonged labor, ruptured membranes, urgent

Table 15-2 Treatment Regimens for Postpartum Endometritis

Agent	Dosage	Comments
PPE ≤48 h		
Ampicillin	2 g q6h	
+		
Gentamicin	1.75 mg/kg q8h or 5 mg/kg q24h	Efficacy of once-daily dosing confirmed by recent study
+		
Clindamycin	600 mg q6h	
or		
Cefoxitin	2 g q6–8h	Regimens 1 to 3 may be used for PPE at 48 h to 7 days
+		
Doxycycline	100 mg q12h	
or		
Unasyn alone (ampicillin sodium and sulbactam sodium)	2 g q6h	
or +		
Gentamicin or doxycycline		
PPE at ≥1 week		
Doxycycline	100 mg po bid	Treat chlamydia for 14 days
+		
Flagyl (metronidazole)	500 mg po tid	
Azithromycin (being studied)		

surgery, diabetes mellitus, obesity, preoperative shaving, and postoperative drains. Diagnosis is made by detection of an erythematous swollen wound or aspiration of purulent drainage. Wounds must be opened, and debridement may be necessary. Serious sequelae of wound infection include wound dehiscence, synergistic bacterial gangrene, and necrotizing fasciitis.

Episiotomy infection occurs after 1% to 2% of deliveries. An infection is a *simple episiotomy infection* when limited to the skin and superficial fascia along the site of incision. *Superficial fascial infection* is an infection no longer limited to the area immediately adjacent to the incision. *Superficial fascial infection with necrosis* is seen when infection of the superficial tissues spreads to the fascial planes below. Treatment in all cases is with broad-spectrum antibiotics and debridement; the extent of debridement depends on the severity of infection.

Necrotizing fasciitis, which can complicate both episiotomy and wound infections, may have a rapid and fatal course, so early diagnosis is imperative. Initial skin signs of erythema and edema are present but may be minimal if deep infection predominates. Later in infection, as vessels become occluded, the formation of vesicles and bullae is followed by blue-gray skin changes and necrosis. Marked systemic signs, including fever, leukocytosis, anemia, hypocalcemia, hypotension, and DIC, may be present. The most frequent inciting agents are group B hemolytic streptococci and anaerobes, followed by nonhemolytic streptococci and staphylococci. Wound exploration under anesthesia is required for diagnosis, and debridement should be done immediately for necrotic tissue. Even with appropriate antibiotic therapy, necrotizing fasciitis is uniformly fatal in the absence of debridement. Myonecrosis is an infection involving the muscle beneath the deep fascia, and treatment for it is similar to that for necrotizing fasciitis. Because clostridia may be an etiologic agent in myonecrosis, penicillin (in addition to extensive debridement) is required.

Breast Infection

Postpartum breast infections occur almost exclusively in lactating women or in women who breastfed briefly and then stopped. Most occur in the first 2 to 3 weeks postpartum, and *Staphylococcus aureus* is the etiologic agent in 95% of cases. Occasionally, other gram-positive cocci and skin flora are present. The epidemic form of postpartum breast infection is related to hospital-acquired *S. aureus*, and the more common endemic form results from exposure of breast tissue to the oropharynx of a colonized infant. It is thought that the organism is introduced through fissures and through negative pressure with sucking and that milk stasis may be a contributing factor.

Localized pain usually begins in one quadrant of the breast, which becomes red, swollen, and tender and takes on a cellulitis-like appearance. Body temperatures of 102 to 105°F can develop rapidly, and associated toxic shock syndrome has been reported in sporadic cases. Mastitis should cause only local swelling and erythema; abscess should be suspected if swelling or fluctuance is seen. Aspiration of fluctuant masses and culture of expressed breast milk are indicated.

Treatment involves antibiotic therapy with penicillin-resistant agents (dicloxacillin or first-generation cephalosporins) and local measures. In mastitis, it is important to continue breastfeeding to prevent stasis; if severe tenderness is present, gentle manual production of breastmilk is a good alternative. Adequate treatment of breast abscess requires surgical drainage and discontinuation of breastfeeding.

Septic Pelvic Thrombophlebitis

Puerperal ovarian venous thrombosis may occur in the setting of postpartum infectious complications. It should be sought when continued fever and pain are seen after treatment for PPE and no evidence of abscess or soft tissue infection is present. The presentation of this thrombosis can mimic that of pyelonephritis because pain is often localized to the flank, most often on the right side. Diagnosis is made with CT or MRI, and treatment should be given as described in Chapter 8.

Postpartum Medical Disorders

Cardiovascular Disease

Cardiac disease, preeclampsia, pre-existing heart disease and peripartum cardiomyopathy are causes of congestive heart failure in the postpartum period. Postpartum volume changes associated with decreased oncotic pressure and capillary leak may contribute to cardiac decompensation. In one series (11), 20 of 28 women with peripartum cardiomyopathy did not have symptoms until the postpartum period, and 93% had persistent or progressive disease. The onset of heart failure may not present until as late as 5 months postpartum, but the mean time from delivery to onset of symptoms in one series was 35 days (12). Risk factors for peripartum cardiomyopathy include obesity, multiparity, black race, and age greater than 30 years, and peripartum cardiomyopathy has been associated with cesarean section, multiple gestations, preeclampsia, and chronic hypertension.

Acute myocardial infarction may, rarely, present in the postpartum period in women without risk factors for coronary artery disease due to coronary dissection, thrombus, or coronary spasm (13). In one review, 75% of patients with acute myocardial infarction in the peripartum period were reported to have no evidence of atherosclerotic disease and were significantly younger (mean age, 29 years) than women with infarction in the antepartum period. The maternal mortality rate was also greater in the postpartum period. Hypercoagulability is augmented at the time of separation of the placenta, and changes in the arterial walls during gestation may increase risk for dissection. Increased hemodynamic load (due to enhanced return of venous blood to the heart) with relief of caval compression and shift of blood from the contracting emptied uterus into the systemic circulation, as well as the threefold increase in oxygen consumption, may contribute to the poorer prognosis seen in postpartum women (13).

Renal and Hypertensive Disorders

Women in whom hypertension is noted for the first time during pregnancy are often misdiagnosed as having preeclampsia alone. In approximately 50% of patients with mild-to-moderate hypertension, blood pressure is normalized by the second trimester (14). Therefore, when a physiologic increase in blood pressure is seen near term, these women may be incorrectly thought to have developed preeclampsia. In addition, women with proteinuric renal disease can be expected to have a substantial increase in protein excretion accompanied by edema, often into the nephrotic range (15). An increase in blood pressure near term accompanied by increased proteinuria and edema may easily be misdiagnosed as preeclampsia alone. In a series of 176 pregnant hypertensive women who were thought to have preeclampsia alone (16), 25% of primigravidas and 65% of multigravidas were misdiagnosed, according to renal biopsy results. In another series (17), nearly two thirds of primigravidas and multigravidas who presented with hypertension before term had renal abnormalities on biopsy that were inconsistent with preeclampsia alone. These abnormalities included essential hypertension, IgA nephropathy, membranous glomerulonephritis, and reflux nephropathy. Therefore, women previously diagnosed with preeclampsia require close follow-up during the postpartum period to ensure that blood pressure normalizes and proteinuria resolves.

Normalization of a blood pressure increase caused by preeclampsia alone may take several weeks, and complete normalization of the underlying renal lesion make take several months if preeclampsia is severe (18). The degree of proteinuria is often related to the extent of renal dysfunction in preeclampsia. Although the glomerular deposits of various hemostatic factors resolve fairly quickly, the endothelial swelling and subendothelial enlargement may persist for a considerable time (18). In a series of 269 pregnancies complicated by hypertension that were monitored in the postpartum period with twice-daily blood pressure readings (19), patients with preeclampsia did not attain normal blood pressure for up to 45 days (mean, 16 days). Women with a history of "gestational" hypertension without proteinuria took up to 25 to achieve normal blood pressure (mean, 6 days).

Patients who receive a diagnosis of preeclampsia or superimposed preeclampsia should have their blood pressure checked at least weekly if they are discharged while using antihypertensive medications. This is because medication requirements may change rapidly. If the blood pressure remains elevated 2 to 3 months postpartum, the patient probably has chronic hypertension. Multigravidas who have elevated blood pressure during pregnancy are more likely to have underlying hypertension and should be monitored for the development of hypertension for several years. Preeclampsia alone does not increase risk for subsequent hypertension, but gestational hypertension may be a harbinger of subsequent chronic hypertension. Chronic hypertension or chronic hypertension with superimposed preeclampsia is often misdiagnosed as preeclampsia alone, and a higher incidence of women who receive this misdiagnosis have elevated blood pressure 5 to 6 years postpartum (20).

Patients with severe early-onset preeclampsia (defined as preeclampsia with or without HELLP [*h*emolysis, *e*levated *l*iver enzyme levels, and *l*ow *p*latelet count] syndrome, necessitating delivery before 34 weeks of gestation) have a significant incidence of underlying coagulopathies, chronic hypertension, and renal disease. As is the case with recurrent unexplained fetal loss or stillbirth, there is a much higher incidence of antiphospholipid antibodies, factor V Leiden mutation, an abnormal prothrombin gene, or other coagulation disturbances. In a series of 101 patients who met the criteria for severe, early-onset preeclampsia (with or without eclampsia) (21), one third of patients had chronic hypertension. Of the patients tested at least 10 weeks postpartum for coagulation disturbances, 30% had antiphospholipid antibodies; 25% had protein S deficiency; 16% had activated protein C resistance; and 18% had a positive result on a methionine loading test, suggestive of hyperhomocysteinemia. Given that these diagnoses may have significant implications for the health of the mother, including her risk for thromboembolism with use of oral contraceptives, clinicians should test for these coagulation disturbances postpartum in women who have presented with severe, early-onset preeclampsia. In one series in southern Italy (22), 65% of women with severe preeclampsia, abruptio placentae, intrauterine growth restriction, or stillbirth and 18% of controls were found to have a hypercoagulable state.

Postpartum hemolytic uremic syndrome, characterized by hemolytic anemia, acute renal failure, and renal thrombosis or microangiopathy, typically follows a normal delivery and can occur up to 10 weeks postpartum (23). It is more common in primigravidas and can be confused with severe postpartum preeclampsia or thrombotic thrombocytopenic purpura. Antithrombin III levels and the aPTT are usually normal, and immediate diagnosis is essential because early dialysis, aggressive control of hypertension, and plasma exchange or prostacyclin infusion may improve prognosis.

Neurologic Disorders

Headaches, Seizures, and Central Nervous System Disorders

In the postpartum period, it is common for patients with migraines to have worsening of their headaches; this may be due in part to decreases in estrogen (24). In one series (25), nearly 40% of patients had a migraine headache within the first week postpartum. The added stressors of sleep deprivation, irregular eating habits, and anxiety related to caring for a newborn probably play a significant role in the exacerbation of migraines postpartum. Headaches that require immediate investigation and that may be increased in incidence in the postpartum period include those related to preeclampsia and eclampsia, cerebral venous thrombosis, and subarachnoid hemorrhage from arteriovenous malformation or ruptured aneurysm (26). An estimated one fourth of pregnancy-related strokes occur during the first week postpartum.

In one study, a history of severe headache or visual disturbance preceded 54 cases of late postpartum eclampsia in which convulsions occurred 1 to 23 days postpartum (27), and only 56% of women had been identified as preeclamptic before seizing. Women with epilepsy may have a worsening of seizures postpartum, especially because sleep deprivation may lower the seizure threshold. However, postpartum eclampsia must remain prominent in the differential diagnosis during the postpartum period. Cerebral venous thrombosis is definitely more common in the 4-week postpartum period and can present with seizures, but headache is an almost universal symptom because of inflammation within the veins (28). Risk factors for cerebral venous thrombosis include cesarean section, dehydration, infection, hyperviscosity, and hypercoagulable states. This thrombosis can be missed on CT, so MRI or MRV is recommended (29).

Neuropathies

Bell palsy more often presents in the third trimester but may occur postpartum. Women who develop Bell palsy during pregnancy usually have a gradual recovery within 3 months postpartum. Injury to the lumbosacral plexus may occur during vaginal delivery, but the pain may be blunted by immediate postpartum sedation or anesthesia. The neurologic deficit occurs predominantly in the sciatic distribution, with a predilection for the territory of the peroneal nerve (30). Risk factors include prolonged labor, use of forceps, craniopelvic disproportion, and primigravity. Some patients show a complete recovery within weeks, and others have a persistent deficit after 2 years. Peroneal neuropathy and lateral femoral cutaneous neuropathy may occur for the first time in the postpartum period. Classic symptoms of the carpal tunnel syndrome may occur during pregnancy and the postpartum period, and a lactational carpal tunnel syndrome has been described in which symptoms persist during lactation and resolve 2 to 3 weeks after weaning (30).

Autoimmune Diseases

Myasthenia gravis may be exacerbated in the postpartum period, and in one literature review of 314 pregnancies (31), postpartum exacerbations occurred in 31% of cases. Myasthenic control must be carefully supervised and rest periods must be enforced in the months after delivery. Exacerbations tend to be most sudden and most dangerous in the postpartum period and can be accompanied by respiratory failure (32).

Multiple sclerosis (MS) may improve during pregnancy, but the rate of relapse is clearly increased during the postpartum period (33). Although it is estimated that 20% to 45% of patients with MS have clinical relapse after delivery (34), pregnancy does not seem to contribute to long-term progression. The period of greatest risk is 1 to 3 months postpartum. Women are also at increased risk for presenting for the first time in the postpartum period with symptoms suggestive of MS. Whether patients who present for the first time in the postpartum period with an isolated monophasic demyelination, such as optic neuritis, are more or less likely to eventually develop MS is not yet known.

Venous Thromboembolism

In the United States, women are more likely to die of a pulmonary embolism (PE) after a live birth than of any other cause (35). The risks for deep venous thrombosis (DVT) and PE remain increased up to 6 weeks postpartum. Although the antepartum risk for DVT is at least as great if not greater than the postpartum risk, the largest series of radiographically proven cases of DVT and PE showed that PE was more common postpartum (36). Of note, 82% of PEs were associated with cesarean section, which markedly increases risk for PE, perhaps in part as a result of pelvic vein injury and thrombosis. Other factors that significantly increase thromboembolic risk include increasing age and parity, obesity, prolonged bedrest, surgical procedures, severe venous stasis, and underlying acquired or congenital hypercoagulable states (37). Because pregnant or postpartum women usually have a normal A-a gradient despite documented PE, V/Q scanning should be done on all patients who have symptoms consistent with this diagnosis (38). Women who have had venous thrombosis during pregnancy should be evaluated postpartum for underlying hypercoagulable states, and activated protein C resistance or the abnormal prothrombin gene may be associated with venous thromboembolism in 50% of cases (39–41). Because protein S levels are decreased in pregnancy, the diagnosis is best made at least 6 weeks postpartum (42). Ovarian venous thrombosis predominantly occurs in the postpartum period and is discussed in the context of postpartum infections, given that endometritis is a strong risk factor for its development.

Autoimmune Diseases

Rheumatoid Arthritis
Although rheumatoid arthritis (RA) improves in at least three fourths of pregnancies, it returns by the end of the fourth month postpartum, with rare exceptions. In addition, the chance that a woman will develop new-onset RA is higher in the first year postpartum, and one trial (43) found a fivefold increase in RA during the first 3 months postpartum. After the first year postpartum, the risk for RA is reduced in parous women compared with nulliparous women.

The postpartum period is characterized by active arthritis both for women who have had a gestational remission and those who have not. Recurrence is about 98% by 4 months. A shift in cytokine production during pregnancy (from TH-1 to TH-2) and a shift back again postpartum (from TH-2 to TH-1) may contribute to the pregnancy-induced alleviation and postpartum relapse of RA; increased prolactin levels may have a proinflammatory role (43).

Systemic Lupus Erythematosus

Systemic lupus erythematosus (SLE) has a more variable course in pregnancy. It is thought that cell-mediated autoimmune diseases (such as RA) improve during pregnancy, whereas antibody-mediated autoimmune diseases (such as SLE) may not. Although SLE may flare postpartum, there is debate about whether the postpartum period is associated with a definite increased risk for lupus flares. Of six recent prospective studies (which included control groups for comparison of flare rates), four suggested a higher incidence of lupus activity and flares during the postpartum period and two did not (44). There does not seem to be a justified role for prophylactic prednisone because no data support the premise that corticosteroids prevent SLE flares postpartum (45). Women with or without SLE who have the antiphospholipid antibody syndrome due to recurrent fetal loss, unexplained stillbirth, severe intrauterine growth restriction, or severe preeclampsia should not receive estrogen-containing oral contraceptives and are at future risk for thromboembolism, thrombocytopenia, and valvular heart disease.

Endocrinopathies

Thyroid Disorders

Enhanced T-cell activation postpartum, from a period of immune suppression during which the helper T-cell population declined and the suppressor T-cell population increased, may partly explain the frequency of postpartum exacerbations of Graves disease and of postpartum thyroiditis. Postpartum thyroiditis is a lymphocytic thyroiditis with an overall incidence of 5% in North America (range, 2% in New York to 21% in one Canadian study) (46). Postpartum flares in Graves disease have occurred in up to 75% of women 1 to 4 months postpartum, and the PTU dose may need significant upward adjustment. Not uncommonly, lymphocytic thyroiditis (Hashimoto or postpartum thyroiditis) occurs postpartum in a woman with a history of Graves disease presenting as hypothyroidism with a low-to-normal radioactive iodine uptake scan (47). Women with type 1 diabetes have a threefold increase in risk for postpartum thyroiditis.

Women with postpartum thyroiditis may have a hyperthyroid phase 2 to 4 months postpartum that can present with only emotional lability, palpitations, or heat intolerance. Their condition can be misdiagnosed as an agitated depressive or anxiety disorder. Postpartum thyroiditis may require a short course of symptomatic treatment with beta-blockers. The hypothyroid phase most often does not occur until 4 to 8 months postpartum and often presents with fatigue alone; it may be confused with postpartum depression (see Chapter 3). Thyroxine therapy should be offered to women with this condition (48). Approximately 80% of women become euthyroid 12 months after delivery, but the risk for permanent hypothyroidism is substantial and 20% to 30% of women are hypothyroid 2 to 5 years later (46).

Diabetes

Women who receive a diagnosis of gestational diabetes have up to a 50% chance of developing type 2 diabetes within 5 to 10 years. Risk factors for type 2 diabetes include earlier gestational age at diagnosis, fasting hyperglycemia, insulin requirement, obesity, and positive family history. Of note, one third of a series of 238 patients diagnosed with gestational diabetes fulfilled the criteria of impaired glucose tolerance or type 2 diabetes 6 weeks postpartum on a 75-g oral glucose tolerance test (49). Roughly half of patients were found to have type 2 diabetes, and the other half met the criteria for impaired glucose tolerance. In another study (50), women who met the criteria for impaired glucose tolerance on a 75-g oral glucose tolerance test had an 80% risk for developing type 2 diabetes within 5 years. Gestational diabetes identifies an insulin-resistant population with limited beta-cell responsiveness that is at high risk for type 2 diabetes and may benefit from dietary, lifestyle, and possibly therapeutic interventions to prevent type 2 diabetes. The risk for type 2 diabetes may double with every 10 pounds gained postpartum, and women who lose weight have a lower risk for type 2 diabetes. The American Diabetes Association and the American College of Obstetricians and Gynecologists recommend that women with gestational diabetes have a fasting glucose test 6 weeks postpartum and, if the result exceeds 115, be considered for a 75-g oral glucose tolerance test (51). Women with a history of gestational diabetes should be targeted for primary intervention trials to prevent type 2 diabetes and should be checked annually.

REFERENCES

1. **Reider MJ.** Drugs and Breastfeeding: Maternal-Fetal Toxicology. New York: Marcel Dekker; 1990.

2. **Briggs G, Freeman R, Yaffe S.** Drugs in Pregnancy and Lactation. Baltimore: Williams & Wilkins; 1998.

3. **Huggins K.** The Nursing Mother's Companion. Boston: The Harvard Common Press; 1995.

4. **La Leche League.** The Womanly Art of Breastfeeding. New York: Penguin Books; 1991.

5. **Mabie WC, Barton JR, Sibai BM.** Septic shock in pregnancy. Obstet Gynecol. 1997;90:553-61.

6. **Watts DH, Krohn MA, Hillier SL, Eschenbach DA.** Bacterial vaginosis as a risk factor for post-cesarean endometritis. Obstet Gynecol. 1990;75:52-8.

7. **Zuckerman J, Levine D, McNicholas MMJ, Konopka S, Goldstein A, Edelman RR, McArdle CR.** Imaging of pelvic postpartum complications. AJR Am J Roentgenol. 1997;168:663-8.

8. **Rosene K, Eschenbach DA, Tompkins LS, Kenny GE, Watkins H.** Polymicrobial early postpartum endometritis with facultative and anaerobic bacteria, genital mycoplasmas, and Chlamydia trachomatis: treatment with piperacillin or cefoxitin. J Infect Dis. 1986;153:1028-37.

9. **Eschenbach DA, Rosene K, Tompkins LS, Watkins H, Gravett MG.** Endometrial cultures obtained by a triple-lumen method from afebrile and febrile postpartum women. J Infect Dis. 1986;153:1038-45.

10. **Del Priore G, Jackson-Stone M, Shim EK, Garfinkel J, Eichmann MA, Frederiksen MC.** A comparison of once-daily and 8-hour gentamicin dosing in the treatment of postpartum endometritis. Obstet Gynecol. 1996;87:994-100.

11. **Witlin AG, Mabie WC, Sibai BM.** Peripartum cardiomyopathy: an ominous diagnosis. Am J Obstet Gynecol. 1997;176:182-8.

12. **Medei MG, DeMent SH, Feldman AM, et al.** Peripartum myocarditis and cardiomyopathy. Circulation. 1990;81:922-8.

13. **Roth A, Elkayam U.** Acute myocardial infarction associated with pregnancy. Ann Intern Med. 1996;125:751-62.

14. **Sibai BM, Ardella TN, Anderson GD.** Pregnancy outcome in 211 patients with mild chronic hypertension. Obstet Gynecol. 1983;61:571-6.

15. **Biesenbach G, Zazgornik J.** Incidence of transient nephrotic syndrome during pregnancy in diabetic women with and without pre-existing proteinuria. BMJ. 1989;299:366-7.

16. **Fisher KA, Luger H, Spargo BH, et al.** Hypertension in pregnancy: clinical-pathological correlations and remote prognosis. Medicine (Baltimore). 1981;60:267-76.

17. **Ihle BU, Long P, Oats J.** Early onset preeclampsia: recognition of underlying renal disease. BMJ. 1987;294:79-81.

18. **Suzuki S, Gejyo F, Ogino S, Maruyama Y, Ueno M, Nishi SI, et al.** Postpartum renal lesions in women with preeclampsia. Nephrol Dial Transplant. 1997;12:2488-93.

19. **Ferrazzani S, De Carolis S, Pomini F, Testa AC, Mastromarino C, Caruso A.** The duration of hypertension in the puerperium of preeclamptic women: relationship with renal impairment and week of delivery. Am J Obstet Gynecol. 1994;171:506-12.

20. **Lindeberg S, Axelsson O, Jorner U, Malmberg L, Sandström B.** A prospective controlled five-year follow-up study of primiparas with gestational hypertension. Acta Obstet Gynecol Scand. 1988;67:605-9.

21. **Dekker GA, de Vries JIP, Doelitzsch PM, Huijgens PC, von Blomberg BME, Jakobs C, van Geijn HP.** Underlying disorders associated with severe early-onset preeclampsia. Am J Obstet Gynecol. 1995;173:1042-8.

22. **Kupfermine MJ, Eldor A, Skinman N, Many A, Bar-Am A, Jaffa A, et al.** Increased frequency of genetic thrombophilia in women with complications of pregnancy. N Engl J Med. 1999;340:9-13.

23. **Krane K, Cucuzzella A.** Acute renal insufficiency in pregnancy: a review of 30 cases. J Mat Fet Med. 1995;4:12-8.

24. **Welch KMA.** Migraine and pregnancy. In: Devinsky O, Feldman E, Hainline B, eds. Neurological Complications of Pregnancy. New York: Raven Pr; 1994:77-81.

25. **Stein GS.** Headaches in the first post-partum week and their relationships to migraine. Headache. 1981;21:201-5.

26. **Simolke GA, Cox SM, Cunningham FG.** Cerebrovascular accidents complicating pregnancy and the puerperium. Obstet Gynecol. 1991;78:37-42.

27. **Lubarsky SL, Barton JR, Friedman SA, Nasreddine S, Ramadan MK, Sibai BM.** Late postpartum eclampsia revisited. Obstet Gynecol. 1994;83:502-5.

28. **Donaldson JO, Lee NS.** Arterial and venous stroke associated with pregnancy. Neurol Clin. 1994;12:583-99.

29. **Lanska DJ, Kryscio RJ.** Peripartum stroke and intracranial venous thrombosis in the national hospital discharge survey. Obstet Gynecol. 1997;89:413-8.

30. **Rosenbaum RB, Donaldson JO.** Peripheral nerve and neuromuscular disorders. Neurol Clin. 1994;12:461-78.

31. **Plauche WC.** Myasthenia gravis in mothers and their newborns. Clin Obstet Gynecol. 1991;34:82-99.

32. **Gilchrist JM.** Muscle disease in the pregnant woman. In: Devinsky O, Feldman E, Hainline B, eds. Neurological Complications of Pregnancy. New York: Raven Pr; 1994: 193-208.

33. **Abramsky O.** Pregnancy and multiple sclerosis. Ann Neurol. 1994;36(suppl):S38-41.

34. **Roullet E, Verdier-Taillefer MH, Amarenco P, Gharbi G, Alperovitch A, Marteau R.** Pregnancy and multiple sclerosis: a longitudinal study of 125 remittent patients. J Neurol Neurosurg Psychiatry. 1993;56:1062-5.

35. **Atrash HK, Koonin LM, Lawson HW, et al.** Maternal morbidity in the United States 1979-1986. Obstet Gynecol. 1990;76:1055-60.

36. **Rutherford S, Montoro M, McGehee W, et al.** Thromboembolic disease associated with pregnancy: an 11 year review [Abstract]. Am J Obstet Gynecol. 1991;164:286.

37. **Barbour LA, Pickard J.** Controversies in thromboembolic disease during pregnancy: a critical review. Am J Obstet Gynecol. 1995;173:1869-73.

38. **Powrie RO, Larson L, Rosene-Montella K, Abarca M, Barbour LA, Trujillo N.** Alveolar-arterial oxygen gradient in acute pulmonary embolism. Am J Obstet Gynecol. 1998;178:394-6.

39. **Dizon-Townson DS, Nelson LM, Jang H, Varner MW, Ward K.** The incidence of the factor V Leiden mutation in an obstetric population and its relationship to deep venous thrombosis. Am J Obstet Gynecol. 1997;176:883-6.

40. **Hallak M, Senderowicz J, Cassel A, Shapira C, Aghai E, Austender R, et al.** Activated protein C resistance (factor V Leiden) associated with thrombosis in pregnancy. Am J Obstet Gynecol. 1997;176:889-93.

41. **Grandone E, Margaglione M, Colaizzo D, D'Andrea G, Cappucci G, Brancaccio V, DiMinno G.** Genetic susceptibility to pregnancy-related venous thromboembolism: roles of factor V Leiden, prothrombin G20210A, and methylenetetrahydrofolate reductase C677T mutations. Am J Obstet Gynecol. 1998;179:1324-8.

42. **Faught W, Garner P, Jones G, Ivey B.** Changes in protein C and protein S levels in normal pregnancy. Am J Obstet Gynecol. 1995;172:147-50.

43. **Nelson JL, Ostensen M.** Pregnancy and rheumatoid arthritis. Rheum Dis Clin North Am. 1997;23:195-212.

44. **Khamashta MA, Ruiz-Irastorza G, Hughes GRV.** Systemic lupus erythematosus flares during pregnancy. Rheum Dis Clin North Am. 1997;23:15-31.

45. **Petri M.** Systemic lupus erythematosus and pregnancy. Rheum Dis Clin North Am. 1994;20:87-118.

46. **Browne-Martin K, Emerson CH.** Postpartum thyroid dysfunction. Clin Obstet Gynecol. 1997;40:90-101.

47. **Momotani N, Noh J, Ishikawa N, et al.** Relationship between silent thyroiditis and recurrent Graves disease in the postpartum period. J Clin Endocrinol Metab. 1994;79: 285-9.

48. **Burrow GN.** Thyroid dysfunction in the recently pregnant: postpartum thyroiditis. Thyroid. 1994;4:3363-5.

49. **Greenberg LR, Moore TR, Murphy H.** Gestational diabetes mellitus: antenatal variables as predictors of postpartum glucose intolerance. Obstet Gynecol. 1995;86:97-101.

50. **Kjos SL, Peters RK, Xiang A, Henry OA, Montoro M, Buchanan TA.** Predicting future diabetes in Latino women with gestation diabetes: utility of early postpartum glucose tolerance testing. Diabetes. 1995;44:586-91.

51. **American Diabetes Association.** Summary and recommendations of the 3rd International Workshops—Conference on Gestational Diabetes Mellitus. Diabetes Care. 1995; 18(Suppl 1):24-5.

Index

hypothyroidism and, 274-275
nodules and, 282-283
normal function and
  fetal, 273-274
  maternal, 272-273
  postpartum, 281-282, 819-820
preconception counseling about, 8
radiation exposure and, 111
Thyroid storm, 280
Thyroidal radioiodine, fetal exposure to,
  109
Thyroiditis, postpartum, 281-282, 819-
  820
Thyroid-stimulating hormone
  anterior pituitary and, 287
  hypothyroidism and, 275
  normal function and, 273
Thyroid-stimulating immunoglobulin,
  273
Thyrotropin-secreting adenoma, 292-293
Thyroxine
  fetus and, 274
  hyperthyroidism and, 277
  hypothyroidism and, 274-275
  normal function and, 272-273
Thyroxine-binding globulin, 272
Tissue plasminogen activator, 438
Tobacco use, 161-165
Tocolytic therapy, 406
Topoisomerase inhibitors, 621
TORCH infection, 11
Total parenteral nutrition, 556-561
Total peripheral resistance, 349
Toxemia; see Preeclampsia
Toxicity, drug
  of chemotherapy, 622
  fetal, 80
  maternal, 82
Toxicology testing for drug use, 149-150
Toxin
  environmental, 773-778
  food-borne, 774-776
Toxoplasmosis, 764-768
  clinical course of, 765-766
  diagnosis of, 766-767
  epidemiology of, 768
  management of, 767-768
  risks of, 705
Transabdominal approach for chorionic
  villus sampling, 101
Transcervical approach for chorionic
  villus sampling, 100-101

Transfusion
  platelet, 465-466
  sickle cell disease and, 492, 495-496
Transient hypertension of pregnancy,
  189
Transient vasopressin-resistant diabetes
  insipidus, 295-296
Transition stage of labor, 48
Transmission of infection
  American trypanosomiasis, 784-785
  hepatitis A, 565
  hepatitis B, 569-571
  hepatitis C, 574-575
  hepatitis E, 578
  hepatitis G, 578-579
  HIV, 732-733
  influenza, 746
  toxoplasmosis, 765
Transplant
  cardiac, 366-367
  liver, 595
  preconception counseling about, 4,
    10-11
  renal, 228-229
Transposition of great arteries, 361-362
Trans-sphenoidal surgery, 299
Trauma
  domestic violence causing, 173-178
  falls causing, 62
Travelers diarrhea, 764
Trendelenburg sign, 64
Treponema pallidum, 724-725
Triazole for fungal infection, 786-787
Trichinosis, 769
Trichomoniasis, 719, 721
Tricuspid valve in Ebstein anomaly,
  360-361
Tricyclic antidepressant, 129
  breastfeeding and, 136
Triiodothyronine
  fetus and, 274
  normal function and, 272-273
Trimethoprim-sulfamethoxazole, 760
Tripelennamine, 393
Triple bolus test of pituitary function,
  288
Trisomy 21, 35-36
Trophoblastic disease, 278
Trypanosomiasis
  African, 784
  American, 784-785
  risks of, 705